HANDBOOK OF NEUROTOXICOLOGY

Section Editors

Patricia A. Broderick

CUNY Medical School and NYU School of Medicine,
New York, NY

Joel L. Mattsson

Dow AgroSciences LLC, Indianapolis, IN

James L. Schardein

Independent Consultant, Mansfield, OH

Thomas E. Schlaepfer

The Johns Hopkins Hospital, Baltimore, MD

HANDBOOK
OF NEUROTOXICOLOGY
Volume II

Edited by

EDWARD J. MASSARO

The National Health and Environmental Effects Research Laboratory, Research Triangle Park, Durham, NC

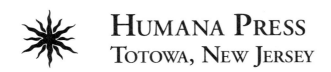

HUMANA PRESS
TOTOWA, NEW JERSEY

Cover illustration: Figure 2B from Volume 1, Chapter 2, "Organophosphate-Induced Delayed Neuropathy," by Marion Ehrich and Bernard S. Jortner.

Production Editor: Jessica Jannicelli.
Cover design by Patricia F. Cleary.

For additional copies, pricing for bulk purchases, and/or information about other Humana titles, contact Humana at the above address or at any of the following numbers: Tel.: 973-256-1699; Fax: 973-256-8341; E-mail: humana@humanapr.com or visit our website: http://humanapress.com

This publication is printed on acid-free paper. ∞
ANSI Z39.48-1984 (American National Standards Institute) Permanence of Paper for Printed Library Materials.

Printed in the United States of America.   10 9 8 7 6 5 4 3 2 1

Library of Congress Cataloging-in-Publication Data

Handbook of neurotoxicology / edited by Edward J. Massaro.
    p. cm.
  Includes bibliographical references and index.
  ISBN 0-89603-796-7 (alk. paper)
    1. Neurotoxicology--Handbooks, manuals, etc. I. Massaro, Edward J.

RC347.5 .N4857 2001
616.8'047--dc21

2001039605

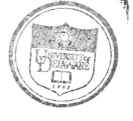

RC
347
. 5
. H343
2002
v. 2

PREFACE

Neurotoxicology is a broad and burgeoning field of research. Its growth in recent years can be related, in part, to increased interest in and concern with the fact that a growing number of anthropogenic agents with neurotoxic potential, including pesticides, lead, mercury, and the polytypic byproducts of combustion and industrial production, continue to be spewed into and accumulate in the environment. In addition, there is great interest in natural products, including toxins, as sources of therapeutic agents. Indeed, it is well known that many natural toxins of broadly differing structure, produced or accumulated for predatory or defensive purposes, and toxic agents, accumulated incidentally by numerous species, function to perturb nervous tissue. Components of some of these toxins have been shown to be useful therapeutic agents and/or research reagents. Unfortunately, the environmental accumulation of some neurotoxicants of anthropogenic origin, expecially pesticides and metals, has resulted in incidents of human poisoning, some of epidemic proportion, and high levels of morbidity and mortality. Furthermore, an increasing incidence of neurobehavioral disorders, some with baffling symptoms, is confronting clinicians. It is not clear whether this is merely the result of increased vigilance and/or improved diagnostics or a consequence of improved health care. In any case, the role of exposure to environmental and occupational neurotoxicants in the etiology of these phenomena, as well as neurodegenerative diseases, is coming under increasing scrutiny and investigation.

Recognition and utilization of environmental (in the broadest sense) information comprise the currency of life. Therefore, the effects of perturbation of these critical capacities deserve thorough investigation. The acquisition of information, and its processing, storage, retrieval, and integration leading to functional outputs, are fundamental nervous system functions. It should not be surprising, then, that structural, functional, and evolutionary research has revealed that even "simple" nervous systems are immensely complex. On the systems level, the intact nervous system is an exquisite example of integration within the context of a continuously evolving, apparently infinitely programmable and regulatable hierarchical input/output system of complex chemical structure. However, as the complexity of nervous systems has increased, so has their vulnerability to chemical and physical insult. In part, this is a consequence of loss of regenerative capacity.

Living systems have evolved to function within relatively narrow ranges of environmental conditions. Perturbation beyond the limits of the range of a given system can result in irreversible damage manifested as loss of function or viability. Also, the nervous tissue of more highly evolved organisms is particularly refractory to regeneration. But, with complexity has come an increased capacity for compensability. Albeit often limited and difficult to achieve, through learning and recruitment, compensation can bypass irreversible damage allowing, to varying degrees, recovery of function. The developing brain, in particular, is endowed with immense plastic potential. Unfortunately, the efficiency of both homeostatic and compensatory mechanisms progressively diminishes as a function of aging. Indeed, a large body of literature indicates that humans generally lose memory with age and the magnitude and rate of loss are highly variable among individuals. In addition, data obtained through the medium of testing protocols, and supported by evidence obtained from functional neuroimaging studies, indicate that not all types of memory are affected equally. Depending on the task, such studies show that, compared with younger adults, older adults can display greater or lesser activity in task-associated brain areas. Conceivably, the increases in activity may be the result of the input from compensatory mechanisms. In any case, age-related diminished mental capacity is a complex function of the interaction of genetic constitution and environmental factors. The type, magnitude, duration, and period of exposure in the life cycle to the latter can impact the functional status of the aging nervous system. Major windows of vulnerability occur during development, when target sizes are small and defense mechanisms immature, and in post-maturity, following decline of the functioning of compensatory and defense mechanisms along with increased duration of exposure.

Intellectually, we may appreciate that thermodynamics dictates that, as a function of population size, environmental pollution will increase. However, do we appreciate that, in the short-run, if a connection between environmental pollution and nervous system damage exists, the incidence of nervous system damage will increase as the population increases? Likewise, as life span increases, exposure to neurotoxicants will increase and, it is not unreasonable, therefore, to predict that the incidence of neurodegenerative diseases also will increase. Are these phenomena self-limiting? If not, can we estimate the magnitude of these problems that ensuing generations will have to face? With time, sufficient funding, and manpower, it may be possible to solve many of these problems. Indeed, we must. If not, the consequences border on the Orwellian.

With an eye to the future, the *Handbook of Neurotoxicology* has been developed to provide researchers and students with a view of the current status of research in selected areas of neurotoxicology and to stimulate research in the field. Obviously, the field is enormous and all areas of interest could not be covered. However, if the *Handbook of Neurotoxicology,* volumes 1 and 2 prove useful, other volumes will be forthcoming. Therefore, we invite your comments and suggestions.

Edward J. Massaro

Contents

I. DEVELOPMENTAL NEUROTOXICOLOGY

James L. Schardein, Section Editor

II. DRUGS OF ABUSE

Patricia A. Broderick, Section Editor

III. IMAGING

Thomas E. Schlaepfer, Section Editor

IV. NEUROBEHAVIORAL ASSESSMENT METHODS

Joel L. Mattsson, Section Editor

CONTENTS OF THE COMPANION VOLUME

Neurotoxicology Handbook

Volume I

CONTRIBUTORS

JAMES W. ALBERS • *Department of Neurology and the Neurobehavioral Toxicology Program, University of Michigan Medical School, Ann Arbor, MI*

KENNETH R. ALPER • *Brain Research Laboratories, Department of Psychiatry, and NYU Comprehensive Epilepsy Center, Department of Neurology, NYU School of Medicine, New York, NY*

MATTHEW BAGGOTT • *University of California at San Francisco, San Francisco, CA*

STANLEY BERENT • *Division of Neuropsychology, Departments of Psychiatry, Neurology, Occupational Medicine, and Psychology, University of Michigan, Ann Arbor, MI*

KATHERINE R. BONSON • *Controlled Substance Staff, Food and Drug Administration, Rockville, MD*

CHRISTIE BRANNOCK • *Molecular Neuropsychiatry Section, National Institute on Drug Abuse, Baltimore, MD*

PATRICIA A. BRODERICK • *Department of Physiology and Pharmacology, The Sophie Davis School of Biomedical Education, CUNY Medical School; and Departments of Biology and Psychology, CUNY Graduate School; and Department of Neurology, NYU School of Medicine, NYU-Mt. Sinai Comprehensive Epilepsy Center, New York, NY*

JEAN LUD CADET • *Molecular Neuropsychiatry Section, Intramural Research Program, National Institute on Drug Abuse, Baltimore, MD*

GREGG D. CAPPON • *Pfizer Global Research and Development, Groton, CT*

MARK DAGLISH • *Psychopharmacology Unit, University of Bristol, UK*

GAYLORD ELLISON • *Department of Psychology, University of California at Los Angeles, Los Angeles, CA*

CORY S. FREEDLAND • *Department of Physiology and Pharmacology, Wake Forest University School of Medicine, Winston-Salem, NC*

ELIOT L. GARDNER • *Intramural Research Program, National Institute on Drug Abuse, Baltimore, MD*

JUDITH W. HENCK • *Parke-Davis Pharmaceutical Research Division of Warner-Lambert Company, Ann Arbor, MI*

E. ROY JOHN • *Brain Research Laboratories, Department of Psychiatry, NYU School of Medicine, New York, NY; and Nathan S. Kline Research Institute, Orangeburg, NY*

SHARON C. KOWALIK • *Brain Research Laboratories, Department of Psychiatry, NYU School of Medicine, New York, NY*

DONALD M. KUHN • *Cellular and Clinical Neurobiology Program, Department of Psychiatry and Behavioral Neurosciences and NIEHS Center for Molecular and Cellular Toxicology, Institute of Chemical Toxicology, Wayne State University School of Medicine; and The John D. Dingell VA Medical Center, Detroit, MI*

SHARON R. LETCHWORTH • *Department of Physiology and Pharmacology, Wake Forest University School of Medicine, Winston-Salem, NC*

DAVID J. LYONS • *Department of Physiology and Pharmacology, Wake Forest University School of Medicine, Winston-Salem, NC*

EDWARD J. MASSARO • *Environmental Protection Agency, Research Triangle Park, Durham, NC*

JOEL L. MATTSSON • *Dow AgroSciences LLC, Indianapolis, IN*

UNA D. MCCANN • *Department of Psychiatry and Behavioral Sciences, The Johns Hopkins School of Medicine, Baltimore, MD*

DIANE B. MILLER • *Centers for Disease Control and Prevention, National Institute for Occupational Safety and Health, Morgantown, WV*

MICHAEL A. NADER • *Department of Physiology and Pharmacology, Wake Forest University School of Medicine, Winston-Salem, NC*

KEVIN NOGUCHI • *Department of Psychology, University of California at Los Angeles, Los Angeles, CA*

DAVID NUTT • *Psychopharmacology Unit, University of Bristol, UK*

JAMES P. O'CALLAGHAN • *Centers for Disease Control and Prevention, National Institute for Occupational Safety and Health, Morgantown, WV*

GODFREY D. PEARLSON • *Department of Psychiatry and Behavioral Sciences, The Johns Hopkins University School of Medicine, Baltimore, MD*

LINDA J. PORRINO • *Department of Physiology and Pharmacology, Wake Forest University School of Medicine, Winston-Salem, NC*

LESLIE S. PRICHEP • *Brain Research Laboratories, Department of Psychiatry, NYU School of Medicine, New York, NY; and Nathan S. Kline Research Institute, Orangeburg, NY*

GEORGE A. RICAURTE • *The Johns Hopkins School of Medicine, Baltimore, MD*

SUSAN A. RICE • *Susan A. Rice and Associates, Inc., Grass Valley, CA*

MITCHELL S. ROSENTHAL • *Phoenix House Foundation, New York, NY*

JOSEPH F. ROSS • *Human and Environmental Safety Division, Miami Valley Laboratories, Cincinnati, OH*

JAMES L. SCHARDEIN • *Independent Consultant, Mansfield, OH*

THOMAS E. SCHLAEPFER • *Department of Psychiatry and Mental Hygiene, The Johns Hopkins Hospital, Baltimore, MD*

DONALD G. STUMP • *WIL Research Laboratories Inc., Ashland, OH*

ZSOLT SZABO • *The Johns Hopkins School of Medicine, Baltimore, MD*

HUGH A. TILSON • *Research Planning and Coordination Staff, US Environmental Protection Agency, Research Triangle Park, NC*

CHRISTINE L. TRASK • *NeuroBehavioral Resources, Inc., Ann Arbor, MI*

COLOR PLATES

Color plates 1–11 appear as an insert following p. 368.

PLATE 1   Fig. 2. Group average (*n* = 13) QEEG VARETA 3D images at 1.95 Hz. (*See* full caption and discussion in Chapter 5, p. 140.)

PLATE 2   Fig. 3. The known serotonergic neurotoxicant, 5,7-dihydroxytryptamine (5,7-DHT) causes a silver degeneration-staining pattern in cortex characterized by the presence of argyrophilic debris (upper right panel) and the induction of hypertrophied astrocytes characteristic of gliosis (lower right panel). (*See* full caption and discussion in Chapter 11, p. 283.)

PLATE 3   Fig. 6. Degeneration in FR induced by nicotine. (*See* discussion in Chapter 12, p. 317.)

PLATE 4   Fig. 3A. Schematic diagram of anatomic dopamine (DA) tracts in the rat brain, represented longitudinally. Adapted with permission from ref. *(108)*. (*See* full caption and discussion in Chapter 13, p. 331.)

PLATE 5   Fig. 3B. Schematic diagram of anatomic dopamine (DA) tracts in the rat brain, represented sagittally. Adapted with permission from ref. *(108)*. (*See* full caption and discussion in Chapter 13, p. 332.)

PLATE 6   Fig. 2. Illustration of the region specific effects during the acute administration of ethanol. (*See* full caption and discussion in Chapter 14, p. 376.)

PLATE 7   Fig. 1. Six transverse slices of a PET scan showing (11C)-Diprenorphine binding in the brain of a normal volunteer. (*See* discussion in Chapter 15, p. 401.)

PLATE 8   Fig. 2A,B. (A) Areas of increased rCBF in response to opioid-related stimuli. (B) Area of increased rCBF correlated with subjective opioid craving. (*See* discussion in Chapter 15, p. 408.)

PLATE 9   Fig. 1. Distribution of [3H] cocaine in coronal sections of a squirrel monkey brain. Adapted with permission from ref. *(47)*. (*See* full caption and discussion in Chapter 16, p. 416.)

I
DEVELOPMENTAL
NEUROTOXICOLOGY

1

Developmental Neurotoxicology

Testing and Interpretation

Judith W. Henck

1. INTRODUCTION

1.1. Overview

Developmental neurotoxicology is the study of adverse effects on the nervous system resulting from exposure to a toxicant during development. The scientific discipline of developmental neurotoxicology integrates the principles and methods of neurotoxicology with those of developmental toxicology; concepts and techniques from developmental neuroanatomy, neurobiology, and experimental psychology are also highly applicable. In addition, developmental neurotoxicology research over the past 50 years has led to concepts and methodologies unique to this discipline. The developing nervous system is highly susceptible to toxic insult, and exposure to toxic agents may result in adverse effects at doses lower than those required to produce the same effect in adults *(1)*. Enhanced sensitivity of the developing nervous system (in particular the central nervous system [CNS]) to disruption is due to factors such as a prolonged course of development, immaturity of the blood-brain barrier (BBB), and lack of regeneration of damaged CNS neurons. One of the more insidious aspects of developmental neurotoxicity is that its functional manifestations may not be readily apparent at birth or in infancy, but rather, become evident during adulthood when the nervous system is mature and possibly even senescent.

Of primary importance in the study of developmental neurotoxicity are the functional consequences of abnormal nervous system development, which are often manifested as changes in behavior, the end result of net sensorimotor and integrative processes in the nervous system *(2)*. Alterations in behavior are considered relatively sensitive indicators of neurotoxicant exposure, and behavioral measures have been used extensively in the identification and characterization of developmental neurotoxicants.

CNS morphology, physiology, and biochemistry may be adversely affected by neurotoxicants, and may in turn lead to adverse behavioral outcomes. The primary focus of this chapter is developmental neurotoxicity testing and interpretation, which in the majority of cases has involved behavioral paradigms. However, alternative means

From: Handbook of Neurotoxicology, Vol. 2
Edited by: E. J. Massaro © Humana Press Inc., Totowa, NJ

Table 1
Human Developmental Neurotoxicants[a]

Carbon monoxide	Quinine
Cocaine	Retinoic acids
Ethanol	Rubella, cytomegalovirus
Heroin	Cigarette smoking
Lead	Thalidomide
Methadone	Toluene
Methamphetamine	Warfarin
Methylmercury	Valproic acid
Phenytoin	X-irradiation
Polychlorinated biphenyls	

[a]Adapted with permission from refs. *36, 131*, and *180.*

of testing, including morphometry, electrophysiology, and neurochemistry, will be addressed briefly and discussed more fully in the following chapter. Historically, developmental neurotoxicity testing has primarily been conducted in rodents, and in particular, rats. Excellent work characterizing specific developmental neurotoxicants has been conducted in other species, including mice, guinea pigs, and nonhuman primates. However, because an extensive historical database has been developed in the rat, and it is the species of choice of regulatory agencies that require developmental neurotoxicity testing, the majority of examples discussed subsequently will be from the rat.

1.2. Scope of Developmental Neurotoxicology

Excellent reviews on the history of developmental neurotoxicology, a scientific discipline in which research has been actively conducted since the 1940s, have been published by Hutchings *(3)* and Butcher *(4)*. In the mid-1970s, Japan and Great Britain issued revised regulations for testing of adverse effects on reproduction and development, which included evaluations of behavioral development *(4)*. With the issuance of these regulations, further emphasis was placed on developmental neurotoxicology as both an applied science and a basic science, which further increased the level of interest in this rapidly developing field. In recent years, additional regulatory requirements for developmental neurotoxicity testing have accelerated the pace of the applied-science component by increasing the need for sensitive and reliable test methods, and advances in in vitro methodology and molecular biology have added an exciting new aspect to the basic science component.

Human populations have demonstrated susceptibility to agents that produce damage to the developing nervous system. A list of human developmental neurotoxicants is provided in Table 1, and representative examples are discussed subsequently. Ethanol is considered the largest environmental cause of developmental neurotoxicity *(5)*, and was the first human developmental neurotoxicant to be studied extensively. Ethanol neurotoxicity, manifested as Fetal Alcohol Syndrome (FAS), is characterized by effects on psychological functioning, growth, facial morphology, and structural development of major organs, and currently occurs at a rate of from 1/700 to 1/1000 births in the United States *(5)*. Developmental neurotoxicity resulting from ethanol exposure has been shown to occur concomitantly with, or in the absence of, physical defects (including growth retardation and CNS malformations), on a continuum ranging from mild to severe. Functional consequences resulting from damage to the nervous system include a neonatal abstinence syndrome, mild to severe cognitive deficits, hyperactivity, distractibility, deficits in attention and reaction time, learning disabilities, and state lability in infants *(3,5)*. Heroin and methadone are also human developmental neurotoxicants, which, unlike ethanol, do not cause CNS malformations. The most distinctive developmental feature of these agents is a neonatal abstinence syndrome with two apparent phases. The first phase is acute narcotic withdrawal characterized by hyperreflexia, tremors, irritability, excessive high-pitched crying, disturbed sleep, and hyperactivity, while the second long-term phase is characterized by impaired organizational and perceptual abilities, poor self-adjustment, heightened activity in situations requiring motor inhibition, and increased risk for poor fine motor coordination and Attention Deficit Disorder (ADD) *(3,6)*. Identification of cocaine as a developmental neurotoxicant has historically been met with some skepticism. A review by Hutchings *(7)* outlined the major concerns: teratogenic effects of cocaine were produced only in infants exposed to the highest doses reported in the literature, and effects on growth and neurobehavioral development might be only marginal and transitory. However, recent studies in infants and children exposed to cocaine prenatally have demonstrated that it may adversely affect neuropsychological functions related to arousal and attention, and laboratory animal studies have identified deficits in dopaminergic neuronal systems associated with an impaired ability to respond to environmental stressors, as well as deficits in attentional processing *(8,9)*.

Several environmental contaminants have been identified as human developmental neurotoxicants. Blood lead concentrations as low as 10–15 μg/dL in children are associated with hyperactivity, poor fine motor control, decreased gestational age, low birth weight, poor academic achievement, and intelligence deficit *(10)*. Acute lead encephalopathy may be produced at higher concentrations, and is more severe in children than in adults; motor peripheral neuropathy may also be seen as a functional consequence *(10)*. Methylmercury was established as a human developmental neurotoxicant following contamination of Minamata Bay in Japan in 1952. Clinical signs of toxicity resulting from *in utero* exposure included cerebral palsy (CP), malnutrition, blindness, delayed speech development, severe hearing impairment or deafness, motor impairment, tremors, convulsions, abnormal reflexes, mental retardation, abnormal EEGs, excessive crying and irritability, and pathologic changes in the CNS *(10–12)*. Most methylmercury-exposed mothers with affected infants showed no symptomatology, in contrast to clinically ill mothers of infants involved in outbreaks of polychlorinated biphenyl (PCB) poisoning in Asia. Children of these mothers exhibited effects on motor and mental function, as well as developmental and behavioral problems *(2)*. Children exposed *in utero* to lower levels of PCBs in Michigan and North Carolina exhibited smaller birth and neonatal size; weak reflexes; were less responsive to stimuli; had more jerky, unbalanced movement and more startles; were hypotonic; had deficits in gross- and fine-motor coordination; and had poorer visual-recognition memory performance *(2)*. These changes were presumed to be in the absence of maternal effects.

CNS anomalies ranging from mild learning disabilities to mental retardation have been estimated to occur in 10–20% of all births *(13)*. A 1991 review by Nelson *(14)* on evidence for behavioral teratogenicity in humans indicated that the overall incidence of birth defects in the United States is 2–3% in liveborn infants, with another 7–8% of infants having malformations or mental deficiencies identified between birth and 1 yr of age. This review speculated that the incidence would be higher if other behavioral dysfunctions for which prenatal factors may play contributory roles were added to the total, such as seizure disorders, autism, childhood schizophrenia, early onset emotional disorders, and ADD. Although the total contribution of toxic insult to the incidence of anomalies of the nervous system cannot be ascertained, CNS defects attributed to developmental insult are now considered to constitute the largest category of birth defects known to arise from exposure to toxicants *(13)*. Only a small fraction of drugs and industrial chemicals currently in use have been evaluated for developmental neurotoxicity (*see* Chapter 3 by Cappon and Stump). However, the positive identification of human developmental neurotoxicants has necessitated the development of predictive animal models. Human developmental neurotoxicants have shown positive responses in various animal models, and the concordance between human and animal responses will be discussed subsequently. It is apparent, however, from the adverse consequences on the nervous system resulting from human developmental exposure, that developmental neurotoxicity must continue to be the subject of research for applied and basic scientists, and an area of concern for safety and risk evaluation.

1.3. Principles of Developmental Neurotoxicology

James Wilson proposed six scientific principles that sought to explain the roles played by critical periods of development, genotype, dose-response relationships, various manifestations of abnormal development, access of agents to developing tissues, and mechanisms, in developmental toxicity *(15)*. These principles were revised and enhanced by Vorhees and Butcher *(5,16)* to make them applicable to developmental neurotoxicology. These revised principles serve as the basis for the subsequent discussion of factors that may influence the susceptibility of the developing organism to neurotoxic insult, and govern the response of the organism to that insult.

1.3.1. Sensitive Periods

While most major organ systems complete their structural development during the period of organogenesis (the major period of organ development), development of various components of the nervous system may occur from the initiation of organogenesis through weaning and into young adulthood. Figure 1 shows the major features of development in the rat, with particular emphasis on development of the CNS. The relevance of this example lies in the fact that rodents are often used as experimental models of developmental neurotoxicity, and that the sequence of nervous-system development is similar across mammalian species. During nervous-system development, the phases that incorporate organogenesis, differentiation, growth, and functional organization are all prolonged. The first phase of neuronal development is neurogenesis, in which a normal number of neurons is produced from precursor cells called neuroblasts within a defined neuronal population. This phase is followed by, or concurrent with, neuronal migration, differentiation, and organization within a final target area, dendrite proliferation and axon orientation along specific pathways, neuronal maturation, gliogenesis (glial cells originate after neurons in specific brain regions), synaptogenesis (formation

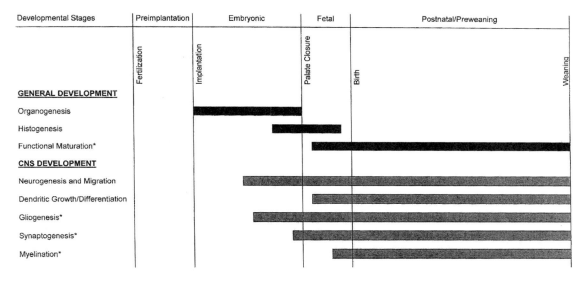

Fig. 1. Approximate timing of key developmental events in the rat. Organogenesis, the period of major organ development, begins at the time of implantation and is essentially complete at the time of palatal closure. Known as the embryonic stage of development, it is the period of greatest susceptibility for structural malformations induced by toxicants. The fetal period is characterized by histogenesis and functional maturation; toxicant insult during this period, as well as neonatally, is associated with growth retardation and functional abnormalities. Development of the CNS occurs throughout these periods. Neurogenesis, the first stage of neuronal development, begins midway through the embryonic stage, and in some neuronal populations, is not complete until weaning. Additional stages of CNS development are also prolonged, and proceed in rats until well after birth. Stages with a "*" continue beyond weaning and into adulthood. Toxicant exposure at any stage during this prolonged development can lead to adverse consequences. Adapted with permission from refs. *5,15,18.*

of synaptic connections with specific targets), development and maturation of neurotransmitter systems, and myelination (following proliferation of glial cells) *(10,17–19)*. Maturation of the BBB, considered a diffusion barrier to most large and/or polar molecules, proceeds at different rates in different brain regions, but is complete in rats at approx postnatal wk 3 and in humans at approx 6 mo of age *(13)*. The components of the BBB, including the capillary-cell membrane, basement membrane, and glial-cell layer, are thinner during development *(1)*; thus, the developing nervous system is vulnerable to diffusible substances *(13)*.

Neural mechanisms underlying different types of function may be subject to injury throughout development, and specific functional impairment is dependent on the state of development of the nervous system at the time of toxic insult. The prolonged period of sensitivity of the developing nervous system reflects such characteristics as architectural complexity, prolonged development, vulnerability of undifferentiated neural cells relative to developed neurons, dependence of neural function on the position to which neuronal cells must migrate, and the inability of the brain to replace lost neurons *(20)*. Neurons are not self-renewing; the capacity of neuronal precursors to divide is exhausted during neurogenesis, and culminates in differentiated neurons that do not undergo further division *(20)*. This inability to produce new neurons, coupled with the interdependency of multiple connections in the nervous system, means that even subtle forms of injury can result in impaired function *(1)*. However, a great deal of structural redundancy exists within the interconnections of the nervous system, such that functions controlled by a damaged population of neurons may conceivably be taken over by another population of related, undamaged neurons. Due to this property of the nervous system, known as plasticity, considerable loss of neurons can occur without evidence of changes in function or behavior *(1)*. However, even this plasticity can be compromised by challenges such as further injury, pharmacological agents, stress, or age.

The greatest period of vulnerability for structural malformations of the nervous system appears to be early organogenesis *(21)*, while that for functional changes appears to range from mid to late organogenesis through histogenesis *(21,22)*, although behavioral effects in rats have resulted from preimplantation (predifferentiation) exposure *(3)*. Dobbing *(23)* advanced the hypothesis that developmental processes in the CNS are most vulnerable to insult during the time of their most rapid growth, i.e., during the "brain growth spurt" that occurs in the rat from birth to weaning (peaking at approximately postnatal day [PND]10). Gottlieb et al. *(24)* have demonstrated that at least three periods of rapid growth occur postnatally in the rat brain, from PND 0–6, 8–12, and 17–23 and Morgane and coworkers *(18)* have further suggested that each brain region has its own growth-spurt period. These regional velocity curves may include events such as early gliogenesis, macroneurogenesis, and early glial and neuronal migrations that occur prior to the overall brain-growth spurt, and thus confer sensitivity early in development. Using behavior as the major functional endpoint of developmental neurotoxicity, Rodier *(17)* constructed a chronology of behaviors affected by cell loss at different stages of development. As an example, hyperactivity in the mouse resulted from toxicant exposure during the middle part of neuron production (approx gestation days [GD]13–18), while exposure before and after tended to result in hypoactivity (approx GD 11–13 and GD 18–PND 7). Because portions of the nervous system controlling various aspects of behavior form at different stages of development, Rodier concluded that many critical periods exist for the induction of behavioral changes, rather than just one, as may be the case with other organ systems.

1.3.2. The Role of Genetics

Genetic makeup of a developing organism determines the susceptibility of that individual to teratogenesis *(15)*. The genotype of the conceptus may affect the response to an agent that crosses the placenta, and differences in reaction to the same insult among individuals, strains, and species may be the result of differences in genetic makeup. Vorhees *(5)* has suggested that, given the relationship of structural defects to behavioral defects, an influence of genetic background on behavioral teratogenicity would not be unexpected. Also of great importance is the manner in which genotype interacts with environmental factors; responses may be due to genetic or environmental factors, or to varying blends of these factors *(5)*.

The importance of genetics in determining the nature of response to a developmental neurotoxicant may be extended to include the maternal animal, since the genotype of the mother determines what will be delivered to the placenta, and ultimately the conceptus *(22)*. Morphine is considered an example of female-mediated behavioral mutagenesis in mice, in that trans-generational effects on behavior result from exposure for several weeks prior to mating *(5)*. Although treatment prior to the initiation of organogenesis could lead to adverse behavioral effects by acting directly on the blasto-cyst, such effects might also be induced by changes in the maternal environment or delayed clearance from embryonic or maternal fluid *(3)*.

Paternally mediated neurobehavioral effects have also been demonstrated. Agents found to produce behavioral changes experimentally in offspring from treated males include cocaine, cyclophosphamide, ethanol, ethylene dibromide, lead, methadone, and 2-methoxyethanol *(25,26)*. Trans-generational effects on activity and learning in off-spring of male rats treated with cyclophosphamide, an agent known to cause genetic damage, lend support to the idea that behavioral effects may be related to the induction of mutations in paternal germ cells *(27)*.

The role of genetics in determining functional consequences of exposure to develop-mental neurotoxicants is often readily apparent in the course of data interpretation. Outcomes may be influenced by individual variation in expression of effects, which leads to increased variance in measured functional parameters *(13)*. If behavior is used as a functional endpoint, genetic differences can be evaluated by measuring various types of behaviors and comparing the same behaviors using multiple species and/or strains of experimental animals.

1.3.3. Response to Developmental Neurotoxicant Exposure

Final manifestations of abnormal development induced by toxicant exposure are death, malformation, growth retardation, and functional disorder *(15)*. Although all of these potential outcomes must be considered in the study of developmental neurotoxic-ity, growth retardation, and functional disorder are probably of the greatest impor-tance, and have been shown to occur at doses below those required to produce CNS malformations. If behavioral change is considered a primary consequence of develop-mental neurotoxicity, these manifestations may be further described as impaired cogni-tive, affective, social, arousal, reproductive, and sensorimotor behavior; delayed behavioral maturation of these capabilities; or other indices of compromised behav-ioral competence *(5)*. Developmental neurotoxicity is usually not expressed as a single type of adverse effect, but rather, may be manifested as a continuum of effects, such as those exerted by ethanol.

Basic dose-response principles dictate that effect is dependent on the dose reaching the target organ. Developmental neurotoxicants such as vitamin A, ethanol, methylazoxymethanol, hydroxyurea, and phenytoin exert their effects in a dose-depen-dent manner; the nature of those effects depends on the dose reaching the target organ *(5)*. It should be noted, however, that in some cases the dose of the agent administered to the maternal animal is not as important as the actual blood levels to which the devel-oping animal is exposed. As an example, lead produces nonmonotonic (U-shaped) dose-response curves for behavioral deficits in offspring exposed during development, rendering species comparisons difficult. However, when exposure (blood lead levels) is considered, the lowest levels at which developmental neurotoxicity has been observed are similar among species: 10–15 µg/dL in children, < 15 µg/dL in primates, and < 20 µg/dL in rodents (28).

The importance of maximum concentration (C_{max}) vs total exposure (area under the blood concentration time curve; AUC) in determining the outcome of developmental neurotoxicity depends on the agent. It has been demonstrated in animal studies with various drugs and chemicals, including ethanol and lead, that brief peaks in blood concentration can cause greater behavioral impairment than long-term lower level exposures *(29)*. Transfer of the agent across the BBB is also of importance, and may be one of the requirements for induction of developmental neurotoxicity. In a study of eight radiolabeled drugs administered to rat dams during late gestation, and to their pups during the first 2 wk of life, Watanabe and coworkers *(30,31)* determined that drugs with high lipid solubility were readily transferred across the BBB of the pups and induced developmental neurotoxicity.

Route of administration can impact pharmacokinetic and pharmacodynamic factors in the maternal animal, as well as in the conceptus and neonate. The desirable route of administration for drugs is that which will be used clinically, while the oral route of administration is generally recommended for environmental contaminants. In standard testing regimens recommended by regulatory agencies (*see* Subheading 2.1.), the maternal animal is typically administered the test agent, which means that the conceptus and neonate are exposed indirectly via placental transfer or in the milk.

Although many developmental neurotoxicants demonstrate typical dose-response relationships, U-shaped dose-response curves are not uncommon. A precedent exists for this in behavioral changes induced in adults by depressants and stimulants, which are characterized by a U-shaped dose-response relationship between behavioral efficiency and arousal. In large doses, barbiturates suppress ongoing behavior and induce sleep (depressed arousal), while in smaller doses behavioral output is actually increased by eliminating irrelevant stimuli *(32)*. Conversely, amphetamine progressively increases arousal until eventually the dose is so high as to be incompatible with efficient behavior *(32)*; at this point stereotyped behavior emerges at the expense of increased locomotor activity. In the CNS, numerous systems interact on different levels to produce a response, so it is not unexpected that exposure during the development of these systems could produce nonlinear dose-response curves. One theory that has been advanced to explain greater differences from control in low- than in high-dose groups is that higher-dose groups may produce increased mortality in susceptible fetuses, yielding more resistant survivors that do not manifest the effects seen in lower dose groups *(22,33)*.

1.3.4. Physiologic and Environmental Influences

Manifestations of developmental neurotoxicity can occur in the absence of overt maternal or developmental toxicity, as is the case with PCBs, which produce similar neurological or behavioral effects across species, often in the absence of decreased body weight or gross signs of intoxication *(2)*. When maternal and/or developmental toxicity are present, they can confound interpretation of results. Abel *(22)* stated that maternal factors such as pharmacokinetics, biological rhythms, age, parity, stress, social environment, and diet; and placental factors such as blood flow and thickness, surface area, and permeability of membranes can greatly influence the access of the agent to the developing nervous system of the offspring, and that the physiological, pathological, and psychological status of the mother can affect susceptibility to teratogens or actually induce teratogenesis or behavioral effects. These effects might mistakenly be attributed to a direct effect on the developing organism, rather than to a secondary effect resulting from maternal toxicity. As an example, effects on activity, learning, and memory were observed in animal studies with cannabis that failed to take maternal nutritional factors into account; these effects were not observed in studies in which pair-fed controls and surrogate fostering to untreated dams were used *(34)*. Current developmental neurotoxicity testing guidelines require that a certain level of maternal toxicity be achieved at the highest dose tested, and this is therefore an issue that must be dealt with on a continuous basis. However, participants in a workshop on the qualitative and quantitative comparability of human and animal developmental neurotoxicity concluded that while maternal toxicity during pregnancy and/or lactation may confound interpretation of effects observed in offspring experimentally, these effects should be presumed relevant to potential risk in humans *(35)*.

Concurrent toxicity and environmental influences may be confounding factors in the response of animals exposed to developmental neurotoxicants. The question invariably arises as to whether altered responses are due to a direct effect of the agent or are secondary to other factors. Behavior is sensitive to many postnatal variables, most of which are capable of producing changes similar to those induced by a developmental neurotoxicant *(22)*. Potential secondary effects on behavior of offspring may be caused by such factors as neonatal undernutrition, species and strain, gender, stress, handling, and body temperature, and these factors must be considered in data interpretation. The ways in which environmental variables may influence the outcome of developmental neurotoxicity testing are discussed in Subheading 3.3.

1.3.5. Mechanisms

Mechanisms of developmental neurotoxicity may involve behavioral, anatomical (cellular), neurophysiological, biochemical (neurochemical), and/or molecular endpoints. The multifactorial nature of most mechanisms of developmental neurotoxicity often renders correlations between these different types of endpoints difficult, which points to the need for mutidisciplinary studies in which toxicant-induced changes at the cellular or molecular level may be linked to alterations at the functional or behavioral level *(19)*.

Cell death and altered differentiation, which may be characterized by decreased proliferation and migration of cells (resulting in abnormal architecture and interconnections of neural systems), structural damage to tissues, changes in the frequency of cell death, altered synaptogenesis, and altered myelination, are changes by which agents may interfere with CNS development on a cellular level *(22,36)*. Cellular damage may be reflected as changes in membrane-ion channels, second-messenger systems, protein sythesis, axonal transport, conduction of action potentials, synaptic transmission, maintenance of the myelin sheath, and general intracellular integrity of the axolemma *(1)*. Changes in neuronal number may result from agents that interfere with DNA synthesis, inhibit mitosis, or preferentially kill migrating cells; in addition to the death of migrating cells, the position or orientation of migrating cells may be changed, as in the case of ectopic cells, which may occur in conjunction with neuronal-cell loss *(37)*. Abnormal synaptogenesis may result in deleterious changes in neuronal connections, while changes in supporting tissues of neurons such as glia may lead to deficiencies in myelination *(37)*.

Although functional or behavioral endpoints are considered appropriate measures of damage to the multiple, interrelated pathways of the CNS, the importance of mechanistic studies using biochemical methodology is clear. Reuhl and coworkers *(38)* established the importance of changes in cell-adhesion molecules involved in neural-tube formation, neuron migration, postmigratory differentiation, and maintenance of mature neural structure, as pivotal molecular events dictating developmental consequences of neurotoxicant exposure. Methylmercury has been shown to inhibit the activity of selected aminoacyl tRNA synthetases prior to the onset of clinical neurotoxicity resulting from cytotoxicity; mechanisms of methylmercury-induced developmental neurotoxicity are considered to be multifactorial, however, as inhibition of these enzymes alone is not cytotoxic in the short term *(19)*. DiLuca and coworkers *(39)* evaluated the role of protein phosphorylation changes in rats exposed to methylazoxymethanol during gestation, and correlated these changes with effects on behavior. Exposure on GD 15 resulted in effects on protein B-50 phosphorylation in the hippocampus and cortex, coupled with alterations in maze learning and passive avoidance, while exposure on GD 19 resulted in effects on phosphorylation of B-50 in the hippocampus only, coupled with alterations in active avoidance. Work by Balduini and Costa *(40–42)* has helped to elucidate the role of muscarinic receptor-stimulated phosphoinositide metabolism in developmental neurotoxicity induced by ethanol during the postnatal brain growth spurt. The cholinergic system is especially susceptible to the effects of ethanol, and muscarinic receptors in the brain are coupled with the phosphoinositide system, which is thought to play a role in cell differentiation and synaptogenesis via increasing intracellular free calcium, particularly during the brain growth spurt *(42)*. Inhibitory effects on phosphoinositide hydrolysis were maximal in the cerebral cortex and hippocampus, with somewhat lower inhibition in the cerebellum, when ethanol was given to rats on PND 7; these three brain regions are thought to be the most sensitive to the developmental neurotoxicity of ethanol *(41)*.

2. DEVELOPMENTAL NEUROTOXICITY TESTING

2.1. Testing Strategies

Laboratory animal testing strategies for developmental neurotoxicity require evaluation of multiple aspects of nervous-system functioning to fully characterize adverse effects in the CNS. This is best accomplished using an apical-testing strategy, which is designed to identify deficiencies in the integrated components of the nervous system, and is the basis for screening test batteries currently used in both clinical and laboratory animal testing to identify behavioral changes. The test subject is required to draw on several functions, such as sensory modalities plus cognitive and/or motor capabilities, to perform a test successfully *(16)*. If the subject's performance is impaired on a given task or in an overall test battery, this is evidence of a deficit in the integrated system; however, higher-level testing is then required to identify and characterize the specific functions that are affected. This represents a global strategy, which includes a series of increasingly specific, sensitive determinations *(43)*. Adams *(36)* has stated that the probability of detection of adverse neurobehavioral outcome varies with the method of measurement (to be discussed subsequently) and the age at measurement. In some cases, the detection of adverse outcomes may increase with age at measurement, although cases also exist in which the incidence of adverse outcomes declines with

Table 2
Automated Behavior Tests[a]

Neuromuscular function	Motor activity/arousal	Sensory function	Learning and memory
Rotorod	Running wheel	Auditory startle	Passive avoidance
Grip strength	Activity monitor	Reflex modification	Active avoidance
	Hole board/head dipping	Tactile startle	Habituation
	Residential maze	Hot plate	Water mazes
	Figure-8 maze	Tail flick	Radial-arm maze
	Contrast-sensitive		Spontaneous alternation
	video tracking		Taste/odor aversion
			Operant conditioning

[a]A selection of tests for which electronic-data capture is available, either commercially or through the efforts of individual investigators. If testing is conducted for regulatory agencies, equipment using electronic data capture must be validated to ensure reliability of operation.

age. However, the fact that adverse effects may increase with age points to the value of longitudinal testing, in which tests are administered repeatedly over time. Sobrian and Pappas *(44)* have stated that there are difficulties inherent in conducting longitudinal testing over the lifespan of an animal: It requires substantial resources, is time-consuming, and may involve large numbers of animals. However, they note that advantages appear to outweigh disadvantages: The possibility of detecting altered function is maximized, information is provided on rates of maturation and decline of function, and the nature of functional alterations can be highlighted by periodic evaluation. An additional advantage to longitudinal testing is that reversibility of functional deficits can be evaluated.

Observational tests are useful because they are capable of describing the nuances of behavioral change. However, they are also subjective, which may confer a certain degree of observer bias. The primary way in which observer subjectivity has been minimized is by the use of electronic-data capture. Many systems are currently on the market or have been created by investigators in their own laboratories that capture aspects of neuromuscular function, activity, sensory acuity, and learning and memory without the intervention of an experimenter. Commonly used tests that are capable of employing electronic data capture are listed in Table 2. Because these systems are computerized, they must be adequately validated, i.e., it must be demonstrated that each system is performing its intended function accurately and reliably.

In addition to validation of electronic data capture systems, evaluation of positive control agents can provide an indication of the ability of a test system to detect changes from baseline in either the positive or negative direction. The use of the plural in this regard is intentional, in that no one agent has been identified that affects the most commonly evaluated aspects of behavior in developmental neurotoxicity-screening batteries: physical growth and development, neuromotor development, sensory function, activity/reactivity, and learning and memory *(45)*. Thus, the best approach would be to select two or more agents that are known to reliably alter behavior in specific ways. One of the most commonly used positive control agents is methimazole: a goitrogen that produces reversible functional thyroidectomy in rats as a result of perinatal exposure. Methimazole induces developmental delay, impaired neuromuscular function, increases or decreases in motor activity, deficits in learning and memory, and impaired or enhanced responding to auditory stimuli when given to the maternal rat during the last week of gestation through the first half of lactation *(46–50)*. Developmental delays are consistently induced by methimazole; however, behavioral effects are not always consistent, and have been reported to occur in opposite directions. Behavioral effects were induced by perinatal administration of methylmercury in five laboratories participating in the Collaborative Behavioral Teratology Study; however, despite attempts made to standardize experimental methods in this study, not all behavioral effects were consistent *(51,52)*. Examples exist of agents such as diazepam and *d*-amphetamine that were reported as developmental neurotoxicants in the literature, or were positive in range-finding studies, but that failed to induce developmental neurotoxicity in definitive positive control studies *(50,53)*. Other positive control agents that have been used include chlorpromazine, ethanol, fenfluramine, hydroxyurea, inorganic lead, methylazoxymethanol, phenylalanine, prochlorperazine, propylthiouracil, and retinoic acid *(54–58)*.

Lack of reproducibility with positive control agents has been attributed in part to inadequate sample size and thus, insufficient power *(59)*, so it is essential to ensure that the design of a positive control study allows for adequate group sizes, and employs agents that do not induce excessive mortality. It is also essential to identify the purpose of the validation. A pre- and postnatal study design is essential in determining if the test battery used to evaluate developmental neurotoxicity is capable of detecting differences from baseline. However, a great deal of effort may be necessary to reproduce the conditions cited for each agent in the scientific literature, and the methodology may be dissimilar to that recommended by regulatory agencies for routine screening. The U.S. Environmental Protection Agency (U.S. EPA) recommends that positive control data be generated by a given laboratory to demonstrate sensitivity of methods *(60)*. However, the agency indicates that positive control studies do not need to employ perinatal exposure as long as they demonstrate competency of the laboratory in evaluating effects in neonatal animals perinatally exposed to chemical and establish norms for the appropriate age group.

If the purpose of the validation is only to determine if electronic data capture by a given behavioral system is accurate, the investigator may wish to consider validating that system in adult animals using single doses of pharmacologic agents with known properties (e.g., *d*-amphetamine for increasing activity and phenobarbital for decreasing activity). This type of validation is accomplished rapidly, avoids excessive mortality due to long-term toxicity, ensures that increases and decreases in responding can be detected, and reduces resource expenditure *(50)*.

2.2. Behavioral Test Methods

Several standardized test batteries in laboratory animals that incorporate basic neurobehavioral functions such as activity, sensory function, neuromuscular function, and learning and memory have been used successfully, including, but not limited to, the Barlow and Sullivan battery *(61)*, the Cincinnati Psychoteratogenicity Screening

Table 3
Study Designs Recommended by the International Conference on Harmonization (65) and the US Environmental Protection Agency (60) to Evaluate Developmental Neurotoxicity

Parameter	ICH[a]	EPA[b]
# Litters/group	16–20	≥20
Treatment period	Implantation to weaning	GD 6 through LD 10
Maternal observations		
Clinical signs	Daily	Daily
Body weight	≥Twice weekly	At least weekly, day of delivery, LD 11 and 21
Offspring observations		
Clinical	Daily	Daily
Developmental landmarks	Vaginal opening, preputial separation	Vaginal opening, preputial separation
Body weight	PND 0, and during preweaning and postweaning periods	PND 0, 4, 11, 17, 21, and at least every 2 wk thereafter
Behavior testing		
# Offspring tested	1/sex/litter	1/sex/litter
Motor activity	Test, method, and test days not specified	PND 13, 17, 21, 60 ± 2, method not specified
Sensory functions	Test, method, and test days not specified	Auditory startle habituation, PND 22, 60 ± 2; prepulse inhibition recommended
Learning and memory	Test, method, and test days not specified	Associative learning and memory, PND 21–24, 60 ± 2; suggested tests: delayed-matching-to-position, olfactory conditioning, schedule-controlled behavior
Neuropathology	Not required	6/sex/dose; PND 11 and study end
Brain weights	Not required	10/sex/dose; PND 11 and study end

GD, Gestation day; LD, Lactation day; PND, Postnatal day.

[a]The design of this study is intended to investigate test agent effects on pre- and postnatal development. This list of parameters includes those most relevant to developmental neurotoxicity testing.

[b]Parameters apply if developmental neurotoxicity is evaluated in a separate study. The testing protocol may also be incorporated concurrently with or as a follow-up to a standard developmental toxicity study or may be incorporated into the second generation of a multigeneration study (181).

battery (62), the National Center for Toxicological Research (NCTR) Collaborative Behavioral Teratology Study battery (63), and the U.S. EPA's Office of Toxic Substances battery (precursor to the current EPA regulations) (64). Some batteries emphasize ontogeny of reflexes and behaviors, while others emphasize adult behavior in developmentally exposed animals, including longitudinal testing at various ages. Table 3 provides an indication of the experimental design of pre- and postnatal development studies that include developmental neurotoxicity testing, as required by the International Conference on Harmonisation (ICH) and the U.S. EPA. These regulatory guidelines are relatively nonspecific about the exact tests to be utilized, but recommendations do suggest an apical testing approach. In a guidance issued by ICH (and adopted by the U.S. Food and Drug Administration [FDA]), no specific behavioral test methods or ages at testing are recommended, but rather, the guidance document recommends that tests should be included for evaluation of motor activity, sensory functions, and learning and memory *(65)*. Suggestions of general types of neurobehavioral tests to evaluate specific areas of function are made in EPA developmental neurotoxicity guidelines *(60)*, including requirements for testing at specific ages, and the overall experimental approach is more systematic and comprehensive than that of ICH. According to EPA guidelines, evaluation of developmental neurotoxicity should include observations to detect gross neurologic and behavioral abnormalities, determination of motor activity, response to auditory startle, assessment of learning and memory, neuropathological evaluation, and brain weights. Developmental neurotoxicity may be evaluated in a separate study, as a follow-up to a standard developmental-toxicity study, or as part of a two-generation reproduction study. These testing batteries provide useful information on the effect of a toxicant on the integrated components of the developing nervous system. However, it must be emphasized that test batteries identify that developmental neurotoxicity exists, but they do not characterize the exact nature or cause of specific effects. A two-tiered approach is required, in which functional deficits identified in the screening battery are characterized by more complex and specific tests.

A word of caution has been sounded by Lochry *(66)* regarding the use of behavior testing in studies designed to evaluate other aspects of reproductive and developmental toxicity. Behavioral tests traditionally used in psychopharmacology may not be appropriate: High levels of shock in some avoidance paradigms may influence body weight or produce adverse clinical signs, tests requiring food or water deprivation such as schedule-controlled operant behavior and appetitive maze learning tasks may negate body weight and food consumption measures, and tests that introduce a second chemical such as *d*-amphetamine challenge in motor activity paradigms may confound test-agent effects.

The following sections provide an indication of the types of behavioral tests currently available to evaluate developmental neurotoxicity in rats. Detailed methodology is not provided, but the reader is encouraged to consult the references cited for specific direction.

2.2.1. Physical Growth and Development

Physical growth is considered an indicator of health status, and is usually evaluated as body-weight gain. From an historical database of 3500 control rats from developmental-toxicology studies, Lochry *(66)* determined that body weight is consistently a more sensitive indicator of developmental status, and frequently detects changes not revealed by developmental landmarks. With the exception of landmarks of sexual maturation, a strong correlation was found between developmental landmarks and pup body-weight data. Because body weight is related to general health status, periodic measurement can indicate if animals continue to be in poor health, or are actually recovering. Knowledge of body weight at the time of behavior testing is crucial to data interpretation because body-weight changes can confound behavioral results. An animal with treatment-related body-weight reduction may act differently, and it may be unclear as to whether the change in behavior is a result of the diminished health of the animal, a direct effect on the CNS, or some combination.

Structural malformations may affect the ability of an animal to perform certain behaviors; some laboratories choose to cull malformed animals at birth to eliminate this potential confounder. Clinical signs in offspring are also of relevance to interpretation of behavior data because they provide an early indication of CNS toxicity, as well as an indication of the overall health status of the animal. Buelke-Sam and Kimmel *(55)* have stated that diarrhea may impair behavioral performance under some conditions more than an actual hearing deficit. Excessive clinical signs may also affect the ability of an animal to perform certain behaviors.

Neonatal mortality is a parameter evaluated in all pre- and postnatal developmental-toxicity studies. It is important to try to ascertain if excessive mortality is due to overt toxicity, behavioral impairment in the pup, or impaired maternal behavior or lactating ability. Holson and coworkers *(67)* described an interesting situation in which damage to the CNS induced by all-*trans* retinoic acid given to the dam on GD 11–13 prevented pups from suckling and thus resulted in their death within 2 d of birth. Pups from treated dams were delivered by cesarean section and fostered onto untreated dams, but initially had difficulty breathing without assistance and could not attach to the nipple, despite being able to locate and mouth the nipple. Abnormalities were found in these pups in the inferior olive, a brain region known to be involved in coordinating rhythmic tongue movements in the adult, and in the area postrema, implicating CNS damage as the reason for pup mortality.

The Chernoff-Kavlock assay was designed as a postnatal screen for developmental toxicants, and evaluates neonatal viability and body weight up to PND 3 *(68)*. The assay has identified agents that cause developmental toxicity, and has good concordance with more comprehensive studies. Goldey et al. *(69)* conducted a review of the literature to determine if parameters evaluated in the Chernoff-Kavlock assay could adequately identify developmental neurotoxicants. They determined that only 65% of developmental neurotoxicants affected at least one of the neonatal endpoints in the assay. Thus, while neonatal viability and growth are important components to evaluate in developmental neurotoxicity studies, they must be accompanied by other components of a testing battery in order to identify developmental neurotoxicants, and to prevent false-negatives.

2.2.2. Ontogeny of Reflexes and Behavior

A rodent is born with limited behavioral ability and then rapidly acquires various reflexes and behaviors. Because simple reflexes are generally acquired prior to specific behaviors, they are among the earliest parameters tested in the postnatal period. Ontogeny of some of the more common of these, as well as developmental landmarks and some behaviors, is provided for Sprague-Dawley (SD) rats in Table 4. Most reflexes become stronger and show superior behavioral integration with age, but one exception is the rooting reflex. This reflex is displayed at birth, is characterized by head turning toward a tactile stimulus presented to the snout of a pup, and is required for nursing *(70)*. If this reflex does not diminish after birth, it could be indicative of damage to the

Table 4
Ontogeny of Developmental Landmarks, Reflexes, and Behaviors in Sprague-Dawley Rats[a]

Landmarks	PND	Reflexes	PND	Behaviors	PND
Pinnae detachment[b]	3–7	Righting reflex (surface)[b]	2–6	Crawling	6
Upper incisor eruption	10–13	Bar grasp	6–7	Olfactory discrimination	8
Lower incisor eruption	11–15	Cliff avoidance	12	Forelimb placing	9–10
Eye opening[b]	15–18	Negative geotaxis	8–14	Walking	15
Testes descent[b]	18–26	Auditory startle[b]	12–13	Hindlimb placing	16
Vaginal patency[b]	31–37	Pinna reflex	14	Active avoidance	51
Preputial separation[b]	45–47	Righting reflex (air drop)	15–16		

[a]Data expressed as the range of postnatal days (PND) of acquisition obtained from a variety of references (50,51,102,163,182–184). Data are combined for males and females, since the majority of these parameters do not display sexual dimorphism in acquisition.

[b]Most commonly used evaluations according to a survey of 51 companies that performed developmental toxicity testing of pharmaceuticals (81).

cerebral cortex, and thus could conceivably be used to identify damage early in the postnatal period.

The usual direction of change observed in ontogeny of landmarks, reflexes, and behavior is a delay. However, agents can affect individual parameters in different ways, and it is therefore wise to apply a two-tailed statistical analysis to these measures. Methimazole is a classic agent for inducing developmental delay, and numerous investigators have demonstrated delays in the acquisition of developmental landmarks and reflexes (46–50). Mixed effects were observed in offspring of dams treated with the antihistamine diphenhydramine on GD 0–21: pinnae unfolding and eye opening were accelerated, testes descent and vaginal opening were delayed, and surface righting and negative geotaxis were accelerated (71). Eye opening, incisor eruption, vaginal opening, and preputial separation were accelerated with recombinant human epidermal growth factor$_{1-48}$ given in the early postnatal period, but acquisition of negative geotaxis, wire maneuver, acoustic startle, and visual placing were delayed (72).

2.2.3. Observational Testing

The functional observational battery (FOB) comprises a series of observational tests designed to evaluate neurobehavioral capabilities of rodents and has been likened to a clinical neurological examination in humans, in that the presence and, in some cases the severity, of behavioral and neurological signs is rated (73). It was originally described in detail in mice by Irwin (74), and since then has been modified in many different ways to enhance efficiency and eliminate excessive redundancy. Table 5 lists some of the more commonly used endpoints in a FOB, including those that may be useful for neonatal rats. A FOB is required by the EPA in adult neurotoxicity testing (75), and most of the published literature describes data obtained from adult rodents.

Table 5
Observational Assessment in Developmental Neurotoxicity Testing[a]

General observation	Reflexes	Neuromuscular function	Motor activity/arousal	Sensory function	Learning and memory	Social interaction/ emotional responsivity
Convulsions/ tremors	Surface righting	Forelimb placing	Ontogeny of adult locomotion	Acoustic startle	Water mazes	Measures of juvenile play
Palpebral closure	Air righting[b]	Hindlimb placing	Mobility	Tail/toe pinch	Spontaneous alternation (T-maze or Y-maze)	Adult social interaction
Lacrimation	Pupil response[b]	Grip strength	Horizontal locomotion	Visual placing	Olfactory discrimination	Open field activity
Piloerection	Negative geotaxis	Rope descent	Rearing	Olfactory discrimination	Visual discrimination	Elevated plus-maze exploration
Salivation	Pinna reflex	Inverted screen	Gait		Biel maze	Ultrasonic distress vocalizations
Vocalization	Cliff avoidance	Wire maneuver	Stereotypy			
Urination		Landing foot splay	Ataxia[b]			
Defecation			Swimming ontogeny			
Bizarre behavior			Figure-8 maze			
			Step-down latency[b]			
			Wall climbing			

[a] Applicable to adults and neonates, with the exceptions noted in [b]; adapted from refs. 76, 163, 185.
[b] Not applicable to neonates, as per Moser and Padilla (76).

However, Moser and Padilla *(76)* applied a FOB to Long-Evans rats successfully on PND 17. This was the youngest age at which they felt the FOB could be successfully applied because the animals had finally achieved eye opening. Modification of some tests was required (e.g., the number of grades for scoring of gait and tremor was reduced), surface righting was used instead of air-drop righting, and some tests (ataxia, pupil constriction, rectal temperature, and hindlimb foot splay) were actually eliminated to accommodate the incomplete development of the rat pups.

Some of the observational tests applied to neonates have the ability to measure relatively sophisticated functions. As an example, olfactory discrimination is an observational test of sensory function that evaluates a rat pup's ability to discriminate between the odor of the home cage and a novel odor. The pup is placed in a rectangular apparatus containing clean bedding on one side and soiled bedding from the home cage on the other. Orientation to the home bedding and the time required to ambulate to it are measured, and are considered to represent sensory discrimination and locomotor skill *(70)*. Olfactory discrimination can also be used as a test of learning and memory through manipulation of the odor.

Observational tests are subjective, and it is therefore important to have well-trained observers to administer the test battery. Mattsson and coworkers *(77)* have suggested establishing a FOB performance standard for adult rats that includes training observers using known reference agents (saline, chlorpromazine, atropine followed by physostigmine, and amphetamine), followed by testing of the observer, with comparison of scores to a standard. This system provides for observer competency and interobserver reliability, and could be readily applied to functional observations of neonates as well. In conducting observational tests, the experimenter should be blind to treatment group to avoid unintentionally impacting the outcome of the study. As an example, experimenter effects made possible by knowledge of the test conditions could produce unintentional effects in handling, even in the case of automated tests *(78)*.

2.2.4. Neuromuscular Function

Although neuromuscular function is often evaluated observationally, few tests exist that actually quantify it. Commonly reported tests are rotorod performance, Meyer forelimb-hindlimb grip strength *(79)*, and the Coughenour inverted-screen apparatus. The inverted screen apparatus is used more frequently with mice *(70)*; it appears from experiments in our laboratory that the weight of adult rats often causes them to fall spontaneously from the inverted screen. The forelimb-hindlimb grip strength apparatus measures flexor response using strain gauges, and provides a value for pull of the forelimbs and push of the hindlimbs. Ross and coworkers *(80)* recently proposed an additional test of grip strength to measure hindlimb extensor response in rats; this device also uses a strain gauge, from which data can be captured electronically. Use of both procedures provides an indication of impaired flexor and extensor responses, which are controlled by different brain regions, and which respond differently to pharmacological challenge.

Rotorod performance is a standard measure of neuromuscular function in behavioral pharmacology testing, but is not frequently employed in developmental neurotoxicity testing. In a survey of 25 laboratories that perform developmental-toxicity testing of pharmaceuticals in the United States and Europe, Lochry et al. *(81)* found that rotorod had been tried by 48% of the laboratories sampled, and retained by only half of those, who rated the test "poor" on a scale for sensitivity. One issue that surrounds rotorod testing is that it is not a "pure" test of neuromuscular function—it requires adequate sensory function (visual cues help to prevent falling from the rotorod), vestibular function, learning and memory if multiple trials are utilized, and motor abilities. If a deficit is observed in rotorod performance, it is difficult to know if it was a result of impaired neuromuscular function, or another behavioral component. Asano and coworkers *(82)* evaluated rotorod performance in Sprague-Dawley and Wistar rats at 19, 20, 21, 22, and 23 d of age, and noted that adequate performance did not begin until eyes were open. Ambulation and rearings were greater in Sprague-Dawley than in Wistar rats, but rotorod performance was poorer. The authors concluded that deficits in rotorod performance were not likely due to motor incoordination, but rather to an increase in exploratory behavior.

A novel test of neuromuscular function used in neonates is rope descent. Rat pups exposed to triethyltin were tested on PND 21 and 22; they were placed on a rope with the head pointing upward, and were then evaluated for their ability to either descend the rope in a head-up or head-down position, or cling to the rope for the duration of the 180-s test session *(83)*. Performance was unsuccessful (i.e., the animal lacked motor coordination or muscle strength) if the animal slid from the rope, which occurred with triethyltin-exposed animals. Another novel observational test was employed in a study of cocaine given to rats via a stock milk solution on PND 4–9, who were then tested for balance using parallel bars and walking gait *(84)*. Rats were required to traverse two parallel aluminum rods for 20 cm with the left paws on one bar and the right paws on the other; distance between the rods was varied by 4-mm increments. Animals were also evaluated for walking gait down a straight acrylic runway, which included stride length, stance width, and step angle. Cocaine exposure impaired performance on the parallel bars, and induced gait disturbance.

2.2.5. Motor Activity/Arousal

Locomotor activity is one of the most extensively studied behaviors in pharmacology and toxicology, largely because of the fact that it is behavior that occurs naturally and is not manipulated by the experimenter. Most animals explore their environment and interact with various components of it; motor activity reflects functional output of the CNS, and it is behavior that is relevant to survival *(85)*. Locomotor activity is movement from one place to another, and is comprised of horizontally directed locomotion (ambulation) and vertically directed locomotion (rearing) *(85)*. The rearing component is particularly useful for identifying peripheral neuropathies. The ontogeny of motor activity in rats has been well-characterized, and is known to be disrupted by neurotoxicants. Motor activity can be evaluated observationally, and is also amenable to electronic-data capture, using a variety of different tests. Tables 4 and 5 list some of the more commonly used automated and observational tests. It is important to note that tests must be capable of detecting an increase or a decrease in activity, as both have been produced by developmental neurotoxicants.

In ontogeny of locomotion, development of quadruped locomotion begins with pivoting (PND 8 in Wistar rats), progresses to crawling (PND 14), and finally, to walking (PND 16) after the eyes are open *(86)*. Forward locomotion progresses with initial elevation of the head, then elevation of the forelimbs and shoulders associated with functional maturation of the forelimbs, and finally elevation of the hindlimbs, associated with maturation of the hindlimbs *(86)*. Randall and Campbell *(87)* observed a sharp increase in locomotion from PND 5–15 in rats separated from their home environment, followed by a rapid decline from PND 15–30; this pattern could be disrupted by various psychoactive agents and was thought to represent maturation of various neurotransmitter systems. In the context of the normal litter environment, however, this developmental pattern was disrupted: pups were relatively inactive during the first 15 d of life, and then showed a gradual increase in activity during the next 15 d. Thus, the initial pattern observed was thought to be a result of isolation distress, rather than just maturational changes in the brain. This "home cage" pattern has also been observed in studies of the ontogeny of figure-8 maze activity; pups initially display a burst of activity during the first 5 min of the test session that soon subsides, but by PND 20 activity becomes more continuous across the test session *(70)*.

Ontogeny of locomotion has been used by Vorhees et al. *(62)* to evaluate early signs of developmental neurotoxicity. In this evaluation, locomotion of neonatal rats is monitored from the most primitive form, pivoting, to forward locomotion with the head and body low, to forward locomotion with the body raised and head low, to adult locomotion with the head and body raised. These stages are achieved on approx PND 2–4, 6–8, 10–11, and 14–15, respectively *(62,72)*. Ontogeny of swimming can also be used to assess neonatal activity, evaluating such endpoints as direction, angle in the water (or head position), and use of limbs *(62)*. Another early behavior that has been evaluated is wall climbing. This behavior is specific to PND 7–17, can be easily evaluated in a standard open field during a 30-min test session, and is disrupted by chemicals inducing aberrant motoric effects *(70)*.

One of the most commonly used observational tests of motor activity is the open field, which can be observational, or can be bounded by photobeams that facilitate electronic-data capture. An open field usually consists of an area greater than the home cage that is bounded by walls and divided into subsections. When placed into the novel environment of an open field, the tendency of a rat is to freeze momentarily, and then to begin exploration. Agents can impact the initial freezing response, so the initial measure of latency is important. As time progresses in the open field, novelty ceases to become a relevant stimulus, and the animal spends most of its time in "wall-hugging" behavior, also known as thigmotaxis. Thigmotaxis is considered an indicator of emotional state (related to avoidance of predators and importance of vibrissae contact), and can also be disrupted by neuroactive compounds *(88)*. Parameters measured include latency to first movement, total number of crossings of the subsections, and number of rearings *(85)*. Many more parameters can be measured, but these are the most common. In addition to locomotor activity, movement in an open field can be used to evaluate fear of novelty. A novel object can be placed in the open field, and the animal can then be assessed for the frequency and duration of wall rearing, sniffing, grooming, face washing, immobility, and contacts with the novel object *(89)*. Although number of urinations and defecations has been used as a measure of emotionality in the open field, the validity of this concept has been questioned due to lack of correlation with measures of emotionality obtained in other behavioral tests such as cage emergence and active avoidance *(90)*. It appears that the pattern of response to novel environments such as an open field, and emotional behavior such as increased heart rate on handling or escape responses following electric shock, may be better indicators of the emotional state of the animal *(90)*.

The most successful and reliable measures of locomotor activity are from devices using infrared photobeams; they are relatively trouble-free, easily calibrated and standardized, and they provide no feedback to the animal. EPA requires motor activity testing in developmental-neurotoxicity evaluations, using a device that can detect both increases and decreases in activity *(60)*. The open field type of test is not the only automated means of measuring locomotor activity. Additional systems include field detectors to measure nonspecific movements, activity wheels attached to the home cage, photocell-based systems (which can include a more complex environment such as a figure-8 maze or residential maze), stabilimeters, and video-based systems to evaluate different types of locomotion and topography of locomotion *(70,84,91)*. The advantage to automated testing is that it provides an objective measure of activity; however, there is one crucial element missing. Because the experimenter is not directly observing the animal, such treatment-related effects on activity as gait abnormalities and stereotypies could be missed. Although some automated open field devices can measure repetitive movement that is designated as stereotypy, the true nature of stereotypic behavior should be described to allow for complete data interpretation. Therefore, automated measures of locomotor activity should be accompanied by observations of clinical signs in the same animals, or at the very least, in animals exposed to the same treatment regimen.

The open-field environment can also be used in further testing of the response to novelty using the hole-board/head-dipping test. Holes can be placed strategically in the floor or sides of an open field, and number of different holes and visits to each hole are recorded *(89)*. Abel *(92)* has shown that ambulation and head dipping are different behaviors, rather than different manifestations of the same behavior—exploration— and thus are under the influence of different brain functions. Consequently, these two behaviors could be differentially affected by a test agent.

One question that frequently arises is the appropriate duration for a test session to evaluate locomotor activity. Observational tests tend to be shorter in duration (≤10 min), while automated tests are either 30 min–1 h, or longer if a residential maze is used or cageside video monitoring is conducted. Short test sessions are considered suitable for evaluation of effects on emotionality or exploration, but may be more susceptible to environmental confounders such as handling, familiarity of the animal with the test chamber, and contributions of behaviors related to attempts to escape *(88)*. Short-duration tests are not acceptable to EPA, which requires that the test session be long enough for motor activity to approach asymptotic levels by the last 20% of the session for untreated control animals *(60)*. In addition to evaluating ambulation and other parameters, tests of 10–60 min duration can also be useful in evaluating habituation of activity. Habituation is defined as decreased response to repeated stimulation, and is considered a form of simple learning, or behavioral plasticity *(93,94)*. As the novelty of the open field declines as a relevant stimulus, the animal learns to respond less to the environment, unless the habituation phenomenon is disrupted by a neurotoxicant. Residential tests can be useful in studying the effects of agents over a prolonged period, and on circadian cycles of activity.

2.2.6. Sensory Function

The most commonly used test of sensory function involves elicitation of the startle reflex in response to a stimulus belonging to a given sensory modality. Although stimuli may be visual or tactile, auditory stimuli are used to the greatest extent. The auditory startle reflex (ASR) is present at an early age in rats (*see* Table 4), and its ontogeny is easily tested by placing a neonate in a sound-attenuated enclosure and then using some means to generate a sharp noise stimulus, such as a "clicker" toy. The response is generally a flicking of the ears, flinching, and/or jumping. The auditory startle neuronal circuit is relatively simple, and involves the auditory nerve, spinal cord, 3–5 central synapses, motor neurons, and the neuromuscular junction *(95)*. It is disrupted by a variety of developmental neurotoxicants, and can be either increased or decreased in magnitude and/or latency. Developing mammals are known to be more sensitive to ototoxicity induced by noise, chemicals, and drugs than are adults, and the period of maximum sensitivity corresponds to the periods of anatomical and functional maturation of the cochlea *(96)*.

The clicker test is considered relatively insensitive, and can be easily confounded by environmental variables such as sound in the testing room. Therefore, the majority of startle testing involves automated equipment. Fukumura et al. *(97)* conducted a comparative study of the observational clicker test in adult rats treated with the neurotoxicant 3,3'-iminodipropionitrile (IDPN). For observational testing a metal clicker with a resonant frequency of 5 kHz, rise time of 50 ms, and amplitude of 100 dB(A) was placed above the rat's head and activated. Scoring of the response was 1 = no response, 2 = small response (evidence sound was heard, e.g., pinna flick), 3 = muscle flinch or noticeable startle response, 4 = more energetic response (movement or small jump), and 5 = extreme response (jump or biting response). Automated equipment was an SR-Pilot portable startle reflex system (San Diego Instruments) that delivered a 115 dB (relative to A scale) broad-band, mixed-frequency, noise-burst stimulus of 40 milliseconds duration, with a rise time of ≤40 ms. While both methods detected a decrement in auditory-startle responding, the automated method was more sensitive and, the authors concluded, more efficient.

Habituation (i.e., decrement in response) occurs upon repeated presentation of a startle stimulus, and can be used to evaluate disruption of plasticity by developmental neurotoxicants. EPA regulations for developmental neurotoxicity testing require evaluation of habituation to an auditory stimulus *(60)*. Both within- (short-term) and between-session (long-term) habituation can be evaluated, as demonstrated in a study of cocaine given to rats on PND 1–10 or 11–20, who were then tested for auditory startle (116 dB white noise for 116 trials) on two consecutive days *(98)*. Treatment on PND 1–10 resulted in an increase in startle responding on D 2 of testing with no effect on within-session habituation. In contrast, treatment on PND 11–20 produced no effects on ASR or habituation. It was therefore concluded that the critical period for cocaine-induced disruption of long-term habituation to auditory stimuli is PND 1–10, and that PND 11–20 may be after the critical period of development. Although not routinely evaluated in toxicity testing, sensitization is another property associated with ASR. Persistent exposure to a low-level stimulus may actually result in an enhanced response to a startle stimulus. Presentation of repeated startle stimuli can engage both habituation and sensitization, so if an agent induces a response decrement, it may not be entirely due to interference with habituation, but rather could also be from increased sensitization *(95)*.

Response to a startle stimulus relies on adequate motivation and neuromuscular function; if a deficit in startle response is induced by a developmental neurotoxicant, it is important to identify if the effect is due to injury to a specific sensory modality or to a deficit in the motivation or ability to respond. One way of dealing with this issue is to evaluate reflex modification of the startle response *(99)*. The amplitude of the startle response can be depressed for about 1 s by preceding the startle stimulus with a brief light flash, noise burst, or tactile stimulus, even though the magnitude of these prepulse stimuli is not sufficient to elicit the startle response *(95)*. Prepulse inhibition occurs across species, and is considered to represent a primitive form of responsivity to stimulus input and a fundamental form of behavioral plasticity *(100)*. In evaluations of ototoxicity, prepulse inhibition is actually considered a more sensitive indicator than is the response elicited by a single auditory stimulus *(101)*. Prepulse inhibition increases with postnatal age, and is developed by about the third week of life in rats *(100)*. Because the animal must be able to detect the prepulse stimulus in order to demonstrate an attenuated startle response, the sensory modality is being tested, rather than the ability of the animal to physically respond. Shifts in sensory thresholds can be determined, as in the case of perinatal treatment of rats with propylthiouracil, in which exposed offspring demonstrated a dose-dependent deficit in auditory threshold at multiple frequencies when tested as adults *(57)*.

Using automated equipment, a substantial amount of information can be collected on the startle response during one test session. In our laboratory, three 90 dB prepulse trials are alternated with three 120 dB startle trials to evaluate prepulse inhibition, and then 50 additional startle trials are presented at 120 dB each to evaluate habituation; the entire test session takes approx 25 min. Other laboratories conduct separate sessions for habituation and prepulse inhibition, and vary the prepulse stimulus at different frequencies and/or amplitudes to evaluate range of hearing loss by establishing an auditory threshold *(57)*. Weir and coworkers *(102)* have combined auditory startle, tactile startle, and prepulse inhibition into a single test session of 5 "no stimulus," 5 auditory, 5 tactile, and 5 prepulse trials, for a total testing duration of 5 min.

Automated equipment used to measure startle responding employs displacement of a platform due to the crouching and/or jumping of the animal, or some other means to translate changes in force exerted by the movements of the animal to voltage readable by dedicated software. The nature of these devices indicates that their output may not only depend on neuromuscular tone, but also on the weight of the animal. Hutchings et al. *(103)* conducted an experiment in which rats treated perinatally with methadone were evaluated for 121 ASR trials on PND 21–23. No treatment-related effect was observed with unadjusted ASR data. However, when body weight was used as a covariate in data analysis, startle responding of methadone-exposed animals, who weighed less than controls, exceeded that of controls. There are different schools of thought regarding the use of a parameter as a covariate in statistical analysis that is also capable of being affected by treatment. However, even if analysis of covariance is not used, interpretation of ASR data must take into account potential body-weight effects. This is important in light of the fact that food deprivation with resultant suppression of body weight is known to depress startle *(95)*.

2.2.7. Learning and Memory

US EPA guidelines for developmental neurotoxicity testing require that tests of associative learning, and memory, be conducted *(60)*. Tests for associative learning are those in which behavior changes as a function of relations that are arranged between two or more events *(104)*. Examples of associative learning are classical Pavlovian conditioning, in which one stimulus is followed temporally and contingently by another, and instrumental learning (operant conditioning), in which there is a temporal, contingent relationship between a response of the subject and subsequent stimulus outcome. While tests of this level of sophistication are normally conducted in adult animals, an olfactory discrimination test that employs Pavlovian conditioning has been used successfully in neonates, and relies on the fact that chemical senses can guide behavior earlier in postnatal development than can auditory and visual senses *(104)*. In this test, olfactory stimuli are paired with footshock; the pup is trained in a two-compartment box (with no movement between compartments) to associate one type of odor with footshock and another with no adverse consequence. The pup is then placed in another apparatus with the same two odors and free passage between the compartments, and is required to choose between compartments. This test can not only be used for acquisition, but is also suitable for evaluating long-term retention. Moderately food-deprived rat pups can be trained in a T-maze task for food reward as early as PND 7, in an example of instrumental learning *(104)*.

US EPA advises that if a treatment-related effect is seen, additional tests should be conducted to rule out alterations in sensory, motivational, and/or motor capacities as potential causes *(60)*. Eckerman and Bushnell *(105)* advocate the use of a test-battery approach to identify specific effects on learning and memory, employing not only assessments of associative learning, but also nonassociative learning (such as habituation) and selective learning (such as reinforcement of operant behavior). These authors indicate that if a neurotoxicant affects persistence of a behavioral change, then it is more appropriate to describe the effect as a change in memory rather than a change in learning; however, the division between learning and memory is not entirely clear-cut, and neurotoxic effects on both are usually comingled *(105)*. This concept is reflected in the US EPA guidelines, which state that effects on memory (short-term or long-term) cannot be evaluated in the absence of a measure of acquisition obtained from the same test *(60)*.

Many tests of learning and/or memory are available, as indicated in Tables 4 and 5. One of the tests used most frequently in developmental neurotoxicity screens is passive avoidance *(81)*, which basically requires a rat to learn to remain in a lighted chamber rather than enter a preferred dark chamber in which it has received footshock. Acquisition can be accomplished in one trial, or shock levels can be lowered and acquisition measured over repeated trials; retention over a delay can also be evaluated as an indication of memory *(105)*. Navigation of mazes is also popular for evaluating learning and memory; the most commonly used of these are simple two-choice mazes in which the rat is required to select the arm with a food reward or an escape from water; the M-maze (either spatial or visually cued), which requires the rat to choose the appropriate side in order to escape from water; the Biel and Cincinnati water mazes, which also require the rat to make a correct choice to escape and can evaluate performance on both a forward and reverse path; the eight-arm radial maze, in which the rat is required to locate specific arms baited with food; and the Morris maze, in which the rat is required to use visual cues to locate an escape platform in a water tank *(49,81,106)*.

Other tests of learning and memory of increased complexity such as active avoidance and operant conditioning have been used extensively in neuropharmacology testing, but are not routinely used in test batteries to evaluate developmental neuotoxicity, largely because they are considered inefficient in the context of a screen. Peele and Vincent *(107)* stated that there appears to be an inverse relationship between number of subjects and number of sessions required to complete an experiment in learning and memory. This can be difficult to justify from a resource standpoint if a large number of agents must be tested. However, more complex tests are used in the characterization of effects on learning and memory. Burbacher and associates *(108)* provide an interesting argument for the use of a more sensitive test, in that the lowest dose of methylmercury required to disrupt active avoidance responding in rats was over 100 times greater than the effective dose for differential reinforcement of high rates of responding. One advantage of a testing paradigm such as schedule-controlled behavior is that it affords precise control over behavior that can be maintained over long periods of time *(107)* and thus is amenable to longitudinal testing.

Ultimately, which tests of learning and memory are best to include in developmental neurotoxicity batteries remains unclear. A survey of pharmaceutical companies conducting developmental neurotoxicity testing revealed that although water mazes were used more often, passive avoidance received a higher degree of satisfaction for practicality, variability, and sensitivity *(81)*. However, in a study of rat offspring from dams treated with methimazole or phenytoin, Weisenburg et al. *(49)* determined that the Cincinnati water maze, spatial M-maze, and passive avoidance with one learning trial detected drug effects (listed in order of decreasing sensitivity), whereas the visually cued M-maze and passive avoidance with multiple learning trials did not. Given this variation, it is difficult to imagine that a "gold standard" for evaluating learning and memory in screening tests will be identified in the near future.

2.2.8. Social Interaction/Emotional Responsivity

The many facets of social interaction in general negate the use of automated data collection; thus, testing is usually observational and takes advantage of the fact that animals are engaging in natural behaviors, and not behavior shaped by the investigator *(109)*. Rather, social behavior in rodents is highly dependent on the stimulus value of littermates and the maternal animal *(110)*. General categories for investigation in rodents include flight or submissive, social grooming, sexual, aggressive, and investigative/exploratory behaviors. Bekkedal and coworkers *(111)* have developed a battery of tests to evaluate social behavior in rats that includes juvenile play, adult social investigation, and the elevated plus maze. In the juvenile play paradigm, rat pups isolated from their littermates for 2–3 h are placed in pairs in an open field and evaluated for dorsal contacts (scored when one partner touches the dorsal surface of the other with its front paws) and pins (scored each time one partner holds the other down on its dorsal surface). Social investigation is evaluated in adults by placing animals in two transparent acrylic boxes oriented end to end, with one end facing the other box and one end facing a bare wall. A hole located at the end of each box allows the animal to stick its nose through and to face the other; social contacts are measured during a 30-min test session. The elevated plus-maze evaluates emotional responsivity in a maze in which two arms are surrounded by walls and two arms are open. The animal is placed in the center of the maze with access to all four arms, and the frequency and duration of episodes in which the open arms are traversed are measured.

One means of evaluating social behavior in neonates is through interactions with the maternal animal. Ultrasonic distress vocalizations have been measured by placing a rat pup in a glass cylinder containing bedding from the home cage. Ultrasonic vocalizations from the pup at 40 kHz are then measured during a 1-min test session. Maternal behavior toward the pups can influence functional outcome and is also of interest. Dams can be evaluated observationally for nest construction, pup retrieval, and grooming and nursing of pups, and at the same time, exploratory behavior of the pups in the home cage can be assessed *(109)*. Ultrasonic vocalizations were found to be altered by prenatal exposure of rats to methylmercury: development of calls was delayed, number of calls was decreased, the base interval and call duration were shortened, and the frequency distribution was flattened and shifted to a higher frequency *(112)*.

The maternal animal provides nutritional and hydrational needs, maintenance of body temperature, and sensory stimulation; disruption of these functions can adversely affect offspring development, including effects on later social and sexual behavior *(113)*.Various aspects of maternal behavior have been characterized experimentally *(67)*, and observational methods or scoring of maternal behavior have proven useful in developmental neurotoxicity studies to interpret subsequent effects on health and behavior of offspring *(67,71)*.

2.3. Additional Test Methods

While behavioral methodology is primarily used to evaluate developmental neurotoxicity, an excellent body of work exists on toxicant-induced changes in morphology, neurochemistry, and electrophysiology. A relatively new and exciting area is the application of molecular biology to developmental neurotoxicology. With the exception of brain histopathology required by EPA *(60)*, these techniques are not routinely used to investigate developmental neurotoxicity in studies conducted according to regulatory guidelines. However, they are of great benefit in characterizing responses identified in preliminary neurobehavioral screens, and in elucidating the mechanisms by which toxicants disrupt the developing nervous system.

A great deal of information is currently known about the development of the brain, as discussed in Subheading 1.3., and of the functional consequences that can arise from toxicant-induced damage to brain structures. Brain pathology in the developing organism is different in nature from that of the adult, and often involves interference with developmental processes rather than destruction of tissue. Rodier *(37)* has detailed specific categories of defects that characterize many developmental neurotoxicants: changes in neuron number, position, or orientation, changes in neuronal connections, and changes in supporting tissues of neurons such as myelin. The nature of these changes is largely quantitative, and they may not be readily apparent on morphologic examination of brain tissue, arguing for the use of quantitative techniques in identification of CNS changes induced during development *(37)*.

Neurotransmitters are present at very early stages of brain development and not only mediate behavioral and physiological responses of the immature animal, but also have trophic effects on maturation of target organs that, if disrupted, can induce reorganization of structures in the adult brain *(114)*. Tissue-culture studies using neurons from various brain regions and microinjections into discrete brain regions have shown that monoamines (norepinephrine [NE], 5-hydroxytryptamine [5-HT], and dopamine [DA]), inhibitory amino acids (γ-amino butyric acic [GABA]), and excitatory amino acids (glutamate, *N*-methyl-D-aspartate [NMDA], quisqualate, and kainate) influence neuronal differentiation via either trophic or degenerative processes *(115)*. The biogenic amines are among the first neurotransmitters present during early stages of brain development, and are functionally mature at birth; other neurotransmitters develop and mature within the first 3 wk after birth in the rat, which is a period of vulnerability to toxicants *(114)*. This is the period of the brain growth spurt, during which brain weight and DNA content increase dramatically *(23,24)*. Many developmental neurotoxicity studies have correlated changes in specific neurotransmitters with functional deficits. Elsner et al. *(116)* participated in a collaborative study in which behavior, proteins indicative of glial damage, and brain weight were evaluated in offspring from rat dams treated with methylmercury on GD 6–9. Treatment-related deficits were observed in swimming behavior, spatial alternation, visual discrimination, and activity, with an increase in auditory startle amplitude. These changes were accompanied by an increased concentration of glial fibrillary acidic protein (GFAP) in the cerebellar vermis and increased cerebellar vermis weight, indicative of hypertrophy or proliferation of astroglial cells in response to injury, and decreased S-100 protein in the hippocampus, indicative of a deleterious effect on normal astroglial status.

In issuing guidelines on neurophysiology, sensory-evoked potentials *(117)*, EPA acknowledged the importance of evaluating dysfunction of auditory, somatosensory, and visual sensory systems by a means other than behavior. Although these guidelines apply to neurotoxicity testing of adult animals (42–120 d of age), the techniques are also applicable to offspring from developmental neurotoxicity studies. This technique requires recording of brain electrical potentials from temporarily or permanently affixed electrodes following stimuli of various sensory modalities. One of the advantages of neurophysiological measures is that the degree of comparability between laboratory animal species and humans is higher than for most behavioral measures *(118)*. Mattsson and coworkers *(119)* developed a neurophysiology battery that appears to be sensitive, comprehensive, and practical, and is used in concert with a functional observational battery, grip performance, body temperature, and comprehensive neuropathology to identify neurofunctional and neuropathological deficits induced by a neurotoxicant. This battery includes flash-evoked potentials, auditory brainstem response to clicks, auditory brainstem response to tone pips, somatosensory-evoked potentials, and caudal nerve-action potentials, and has been shown to successfully identify neurotoxic potential.

In a developmental neurotoxicity study, Yargicoglu et al. *(120)* successfully evaluated flash-evoked potentials in offspring from female mice treated with cadmium chloride during gestation or during gestation and lactation. Mean latency and amplitudes of peaks associated with flash-evoked potentials were lower than those of controls for both exposure conditions, indicating that cadmium was toxic to the developing visual system. Kremer and coworkers *(121)* evaluated the effect of maternal exposure to two PCB congeners on the flash-evoked electroretinogram (ERG) of adult rats, and determined that the amplitudes of ERG were reduced in females but not males, in what was apparently the first experimental report of PCB effects on visual processes. Brainstem auditory evoked potentials elicited by click stimuli were employed by Church and Overbeck *(122)* to evaluate hearing in rat offspring prenatally exposed to cocaine. Testing was conducted on PND 35 and at 6 mo of age; prolonged latency of peaks associated with brainstem-evoked potentials and reduced amplitude were observed on PND 35 only, leading to the conclusion that the effect was a developmental delay that dissipated with age.

Several examples are given in Subheading 1.3.5. of the ways in which biochemistry and molecular biology are contributing to the field of developmental neurotoxicology. A great deal of recent work has investigated the role of various proteins, second messengers, and oxygen radicals in toxicant-induced damage. In the previous example on visual-evoked potentials from the laboratory of Yargicoglu and coworkers *(120)*, thiobarbituric acid reactive substances (TBARS) were measured in brain homogenates as an indication of lipid peroxidation. Peroxidative damage of membrane structure and changes in associated enzymes, receptors, and physiological function may ultimately result in disturbances of neuronal function, and this type of damage was associated with effects on visual function.

In vitro experiments with neuronal cell cultures, as described previously for studies with neurotransmitters, as well as work with specific cell lines, are also ongoing. The purpose in designing an in vitro model of developmental neurotoxicity is to explore the mechanisms underlying adverse effects found in in vivo studies in a setting in which the cellular environment is controlled, and to uncover new, unsuspected targets that can be subsequently examined in animals. In a study of the developmental effects of the insecticide chlorpyrifos, Song and coworkers *(123)* used a rat pheochromocytoma (PC12) cell line to investigate the means by which it affects cell acquisition through a mixture of cholinergic and noncholinergic mechanisms. The cloned PC12 cell line initially resembles sympathetic neuronal precursor cells, but then differentiates (under the induction of nerve-growth factor) to resemble sympathetic neurons morphologically, physiologically, and biochemically. Chlorpyrifos was found to exert disruption in three different contexts: effects during cell replication, effects on early stages of differentiation, and effects on neurite extension. Inhibition of macromolecule synthesis was found to be the basic mechanism underlying deficits in cell acquisition and differentiation. Hippocampal and cortical slices have also been used in recent years to investigate mechanisms. In a study of lead given to nursing female rats, following treatment with the nitric oxide (NO)-generating inhibitor nitroprusside, long-term potentiation, considered a form of synaptic plasticity and an important component of learning and memory, was evaluated in young adult offspring *(124)*. A single hippocampal slice was taken from each animal, a recording electrode was placed in the dendrites of pyramidal cells in area CA1 or CA3, tetanic stimulation was given, and excitatory postsynaptic potentials were recorded. Lead caused an increase in long-term potentiation, and the authors concluded that NO could be a messenger molecule in these areas of the hippocampus.

3. DATA INTERPRETATION

3.1. Relevance of Animal Models

A common question is whether developmental neurotoxicity testing in animals provides a reasonable prediction of what will occur in humans. One issue surrounding extrapolation of rodent data to humans is that behavior in particular is highly species-specific and exquisitely adapted to the survival needs of the individual and its species; structural differences exist between rodent and human brains, and behavioral repertoires differ *(125)*. In addition, while the sequence of development of the CNS is very similar across species, the timing of events is not; as an example, a great deal of functional maturation of the nervous system occurs postnatally in the rat, while many of the maturational processes occur in late gestation in the human. However, there are correlates between animals and humans for many nervous-system functions, and testing may include such commonalities as reflex development, sensory-motor function, reactivity and/or habituation, locomotor activity, and learning and memory, as well as reproductive behavior and other behaviors such as aggression and socialization. Good animal models exist that duplicate effects seen with the developmental neurotoxicants ethanol, lead, and methylmercury. These animal models have also implicated over 200 agents, based on lists of developmental neurotoxicants identified experimentally *(16,58)*.

In 1989, the EPA and the National Institute on Drug Abuse (NIDA) cosponsored a workshop on the comparability of human and animal developmental neurotoxicants, which involved discussions of agents known to affect humans and laboratory animals, including ethanol, methylmercury, lead, ionizing radiation, selected agents of abuse, PCBs, and phenytoin; comparability of data related to motor development and function, sensory function, cognitive function, motivation/arousal behavior, and social behavior was evaluated. Various work groups were asked to discuss comparability of endpoints, test methods used in human risk assessment, weight of evidence and quantitative evaluation of developmental neurotoxicity data, and triggers for developmental neurotoxicity testing; a summary of these proceedings is provided in Rees et al. *(126)*. Workshop participants concluded that comparable measures of function are available across species, but that data for each species are not always available; dose-response comparisons usually cannot be made across species because data are often not available for multiple dose levels or similar functions *(127)*. In general, it was recognized that comparable changes in motor development and function are observed between rodents and humans, and, with the exception of some drugs of abuse, effects on cognitive function were also comparable; the minimal data available for sensory systems at that time also revealed good concordance *(126)*. The database for social behavior was considered too limited to draw conclusions.

Consideration of well-characterized developmental neurotoxicants in general reveals concordance between human and animal effects; there are some exceptions, however. For moderate doses of ethanol, there is a good deal of congruence with respect to qualitative endpoints: general functional categories such as deficits in learning and memory, inhibition, attention, regulatory behaviors, and motor performance are affected in both laboratory animals and children, and are in general dose-related in magnitude *(128)*. Qualitative similarities between human and animal findings also occur for lead and involve relatively complex behavioral processes such as cognition and learning *(28)*. Convergence is not as good for other neurobehavioral endpoints; as an example, perseverative tendencies and increased variability in individuals' responses have been noted in rodent and primate experiments, but not in human epidemiology studies. Davis and coworkers *(28)* state that the primary effects on learning and memory with lead would argue for using more complex schedules in operant conditioning tasks in an experimental test battery, rather than simple discriminations or other schedules that might not adequately tax an animal's capabilities. With PCBs, allowing for differences in testing, effects are roughly similar across species; however, for the most part tests of higher cortical function are affected in laboratory animals, while observed delays in development in children are predominantly motor, although it is difficult to assess higher cortical function in infants *(129)*. Methylmercury-induced pathology appears to exhibit species-related differences: in humans cell loss, reduced myelin, and ectopic cell masses in the cortex with disorganization of cell layers occurs, while in rodents myelin deficiency is observed in the absence of ectopic cells *(130)*. At very high doses behavioral effects in animal models are similar to humans, but at lower doses comparison of specific endpoints does not demonstrate many similarities across species.

Results with these agents tend to support the statement by Rees et al. *(64)* that the type of functional impairment is generally predictive, rather than specific endpoints. Multiple factors must be weighed in determining the relevance of animal models to human risk, including time and duration of exposure, route of exposure and dose level, and species or genotype; also important are the number of species exhibiting adverse developmental effects, how this was manifested, and the conditions under which they were induced, as well as frequency and dose responsiveness *(131)*. Species differences in response can result from intrinsic genetic characteristics, differences in pharmacokinetic and metabolic capabilities, physiological and morphological differences in pregnancy and fetal development, and extrinsic environmental factors *(131)*; control of as many of these factors as possible is essential for adequate extrapolation of laboratory animal data to humans.

3.2. Relevance of Test Methods

In humans, multiple aspects of nervous system functioning are evaluated by testing for sensory abilities, motor skills and coordination, sensory-motor integration, language-based abilities, accumulated knowledge, attention, reasoning ability, and other aspects of cognition. Correlates for many of these functions exist in laboratory animals in reflex development, sensory-motor function, reactivity and/or habituation, locomotor activity, and learning and memory, as well as reproductive behavior and other behaviors such as aggression and socialization *(132,133)*. In addition to behavior testing, functional assessments in the laboratory setting may also include evaluations of neurochemistry, neuropathology, and neurophysiology, which in turn may be correlated with behavioral function and, particularly in the case of neurophysiology, may be correlated with human data *(see* Chapter 2 by Rice). Neurochemical assessments may include changes in neurotransmitter levels, turnover rates, and receptor binding, CNS metabolic profiles, and activities of developmental markers. Evaluation of structural alterations may include whole and regional brain weights; histologic assessments; electron microscopy; quantitative assessment of neuronal and glial proteins, which signal damage within the nervous system, and morphometry *(13)*. Neurophysiologic measures offer good opportunities for cross-species comparison between humans and laboratory species with minimal modification to the tests, and may include flash-evoked potentials, auditory brainstem response, and somatosensory-evoked potentials, as well as experimental measurement of caudal nerve action potentials *(118,119)*.

A survey conducted by Kimmel and Buelke-Sam of academic and industrial laboratories found a total absence of consensus on acceptable test methods, with approx 100 individual tests being conducted in 14 major categories of behavioral functioning *(55)*. The majority opinion expressed in a workshop on test methods *(132)* indicated that it was inappropriate to assemble a final list of test procedures for use in every situation, but rather, a list of functions such as those indicated previously should be tested. This is in keeping with the ICH guidance for reproductive toxicity testing, which indicates that all persons involved in protocol design should be willing to discuss and consider variations in test strategy according to the state-of-the-art and ethical standards in human and animal experimentation *(65)*. Thus, creativity is encouraged in designing testing strategies. Publication of results using a variety of tests should be encouraged to build an adequate historical database for developmental neurotoxicology test batteries. There are bound to be some differences in behavior data generated by different laboratories due to environmental influences, and genetic drift may be a factor to consider in comparing study data with historical reference ranges, but having a standard range of values with which to compare ongoing testing can be a valuable asset in data interpretation. Interlaboratory comparisons of developmental neurotoxicity data can help to increase comfort levels with the reliability and sensitivity of tests. Reliability is the ability of a test to produce a consistent pattern of results within the same laboratory concurrently and over time, and across different laboratories *(134)*. Note that this indicates a consistent pattern of results, but not necessarily the identical values. Sensitivity is considered to relate to CNS functional integrity in relation to other methods of detecting developmental toxicity, the ability of the test to respond to particular types of dysfunction, or the detection sensitivity of measurement based on error variance *(134)*. Validity of tests, concerned with the parameter measured by a test and how well the test measures this parameter, is also an important consideration, in that statistically significant findings with invalid tests can impede or prevent the development of important agents that are safe *(52)*.

3.3. Factors That Can Influence the Outcome of Testing

Many intrinsic and extrinsinc factors can influence the outcome of developmental neurotoxicity testing, and thus should be carefully considered in designing test batteries and testing facilities, and in data interpretation. The ultimate question, and one which is not easily answered with general test batteries, is whether behavioral changes are due to direct effects on the CNS, or are secondary to a number of factors, including the following.

3.3.1. Overt Toxicity

There are many factors that can influence the outcome of behavior testing, and that have to be taken into account when interpreting data. A positive effect in a testing battery may or may not be indicative of a direct effect on the CNS. Overt toxicity to the exposed adult or neonate can certainly change behavior. Maternal toxicity can also confound interpretation in a developmental study; such factors as maternal malnutrition and stress can exert a negative impact on the behavioral development of the offspring.

In a review on neurobehavioral aspects of developmental toxicity testing, Ulbrich and Palmer *(135)* examined 197 reported pre- and postnatal studies that included behavioral assessment of offspring. One aspect of this review was a comparison of the incidences of maternal toxicity, pregnancy duration, pup mortality, pup body weight, and developmental effects in studies in which behavioral effects were manifested, vs those in which no behavioral effects were observed. Behavior was affected in offspring in 64 of these studies, and was unaffected in 133 studies. Maternal toxicity and increased pup mortality occurred in approx half of the studies, with essentially no difference between studies in which offspring behavior was affected or unaffected. There also was no distinction between studies with behaviorally affected or unaffected offspring for increased pregnancy duration or developmental effects, which occurred in approx 20 and 30% of studies, respectively. The only parameter that was distinctly different was reduced pup weight, which occurred in 59% of studies in which offspring behavior was unaffected, but occurred in 70% of those in which behavior was affected. This difference was borne out in comparisons conducted for fertility studies and teratology studies, which included behavioral testing of offspring.

Nelson *(136)* discussed the impact of prolonged exposure on overt toxicity to offspring in developmental neurotoxicity testing, and proposed that reduction in exposure duration might unmask behavioral deficits that could be confounded by weight reductions induced by long-term exposure. While exposure period is mandated by regulatory guidelines for test batteries conducted to identify developmental neurotoxicity, shorter exposure periods could certainly be considered in subsequent studies conducted to characterize effects.

Regulatory guidelines for developmental neurotoxicity testing mandate that the highest dose tested induce maternal toxicity. Essential measures of maternal toxicity include body weight and weight gain; clinical signs of toxicity, morbidity, or mortality; food/water consumption; and necropsy for gross evidence of organ toxicity *(137)*. Additional parameters may be evaluated as necessary. One issue surrounding maternal toxicity is that the stress caused to the maternal animal can in itself influence offspring behavior and thus be a potential confounder. Mattsson and coworkers *(138)* suggested that the severity of maternal toxicity could be minimized by more careful attention to maternal health through the use of histopathology, organ weight, neurochemistry, neurophysiology, and behavioral evaluations, as well as standard body-weight data.

The paternal animal may also contribute to developmental neurotoxicity through genetic (germ-cell) alterations, toxic or epigenetic effects, seminal-fluid transfer of the toxicant, and hormone alterations in the male *(139)*. Overt toxicity in the male could influence several of these parameters and thus have an impact on the conceptus. However, due to the lack of direct contact between the paternal animal and the conceptus, and the fact that most agents identified so far that induce paternally mediated developmental neurotoxicity do so through genotoxic mechanisms *(27,140)*, overt paternal toxicity does not seem to represent a major potential confounder in data interpretation.

3.3.2. Undernutrition

Nutrition is probably the single greatest environmental influence on the fetus and neonate, and plays a necessary role in maturation and functional development of the CNS *(18)*. Undernutrition/malnutrition can exert adverse effects during any stage of the prolonged development of the nervous system. Undernutrition is an important consideration in interpreting developmental neurotoxicity studies; although developing rat offspring can probably tolerate a 10–15% deficit in maternal body-weight gain without showing neurobehavioral effects *(34)*, undernutrition during the preweaning growth spurt is particularly deleterious to brain development. Prenatal undernutrition is also deleterious, can adversely affect early developmental processes such as neurogenesis, cell migration, and differentiation, and shows little or no "catch-up" potential *(18)*. Undernutrition is one of the biggest confounders of developmental neurotoxicity data. Testing conducted under regulatory guidelines requires that some degree of maternal toxicity be produced in the highest dose tested, and this toxicity is often manifested as reductions in food intake and body-weight gain. Thus, the developing animal could be undernourished from the time of conception through weaning.

Experimental production of undernutrition can be accomplished by nutrient restriction of the dam during pregnancy and/or lactation, and/or by various manipulations of the pups. One means of producing undernutrition in offspring is to manipulate litter size, based on the concept that larger litter sizes require greater energy expenditure. In a study in mice, Wainwright and coworkers *(141)* found that for every additional pup in a litter (considered an indication of diminishing nutrient availability), body growth was retarded by the equivalent of 1.28 d, brain weight by 0.44 d, and behavioral development by 0.07 d. Effects of undernutrition have been studied using a variety of behaviors, and have included increased activity in familiar, nonstressful situations; hyperresponsiveness to aversive and novel kinds of stimulation (including electric shock), delayed habituation of locomotor activity, decreased retention in a visual-discrimination test, poor active avoidance performance, and increased motivation to navigate a maze or lever press for a food reward *(142–146)*.

Many laboratories employ the practice of litter-size reduction (culling) to equal numbers within the first few days following parturition to minimize potential nutritional and behavioral bias resulting from unequal litter sizes. Litter size in rodents appears to be inversely correlated with brain and body weights *(147–150)* the appearance of some developmental landmarks *(151,152)*, and behavioral performance *(148)*. In a study of mice reared in litters of 8 or 16, Nagy and coworkers *(153)* found delays in acquisition of adult-like swimming and spontaneous locomotor activity, and a delay in retention of a T-maze task. The impact of unequal litter sizes on behavior was considered of sufficient importance by the EPA that their guidelines on developmental neurotoxicity testing recommend litter-size adjustment, and state that litters of fewer than seven pups should not be tested *(60)*. It should be noted, however, that early postnatal litter-size reduction is not a universally accepted practice; Palmer and Ulbrich *(154)* caution that the more animals that are removed from the study and the earlier they are removed, the greater the risk of failing to detect some aspect of developmental toxicity, and suggest that reducing the number of animals at weaning might be a reasonable compromise for most known toxicities.

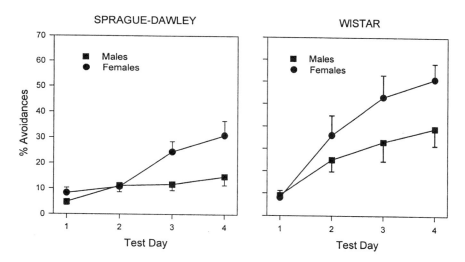

Fig. 2. Strain-related and gender-related differences in acquisition of active avoidance responding are illustrated in these comparative data in Sprague-Dawley and Wistar rats tested at 9–10 wk of age. A two-compartment shuttle box apparatus was used with a combined light-tone (2.5 Hz) conditioned stimulus (CS). The unconditioned stimulus (US) was footshock: 0.33 and 0.22 mA in male and female Sprague-Dawley rats, respectively, and 0.5 and 0.67 mA in male and female Wistar rats, respectively. Footshock levels were optimized in each species to produce a maximum avoidance response, without the "freezing" behavior characteristic of excessive shock levels in avoidance paradigms. Twenty-five consecutive trials were performed each day. The duration of the CS prior to initiation of the United States was 10 s, and the maximum duration of the United States was 10 s. The intertrial interval varied between 2 and 7 s. The maximum avoidance rate achieved on the fourth day of testing in Sprague-Dawley rats was only approx 35%. In contrast, Wistar rats achieved maximum avoidance rate of approx 65% on the fourth day. Females acquired and performed this task at a higher rate than did males in both strains, but female Sprague-Dawley rats did not perform the task as well as did female Wistar rats.

Undernutrition can exert deleterious effects on social behavior. Chronically undernourished animals are also usually understimulated and show altered social and behavioral maturation; they may isolate themselves from learning experiences by withdrawing from interaction with the environment *(18)*.

3.3.3. Species and Strain

Genetic differences in response to a developmental neurotoxicant can be manifested as different deficits in performance of behavioral tasks. Baseline differences in physical maturation and reflex and behavioral ontogeny and performance exist among species and among strains within species, which can make cross-species extrapolation difficult. Because behavioral responses are often the result of genetic and nongenetic influences, it is important to consider both in interpreting data. Crabbe *(155)* evaluated baseline open field activity in 19 inbred mouse strains and found a 2.6-fold difference in the number of crossings from the least to the most active strain. Mice from each strain were then injected with an intraperitoneal dose of 2 g/kg ethanol, resulting in increased activity in two strains, decreased activity in six strains, and no effect in 11 strains. Strain differences in blood-ethanol concentration measured at the time of testing did not appear to correlate in a meaningful way with activity scores, leading to the conclusion that strain-related differences in activity in an open field may have been largely genetically determined.

Since the rat is the species of choice for developmental neurotoxicity testing mandated by regulatory agencies, strain differences are of the greatest interest among researchers conducting developmental neurotoxicity screening batteries. Figure 2 provides an example of strain-related differences in the acquisition of active avoidance behavior. Experiments were conducted in our laboratory to optimize active avoidance testing in SD rats, and to then repeat this optimization when we began using Wistar rats. In the course of testing it was very apparent that a strain-related difference in performance existed. Sprague-Dawley rats can be poor performers in an active-avoidance paradigm *(156)*, and this is apparent in the example given. For each gender, maximum avoidance responding achieved on the fourth day of testing by SD rats was approx half that achieved by Wistar rats. In developmental neurotoxicity testing, the majority of agents that affect learning and memory cause impairment rather than facilitation. Thus, impairment of learning and memory would be more difficult to detect in a rat strain with low baseline performance, such as the SD rat, and would be a consideration in the selection of strain or of behavioral test (e.g., SD rats perform better in passive- than active-avoidance paradigms).

Most laboratories that conduct developmental-neurotoxicity testing do so with the same rat strain, so strain differences would not be a confounder in data interpretation. However, differences in baseline behavior can even occur within a given rat strain. Poor performance in an active-avoidance paradigm by SD rats was shown by Rech to be characteristic of approx half the animals tested *(156)*. Expanding on this difference, Ohta and coworkers *(157)* bred SD rats selectively to produce high (HAA) and low (LAA) shuttle avoidance performers, and compared results from these animals to standard SD rats. Dams were treated with methylnitrosourea (MNU) on GD 13 to induce micrencephaly, and offspring were then tested in the Biel maze, and for shuttle-avoidance and wheel-cage activity at 6–9 wk of age. Of particular interest is the fact that shuttle avoidance of HAA, LAA, and SD rats was unaffected by MNU exposure, despite markedly different response rates in controls. Although errors were increased in the Biel maze in MNU-exposed offspring, no differences were apparent among the three types of SD rats. Despite large differences among the three types of SD rats in baseline wheel running, MNU-induced deficits were apparent in all three types.

3.3.4. Gender

Sexual dimorphism of the brain is an important aspect of CNS development. Both masculinization and feminization of the brain depend on differing levels of estrogenic stimulation, and the cerebral cortex contains substantial levels of estrogen receptors and estrogen-containing cells during late gestation and the early postnatal period *(13)*. It is well-known that gender-related differences exist in spontaneous behaviors, and these differences could be magnified by perinatal exposure to a neurotoxicant. This underscores the importance of including males and females in developmental neuro-toxicity test batteries, and of not discounting an effect if it is observed in only one gender. Indeed, sex-related differences in response are not uncommon in developmental neurotoxicity. As an example, Schantz and coworkers *(158)* found a sex-related difference in response in a working/reference memory task following developmental exposure of rats to three PCB congeners; females, but not males, demonstrated slower acquisition of the task. The authors speculated that the sexually dimorphic response might be related to changes in the hormonal milieu during development involving gonadal and thyroid function, as changes in these hormones during brain development have been shown to affect learning and memory in males and females differentially. Some researchers have not used females due to the potential confounding factor of the estrous cycle. While estrous cycle-related changes have been observed in the running wheel, in other devices that measure activity the differences are small or nonexistent *(85)*. Because testing in only one sex could produce a false-negative response, using both is highly recommended.

Gender-related differences in baseline performance occur in behavioral tests that employ shock as a negative reinforcer. Female rats generally have lower thresholds for, and shorter escape latencies from, shock presentation than males *(159)*. In the example given in Fig. 2, for each strain, a higher footshock level was required to elicit avoidance responding in males than in females, and performance was better in females than in males. Beatty and Beatty *(160)* observed a similar gender-related difference in Holtzman rats in an active avoidance paradigm, and determined that it was not due to the difference in body weight between males and females. This difference is determined early in life: gonadectomy in adulthood has no effect on avoidance, but neonatal castration of males or neonatal androgenization of females reverses behavioral differences observed in intact males and females *(159,160)*. This is also true for baseline locomotor activity, which is higher in females than in males *(85,159,161)* due to increased perseverative activity *(162)*, and is reversed by gonadectomy during the neonatal period, but not adulthood *(159)*. Males also habituate more rapidly than females, with respect to motor activity *(162)*.

Onset of puberty may impact baseline behaviors. In a study comparing preweaning and postweaning activity of Fischer 344 (F344) and SD rats, Vorhees *(163)* determined that ontogeny of behavior in F344 rats was slower than that for SD rats, and that F344 rats were less active than SD rats. The question was raised whether delayed sexual maturation in F344 rats could be the cause of the differing responses (vaginal opening is achieved in F344 rats on PND 44–46 and in SD rats on PND 31–37). This question was of sufficient concern that the EPA recommended not using the Fischer 344 rat for developmental neurotoxicity testing due to differences in timing of developmental events relative to other rat strains *(60)*. Figure 3 provides an example of the potential influence of the onset of puberty on behavioral performance, in this case in rotorod performance. Male rats achieved stable performance levels by PND 28, but females had a decline in performance from PND 28–35, with increased performance on PND 42. Since PND 35 is approximately the age of puberty in female SD rats, we postulated that the change in hormonal milieu during this time might lead to disruption of rotorod performance. More work is needed to evaluate the effects of onset of puberty on behavior, including hormone measurements, and studies in males as well as females.

Interrelationships can exist between gender differences and environmental stressors. Baseline and *d*-amphetamine-induced stimulation of locomotor activity was evaluated in an experiment with adult Sprague-Dawley rats, in which half of the males and

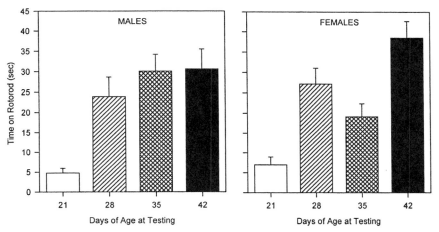

Fig. 3. Effect of age at testing is illustrated in this experiment, conducted to optimize rotorod performance as part of a test battery used to evaluate developmental neurotoxicity. Twenty litters of Sprague-Dawley rats were reduced to 4 male and 4 female offspring each, and 1 male and 1 female from each litter were evaluated for rotorod performance on Postnatal Day (PND) 21, 28, 35, or 42. Bars represent group mean and standard error time spent on a rotorod set to deliver 10 RPMs, to a maximum of 60 s/trial. The value from each animal used to construct the mean was a mean of three test trials. It is apparent that performance was not adequate in either gender at 21 d of age, but that performance was essentially comparable in males at 28–42 d of age. Males and females performed at essentially the same level on PND 28 and on PND 42, but not on PND 35. Reduced rotorod performance in females on PND 35 may have been related to the onset of puberty (approx PND 32–34 in Sprague-Dawley rats) and resultant changes in activity levels.

females were handled for 5 d prior to testing (considered a stressor), and half were not *(164)*. Handling and amphetamine increased activity, and effects were larger in males than females; there were no gender-related differences in baseline motor activity, contrary to previous reports in the literature. The authors concluded that gender-related differences in behavior may be influenced by previous experience, and speculated that the larger effect in females may be related to a larger neuroendocrine response to stressors.

3.3.5. Age

As mentioned previously, developmental age at the time of exposure to a neurotoxicant can have a profound impact on function. Maternal dosing periods described in regulatory guidelines are designed to encompass the prolonged period of development over which the CNS is formed, allowing for maximum exposure of the postimplantation conceptus and neonate. Because these exposure periods are so prolonged, it is often difficult to determine at exactly which stage of development insult has led to impaired function. Specificity of timing is well illustrated by the case of triethyltin (TET). TET was given directly to neonatal rats by intraperitoneal injection on PND 1, 5, 10, or 15 to coincide with different stages of rapid brain growth in a study conducted by Ruppert and coworkers *(83)*. Mortality, body and brain weight, and various behavioral functions previously shown to be sensitive to TET (rope descent, motor activity, and ASR) were evaluated. Treatment-related effects occurred from exposure on PND 5, and included decreased rope descent and increased activity in a figure-8 maze. TET-induced effects on behavior on PND 5 are not unexpected, since TET given at this time produces persistent effects on myelin, neuronal development, and neurochemical processes occurring at this postnatal stage of development (*see* Fig. 1). It is unknown why these effects did not occur on surrounding days, but it does reinforce the concept that damage from toxicant insult that occurs during the brain growth spurt is not universal across its entire range.

Timing of gestational exposure can also be critical. Holson and coworkers *(165)* gave all-*trans* retinoic acid to pregnant rats during GD 8–10 (period of maximum sensitivity to retinoic acid-induced malformations), 11–13, or 14–16, and then subjected their offspring to a battery of behavioral tests as young adults. There was a reduction in *d*-amphetamine-stimulated motor activity, resulting from exposure at all timepoints. However, other behavioral effects were phase-specific: impaired rotorod performance resulted from exposure during GD 14–16 only, and increased daytime activity in residential running wheels occurred from exposure during GD 11–13 only.

Not only is the age at exposure important, but also the age at testing. Testing at only one specific age could prevent detection of a toxicant-induced behavioral effect; the importance of this lies in the fact that it is not unusual in developmental neurotoxicity to see injury that occurs early but is not expressed until some later stage in life *(166)*.

Unless the purpose of testing is to evaluate the effects of an agent on ontogeny of behavior, it is important to conduct specific behavioral tests at an age at which the animal is capable of performing them. Table 4 lists the age of acquisition of various developmental landmarks, reflexes, and behaviors; for screening batteries, a general rule is to conduct testing after the ages indicated to ensure optimal performance. However, one testing strategy is to conduct behavior testing in the neonatal animal at a time when the major neurotransmitter systems are maturing. As an example, periadolescent animals differ markedly in behavior and sensitivity to drugs affecting catecholaminergic systems, compared with younger or older animals; animals at PND 30–42 exhibit a markedly attenuated response to *d*-amphetamine and increased sensitivity to haloperidol *(167)*. It appears that this may be due to the development of DA autoreceptors, which may temporarily decrease DA-mediated activity in the brain. Examination of this specific developmental period provided useful information on the characterization of functional maturation of DA systems.

Conversely, testing in young adults only may not identify behavioral effects that could be uncovered as the animal ages and the functional reserves of the CNS are diminished. As an example, hyperactivity is a typical behavioral effect of exposure to antimitotic agents during the midfetal period, and is seen when animals reach puberty, but not before *(166)*. These examples provide evidence that testing can be valuable at specific ages; however, with an untested agent, specific age is usually unknown and longitudinal testing would be the best way to identify critical periods.

3.3.6. Handling

Previously mentioned factors that might influence the outcome of developmental neurotoxicity testing are essentially beyond the control of the experimenter. Subsequent factors discussed are within the realm of control. Differences in early experience can alter behavior in later years. Meaney and coworkers *(168)* conducted a study in which infant rats handled throughout the lactation period with the dam removed from the cage were compared to nonhandled infants. At all subsequent ages, nonhandled rats secreted more glucocorticoids in response to stress than handled rats and had higher baseline levels with aging. Increased exposure to glucocorticoids can accelerate hippocampal neuron loss and cognitive impairments in aging, and this was observed in the nonhandled rats only in this study. Handling can be a positive experience for neonatal rats, and indeed has been used as enrichment, in combination with social experience, synthetic fur and balsa wood to chew on, extra warmth, and anogenital stimulation. These enrichment techniques have been shown to slightly accelerate eye opening *(146)*.

Conversely, tail handling was shown to be aversive to adult male rats tested in a step-through latency apparatus, in that it suppressed exploratory behavior when handling was temporally close to testing *(169)*. These examples would seem to indicate that rats unaccustomed to being handled react in an aversive way, but that continual handling from infancy has a more positive outcome.

One concern that has been raised regarding developmental neurotoxicity test batteries is whether early reflex testing and handling can influence later postweaning behavior testing. In a comparative study of SD and Fischer 344 rats, Vorhees *(163)* found an effect of prior experience on activity only; the increase in activity observed was not unexpected as it is known to be a consequence of early handling. The effect was modest, and no other postweaning tests were affected, so it was concluded that extensive early experience did not influence postweaning performance.

3.3.7. Temperature

Increased or decreased body temperature can affect the developing nervous system. Maternal hyperthermia during pregnancy has been associated with damage to the CNS of the embryo, and it has been demonstrated experimentally that immersion of pregnant mice in heated water during GD 12–15 results in reduced postnatal open-field activity and delayed acquisition of a T-maze task and shuttle avoidance *(170)*. Hutchings *(34)* found that hypothermia, which can result from handling or other stressors in neonatal rats, produces enhanced growth, precocious development, and increased resistance to stress. While these do not necessarily represent adverse effects, they still may confound developmental neurotoxicant-induced effects.

3.3.8. Circadian Rhythms

Most laboratories employ a light cycle in which lights are on for 12 h and off for 12 h. Baseline behavior of rodents changes in fairly typical ways throughout the 24-h cycle. In a residential maze, rats were more active in the 12-h dark period than in the light as early as PND 23 *(171)*. Although females greater than 5 wk of age were more active in both the light and dark phases than males, a ratio of nocturnal:diurnal behavior showed the same trends in both genders. Activity also shows peaks and valleys within the light or dark cycle, with the highest activity shortly after onset of the dark cycle and before onset of the light cycle *(172,173)*. It is not always possible in a screening situation to test animals at the same time during the day. However, testing on a given study (and across studies as well for historical reference purposes) should be conducted at approximately the same time of day, and as close to the dark cycle as possible.

3.3.9. Additional Environmental Disturbances

Agents that alter the nervous system are likely to alter the ability of an animal to adapt to changing environmental conditions *(174)*; if the testing environment itself is altered in some unexpected way, this can confound data interpretation, and therefore care must be taken to provide as consistent an external environment as possible. As an example, background noise can disrupt most behaviors because it may be perceived as a threat and the animal may "freeze." This could be as simple as the banging of a cage, a person entering the testing room, or conversation. Excessive environmental noise can even exert an adverse effect *in utero*: Tabacova and coworkers *(175)* determined that exposure of pregnant rats to narrow-band noise (105 dB, 1000 Hz) for 4 h/d throughout gestation resulted in increased signs of excitability on PND 9, but decreased locomotor activity on PND 14; these effects were transient, as all pups were normal by PND 21.

The presence of visual cues within or outside of a given testing apparatus can also influence behavoir. Therefore, visual cues should remain consistent. The experimenter may serve as a visual cue, and movement may distract the animal from the task being performed. Because the majority of rat strains used in developmental neurotoxicity testing are albino, they tend to avoid bright light, so test equipment should be covered with opaque material, the room lights dimmed, or red light used. The scent of another animal, and particularly pheromones from the opposite sex, can influence behavior; thus, testing chambers should be dedicated to one gender, if possible, and chambers should be cleaned between each animal. Knowledge of the many environmental conditions that can influence experimental results leads to the conclusion that testing conditions should be held as constant as possible among animals and testing days. If a change in environment occurs, it must be taken into consideration in data interpretation.

3.4. Implications for Safety Evaluation

One of the key factors in data interpretation is the use of statistical analyses to identify changes from control that do not occur merely by chance. Review of the developmental neurotoxicity literature reveals a variety of appropriate means by which data may be analyzed. Observational data tend to be discontinuous, and are usually quantal or ranked; these types of data are most often analyzed by a contingency table, such as a chi-square or Fisher's exact test, analysis of variance (ANOVA) with an appropriate post-hoc test, or a rank sum test such as the Mann-Whitney U-test *(176)*. Continuous, or quantitative data, are usually expressed as a group mean with an associated measure of variability around the mean, such as standard deviation or standard error. Group mean comparisons are most often conducted using t-tests, ANOVA, or the trend test, which has become increasingly popular in toxicology in recent years. Caution needs to be used in applying the trend test to behavior data, however. As mentioned previously, it is not unexpected to find U-shaped or inverted U-shaped dose-response curves with behavior data. Since the trend test relies on a monotonic relationship between doses, significance could potentially be masked in situations in which the dose-response relationship is nonmonotonic, and thus a test such as Dunnett's t-test might be of more value. For evaluating rates of habituation, tests of parallelism have proven useful.

Another word of caution involves the multiplicity of parameters generated in a typical pre- and postnatal development study that includes evaluation of developmental neurotoxicity. The use of multiple t-tests applied to the same dataset can result in an inflated false positive rate. Weissman *(52)* states that every time a test of significance is performed, the probability of a false-positive will be increased above the nominal level, such that if 72 independent tests were performed at the 5% level, at least one Type I (false-positive) error would occur with approx 98% certainty. It is therefore important to adjust the significance level to account for multiple observations in the same animal using a correction factor such as the Bonferroni test, which divides the established significance level by the number of parameters in a distinct class of data; a more liberal approach currently in favor is to divide the significance level by the square root of the number of parameters in a class *(177)*. Use of a correction factor keeps Type I error manageable; however, Type II error can be quite large in behavioral studies, primarily due to small sample size and large variance in dependent variables *(178)*, and has not received the same attention as Type I error. Sample size is a relatively easy issue to address, provided adequate resources are available, but variability is not.

Because behavior data tend to be variable, it is important in statistical analyses to adjust for this inherent variability in order to have the most representative analysis possible, which may require the application of more flexible and/or powerful statistical tests to developmental neurotoxicity data in the future. As an example, some behavioral tests employ a "ceiling," beyond which testing ceases. The rotorod test in our laboratory requires an animal to remain on the rod no longer than 60 s for each trial; if the animal does so, the length of time recorded for that animal is 61 s, and constitutes "censored" data. In such a case, median rather than mean might be a more accurate representation of central tendency. And, rather than employ a typical analysis such ANOVA or the trend test, a more creative solution might be to use the type of survival analysis typically used in bioassays *(179)*. No matter how powerful the statistical testing regime, however, the biological significance of any apparent difference from control must always be considered in the context of historical reference data from the testing laboratory and from the scientific literature.

Developmental neurotoxicity data are ultimately used in the risk-assessment process, in which information generated from laboratory animals is used to evaluate the potential risk to humans from agents which may cause neural deficits in children of exposed parents (*see* Chapter 4 by Tilson). Proceedings from a workshop on maternal and developmental toxicity *(137)* recommended that regulation of chemicals should be based on the most sensitive indicator of toxicity, whether maternal or developmental. This principle can also be extended to establishment of margins of safety for therapeutic agents.

In the EPA- and NIDA-sponsored workshop on comparability of human and animal developmental neurotoxicants, it was concluded that for evaluation of weight of evidence, any adverse developmental neurotoxic effect, including transient effects and/or developmental delays, may be considered relevant, even if other effects such as maternal toxicity are present *(35)*. However, the point was also made that a statistically significant difference in a single endpoint in one test procedure would not necessarily indicate developmental neurotoxicity. The whole picture needs to be considered in evaluating the safety implications of significant test results.

Data from initial test batteries in laboratory animals are sometimes inconclusive and the question is often asked, "What does this mean?" The ideal situation would be a follow-up of these positive results with tests designed to characterize effects, which could be accomplished in some cases with a longitudinal design to investigate changes over time. Investigation of mechanisms would also help to answer difficult questions by correlation of different behavioral effects; of behavioral effects with brain morphology, neurochemistry, electrophysiology, and biochemistry; or of in vivo with in vitro effects. The reality of the situation is, however, that in the context of safety testing, this type of luxury is often not available due to constraints of time and/or resources, and data from behavioral screens must be used to aid in evaluating safety. In the course of safety assessment, a systematic series of questions could be asked to try to explain behavioral effects in the context of the magnitude and direction, effects on other behaviors, overt toxicity to the maternal animal, deficits in growth and development, clinical signs, and expected pharmacologic effects. While the exact nature of behavioral changes will not likely be elucidated, an overall picture of developmental effects on the nervous system (or lack of effects) will emerge. As an example, if a statistically significant reduction in acoustic startle responding occurred as a result of exposure to a test agent, the following series of questions might apply:

1. How profound was the difference from concurrent controls? Were values for concurrent controls within the historical reference range for the laboratory, and if so, were values for the treated group within this historical range? Due to the interrelationship of behavioral effects with environmental variables, the best means of comparison is with concurrent controls. However, reference ranges are useful to determine if control animals are responding in an expected manner.
2. What was the variability around the mean? If the standard error of the affected treatment groups was larger than that of controls, select individuals could have been responsible for the effect, and therefore, a careful examination of individual animal data would be warranted.
3. Was the difference transient, in the case of presentation of multiple stimuli? Did it persist throughout the test session, or did the difference from control increase over time (potentially indicating an effect on habituation)?
4. Was a dose-response relationship demonstrated? Were both genders affected? Neither of these conditions need to be met to have a positive effect, as demonstrated in the developmental neurotoxicity literature. However, lack of a dose-response relationship and/or presence of an effect in only one gender must be carefully considered and explained in the final evaluation of safety.
5. Did maternal toxicity and/or changes in maternal behavior occur at the dose(s) that affected acoustic startle in the offspring, and if so, how profound were the effects? Mild reductions in maternal body weight would not be expected to greatly affect the neurobehavioral development of offspring, but more severe toxicity might be implicated as a possible causative factor.
6. Was overt toxicity evident in offspring, and if so, what was the nature and magnitude? As mentioned previously, many agents identified as developmental neurotoxicants induce body-weight changes in offspring, which could be implicated as a possible reason for behavioral changes. Reduced body-weight gain and delayed developmental landmarks might be indicative of developmental delay, which could also be manifested as nonspecific deficits in behavior. Longitudinal testing could help to decide this question. Also, rats with lower body weight might appear to respond less to an acoustic stimulus in an apparatus that measures startle response by physical displacement.
7. Did changes occur in other behavioral tests? If a deficit was observed in rotorod performance, or animals were hypoactive observationally or in an automated measure of motor activity, it could mean that they were physically incapable of a maximum response to acoustic stimuli, or that they lacked the motivation to respond.

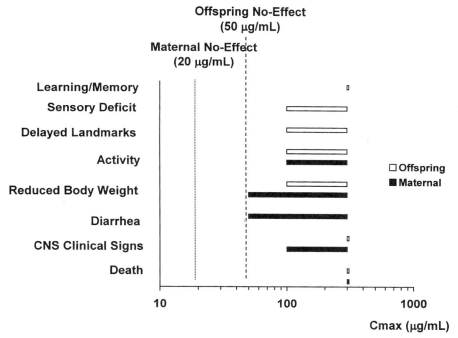

Fig. 4. This safety assessment graphic illustrates a situation in which a no-effect plasma concentration was achieved for both maternal toxicity and developmental neurotoxicity. In this hypothetical situation, a centrally active drug was given to female rats from Gestation Day 6 through delivery and weaning of their offspring. Various maternal parameters were evaluated throughout treatment, and offspring were evaluated for appearance, growth, development, and behavior (including evaluation of activity, sensory function, and learning and memory during young adulthood). Maternal plasma drug concentration was determined during early lactation, and was 20, 50, 100, and 300 µg/mL at the four dose levels tested. Maternal toxicity and developmental delay occurred at 50–300 µg/mL, but not at 20 µg/mL; developmental neurotoxicity occurred at 100 and 300 µg/mL, but not at 20 or 50 µg/mL. Thus, developmental neurotoxicity occurred only at maternally toxic doses, and was not unexpected given the known site of drug action.

8. What were the results of prepulse inhibition testing, or other means of evaluating hearing threshold? If the deficit in acoustic startle responding was not accompanied by a deficit in prepulse inhibition or a shift in hearing threshold, it was likely due to some factor other than ototoxicity, such as a deficit in reactivity. However, if reflex modification was also impaired, then consideration should be given to an effect on hearing.
9. Do the study records indicate any type of environmental influence that could have impacted the response of individual animals to acoustic stimuli?

There are likely additional questions that could be asked in evaluating a positive response to a given test in a developmental-neurotoxicity screen. The important point, however, is that one positive test result cannot be considered in isolation; the entire body of results must be considered in evaluating the implication of a difference from control.

Figures 4–6 illustrate three different safety evaluation scenarios that might occur with developmental neurotoxicity data. Each figure provides hypothetical data from a

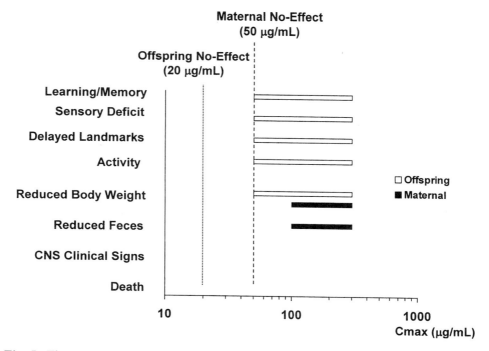

Fig. 5. The experimental outcome illustrated in this safety assessment graphic is the result of a design similar to that in Fig. 4. In this case the drug was not known to be a centrally active drug, and it was unknown prior to the experiment if it crossed the blood-brain barrier. This outcome raises more concerns than that in Fig. 4 because developmental delay and developmental neurotoxicity occurred at a maternal plasma concentration lower than that required to produce maternal toxicity. Because developmental neurotoxicity occurred at the same plasma concentrations as developmental delay (manifested as reduced body weight and delayed achievement of developmental landmarks), it is unknown if some of the behavioral effects observed could be indirect, rather than due to a direct effect on the CNS. The offspring no-effect concentration of 20 μg/mL would be related to the projected human therapeutic concentration to complete the safety evaluation.

pre- and postnatal development study in which a developmental neurotoxicity test battery was employed, and shows maternal and offspring data at doses producing maternal plasma concentrations of 20, 50, 100, and 300 μg/mL. In Fig. 4, behavioral effects were observed in offspring, but only at doses that were maternally toxic and caused developmental delay. While the behavioral effects cannot be discounted, they occurred at maternal plasma concentrations that overtly affected health, and thus could be secondary, rather than primary effects on the CNS. A no-effect plasma concentration was achieved in this case for both maternal and developmental toxicity, and for developmental neurotoxicity, and a safety margin could therefore be calculated relative to known (e.g., environmental contaminant) or proposed (e.g., candidate therapeutic agent) human plasma concentrations. Figure 5 illustrates a situation in which effects on offspring body-weight and developmental landmarks occurred at maternal plasma concentrations below those required to elicit maternal toxicity. While the health of the dam no longer seemed to be an influence at the lowest dose affected in offspring, there was still evidence of overt toxicity to the offspring, which could have impacted develop-

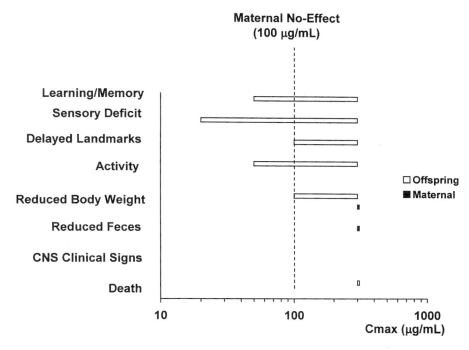

Fig. 6. The experimental outcome illustrated in this safety assessment graphic is also the result of a design similar to that in Fig. 4, and represents what may be considered a "worst-case" scenario. The drug was not known to be a centrally active drug, and it was unknown prior to the experiment if it crossed the blood-brain barrier. Few maternal signs of toxicity were observed, and these only occurred at the highest plasma drug concentration of 300 µg/mL. Although developmental delay occurred at a maternal concentration of 100 µg/mL, effects on activity and learning and memory occurred at 50 µg/mL, and sensory deficit occurred at the lowest concentration tested, 20 µg/mL. A no-effect concentration was not achieved in this study for developmental neurotoxicity, and could result in repetition of the study at lower doses, depending on the robustness of the effect and the projected human therapeutic concentration.

mental neurotoxicity results. As in the previous scenario, a no-effect plasma concentration was achieved for maternal and developmental toxicity, and developmental neurotoxicity. Finally, Fig. 6 illustrates the "worst-case" scenario: A "pure" developmental neurotoxicant, defined by Buelke-Sam and Kimmel *(55)* as an agent that produces behavioral alterations in the absence of any overt maternal or neonatal toxicity. Maternal toxicity occurred at the highest dose in this study, and evidence of developmental delay occurred at the next highest dose. Of greatest concern was the presence of effects on activity, sensory systems, and learning and memory at a dose with no other indication of adverse effects, and the lack of a no-effect dose for sensory deficits. Depending on known or proposed human-plasma concentrations, this agent could represent a real concern in terms of safety.

In the case of an environmental contaminant or industrial chemical, the risk assessment process is crucial for putting developmental neurotoxicity data into perspective, and will be discussed later in Chapter 4 by Tilson. With regard to a candidate therapeutic agent, exposure of susceptible populations can be limited by decisions to not market a drug, or to issue precautionary labeling, depending on the outcome of developmental-neurotoxicity testing relative to proposed human exposure levels and other toxicities. Careful design of developmental neurotoxicity test protocols in evaluation of environmental and industrial agents, as well as pharmaceuticals, can aid in the overall evaluation of safety for the conceptus and neonate. In addition, identification of the nature of potential problems in the developing nervous system can provide information useful in providing support for exposed individuals.

REFERENCES

1. Harry, G. J. (1994) Introduction to developmental neurotoxicology, in *Developmental Neurotoxicology* (Harry, G. J., ed.), CRC Press, New York, pp. 1–7.
2. Tilson, H. A. (1990) Behavioral indices of neurotoxicity. *Toxicol. Pathol.* **18,** 96–104.
3. Hutchings, D. E. (1983) Behavioral teratology: a new frontier in neurobehavioral research, in *Handbook of Experimental Pharmacology* (Johnson, E. M. and Kochar, D. M., eds.), Springer-Verlag, New York, pp. 207–235.
4. Butcher, R. E. (1985) An historical perspective on behavioral teratology. *Neurobehav. Toxicol. Teratol.* **7,** 537–540.
5. Vorhees, C. V. (1986) Principles of behavioral teratology, in *Handbook of Behavioral Teratology* (Riley, E. P. and Vorhees, C. V., eds.), Plenum Press, New York, pp. 3–48.
6. Hutchings, D. E. (1990) Issues of risk assessment: Lessons from the use and abuse of drugs during pregnancy. *Neurotoxicol. Teratol.* **12,** 183–189.
7. Hutchings, D. E. (1993) The puzzle of cocaine's effects following maternal use during pregnancy: are there reconcilable differences? *Neurotoxicol. Teratol.* **15,** 281–286.
8. Dow-Edwards, D., Mayes, L., Spear, L., and Hurd, Y. (1999) Cocaine and development: Clinical, behavioral, and neurobiological perspectives: a symposium report. *Neurotoxicol. Teratol.* **21,** 481–490.
9. Mactutus, C. F. (1999) Prenatal intravenous cocaine adversely affects attentional processing in preweanling rats. *Neurotoxicol. Teratol.* **21,** 539–550.
10. Suzuki, K. and Martin, P. M. (1994) Neurotoxicants and developing brain, in *Developmental Neurotoxicology* (Harry, G. J., ed.), CRC Press, New York, pp. 2–32.
11. Rice, D. C. and Gilbert, S. G. (1992) Exposure to methyl mercury from birth to adulthood impairs high-frequency hearing in monkeys. *Toxicol. Appl. Pharmacol.* **115,** 6–10.
12. Zelikoff, J. T., Bertin, J. E., Burbacher, T. M., Hunter, E. S., Miller, R. K., Silbergeld, E. K., et al. (1995) Health risks associated with prenatal metal exposure. *Fundam. Appl. Toxicol.* **25,** 161–170.
13. Rodier, P. M., Cohen, I. R., and Buelke-Sam, J. (1994) Developmental neurotoxicology: Neuroendocrine manifestations of CNS insult, in *Developmental Toxicology,* Second Edition (Kimmel, C. A. and Buelke-Sam, J., eds.), Raven Press, New York, pp. 65–92.
14. Nelson, B. K. (1991) Evidence for behavioral teratogenicity in humans. *J. Appl. Toxicol.* **11,** 33–37.
15. Wilson, J. G. (1977) Current status of teratology. General principles and mechanisms derived from animal studies, in *Handbook of Teratology* (Wilson, J. G and Fraser, F. C., eds.), Plenum Press, New York, pp. 47–74.
16. Vorhees, C. V. and Butcher, R. E. (1982) Behavioural teratogenicity, in *Developmental Toxicology* (Snell, K., ed.), Praeger, New York, pp. 247–298.
17. Rodier, P.M. (1980) Chronology of neuron development: Animal studies and their clinical implications. *Dev. Med. Child Neurol.* **22,** 525–545.
18. Morgane, P. J., Austin-LaFrance, R., Bronzino, J., Tonkiss, J., Diaz-Cintra, S, Cintra, L., et al. (1993) Prenatal malnutrition and development of the brain. *Neurosci. Biobehav. Rev.* **17,** 91–128.
19. Verity, M. A. (1994) Oxidative damage and repair in the developing nervous system. *Neurotoxicology* **15,** 81–91.

20. Schull, W. J., Norton, S., and Jensh, R. P. (1990) Ionizing radiation and the developing brain. *Neurotoxicol. Teratol.* **12,** 249–260.
21. Vorhees, C. V. (1987) Dependence on the stage of gestation: prenatal drugs and offspring behavior as influenced by different periods of exposure in rats, in *Functional Teratogenesis* (Fujii, T. and Adams, P. M., eds.), Teikyo University Press, Tokyo, pp. 39–51.
22. Abel, E. L. (1989) *Behavioral Teratogenesis and Behavioral Mutagenesis*, Plenum Press, New York.
23. Dobbing, J. (1974) The later growth of the brain and its vulnerability. *Pediatrics* **53,** 2–6.
24. Gottlieb, A., Keydar, I., and Epstein, H. T. (1977) Rodent brain growth stages: an analytical review. *Biol. Neonate* **32,** 166–176.
25. Abel, E.L. (1989) Paternal behavioral mutagenesis. *Neurotoxicology* **10,** 335–345.
26. Adams, P. M., Fanini, D., and Legator, M. S. (1987) Neurobehavioral effects of paternal drug exposure on the development of the offspring, in *Functional Teratogenesis* (Fujii, T. and Adams, P. M., eds.), Teikyo University Press, Tokyo, pp. 147–156.
27. Aurox, M. R., Dulioust, E. J., Nawar, N. N., Yacoub, S. G., Mayaux, M. J., Schwartz, D., and David, G. (1989) Antimitotic drugs in the male rat. Behavioral abnormalities in the second generation. *J. Androl.* **9,** 153–159.
28. Davis, J. M., Otto, D. A., Weil, D. E., and Grant, L. D. (1990) The comparative developmental neurotoxicity of lead in humans and animals. *Neurotoxicol. Teratol.* **12,** 215–229.
29. Schantz, S. (1996) Response to commentaries. *Neurotoxicol. Teratol.* **18,** 271–276.
30. Watanabe, T., Matsuhashi, K., and Takayama, S. (1984) Study on the neuro-behavioral development in rats treated neonatally with drugs acting on the autonomic nervous system. *Folia Pharmacol. Japon.* **84,** 267–282.
31. Watanabe, T., Matsuhashi, K., and Takayama, S. (1990) Placental and blood-brain barrier transfer following prenatal and postnatal exposures to neuroactive drugs: relationship with partition coefficient and behavioral teratogenesis. *Toxicol. Appl. Pharmacol.* **105,** 66–77.
32. Iversen, S. D. and Iversen, L. L. (1981) *Behavioral Pharmacology*, Second Edition, Oxford University Press, New York, pp. 182–200.
33. Nelson, B. K. (1981) Dose/effect relationships in developmental neurotoxicology. *Neurobehav. Toxicol. Teratol.* **3,** 255.
34. Hutchings, D. E. (1985) Issues of methodology and interpretation in clinical and animal behavioral teratology studies. *Neurobehav. Toxicol. Teratol.* **7,** 639–642.
35. Tyl, R. W. and Sette, W. F. (1990) Workshop on the qualitative and quantitative comparability of human and animal developmental neurotoxicity, Work Group III report: weight of evidence and quantitative evaluation of developmental neurotoxicity data. *Neurotoxicol. Teratol.* **12,** 275–280.
36. Adams, J. (1993) Principles of neurobehavioral teratology. *Reprod. Toxicol.* **7,** 171–173.
37. Rodier, P. M. (1990) Developmental neurotoxicology. *Toxicol. Pathol.* **19,** 89–95.
38. Reuhl, K. R., Lagunowich, L. A., and Brown, D. L. (1994) Cytoskeleton and cell adhesion molecules: critical targets of toxic agents. *Neurotoxicology* **15,** 133–145.
39. Di Luca, M., Caputi, A., and Cattabeni, F. (1994) Synaptic protein phosphorylation changes in animals exposed to neurotoxicants during development. *Neurotoxicology* **15,** 525–532.
40. Balduini, W. and Costa, L. G. (1990) Developmental neurotoxicity of ethanol: in vitro inhibition of muscarinic receptor-stimulated phosphoinositide metabolism in brain from neonatal but not adult rats. *Brain Res.* **512,** 248–252.
41. Balduini, W., Cattabeni, F., Reno, F., and Costa, L. G. (1993) The muscarinic receptor-stimulated phosphoinositide metabolism as a potential target for the neurotoxicity of ethanol during brain development, in *Alcohol, Cell Membranes, and Signal Transduction in Brain* (Alling, C., Diamond, I., Leslie, S. W., Sun, G. Y., and Wood, W. G., eds.), Plenum Press, New York, pp. 255–263.
42. Costa, L. G. (1994) Second messenger systems in developmental neurotoxicology, in *Developmental Neurotoxicology* (Harry, G. J., ed.), CRC Press, New York, pp. 77–101.

43. Tilson, H. A. and Wright, D. C. (1985) Interpretation of behavioral teratology data. *Neurobehav. Toxicol. Teratol.* **7,** 667–668.

44. Sobrian, S. K. and Pappas, B. A. (1992) Advantages and disadvantages of longitudinal assessment of offspring function. *Senten Ijo* **32(Suppl.),** S43–S54.

45. Schardein, J. L., York, R. G., and Weisenburger, W. P. (1992) Behavioral testing in the context of reproductive and developmental toxicity screening in the West. *Cong. Anom* **32,** 15–29.

46. Comer, C. P. and Norton, S. (1982) Effects of perinatal methimazole exposure on a developmental test battery for neurobehavioral toxicity in rats. *Toxicol. Appl. Pharmacol.* **63,** 133–141.

47. Szakacs, N. A. and Halladay, S. C. (1983) Behavioral assessment of rats treated perinatally with methimazole: Industrial application of the test battery. *Teratology* **27,** 79A.

48. Rice, S. A. (1989) Startle reflex reactivity of rats perinatally treated with methimazole or prenatally exposed to N_2O. *Teratology* **39,** 508.

49. Weisenburger, W. P., Keller, K. A., and Schardein, J. L. (1991) Perinatal methimazole exposure in the rat: validation of a developmental neurobehavioral battery. *Teratology* **43,** 498.

50. Henck, J. W., Frahm, D. T., and Anderson, J. A. (1996) Validation of automated behavioral test systems. *Neurotoxicol. Teratol.* **18,** 189–197.

51. Buelke-Sam, J., Kimmel, C. A., Adams, J., Nelson, C. J., Vorhees, C. V., Wright, D. C., et al. (1985) Collaborative behavioral teratology study: Results. *Neurobehav. Toxicol. Teratol.* **7,** 591–624.

52. Weissman, A. (1990) What it takes to validate behavioral toxicology tests: a belated commentary on the collaborative behavioral teratology study. *Neurotoxicol. Teratol.* **12,** 497–501.

53. Kosazuma, T., Kobayashi, Y., Shiota, S., Suzuki, M., Inomata, N., and Akahori, A. (1982) Summary of the survey on behavioral teratology study in Japanese pharmaceutical industries. *Cong. Anom.* **22,** 111–125.

54. Butcher, R. E. and Vorhees, C. V. (1979) A preliminary test battery for the investigation of the behavioral teratology of selected psychotropic drugs. *Neurobehav. Toxicol.* **1(Suppl. 1),** 207–212.

55. Buelke-Sam, J. and Kimmel, C. A. (1979) Development and standardization of screening methods for behavioral teratology. *Teratology* **20,** 17–30.

56. Tanimura, T. (1986) Collaborative studies on behavioral teratology in Japan. *Neurotoxicology* **7,** 35–46.

57. Goldey, E. S., Kehn, L. S., Rehnberg, G. L., and Crofton, K. M. (1995) Effects of developmental hypothyroidism on auditory and motor function in the rat. *Toxicol. Appl. Pharmacol.* **135,** 67–76.

58. Goldey, E. S., O'Callaghan, J. P., Stanton, M. E., Barone, S., Jr., and Crofton, K. M. (1994) Developmental neurotoxicity: Evaluation of testing procedures with methylazoxymethanol and methyl-mercury. *Fundam. Appl. Toxicol.* **23,** 447–464.

59. Tachibana, T. (1982) Instability of dose-response results in small sample studies in behavioral teratology. *Neurobehav. Toxicol. Teratol.* **4,** 117–118.

60. U.S. Environmental Protection Agency (1998) Health effects test guidelines OPPTS 870.6300, developmental neurotoxicity study. US EPA 712-C-98-239.

61. Barlow, S. M. and Sullivan, F. M. (1975) Behavioural teratology, in *Teratology: Trends and Applications* (Berry, C. L. and Poswillo, D. E., eds.), Springer, New York, pp. 103–120.

62. Vorhees, C. V., Butcher, R. E., Brunner, R. L., and Sobotka, T. J. (1979) A developmental test battery for neurobehavioral toxicity in rats: a preliminary analysis using monosodium glutamate, calcium carrageenan and hydroxyurea. *Toxicol. Appl. Pharmacol.* **50,** 267–282.

63. Kimmel, C. A., Buelke-Sam, J., and Adams, J. (1985) Collaborative Behavioral Teratology Study: implications, current applications, and future directions. *Neurobehav. Toxicol. Teratol.* **7,** 669–673.

64. Rees, D. C., Francis, E. Z., and Kimmel, C. A. (1990) Scientific and regulatory issues relevant to assessing risk for developmental neurotoxicity: an overview. *Neurotoxicol. Teratol.* **12,** 175–181.

65. International Conference on Harmonisation (ICH) (1994) Guideline on detection of toxicity to reproduction for medicinal products. *Fed. Regist.* **59,** 48746–48752.

66. Lochry, E. A. (1987) Concurrent use of behavioral/functional testing in existing reproductive and developmental toxicity screens: practical considerations. *J. Am. Coll. Toxicol.* **6,** 433–439.

67. Holson, R. R., Gazzara, R. A., Ferguson, S. A., and Adams, J. (1997) A behavioral and neuroanatomical investigation of the lethality caused by gestational day 11–13 retinoic acid exposure. *Neurotoxicol. Teratol.* **19,** 347–353.

68. Chernoff, N. and Kavlock, R. J. (1982) An in vivo teratology screen utilizing pregnant mice. *J. Toxicol. Environ. Health* **10,** 541–550.

69. Goldey, E. S., Tilson, H. A., and Crofton, K. M. (1995) Implications of the use of neonatal birth weight, growth, viability, and survival data for predicting developmental neurotoxicity: a survey of the literature. *Neurotoxicol. Teratol.* **17,** 313–332.

70. Kallman, M. J. (1994) Assessment of motoric effects, in *Developmental Neurotoxicology* (Harry, G. J., ed.), CRC Press, New York, pp. 103–122.

71. Chiavegatto, S., Oliveira, C. A., and Bernardi, M. M. (1997) Prenatal exposure of rats to diphenhydramine: effects on physical development, open field, and gonadal hormone levels in adults. *Neurotoxicol. Teratol.* **19,** 511–516.

72. Henck, J. W., Reindel, J. F., and Anderson, J. A. (2001) Growth and development in rats given recombinant human epidermal growth factor $_{1-48}$ as neonates. *Toxicol. Sci.* **62,** 80–91.

73. Tilson, H. A. and Moser, V. C. (1992) Comparison of screening approaches. *Neurotoxicology* **13,** 1–14.

74. Irwin, S. (1968) Comprehensive observational assessment: Ia. A systematic, quantitative procedure for assessing the behavioral and physiologic state of the mouse. *Psychopharmacology* **13,** 222–257.

75. U.S. Environmental Protection Agency (1996) Health effects test guidelines OPPTS 870.6200, neurotoxicity screening battery. U.S. EPA 712-C–96–238.

76. Moser, V. C. and Padilla, S. (1998) Age- and gender-related differences in the time course of behavioral and biochemical effects produced by oral chlorpyrifos in rats. *Toxicol. Appl. Pharmacol.* **149,** 107–119.

77. Mattsson, J. L., Spencer, P. J., and Albee, R. R. (1996) A performance standard for clinical and functional observational battery examinations of rats. *J. Am. Coll. Toxicol.* **15,** 239–254.

78. Benignus, V. A. (1993) Importance of experimenter-blind procedure in neurotoxicology. *Neurotoxicol. Teratol.* **15,** 45–49.

79. Meyer, O. A., Tilson, H. A., Byrd, W. C., and Riley, M. T. (1979) A method for the routine assessment of fore- and hindlimb grip strength of rats and mice. *Neurobehav. Toxicol.* **1,** 233–236.

80. Ross, J. F., Handley, D. E., Fix, A. S., Lawhorn, G. T., and Carr, G. J. (1997) Quantification of the hindlimb extensor thrust response in rats. *Neurotoxicol. Teratol.* **16,** 405–411.

81. Lochry, E. A., Johnson, C., and Wier, P. J. (1994) Behavioral evaluations in developmental toxicity testing: MARTA survey results. *Neurotoxicol. Teratol.* **16,** 55–63.

82. Asano, Y., Kobayashi, T., and Higaki, K. (1984) Strain differences of postnatal development of righting reflex, traction and motor co-ordination, and emotional behavior in rats. *Cong. Anom.* **24,** 103–110.

83. Ruppert, P. H., Dean, K. F., and Reiter, L. W. (1984) Neurobehavioral toxicity of triethyltin in rats as a function of age at postnatal exposure. *Neurotoxicology* **5,** 9–22.

84. Barron, S. and Irvine, J. (1994) Effects of neonatal cocaine exposure on two measures of balance and coordination. *Neurotoxicol. Teratol.* **16,** 89–94.

85. Reiter, L. W. and MacPhail, R. C. (1982) Factors influencing motor activity measurements in neurotoxicology, in *Nervous System Toxicology* (Mitchell, C. L., ed.), Raven Press, New York, pp. 45–65.

86. Altman, J. and Sudarshan, K. (1975) Postnatal development of locomotion in the laboratory rat. *Anim. Behav.* **23,** 896–920.

87. Randall, P. K. and Campbell, B. A. (1976) Ontogeny of behavioral arousal in rats: effect of maternal and sibling presence. *J. Comp. Physiol. Psychol.* **90,** 453–459.

88. Geyer, M. A. (1990) Approaches to the characterization of drug effects on locomotor activity in rodents, in *Modern Methods in Pharmacology, vol. 6, Testing and Evaluation of Drugs of Abuse*, Wiley-Liss, Inc., New York, pp. 81–99.

89. Calamandrei, G., Pennazza, S., Ricceri, L., and Valanzano, A. (1996) Neonatal exposure to anti-nerve growth factor antibodies affects exploratory behavior of developing mice in the hole board. *Neurotoxicol. Teratol.* **18,** 141–146.

90. Archer, J. (1973) Tests for emotionality in rats and mice: a review. *Anim. Behav.* **21,** 205–235.

91. Vorhees, C. V., Acuff-Smith, K. D., Minck, D. R., and Butcher, R. E. (1992) A method for measuring locomotor behavior in rodents: Contrast-sensitive computer-controlled video tracking activity assessment in rats. *Neurotoxicol. Teratol.* **14,** 43–49.

92. Abel, E. L. (1995) Further evidence for the dissociation of locomotor activity and head dipping in rats. *Physiol. Behav.* **57,** 529–532.

93. Thompson, R. F. and Spencer, W. A. (1966) Habituation: a model phenomenon for the study of neuronal substrates of behavior. *Psychol. Rev.* **73,** 16–43.

94. Groves, P. M. and Thompson, R. F. (1970) Habituation: a dual-process theory. *Psychol. Rev.* **77,** 419–450.

95. Davis, M. (1980) Neurochemical modulation of sensory-motor reactivity: acoustic and tactile startle reflexes. *Neurosci. Biobehav. Rev.* **4,** 241–263.

96. Henley, C. M. and Rybak, L. P. (1995) Ototoxicity in developing mammals. *Brain Res. Rev.* **20,** 68–90.

97. Fukumura, M., Sethi, N, and Vorhees, C.V. (1998) Effects of the neurotoxin 3,3'-iminodipropionitrile on acoustic startle and locomotor activity in rats: a comparison of functional observational and automated startle assessment methods. *Neurotoxicol. Teratol.* **20,** 203–211.

98. Dow-Edwards, D. L. and Hughes, H. E. (1995) Adult reactivity in rats exposed to cocaine during two early postnatal periods. *Neurotoxicol. Teratol.* **17,** 553–557.

99. Fechter, L. D. and Young, J. S. (1983) Discrimination of auditory from nonauditory toxicity by reflex modulations audiometry: effects of triethyltin. *Toxicol. Appl. Pharmacol.* **70,** 216–227.

100. Parisi, T. and Ison, J.R. (1979) Development of the acoustic startle response in the rat: ontogenetic changes in the magnitude of inhibition by prepulse stimulation. *Develop. Psychobiol.* **12,** 219–230.

101. Young, J. S. and Fechter, L. D. (1983). Reflex inhibition procedures for animal audiometry: a technique for assessing ototoxicity. *J. Acoust. Soc. Am.* **73,**1686–1693.

102. Weir, P. J., Guerriero, F. J., and Walker, R. F. (1989) Implementation of a primary screen for developmental neurotoxicity. *Fundam. Appl. Toxicol.* **13,** 118–136.

103. Hutchings, D. E., Zmitrovich, A. C., Brake, S. C., Church, S. H., and Malowany, D. (1993) Prenatal administration of methadone in the rat increases offspring acoustic startle amplitude at age 3 weeks. *Neurotoxicol. Teratol.* **15,** 157–164.

104. Stanton, M. E. (1994) Assessment of learning and memory in developmental neurotoxicology, in *Developmental Neurotoxicology* (Harry, G. J., ed.), CRC Press, New York, pp. 123–156.

105. Eckerman, D. A. and Bushnell, P. J. (1992) The neurotoxicology of cognition: attention, learning, and memory, in *Neurotoxicology* (Tilson, H. and Mitchell, C., eds.), Raven Press, New York, pp. 213–270.
106. Akaike, M, Ohno, H., Tsutsumi, S., and Omosu, M. (1994) Comparison of four spatial maze learning tests with methylnitrosourea-induced microcephaly rats. *Teratology* **49,** 83–89.
107. Peele, D. B. and Vincent, A. (1989) Strategies for assessing learning and memory, 1978–1987: a comparison of behavioral toxicology, psychopharmacology, and neurobiology. *Neurosci. Biobehav. Rev.* **13,** 33–38.
108. Burbacher, T. M., Rodier, P. M., and Weiss, B. (1990) Methylmercury developmental neurotoxicity: a comparison of effects in humans and animals. *Neurotoxicol. Teratol.* **12,** 191–202.
109. Kulig, B, Alleva, A., Bignami, G., Cohn, J., Cory-Slechta, D., Landa, V., O'Donoghue, J., and Peakall, D. (1996) Animal behavioral methods in neurotoxicity assessment: SGOMSEC joint report. *Environ. Health Perspec.* **104(Suppl. 2),** 193–204.
110. Bolles, R. C. and Woods, P. J. (1964) The ontogeny of behaviour in the albino rat. *Anim. Behav.* **12,** 427–441.
111. Bekkedal, M. Y. V., Rossi III, J., and Panksepp, J. (1999) Fetal and neonatal exposure to trimethylolpropane phosphate alters rats social behavior and emotional responsivity. *Neurotoxicol. Teratol.* **21,** 435–443.
112. Elsner, J., Suter, D., and Alder, S. (1990) Microanalysis of ultrasonic vocalizations of young rats: assessment of the behavioral teratogenicity of methylmercury. *Neurotoxicol. Teratol.* **12,** 7–14.
113. Birke, L. I. A. and Sadler, D. (1987) Differences in maternal behavior of rats and the sociosexual development of offspring. *Dev. Psychobiol.* **20,** 85–99.
114. Mirmiran, M. and Swaab, D.F. (1986) Central neurotransmitter disturbances underlying developmental neurotoxicological effects. *Neurotoxicology* **7,** 95–102.
115. Meier, E., Hertz, L., and Schousboe, A. (1991) Neurotransmitters as developmental signals. *Neurochem. Int.* **19,** 1–15.
116. Elsner, J., Hodel, B., Suter, K. E., Oelke, D., Ulbrich, B., Schreiner, G., et al. (1988) Detection limits of different approaches in behavioral teratology, and correlation of effects with neurochemical parameters. *Neurotoxicol. Teratol.* **10,** 155–167.
117. U.S. Environmental Protection Agency (1996) Health effects test guidelines OPPTS 870.6855, neurophysiology sensory evoked potentials. US EPA 712-C–96–242.
118. Winneke, G. (1992) Cross species extrapolation in neurotoxicology: neurophysiological and neurobehavioral aspects. *Neurotoxicology* **13,** 15–25.
119. Mattsson, J. L., Albee, R. R., Yano, B. L., Bradley, G. J., and Spencer, P. J. (1998) Neurotoxicologic examination of rats exposed to 1,1,2,2-tetrachloroethylene (perchloro-ethylene) vapor for 13 weeks. *Neurotoxicol. Teratol.* **20,** 83–98.
120. Yargicoglu, P., Agar, A., Oguz, Y., Nimet Izgut-Uysal, V., Senturk, U. K., and Oner, G. (1997) The effect of developmental exposure to cadmium (Cd) on visual evoked potentials (VEPs) and lipid peroxidation. *Neurotoxicol. Teratol.* **19,** 213–219.
121. Kremer, H., Lilienthal, H., Hany, J., Roth-Harer, A., and Winneke, G. (1999) Sex-dependent effects of maternal PCB exposure on the electroretinogram in adult rats. *Neurotoxicol. Teratol.* **21,** 13–19.
122. Church, M. W. and Overbeck, G. W. (1990) Prenatal cocaine exposure in the Long-Evans rat: III. Developmental effects on the brainstem auditory-evoked potential. *Neurotoxicol. Teratol.* **12,** 345–351.
123. Song, X., Violin, J. D., Seidler, F. J., and Slotkin, T. A. (1998) Modeling the developmental neurotoxicity of chlorpyrifos *in vitro*: macromolecule synthesis in PC12 cells. *Toxicol. Appl. Pharmacol.* **151,** 182–191.
124. Xu, Y-Z., Ruan, D-Y., Wu, Y., Jiang, Y-B., Chen, S-Y., Chen, J., and Shi, P. (1998) Nitric oxide effects LTP in area CA1 and CA3 of hippocampus in low-level lead-exposed rat. *Neurotoxicol. Teratol.* **20,** 69–73.

125. Weiss, B. and Elsner, J. (1996) The intersection of risk assessment and neurobehavioral toxicity. *Environ. Health Perspec.* **104(Suppl. 2),** 173–177.
126. Rees, D. C., Francis, E. Z., and Kimmel, C. A. (1990) Qualitative and quantitative comparability of human and animal developmental neurotoxicants: a workshop summary. *Neurotoxicology* **11,** 257–270.
127. Stanton, M. E. and Spear, L. P. (1990) Workshop on the qualitative and quantitative comparability of human and animal developmental neurotoxicity in humans and laboratory animals. *Neurotoxicol. Teratol.* **12,** 261–267.
128. Driscoll, C. D., Streissguth, A. P., and Riley, E. P. (1990) Prenatal alcohol exposure: comparability of effects in humans and animal models. *Neurotoxicol. Teratol.* **12,** 231–237.
129. Tilson, H. A., Jacobson, J. L., and Rogan, W. J. (1990) Polychlorinated biphenyls and the developing nervous system: cross-species comparisons. *Neurotoxicol. Teratol.* **12,** 239–248.
130. Burbacher, T. M., Rodier, P. M., and Weiss, B. (1990) Methylmercury developmental neurotoxicity: a comparison of effects in humans and animals. *Neurotoxicol. Teratol.* **12,** 191–202.
131. Schardein, J. L. and Keller, K. A. (1989) Potential human developmental toxicants and the role of animal testing in their identification and characterization. *CRC Crit. Rev. Toxicol.* **19,** 251–339.
132. Geyer, M. A. and Reiter, L. W. (1985) Workshop report: strategies for the selection of test methods. *Neurobehav. Toxicol. Teratol.* **7,** 661–662.
133. Vorhees, C. V. (1985) Comparison of the collaborative behavioral teratology study and Cincinnati behavioral teratology test batteries. *Neurobehav. Toxicol. Teratol.* **7,** 625–633.
134. Vorhees, C. V. (1987) Reliability, sensitivity and validity of behavioral indices of neurotoxicity. *Neurotoxicol. Teratol.* **9,** 445–464.
135. Ulbrich, B. and Palmer, A. K. (1996) Neurobehavioral aspects of developmental toxicity testing. *Environ. Health Perspect.* **104(Suppl. 2),** P407–P412.
136. Nelson, B. K. (1991) Developmental neurotoxicity assessment: selecting exposure parameters. *Cong. Anom.* **32(Suppl.),** S31–S41.
137. Kimmel, G. L., Kimmel, C. A., and Francis, E. Z. (1987) Implications of the consensus workshop on the evaluation of maternal and developmental toxicity. *Teratogen. Carcinogen. Mutagen.* **7,** 329–338.
138. Mattsson, J. L., Eisenbrandt, D. L., and Albee, R. R. (1990) Screening for neurotoxicity: complementarity of functional and morphologic techniques. *Toxicol. Pathol.* **18,** 115–127.
139. Nelson, B. K., Moorman, W. J., and Schrader, S. M. (1996) Review of experimental male-mediated behavioral and neurochemical disorders. *Neurotoxicol. Teratol.* **18,** 611–616.
140. Adams, P. M., Shabrawy, O., and Legator, M. S. (1984) Male-transmitted developmental and neurobehavioral deficits. *Teratogen. Carcinogen. Mutagen.* **4,** 149–169.
141. Wainwright, P., Pelkman, C., and Wahlsten, D. (1989) The quantitative relationship between nutritional effects on preweaning growth and behavioral development in mice. *Dev. Psychobiol.* **22,** 183–195.
142. Wetzel, W., Ruthric, H-L., and Matthies H. (1979). Memory impairment in adult rats after postnatal undernutrition. *Behav. Neural Biol.* **25,** 157–165.
143. Smart, J. L. (1974) Activity and exploratory behavior of adult offspring of undernourished mother rats. *Dev. Psychobiol.* **7,** 315–321.
144. Bush, M. and Leathwood, P. D. (1975) Effect of different regimens of early malnutrition on behavioural development and adult avoidance learning in Swiss white mice. *Br. J. Nutr.* **33,** 373–385.

145. Resnick, O., Miller, M., Forbes, W., Hall, R., Kemper, T., Bronzino, J., and Morgane, P. J. (1979) Developmental protein malnutrition: Influences on the central nervous system of the rat. *Neurosci. Biobehav. Rev.* **3**, 233–246.

146. Smart, J. L., McMahon, A. C., Massey, R. F., Akbar, G.-N. K., and Warren, M. A. (1990) Evidence of non-maternally mediated acceleration of eye-opening in "enriched" artificially reared rat pups. *Dev. Brain Res.* **56**, 141–143.

147. Duff, D. and Snell, K. (1982) Effect of altered neonatal nutrition on the development of enzymes of lipid and carbohydrate metabolism in the rat. *J. Nutr.* **112**, 1057–1066.

148. Fleischer, S. and Turkewitz, G. (1979) Effect of neonatal stunting on development of rats: large litter rearing. *Dev. Psychobiol.* **12**, 137–149.

149. Agnish, N. D. and Keller, K. A. (1997) The rationale for culling of rodent litters. *Fundam. Appl. Toxicol.* **38**, 2–6.

150. Azzam, S. M., Nielsen, M. K., and Dickerson, G. E. (1984) Postnatal litter size effects on growth and reproduction in rats. *J. Anim. Sci.* **58**, 1337–1342.

151. Galler, J. and Turkewitz, G. (1975) Variability of the effects of rearing in a large litter on the development of the rat. *Dev. Psychobiol.* **8**, 325–331.

152. Jen, K.-L., Wehmer, F., and Morofski, J. (1978) Effects of undernutrition and litter size on maternal variables and pup development. *Dev. Psychobiol.* **11**, 279–287.

153. Nagy, Z. M., Porada, K. J., and Anderson, J. A. (1977) Undernutrition by rearing in large litters delays the development of reflexive, locomotor, and memory processes in mice. *J. Comp. Physiol. Psychol.* **91**, 682–696.

154. Palmer, A. K. and Ulbrich, B. C. (1997) The cult of culling. *Fundam. Appl. Toxicol.* **38**, 7–22.

155. Crabbe, J. C. (1986) Genetic differences in locomotor activation in mice. *Pharmacol. Biochem. Behav.* **25**, 289–292.

156. Rech, R. H. (1966) Amphetamine effects on poor performance of rats in a shuttle-box. *Psychopharmacology* **9**, 110–117.

157. Ohta, R., Matsumoto, A., Hashimoto, Y, Nagao, T., and Mizutani, M. (1997) Behavioral characteristics of micrencephalic rats in high and low shuttlebox avoidance lines. *Neurotoxicol. Teratol.* **19**, 157–162.

158. Schantz, S. L., Moshtaghian, J., and Ness, D. K. (1995) Spatial learning deficits in adult rats exposed to ortho-substituted PCB congeners during gestation and lactation. *Fundam. Appl. Toxicol.* **26**, 117–126.

159. Van Haaren, F., van Hest, A., and Heinsbroek, R. P. W. (1990) Behavioral differences between male and female rats: effects of gonadal hormones on learning and memory. *Neurosci. Biobehav. Rev.* **14**, 23–33.

160. Beatty, W. W. and Beatty, P. A. (1970) Hormonal determinants of sex differences in avoidance behavior and reactivity to electric shock in the rat. *J. Comp. Physiol. Psychol.* **73**, 446–455.

161. Archer, J. (1975) Rodent sex differences in emotional and related behavior. *Behav. Biol.* **14**, 451–479.

162. Hyde, J. F. and Jerussi, T. P. (1983) Sexual dimorphism in rats with respect to locomotor activity and circling behavior. *Pharmacol. Biochem. Behav.* **18**, 725–729.

163. Vorhees, C. V. (1983) Influence of early testing on postweaning performance in untreated F344 rats, with comparisons to Sprague-Dawley rats, using a standardized battery of tests for behavioral teratogenesis. *Neurobehav. Toxicol. Teratol.* **5**, 587–591.

164. West, C. H. K. and Michael, R. P. (1988) Mild stress influences sex differences in exploratory and amphetamine-enhanced activity in rats. *Behav. Brain Res.* **30**, 95–97.

165. Holson, R. R., Adams, J., and Ferguson, S. A. (1999) Gestational stage-specific effects of retinoic acid exposure in the rat. *Neurotoxicol. Teratol.* **21**, 393–402.

166. Rodier, P. M. (1986) Time of exposure and time of testing in developmental neurotoxicology. *Neurotoxicology* **7**, 69–76.

167. Spear, L. P., Enters, E. K., and Linville, D. G. (1985) Age-specific behaviors as tools for examining teratogen-induced neural alterations. *Neurobehav. Toxicol. Teratol.* **7,** 691–695.

168. Meaney, M. J., Aitken, D. H., van Berkel, C., Bhatnagar, S., and Sapolsky, R. M. (1988) Effect of neonatal handling on age-related impairments associated with the hippocampus. *Science* **239,** 766–768.

169. Lorenzini, C. A., Bucherelli, C., Giachetti, A., and Tassoni, G. (1990) Inhibition of exploratory behavior in the rat by handling. *Anim. Learning Behav.* **18,** 191–198.

170. Shiota, K. and Kayamura, T. (1989) Effects of prenatal heat stress on postnatal growth, behavior and learning capacity in mice. *Biol. Neonate* **56,** 6–14.

171. Norton, S., Culver, B., and Mullenix, P. (1975) Development of nocturnal behavior in albino rats. *Behav. Biol.* **15,** 317–331.

172. Lemmer, B. and Berger, T. (1978) Diurnal variations in the motor activity of the rat: effects of inhibitors of the catecholamine synthesis. *Arch. Pharmacol.* **303,** 251–256.

173. Reiter, L. (1978) Use of activity measures in behavioral toxicology. *Environ. Health Perspect.* **26,** 9–20.

174. MacPhail, R. C., Crofton, K. M., and Reiter, L. W. (1983) Use of environmental challenges in behavioral toxicology. *Federation Proc.* **42,** 3196–3200.

175. Tabacova, S., Nikiforov, B., Balabaeva, L., and Hinkova, L. (1983) Toxicological implications of chronic noise exposure during gestation, in *Developments in the Science and Practice of Toxicology* (Hayes, A. W., Schnell, R. C., and Miya, T. S., eds.), Elsevier, Amsterdam, pp. 545–548.

176. Gad, S. C. (1989) Screens in neurotoxicity: objectives, design, and analysis, with the functional observational battery as a case example. *J. Am. Coll. Toxicol.* **8,** 287–301.

177. Tukey, J. W., Ciminera, J. L., and Heyse, J. F. (1985) Testing the statistical certainty of a response to increasing doses of a drug. *Biometrics* **41,** 295–301.

178. Tachibana, T. (1982) Instability of dose-response results in small sample studies in behavioral teratology. *Neurobehav. Toxicol. Teratol.* **4,** 117–118.

179. Tarone, R. E. and Ware, J. (1977) On distribution-free tests for equality of survival distributions. *Biometrika* **64,** 156–160.

180. Vorhees, C. V. (1994) Developmental neurotoxicity induced by therapeutic and illicit drugs. *Environ. Health Perspec.* **102(Suppl. 2),** P145–P153.

181. U.S. Environmental Protection Agency (1998) Health effects test guidelines OPPTS 870.3800, reproduction and fertility effects. U.S. EPA 712-C–208.

182. Applewhite-Black, L. E., Dow-Edwards, D. L., and Minkoff, H. L. (1998) Neurobehavioral and pregnancy effects of prenatal zidovudine exposure in Sprague-Dawley rats: preliminary findings. *Neurotoxicol. Teratol.* **20,** 251–258.

183. Henck, J. W., Craft, W. R., Black, A., Colgin, J., and Anderson, J. A. (1998) Pre- and postnatal toxicity of the HMG-CoA reductase inhibitor atorvastatin in rats. *Toxicol. Sci.* **41,** 88–99.

184. Bauer, R. H. (1978) Ontogeny of two-way avoidance in male and female rats. *Dev. Psychobiol.* **11,** 103–116.

185. Bussiere, J. L., Hardy, L. M., Peterson, M., Foss, J. A., Garman, R. H., Hoberman, A. M., and Christian, M. S. (1999) Lack of developmental neurotoxicity of MN rgp120/HN-1 administered subcutaneously to neonatal rats. *Toxicol. Sci.* **48,** 90–99.

2

Manifestations of CNS Insult During Development

Susan A. Rice

1. INTRODUCTION

Abnormalities of anatomy, function, behavior, and cognition may be the manifestations of insult to the central nervous system (CNS) during development. The initiating insult to the vertebrate organism may act at any level of organization from a single molecule to the entire organism. The consequences of insult at any level then may be "passed on" to other levels of organization. For example, the normal function of a macromolecule, such as an enzyme, may be altered and in turn may affect the function of an organelle, the cell containing the affected organelle, the tissue containing the cell, and so on. The consequences of insult to the CNS, if not repaired or eliminated, may be detected as early as the fetal period or may be asymptomatic and manifest only if the organism is challenged by environmental factors, such as neurotoxic solvents.

The ultimate manifestation of any insult is the result of interactions of the developing organism with a myriad of internal processes and internal or external agents or forces. This chapter addresses the complexity of CNS development and the impact it has on the selection of appropriate methods to detect CNS insults in experimental animals induced by chemicals, pharmaceuticals, physical agents (e.g., X-ray), and trauma during development.

2. THE CNS

The CNS and peripheral nervous system (PNS) comprise the nervous system. Functionally, the nervous system is divided into a sensory (afferent) component and a motor (efferent) component. The sensory component receives and transmits impulses to the CNS for processing. The motor component originates in the CNS and transmits impulses to effector organs throughout the body. The motor component is further subdivided into the somatic system and the autonomic system. In the somatic system, impulses that originate in the CNS are transmitted directly, via a single neuron, to skeletal muscles. In the autonomic system, impulses from the CNS are first transmitted to an autonomic ganglion via one neuron and then a second neuron, which originates in the autonomic ganglion, and transmits the impulses to smooth muscles, cardiac muscles, or glands.

From: Handbook of Neurotoxicology, Vol. 2
Edited by: E. J. Massaro © Humana Press Inc., Totowa, NJ

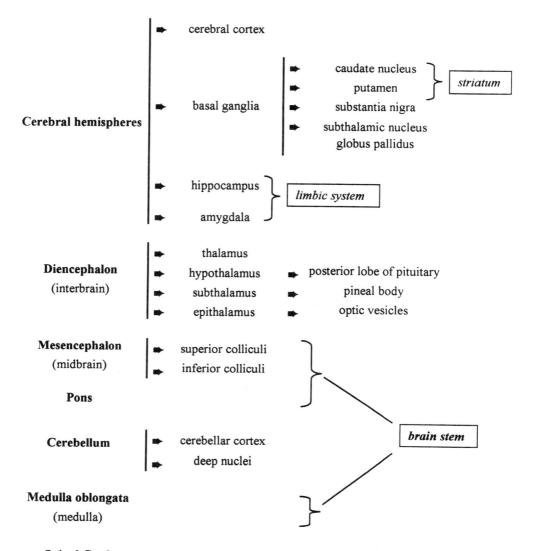

Fig. 1. The Developed CNS. Six major parts of the CNS are shown with their associated structures. The areas shown are selected and many related areas, nuclei, and nerve tracts included. The globus pallidus, one of the basal ganglia, is derived from the diencephalon. *See* text for additional information and Table 1 for a summary of associated functions.

The CNS, which consists of the brain and the spinal cord, is the focus of this chapter. The PNS, which consists of the cranial and spinal nerves, will be addressed indirectly.

2.1. The Developed CNS

The fully developed CNS is bilateral and essentially symmetrical. The brain is composed of nerve cells (neurons) and numerous other cells, which collectively are called neuroglial or glial cells. The spinal cord is composed of gray matter, which consists of the cell bodies and dendrites of neurons and neuroglial cells, and white matter, which

Table 1
Selected Functions in the Developed CNS

Area	Function
Cerebral hemispheres	
Cerebral cortex	Controls cognitive functions; storage and retrieval area
Basal ganglia	Coordinates muscle movement; role in cognitive functions
Hippocampus	Assists cerebral cortex in learning and memory
Amygdala	Acts as relay center; may mediate affective component of odors
Diencephalon	Integrates all information for cerebral cortex
Thalamus	Processes somatic sensory signals (e.g., taste); maintains consciousness; directs movement signals to cortex
Hypothalamus	Controls secretion of hormones from anterior pituitary
Midbrain	Colliculi control ocular reflexes; act as relay in auditory pathway
Pons	Shares some control of vital function with medulla
Cerebellum	
Cerebellar cortex	Indirectly controls posture, balance, and execution of movements
Deep nuclei	Projects output of cortex to descending motor systems of brain
Medulla	Acts as a relay center between spinal cord and rest of brain; regulates respiration, blood pressure, heart beat, reflex movements; other
Spinal cord	Receives sensory information; contains motor neurons for voluntary and reflex movement; controls many visceral functions

consists primarily of axons grouped into tracts. The neurons receive and transmit impulses. The neuroglial cells nourish and support the neurons. The constant interaction of different cell types, and a complex extracellular matrix are necessary to maintain CNS integrity.

The CNS consists of six main parts: the cerebral hemispheres, the diencephalon (interbrain), the mesencephalon (midbrain), the medulla oblongata (medulla), the pons and cerebellum, and the spinal cord. These major parts and selected structures within these parts are listed in Fig. 1. A brief summary of their functions is described in Table 1.

The cerebral hemispheres consist of the cerebral cortex and three deep-lying structures: the basal ganglia, the hippocampus, and the amygdala (amygdaloid nucleus). One of the basal ganglia, the globus pallidus, actually arises from the diencephalon.

The diencephalon is a paired structure on each side of the third ventricle. This structure forms the central core of the cerebrum. The diencephalon contains the thalamus, the hypothalamus, the subthalamus, and the epithalamus.

The midbrain, the pons, and the medulla collectively are called the brain stem. The brain stem has ascending and descending pathways that carry sensory and motor information to and from the higher brain regions[1]. A network of neurons in the brain stem extending through the medulla, pons, and midbrain, called the reticular formation, mediates aspects of arousal.

The midbrain has four rounded eminences, two on each side. The upper pair is referred to as the superior colliculi and the lower pair is referred to as the inferior colliculi. The pons is caudal to the midbrain and consists mainly of massive white matter tracts that serve the cerebellum. The cerebellum lies dorsal to the pons and the medulla and extends laterally, wrapping around the brain stem. The cerebellum consists of two lateral cerebellar hemispheres and a middle portion called the vermis. A specialized process of cytodifferentiation in the cerebellum gives rise to the gray matter of the cerebellar cortex, the internal white matter, and the deep internal nuclei. The medulla is a direct extension of the spinal cord and resembles the spinal cord in both organization and function.

The spinal cord is the most primitive part of the CNS and resembles the embryonic neural tube from which it is derived. It extends from the base of the skull through the first lumbar vertebrae. The spinal nerves are peripheral, not central, nerves. These nerves are involved in reflex actions.

As suggested by the preceding descriptions, neurons in the CNS are diverse in structure, size, neurotransmitters, and receptors. For example, the Purkinje cell is among the largest neurons in vertebrates and its cell body measures approx 80 μm in diameter. In contrast, the granule cell is among the smallest neurons with a cell body 6–8 μm in diameter.

Identification of the area affected by an insult in the developed CNS will help to estimate the likely functional outcome. A functional abnormality, conversely, may help to identify the area of damage. Knowledge of the anatomy of the mature CNS, however, may not be sufficient. Knowledge of the ontogeny of the CNS may be necessary to determine the etiology of an abnormality following physical injury or exposure to a chemical, drug, or physical agent during development. The knowledge of CNS ontogeny may be even more important in accurately interpreting and fully appreciating the implications of an abnormality.

The following section will briefly describe the development of the CNS. The descriptions will be necessarily abbreviated and contain only selected portions of the CNS in an attempt to provide an appreciation for the complexity of the CNS and to give the reader somewhat of a background to follow the information provided later in the chapter.

2.2. Normal Development of the CNS

The ontogeny of the CNS starts with the dorsal ectoderm as shown in Fig. 2. Although the developmental process results in a CNS that is basically the same in all vertebrates, there are significant differences among species in the timing of various developmental events. Table 2 summarizes some reproductive characteristics and developmental events for humans and five species of experimental animals. More complete embryology and timing of organ development of various species (i.e., rat [1,2], mouse

---

[1]Sensory input and motor output of the brain stem is carried by cranial nerves that are concerned with sensation from skin and joints in the head, neck, and face as well as with the special senses.

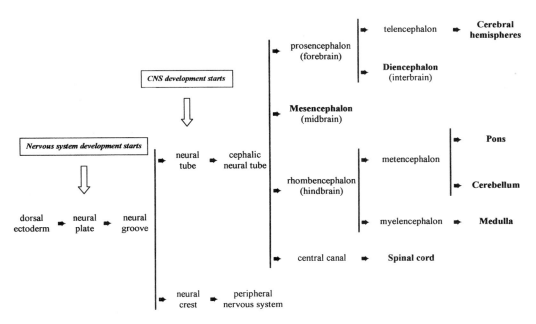

Fig. 2. CNS Development. The ontogeny and organization of the CNS are depicted in an abbreviated form. The areas that are shown in bold represent the six primary parts of the developed CNS, which are shown in Fig. 1. Development is further discussed in the text.

[3–5], hamster *[6]*, rabbit *[1,7]*, guinea pig *[3,8]*, rhesus monkey *[9,10]*, human *[11–13]*, chicken *[14–16]*), are contained in several developmental textbooks.

The ensuing description of the CNS follows the order seen in Fig. 2. The nervous system begins to develop relatively early in gestation. The neural tube is derived from the dorsal ectoderm and ultimately will form the CNS. The stages of development progress from the ectoderm to the neural plate, then to the neural groove, which is a single layer of cells. Fusion of the neural tube begins cervically and proceeds both cranially and caudally. The anterior neuropore closes first and the posterior neuropore follows. Fusion is completed during the fourth week in humans and gestational day (GD) 8.5, 9, 9.5, 11, and 25 for the hamster, mouse, rabbit, rat, and monkey, respectively, by gestational day *(17)*.

The original neural cavity becomes either the brain ventricles or the central canal of the spinal cord. The neural cavity is lined by an ependyma marginal layer, which becomes white matter; neuroepithelium cells of the mantle layer become gray matter. Some of the neuroepithelium are termed neuroblasts because they will give rise to the motor neurons and to the association (internuncial) neurons. Most of the neuroepithelial cells are gliablasts, which give rise to the astrocytes and the oligodendrocytes. The ependyma that does not migrate out from the neural cavity will line the ventricles.

The neural cavity enlarges in the brain to form the brain vesicles (except in the mesencephalon where it narrows to form the aqueduct of Sylvius). Three primary brain vesicles develop in the anterior neural tube. These vesicles are increased to four from which the adult structures are derived (*see* Figs. 1 and 2). At certain sites, the ependyma of the roof of the ventricle and the pia mater are invaded by blood vessels to form the choroid plexus, which forms the cerebrospinal fluid (CSF).

Table 2
Placental Type and CNS Developmental Events in Selected Species[a]

Species	Placenta[b]	Implantation	Primitive streak[c]	Neural plate	3 Brain vesicles[d]	Cerebral hemispheres	Cerebellum	Gestation length
Hamster	Hemotrichorial	4.5–5.0	6.0–7.0	7.5	8.5	9	11	16
Mouse	Hemotrichorial	4.5–5.0	7.0–8.0	7	8	10	12	19–20
Rat	Hemotrichorial	5.5–6.0	8.5–9.0	9–9.5	10.5–12	12–12.3	14	21–22
Rabbit	Hemodichorial	7.0–7.5	7.0–8.0	8	8.3–9.5	11	15	30–32
Macaque	Hemomonochorial	9.0	17.0	20	25	29	36	167
Human	Hemomonochorial	6.0–10	14–20	18–19	26 ± 1	29–33	37	267–270

[a]References (17,21,34).
[b]Internal placental structure is labyrinthine for hamster, mouse, cat, and rabbit.
[c]Start of the embryonic period.
[d]Posterior neuropore closed. Prosencephalon (forebrain), mesencephalon (midbrain), and rhombencephalon (hindbrain).

The growth of the neuroepithelium also causes the neural cavity of the spinal cord to narrow, forming the central canal. The spinal cord is derived from the caudal neural tube. The marginal layer is the white matter that is invaded by ingrowing axons. The mantle layer is subdivided by the sulcus limitans into the alar plate (sensory and association neurons) and the basal plate (motor and association neurons).

The neural crest is also derived from the neural groove. Neural-crest cells are migratory and give rise to most of the PNS, including the sensory neurons in the dorsal-root ganglia and the cranial nerves V, VII, IX, and X.

2.2.1. Neuron Formation and Maturation

Neuron formation and maturation does not occur in all species at the same relative time or in the same chronological order. For example, neurons in the fetal mouse form between gestational day (GD) 10 and 20 and continue to form in the hippocampus, cerebellum, and olfactory bulb through 2–3 wk of postnatal life *(18,19)*. Neurons in the fetal rat brain form principally between GD 13 and 20; neurons in the cerebellum do not appear until about GD 15. Brain development in the rat also continues for several weeks in the postnatal period.

Neurons that are born at the early stages of cortical development end up in the deepest cortical layers, while those born later end up in progressively more superficial layers. The radial glial cells act as substrates for the migration of neurons. In the cerebral cortex, many neurons use radial glial cells to guide migration from the ventricular zones to their final destination.

In the diencephalon, migration of neurons occur in successive waves. The neurons that are more superficial were the last to migrate. The marginal layer gives rise to the white matter, and the mantle layer gives rise to the gray matter. Neuroepithelial cells of the cerebral cortex migrate farther away from the neural cavity and become peripheral; thus, the gray matter is outside the white matter in this area because the neuroepithelium migrated further.

Brain development in most species continues after birth. At birth, the brain of the rat and human, as well as other species, is largely unmyelinated and myelinates slowly until adolescence or later. The reticular formation is the last to be fully myelinated. The complex neural circuitry also continues to be organized postnatally as with the cortical, limbic, and cerebellar regions.

With some knowledge of the normal mature CNS and how it develops, it is possible to consider how abnormal development can occur.

2.3. Abnormal Development of the CNS

Each brain region possesses a characteristic maturational pattern. Perturbation typically results in subsequent abnormalities of cell number, size, and/or organization. Both teratogenic and toxic agents can act directly on the embryo, fetus, or neonate, or indirectly through the mother and the placental system, to adversely affect CNS development.

Susceptibility to CNS insult, subsequent abnormal development, and the severity of an abnormality are dependent on the developmental stage at the time of exposure, the intensity and duration of exposure, and the specificity of the agent for its target cell or tissue. Different combinations of developmental stage, specificity of action, and exposure route, dose, and duration all result in different patterns of effects.

Teratogenesis produces alterations in the formation of cells, tissues, organs, and systems that result in structural, behavioral, or functional abnormalities. In general, susceptibility to teratogenesis decreases as differentiation and organogenesis proceed because the proliferative and morphogenic activities necessary for the formation of tissues and organs become less prominent as the organ develops. Toxicity, however, produces degenerative changes that are not directly related to the formation of cells, tissues, and organs. These degenerative changes result in embryo, fetal, or organ-system growth retardation or other adverse effects, including behavioral and functional abnormalities.

The CNS, as a system, is particularly vulnerable to injury during development simply because of the extended period of time during which the specialized cell populations of the CNS are produced and mature. Histogenesis for several cell populations continues into the neonatal period.

2.3.2. Influence of Genotype

Variations in response among species following exposure to a teratogenic or toxic agent may be due to differences in: timing of exposure; critical periods for different regions of the CNS; active metabolic pathways; developmental patterns; placentation; or the distribution and action of exogenous the agent.

Development of the vertebrate organism is based on the expression of information contained within the genome of embryonic cells. The timing of expression is both triggered by and permitted by signals in the environment of those cells. Different neurologic structures and functions mature at different rates in any single species and the pattern differs among species *(17,20–22)*. Some developmental events are shown in Table 2.

When the exogenous agent is a mutagen, mutations[2] in the genetic information can result in misdirection and partial or complete failure of cell migration or the induction of apoptosis in the developing animal. Cleft palate and defects in neural-tube closure in mice have been associated with mutations of the genome in mice *(23)*. With the use of the knockout approach to the analysis of gene function, neural-tube defects have been found to be associated with genes with roles in oncogenesis, signal transduction, and adult physiology that are not known to be expressed specifically in the embryonic neural folds. Mutations may also result in syndromes of what would otherwise be seen as minor anomalies.

3. IDENTIFYING CNS INSULT

The methodological approaches of many experimental and clinical traditions are used to identify abnormalities resulting from insult during CNS development. Approaches can be thought of as either visualizing a change or measuring a change in the system.

The latter is referred to as a biological marker of effect. For our consideration, a biological marker of effect is a detectable alteration of an endogenous component within the CNS that, depending on the magnitude of endogenous component, can be

---

[2]A mutation is an alteration in the DNA sequence of genes. Germ cells in mature animals can pass changes in genetic information from one generation to the next; somatic cells cannot.

recognized as an indication of potential or actual system impairment or damage. These markers can be qualitative or quantitative. The following sections are not exhaustive compilations of available methods, but rather provide an impetus for individuals to think in very broad terms as to what constitutes a biological marker in the investigation of insult to the CNS during development. The material has been divided into noninvasive and invasive techniques. In vitro techniques, such as cell culture, have not been addressed.

3.1. Noninvasive

3.1.1. Electroencephalogram (EEG) and Sensory-Evoked Potential

There are definite advantages to the use of noninvasive techniques to identify CNS abnormalities. The majority of the noninvasive techniques available, apart from the behavioral, have been designed primarily for diagnostic use in the human clinical situation. These approaches have not been extensively used with laboratory animals because of the relatively small size of rats and mice, which are the most commonly used animals, and the cost of purchasing and maintaining the needed equipment.

The EEG has been used clinically to assess cortical function. The information gathered includes indices to evaluate arousal, wakefulness, sleep, epilepsy, and coma. The EEG records the electrical activity (extracellular current flow) of large groups of neurons in the brain. Macroelectrodes are placed on the surface of the scalp and the recordings measure the potential difference between two electrodes. Primarily, surface recorded potentials reflect the activity (postsynaptic potentials) of cortical neurons in the area underlying the EEG electrode.

When a significant stimulus is presented, such as an auditory stimulus, the component of the EEG that is specifically related to the stimulus is called a sensory-evoked potential. The sensory evoked potential, in essence, reflects the processing of the physical characteristics of the stimulus. The information gathered can help to assess sensory systems and to evaluate the degree of myelination (evoked potential latencies are longer with less myelination).

3.1.2. Imaging

Imaging techniques are used for human diagnosis and are becoming more common for use with laboratory animals, especially the larger species (i.e., primate, dog, and cat). These techniques are X-ray, computerized tomography (CT), positron emission tomography (PET), and magnetic resonance imaging (MRI) *(24)*.

The regional anatomy of the brain may be explored with CT. Much of our understanding of higher brain function depends on refined mapping of neuronal circuits with newer anatomical and imaging techniques. PET and MRI make the functional neuroanatomy of the brain accessible during behavioral experiments.

3.1.3. X-Ray CT, PET, and MRI

Conventional radiography (i.e., X-ray) gives a three-dimensional representation of an object in two dimensions. The X-ray CT scan, in contrast, is an image of a single plane or section of tissue. X-ray CT provides images of brain tissue, CSF, and bone. It can also distinguish the thalamus, basal ganglia, the ventricles, and the gray and white matter of the cerebral cortex. Other techniques, the static CT, may be combined with images of brain structure to produce images of the functioning (dynamics) of the brain.

PET combines the principles of CT and radioisotope imaging to project images of brain function. The PET image reflects the tissue distribution of an injected or inhaled isotope. One application is the mapping of glucose utilization/metabolism of neurons *(25)*. An analog of glucose, 2-deoxyglucose, is taken up by neurons and is phosphory-lated by hexokinase, as glucose-6-phosphate would be; however, phosphorylated deoxyglucose cannot be further metabolized nor can it cross the cell membrane. It accumulates within active brain cells and the positron-emitting isotope of fluorine, ^{18}F, covalently binds to make ^{18}F-labeled deoxyglucose. The positron emissions make it possible to image glucose utilization in small regions of the brain.

Glucose utilization mapping can be very important because the CNS depends almost entirely on glucose for energy and as a starting material for the synthesis of other mol-ecules. The energy requirements of the CNS are high because of activities such as maintaining electric potentials, neurotransmitter reuptake, and neuro-axonal transport.

MRI also uses the principles of CT. Similar to PET, MRI can be used to identify function as well as structure, but MRI has much better spatial resolution. This imaging technique, combined with CT, provides images that localize atomic nuclei. Atomic nuclei align their spin axes in a magnetic field, which is subsequently perturbed by pulsed radio waves. The nuclei absorb energy, and when the radio wave is turned off, the nuclei release energy in the form of radio waves as they return to a lower-energy state. The frequency of the radio wave released is distinctive for each atomic nucleus in each chemical or physical environment. Nuclear magnetic resonance (NMR) is the ability of atomic nuclei to absorb radio waves. The rate of return to lower-energy states is called relaxation and is described by its time constant. Images that give the greatest contrast are derived from time constants that are derived from relaxation times *(24)*.

The MRI scan can reveal all major regions of the CNS, including the ventricular system. For example, it can reveal minute differences in tissue water concentrations and is a sensitive technique for detecting brain lesions. The brain has the smallest ex-tracellular space of all organs (~20% of volume); most structural disease processes expand the extracellular space with brain swelling. Using computer techniques similar to those used in CT and PET, an entire cross-section of the brain can be obtained from information in MRI profiles.

3.1.4. Behavior and Function

Behavior is a reflection of brain function. Brain regions are specialized for different functions (*see* Table 1). One classification scheme for CNS function is sensory, motor, sensorimotor integration, cognition, emotion, and reproductive behavior. Multiple be-havioral end-points can be used to assess CNS function, such as reflex and motor de-velopment, sensory function, reactivity levels, learning and memory, and functioning in neurotransmitter systems. The previous chapter fully addresses the physiologic ba-sis, the rationale, and methodology for behavioral and functional testing to identify CNS insult during development.

As expected, the timing of many of the tests in young animals is critical because there are pronounced changes in brain maturation that are reflected by changes in behavior. Table 3 provides a small sample of the type of information that can be at-tained with this methodology. *See* the previous chapter for many more examples.

Table 3
Examples of Behavior and Function Altered in Selected Experiments[a,b]

Observed effect	Species	Agent and exposure	Comments	References
Activity, residential running wheel: ↑ daytime activity PND 78–91	SD rats	RA: 2.5 mg/kg gavage GD 11–13	↓ Cerebellar weight: 4% male, 14% fem.	(35)
Spontaneous breathing and nursing: difficulty initiating	SD rats	RA: 10 mg/kg gavage GD 11–13	Abnormal areas in cell-dense medial medulla	(35)
Rotorod activity: deficit (robust) PND 26–28	SD rats	RA: 12.5 mg/kg gavage GD 14–16	↓ Cerebellar weight: 11% male, 11% fem.	(35)
Surface-righting reflex: ↑ latency to right PND 3	Wistar rats	Toluene: 1200 ppm 6 h/d GD 6 - PND 17	↓ Birth weight 12.7%; no maternal tox.	(36)
Cognitive function, new learning: ↑ latency to find hidden platform[c] (fem. 3.5 mo)	Wistar rats	Toluene: 1200 ppm 6 h/d GD 6 - PND 17	↓ Birth weight 12.7%; no maternal tox.	(36)

[a]Abbreviations used: abn., abnormal; d, day; fem, female; GD, gestational day; h, hour; mo, month; PND, postnatal day; RA, retinoic acid; tox., toxicity.
[b]Where known, data has been adjusted so that GD 0 is a day a copulatory plug is observed or sperm is identified in the vagina of the animal.
[c]Impaired performance in the Morris water maze has been linked to hippocampal dysfunction in adult rats. The task is sensitive to a variety of experimental insults to the hippocampal formation or closely related structures (37).

67

3.2. Invasive

3.2.1. Imaging

Optical imaging permits a high-resolution spatial record of activity in a neural population by using voltage-sensitive dyes, which change their fluorescence or absorption with changes in membrane potential. Neurons also emit activity-dependent signals based on their intrinsic fluorescence. These techniques require direct visualization of the cortical surface.

3.2.2. Gross Pathology

In the classical approach of teratology, a pregnant animal is treated one or more days during pregnancy, and the offspring are examined near the end of gestation for gross external or internal malformations or variations. Craniofacial examination is usually performed after a specific pattern of cuts is made through the fetal head. These relatively precise cuts are necessary to observe internal structures that are either partially or fully hidden during external examination, such as the palate and eye structure. The status of the lateral ventricles of the cerebrum can also be assessed.[3]

Table 4 gives several examples of the gross effects that have been identified by this technique. Depending on the intended use of the study results, neuropathological assessment of pups at necropsy generally includes, at a minimum, visualization of the following tissues: olfactory bulbs, cerebral cortex, hippocampus, basal ganglia, thalamus, hypothalamus, midbrain, thecum, tegmentum, cerebral peduncles, brain stem, and cerebellum. More areas may be examined as needed. This type of gross approach identifies abnormalities, but visual observation, even by stereomicroscopy, is limited; light and electron microscopy are needed to observe more subtle effects at the tissue and cellular levels.

3.2.3. Cytology

The developing vertebrate embryo and fetus exhibit migration, proliferation, differentiation, and apoptosis. Apoptosis occurs when an internally controlled suicide program is activated that results in cell death. Apoptosis is normally activated during embryogenesis and tissue remodeling to remove aged cells, and during some physiologic processes to eliminate unwanted cells. Apoptosis removes cells with minimal disruption to the surrounding tissue. The chief morphologic characteristic of controlled apoptosis is chromatin condensation and fragmentation.

A cell, under normal physiologic conditions and demands, is in normal homeostasis. Excessive physiologic stress or pathologic stimuli (e.g., hypertrophy) may result in cellular adaptations that are physiologic or morphologic in nature. If adaptation is insufficient or unavailable, then a sequence of events is initiated that is commonly referred to as cell injury. An insult to the developing CNS during the phases of organogenesis and histogenesis may not only cause cell injury, but may produce such a profound effect that either apoptosis or necrosis is initiated. Either of the routes of cell death may not produce such that is immediately evident, but rather, the full extent of any insult will only be manifest when cellular migration is complete.

3.2.3.1. CELL CHARACTERISTICS

Cell injury may be reversible, or irreversible leading to cell death by necrosis or apoptosis. Following an exogenous insult, necrosis (or coagulation necrosis) is more

---

[3]Many techniques require that the head be fixed and decalcified in Bouin's solution.

Table 4
Examples of CNS Malformations in Selected Experiments[a]

Observed effect	Species	Agent and exposure	Comments	References
Exencephaly: ↑; mean litter % 3.6 GD 6.5, 88.3 GD 7.0, 66.2 GD 8.0	C57BL/6 mice	Cd: 4 mg/kg single ip. GD 6.5, 7.0, 7.5, 8.0, 8.5, or 9.0	Evaluated GD 18	(38)
Exencephaly: ↑; mean litter % 0.0 GD 6.5, 4.1 GD 7.0, 27.7 GD 8.0	SWV mice	Cd: 4 mg/kg single ip. GD 6.5, 7.0, 7.5, 8.0, 8.5, or 9.0	Evaluated GD 18	(38)
Hydrocephaly: ↑; mean litter % 7.5 GD 7.0; 6.1 GD 8.5	SWV mice	Cd: 4 mg/kg single ip. GD 6.5, 7.0, 7.5, 8.0, 8.5, or 9.0	Evaluated GD 18	(38)
Hydrocephaly: ↑; mean litter % 3.6 GD 7.0, 8.2 GD 8.0; 17.0 GD 8.5; 20.8 GD 9.0	C57BL/6 mice	Cd: 4 mg/kg single ip. GD 6.5, 7.0, 7.5, 8.0, 8.5, or 9.0	Evaluated GD 18	(38)
Micro-/anophthalmia: ↑; mean litter % 43.8 GD 6.5, 7.1 GD 7.0, 25.0 GD 7.5, 14.9 GD 8.0, 19.8 GD 8.5, 4.9 GD 9.0	C57BL/6 mice	Cd: 4 mg/kg single ip. GD 6.5, 7.0, 7.5, 8.0, 8.5, 9.0	Evaluated GD 18	(38)
Micro-/anophthalmia, distended brain ventricles: ↑; most in 2 litters w/greatest maternal tox.	COBS rat	NMF: 50 or 150 ppm inhal. 6 h/d GD 6–15	↓ fetal wt. 12.2%; embryolethal	(39)
Pituitary agenesis: ↑ 63% (54 fetuses; 11 litters) Holoprosencephaly: 29 of above 54 fetuses Cebocephaly: 26 of above 29 fetuses	Wistar rats	BM15.766[b] 300 mg/kg/d gavage GD 4–7	Embryolethal	(30)

[a]Abbreviations used: Cd, cadmium chloride; GD, gestational day; inhal., inhalation; ip, intra peritoneal; NMF, N-methylformamide; 7DHC reductase, 7-dehydrocholesterol-δ-7-reductase; tox., toxicity; w/, with; wt, weight

[b](4-(2-{1-(4-chlorocinnamyl)piperazin-4-yl}ethyl)-benzoic acid), a 7DHC reductase inhibitor.

69

Table 5
Cytologic Manifestations of CNS Insult[a]

Cell or component	Normal cell	Cell injury	
		Reversible[b]	Irreversible
Nerve cell (neuron)	Great diversity; most polygonal w/concave surfaces	Generalized cellular swelling	Autolysis by lysosomal contents; in necrosis, clumps of dying neurons
Plasma membrane (cell membrane; plasmalemma)	Trilaminar structure, two thin dense lines and inner light area; not visible w/light microscope	Membrane blebs; aggregation of intramembranous particles	Defects in cell membrane; myelin figures; loosening of intercellular attachments
Cell body[c] (soma; perikaryon)	Centrally located nucleus in perinuclear cytoplasm	Hypertrophy; chromatolysis[d]	In necrosis, severe cell swelling or rupture
Cytoplasm, perinuclear	Abundant SER and RER; scattered clumps of Nissl bodies[e]; Golgi, mitochondria, lysosomes	Fewer Nissl bodies; nucleus displaced	In necrosis, denaturation and coagulation of cytoplasmic proteins
Nucleus[f]	Large and pale-staining; amorphous appearance; spherical to ovoid; finely dispersed chromatin[g]	Displaced clumping of nuclear chromatin	Fragmentation of chromatin; nuclear pyknosis, karyolysis, or karyorrhexis
Mitochondrion	Numerous; scattered in perinuclear, dendritic, and axonal cytoplasm; most abundant at axon terminals	Swelling; small phospholipid-rich amorphous densities; and autophagy by lysosomes	Swelling; presence of large densities; autophagy by lysosomes
Endoplasmic reticulum (ER)	Abundant in perinuclear cytoplasm w/many cisternae in parallel arrays	Swelling; disaggregation and dispersion of ribosomes	Swelling; dispersed ribosomes; lysis
Golgi complex	Prominent juxta-nuclear complex; several closely associated cisternae w/ a dilated periphery	Swelling	Swelling; lysis
Lysosome	Small, <1 μm; spherical or ellipsoid; membrane bound	Autophagy of mitochondria may be observed	Autophagy of mitochondria; rupture of lysosomes
Inclusions	Lipofuscin, irregularly shaped yellow to brown granule[h]; melanin granules, in certain regions[i]; lipid droplets	May be increased in number	
Axon[j]	SER extends from soma forming hypolemmal cisternae beneath plasmalemma; no ribosomes	Swelling; axon (and myelin sheath) atrophy or degeneration; phagocytosis of axon (and myelin)	Phagocytosis of denerated axon (and myelin); proliferation of glial cells; formation of glial scar
Dendrite[k]	SER extends from soma; RER present as scattered short or branching cisternae	Degeneration	Degeneration
Boutons (terminal; en passage)	Area of specialized swelling, at end of fine branches of axon/dendrites or along the axon	Degeneration	Degeneration

Table 5 (*continued*)

Cell or component	Normal cell	Cell injury	
		Reversible[b]	Irreversible
Synapse		Glial cells push apart pre- and postsynaptic elements of synapse	Glial cells present; phagacytosis of degenerated synaptic
Glial cells (glia; neuroglia)		Changes organization of synapses on injured neurons	
Macroglia			
Astrocytes	Star shaped cells; cytoplasmic bundles of GFAP; endfeet contact both neurons and capillaries forming tight endothelial junction	May act as phagocyte and remove cell debris	May act as phagocyte and remove cell debris
Oligodendrocytes	Small cells; many processes; in gray matter, surrounds neuronal soma	Processes pull away from soma	Processes pulled away from soma
Microglial cells[l]	Smallest glial cell, rod-shaped nuclei		
Ependymal cells	Cuboidal or columnar cells lining ventricles	Scavenge local neuronal debris	Scavenge local neuronal debris

[a]Abbreviations used: GFAP, glial fibrillar acidic protein; PNS, peripheral nervous system; RER, rough endoplasmic reticulum; SER, smooth endoplasmic reticulum; w/, with.

[b]Regeneration of a severed axon is much less likely in the CNS than in the PNS.

[c]Characteristic for type and location.

[d]Nissl bodies are dispersed and nucleus is displaced.

[e]When stained with basic dyes, polyribosomes appear as clumps of basophilic material called Nissl bodies, which have a characteristic form, shape, and size in each type of neuron.

[f]Mature neurons cannot divide and their chromosomes exist in a relatively uncoiled state; well-defined nucleolus is common.

[g]Smaller neurons may have some inactive heterochromatin (condensed nuclear material often adjacent to inner nuclear membrane).

[h]Most pronounced in aged neurons.

[i]Substantia nigra, locus cereleus, dorsal motor nucleus of vagus, spinal cord.

[j]Varied, dependent on neuron type: 5–150 μm in diameter and up to 100 cm in length.

[k]Cytoskeleton composed predominantly of fibrous polymeric proteins, neurofilaments, microtubules, and microfilaments similar to that of soma.

[l]Embryologic origin is in bone marrow; part of mononuclear phagocytic-cell population.

common than apoptosis. Necrosis is manifest by severe cell swelling and/or cell rupture, denaturation and coagulation of cytoplasmic proteins, and degradation of cell organelles. Axotomy can be used to model the effects of axonal injury on the neuron. Severing an axon or sectioning a tract within the brain results in swelling of both proximal[4] and distal[5] segments. Ca^{2+} enters the swollen segments and may cause further injury by activating proteases or initiating free-radical generation.

[4]The part of the axon connected to the cell body.

[5]The remaining part of the axon.

Both cell-to-cell and cell-to-matrix interactions contribute significantly to the response following injury. As time progresses, distinct microscopic changes may be seen for reversible and irreversible injuries *(26,27)* (Table 5). Normal input to the cell body returns if the regenerated axon makes contact with a new target cell. If successful neuronal regeneration occurs, the cell body usually regains its normal appearance. If a new target cell is not contacted, the neuron will atrophy and die.

The degeneration of one cell type in the CNS can impair the function of cells with which it forms functional contacts. Axonal transport, for example, is crucial to the trophic relationships between neurons and their target cell. If the trophic relationship is interrupted, the target cell will atrophy. It is important to recognize, however, that not all neurons exhibit chromatolysis[6] or regenerative changes after axotomy. For example, the Purkinje cells of the cerebellum do not shrink detectably, whereas the neurons in the thalamus shrink and remain in that state indefinitely.

Transneuronal or transsynaptic changes are those degenerative changes that occur in cells that previously had synaptic contact with an injured neuron. Transneuronal degeneration explains, in part, how injury at one site in the CNS can affect sites at some distance from the lesion. Contact between the terminals and the postsynaptic cell is disrupted by invading glial cells. The terminals withdraw completely from the postsynaptic cell, and the entire distal segment degenerates and is lost. But the process of degeneration may persist for several months depending on the specific species and neuron type.

Glial cells also change the organization of the synapses on injured neurons. Glial cells push apart the pre- and postsynaptic elements of the synapse, which results in a decreased number of presynaptic contacts and correspondingly smaller amplitude of the evoked excitatory synaptic potentials. There also may be a change in excitability as is observed with axotomy where there is an enhanced efficacy of dendritic synapses, possibly due to an increased excitability of dendrites postaxotomy.

More information is obtained at the level of electron microscopy. At degenerating synapses within the CNS, the terminals of some neurons become filled with whirls of neuro-filaments that surround disrupted and swollen mitochondria. Other neuron terminals become filled with electron-dense products of degeneration. Resident microglial cells and astrocytes, not macrophages, remove the cellular debris in the CNS.

3.2.3.2. MORPHOMETRY

Morphometric analysis may take many forms, from weighing the whole brain to determining the density of a certain cell type in a specific region or area, such as the ventricular system or the caudate-putamen.

Weight is one of the simplest measurements to make. Weight of the whole brain, however, is relatively uninformative unless the effects of an insult are pronounced. Weights of specific areas of the brain may be much more informative, but the smaller the area of interest, the greater the probability that differences among samples will be due to the dissection technique and not to actual weight differences.

The cerebellum is a structure frequently chosen for developmental study because of its distinctive morphology, in which proliferating cells are clearly separated from postmitotic cells, and because it has a long period of postnatal development in most

---

[6]Chromatolysis is a sign that a neural axon has been severed. Nissl bodies are seen around the cell margin with injury instead of around the nucleus, as in its uninjured state.

Table 6
Histopathologic and Morphometric Manifestations of CNS Insult[a,b]

Observed effect	Species	Agent and exposure	Comments	Reference
Cerebellum: ↓ weight 4% male, 11% fem.	SD rats	RA: 2.5 mg/kg gavage GD 11–13		(35)
Cerebellum: ↓ weight 11% male, 11% fem.	SD rats	RA: 12.5 mg/kg gavage GD 14–16		(35)
Inferior olive and area postrema: ↓ cell density and/or staining intensity	SD rats	RA: 10 mg/kg gavage GD 11–13	Inability of pups to nurse; eventually died	(40)
Telencephalon, ventricular zone: ↑ pyknotic cells ~12–20% w/↑ dose	ICR mice	BrdU: 25–800 mg/kg single ip. GD 10	Evaluated 24 h post-injection	(41)
Diencephalon, ependymal, & mantle layers: ↑ pyknotic cells ~1–10% w/↑ dose	ICR mice	BrdU: 25–800 mg/kg single ip. GD 10	Evaluated 24 h post-injection	(41)
SDN-POA: ↓ volume 46.1%; ↓ number of neurons 47.8%	SD rats, male	Tamoxifen: 100 µg sc. PND 1–5		(42)
Pituitary agenesis: ↑ 63% (54 fetuses; 11 litters) Holoprosencephaly: 29 of above 54 fetuses Cebocephaly: 26 of above 29 fetuses	Wistar rats	BM15.766[c] 300 mg/kg/d gavage GD 4–7	Embryolethal	(30)

[a]Abbreviations used: BrdU, 5-bromo-2'-deoxyuridine; fem, feminine; GD, gestational day; h, hour; ip., intraperitoneal; PND, postnatal day; RA, retinoic acid; sc., subcutaneous; SDN-POA, sexually dimorphic nucleus of the medial preoptic area.

[b]Where known, data has been adjusted so that GD 0 is day a copulatory plug or sperm is identified in the female animal.

[c](4-(2-{1-(4-chlorocinnamyl)piperazin-4-yl}ethyl)-benzoic acid), a 7DHC reductase inhibitor.

Table 7
Selected Biochemical Indices of CNS Development

Macromolecule or component	*Index of*		
	(Total mg of component/brain area)	*(mg of component/g tissue)*	*(mg of component mg/mg DNA)*
DNA	Number of cells[a]	Cellular density	—
Protein	Brain growth	Protein density	Cell size
Cholesterol	Tissue myelination	Myelin density	Myelination and arborization/cell
Choline acetyl-transferase (ChAT)	Synaptic proliferation	Synaptic density	—
Hemicolinum-3 binding	Synaptic activity	Synaptic density	—

[a]An average of 6.2 pg of DNA is assumed to be present in a single rat diploid nucleus.

species. Table 6 lists several ways in which morphometry has helped to identify injury to the CNS.

3.2.3.3. HISTOCHEMISTRY

There are literally hundreds of procedures that utilize histochemistry to visualize and localize varied biochemical and neurochemical activities (*26–28*). Projections among intact neurons can be traced using the label horseradish peroxidase, autoradiography, and fluorescent dye tracers. Several differential-staining techniques are available for tracing degenerative changes in neurons *(24)*. Other techniques are available for evaluating myelination. For example, chromium salts and hematoxylin only stain-myelinated fiber, demyelinated fibers show as pale regions devoid of staining. Dopaminergic neurons are visualized in light microscopy by labeling with antibodies to tyrosine hydroxylase.

3.2.4. Biochemical and Neurochemical Measurements

There are many biochemical approaches to identifying basic changes in structure and function. One approach is to microdissect a discrete brain area that can then be subjected to one or more microanalytical techniques. Better resolution is thus attained by analysis of a smaller area, such as a nucleus, instead of a more heterogeneous brain region.

3.2.4.1. MACROMOLECULES

Measurement of specific endogenous substances can be used to evaluate development and maturation, both normal and abnormal. Any number of substances, such as amino acids, nucleic acids, proteins, enzymes, hormones, neurotransmitters, and receptors, can be mapped to specific brain areas.

Macromolecular composition of the brain can be determined to evaluate the developmental effect of prenatal treatment. Individual or aggregate samples of specific brain areas may be prepared to analyze macromolecules, such as DNA, protein, and cholesterol. These macromolecules may also serve as indices of brain development. Table 7 shows a few samples of the indices of brain growth and maturation that have been developed.

3.2.4.2. Enzymes

Brain enzyme ontogeny and function is also important in cell survival and development of brain tissues. Several enzymes and their metabolic products, such as ornithine decarboxylase and 7-dehydrocholesterol δ reductase (7DHC reductase) are essential to normal development. Ornithine decarboxylase and its metabolic products, the polyamines, are regulators of macromolecule synthesis during differentiation as well as during replication *(29)*. 7DHC reductase is necessary for normal craniofacial development.

As an example of the profound effects that enzymes have on the developing system, inhibition of 7DHC reductase by blockers, such as BM15.766 (4-(2-{1-(4-chlorocinnamyl)piperazin-4-yl}ethyl)-benzoic acid), induce holoprosencephaly in rats (*see* Table 6) *(30)*. Holoprosencephaly results from a failed diverticularization of the embryonic prosencephalon into the cerebral hemispheres and the diencephalic structures. The etiology is heterogenous, but the primary disorder seems to reside in the prechordal mesenchyma, which is thought to induce both cleavage of the primitive forebrain and development of the median facial structures (orbits, nose, median upper lip, and palate).

Failure of the forebrain to undergo paired symmetrical division along the sagittal plane and diverticularization results in varying degrees of fusion of the cerebral structures. There is a typical association of brain anomalies to facial dysmorphism seen in this malformation sequence. Two subtypes of holoprosencephaly are cyclopia and cebocephaly. Pituitary agenesis is a minor form of holoprosencephaly. In the aforementioned study approx 63% of fetuses exhibited pituitary agenesis. Mid-sagittal sections of the head and neck must be examined with a stereomicroscope to identify the malformation.

The BM15.766 treated dams showed abnormal cholesterol biosynthesis as indicated by low serum cholesterol and accumulation of 7- and 8-dehydrocholesterols (DHC), and trienols. This profile approximates the profile of abnormal cholesterol biosynthesis present in Smith-Lemli-Optiz syndrome (SLOS)-affected children. This example demonstrates that the functionality of enzymes is as important as their ontogeny. In the case of BM15.766, 7DHC reductase was present in the brain tissue, but it was unable to fully participate in cholesterol synthesis.

Several enzymes are essential for normal development. A pattern of prolonged elevation of ODC is known to be associated with an overall delay in the course of cellular maturation.

3.2.4.3. Neurotransmitters

Neurotransmitters play essential roles in the cellular and architectural development of the brain *(31,32)*. They are signaling molecules that serve as first messengers and they act on receptors directly associated with ion channels. Approximately one half of the neurons in the brain are inhibitory and release inhibitory transmitters (e.g., glycine) that hyperpolarize the membrane potential of the postsynaptic cell and thus decrease the likelihood of firing.

Neurotransmitters commonly measured in tissues for developmental study are acetylcholine, dopamine, norepinephrine, glutamic acid, γ-aminobutyric acid (GABA), and

Table 8
Transmitter Systems

Aminergic	Amino acid
Dopamine (DA)	Excitatory
Epinephrine (Epi, E)	Aspartate
Norepinephrine (NE)	Glutamate
	Inhibitory
Cholinergic	γ-aminobutyric acid (GABA)
Choline acetyltransferase[a]	Glycine
Peptidergic	Serotonergic
Carnosine	Serotonin (5HT)
Endorphins	
Enkephalins	Others
Hypothalamic controlling factors	N-acetyl-L-aspartate
Neurotensin	Proline
Pituitary hormones	Serine
Substance P	Taurine
	Tryptamine

[a]Muscarinic and nicotinic receptors.

serotonin. These transmitters are only a few of the transmitters that have been identi-fied. Table 8 lists several of the neurotransmitters that may be evaluated.

During development, receptor stimulation and associated signal cascades control genes that influence cell differentiation, changing the ultimate fate of the cell. The ontogenetic state of the target cell is critical in determining whether the outcome of receptor stimulation affects cell replication, differentiation, growth, apoptosis, or "learning," that is, determining the future set-point for responsiveness of the cell.

According to the tenets of classical teratology, exposure to a teratogen during the first trimester of fetal development is the most critical stage for inducing malforma-tions. The CNS is different from most organ systems, because it is likely to be affected by exposures ranging from the early embryonic stage through adolescence.

It is interesting that morphogenic roles during neuronal growth have also been sug-gested for several neurotransmitters (e.g., AChE involvement in axonal outgrowth) *(31,32)*. Cholinergic stimulation is essential for establishment of cerebrocortical cyto-architecture, and even transient interference with cholinergic input during develop-ment produces permanent structural and behavioral damage *(32)*. For example, administration of cholinergic agonists is known to evoke neurodevelopmental damage because of the inappropriate timing or because of the intensity of stimulation they elicit.

Neurological disorders induced by pre- or postnatal toxicants may be related to spe-cific defects of synaptic functions. For example, neurotransmitter synthesis or degra-dation can be inhibited or enhanced; receptors may be up- or downregulated.

The steady-state turnover of neurotransmitters in vivo can be determined by simul-taneous measurement of endogenous transmitter and its precursor by means of a label (e.g., radioisotope) that can be followed. The activity or actual concentrations of par-

Table 9
Second Messenger Systems

G-Protein coupled receptors (transmembrane, coupled to specific enzymes)
    Adenylate cyclase
    Phospholipases
MAP kinases
    c-jun N-terminal kinases (JNK)
    Extracellular signal regulated kinase (ERK)
Nitric oxide (NO)
Protein kinase C (PKC) family
    Isoforms α, β, γ: activated by Ca^{2+}, diacylglycerol (DAG), and phosphatidylserine
    Isoforms δ, ε, η, μ: activated by DAG and phosphatidylserine
    Isoforms ζ, λ: activated by Ca^{2+} and phosphatidylserine
Protein kinase A (PKA)
    Cyclic AMP
Tyrosine kinase receptors (transmembrane, tyrosine-specific)
    Phospholipase C-γ
    RAS GAP

ticular neurochemical substances alone, however, cannot answer questions regarding the functional significance of those changes *(24)*. Functionality can only be assessed by observation and testing of the whole animal.

3.2.5.2. MISCELLANEOUS FACTORS

Many trophic factors, hormones, and second messengers are directly and indirectly involved in CNS development *(24,33)*. Nerve growth factor (NGF) is one growth factor that is essential to normal development of the CNS. Many roles have been identified for NGF during CNS development. NGF is important in regulating axonal sprouting. It is implicated in preventing neuronal damage and protecting cells from apoptosis, and it is probably involved in neuronal plasticity.

Second messenger systems are no less important and play many roles in development. Table 9 gives a brief list of some of the known second-messenger systems.

4. SUMMARY

The development and maturation of the CNS are extremely complex processes. It is this very complexity that makes the CNS vulnerable to disruption by any prenatal exposure to an exogenous compound. Vulnerability also extends to the introduction of an endogenous compound at an unusual tissue location, at a higher than normal concentration, or at an unusual time.

Investigation of an insult during CNS development calls for the use of multiple approaches. The danger in any multipronged investigation, however, is that it is next to impossible for any one investigator to have in all facets of the planned work. Above all, it must be remembered that the interpretation and extrapolation of experimental results are only as good as the study design, execution, and analysis.

REFERENCES

1. Edwards, J. A. (1968) The external development of the rabbit and rat embryo, in *Advances in Teratology* (Woolam, D. H., ed.), Academic Press, New York, NY.
2. Hebel, R. and Stromberg, M. W. (1986) *Anatomy and Embryology of the Rat*. BioMed Vertag, Worthsee, Germany.
3. Nelson, O. E. (1953) *Comparative Embryology of the Vertebrates*. McGraw-Hill, New York, NY.
4. Snell, G. D. and Stevens, L. C. (1966) The early embryology of the mouse, in *Biology of the Laboratory Mouse* (Green, E. L., ed.), Blakiston, PA.
5. Rugh, R. (1968) *The Mouse: Its Reproduction and Development*. Burgess, Minneapolis, MN.
6. Boyer, C. C. (1953) Chronology of development of the golden hamster. *J. Morphol.* **92**, 1.
7. Waterman, A. J. (1943) Studies on the normal development of the New Zealand White strain of rabbit. *Am. J. Anat.* **72**, 473.
8. Scott, J. P. (1937) The embryology of the guinea pig. 1. Table of normal development. *Am. J. Anat.* **60**, 397–432.
9. Heuser, C. H. and Streeter, G. L. (1941) Development of the macaque embryo. *Contrib. Embryol.* **29**, 15.
10. Hendrickx, A. G. and Sawyer, R. H. (1975) Embryology of the rhesus monkey, in *The Rhesus Monkey*, vol. 2 (Bourne, G. H., ed.), Academic Press, New York, NY.
11. Hamilton, W. J. and Mossman, H. W. (1974) *Hamilton, Boyd and Mossman's Human Embryology*. Williams & Wilkins, Baltimore, MD.
12. O'Rahilly, R. and Muller, F. (1987) *Developmental Stages in Human Embryos*. Publication No. 637. Carnegie Institute, Washington, DC.
13. Larsen, W. J. (1997) *Human Embryology*, 2nd ed. Churchill Livingstone, Inc., New York, NY.
14. Hamburger, V. and Hamilton, H. L. (1951) A series of normal stages in the development of the chick embryo. *J. Morphol.* **88**, 49.
15. Patten, B. M. (1951) *Early Embryology of the Chick*, 4th ed. McGraw-Hill, New York, NY.
16. Arey, L. B. (1965) *Developmental Anatomy*, 5th ed. W. B. Saunders, Philadelphia, PA.
17. DeSesso, J. M. (1996) Comparative embryology, in *Handbook of Developmental Toxicology* (Hood, R. D., ed.), CRC Press, Boca Raton, FL, pp. 111–174.
18. Fish, I. and Noble, A. (1969) Cellular growth in various regions of the developing rat brain. *Pediatr. Res.* **3**, 407–412.
19. Winick, M. and Noble, A. (1965) Quantitative changes in DNA, RNA, and protein during prenatal and postnatal growth in the rat. *Dev. Biol.* **12**, 451–466.
20. Hoar, R. M. and Monie, I. W. (1981) Comparative development of specific organ systems, in *Developmental Toxicology. Target Organ Toxicology Series* (Kimmel, C. A. and Buelke-Sam, J., eds.), Raven Press, New York, NY, pp. 13–33.
21. Rodier, P. M. (1980) Chronology of neuron development: animal studies and their clinical implications. *Dev. Med. Child Neurol.* **22**, 525–545.
22. Rodier, P. M. (1994) Comparative postnatal neurologic development, in *Prenatal Exposure to Toxicants. Developmental Consequences* (Needleman, H. L. and Bellinger, D., eds.), The Johns Hopkins University Press, Baltimore, MD, pp. 3–23.
23. Harris, M. J. and Juriloff, D. M. (1997) Genetic landmarks for defects in mouse neural tube closure. *Teratology* **56**, 177–187.
24. Kandel, E. R., Schwartz, J. H., and Jessell, T. M. (1991) *Principles of Neural Science*, 3rd ed. Elsevier, New York, NY.
25. Sokoloff, L. (1984) Modeling metabone processes in the brain in vivo. *Ann. Neurol.* **15**, S1–S11.
26. Gartner, L. P. and Hiatt, J. L. (1997) *Color Textbook of Histology*. W. B. Saunders Company, Philadelphia, PA.
27. Kerr, J. B. (1999) *Atlas of Functional Histology*. Mosby, St. Louis, MO.

28. Garcia, J. H. (ed.) (1997) *Neuropathology. The Diagnostic Approach.* Mosby, St. Louis, MO.
29. Slotkin, T. A. (1979) ODC as a tool in developmental neurobiology. *Life Sci.* **24,** 1623–1629.
30. Kolf-Clauw, M., Chevy, F., Sillart, B., Wolf, C., Mulliez, N., and Roux, C. (1997) Choles- terol biosynthesis inhibited by BM15.766 induces holoprosencephaly in the rat. *Teratol- ogy* **56,** 188–200.
31. Bigbee, J. W., Sharma, K. V., Gupta, J. J., and Dupree, J. L. (1999) Morphogenic role for acetylcholinesterase in axonal outgrowth during neural development. *Environ. Health Persp.* **107(Suppl. 1),** 81–87.
32. Slotkin, T. A. (1999) Developmental cholinotoxicants: nicotine and chlorpyrifos. *Environ. Health Persp.* **107(Suppl. 1),** 71–80.
33. Slikker, Jr., W. and Chang, L. W. (eds.) (1998) *Handbook of Developmental Neurotoxicology.* Academic Press, San Diego, CA.
34. Beck, F. (1981) Comparative placental morphology and function, in *Developmental Toxi- cology. Target Organ Toxicology Series* (Kimmel, C. A. and Buelke-Sam, M. A., eds.), Raven Press, New York, NY, pp. 35–54.
35. Holson, R. R., Adams, J., and Ferguson, S. A. (1999) Gestational stage-specific effects of retinoic acid exposure in the rat. *Neurotox. Teratol.* **21,** 393–402.
36. Hass, U., Lund, S. P., Hougaard, K. S., and Simonsen, L. (1999) Developmental neurotox- icity after toluene inhalation exposure in rats. *Neurotox. Teratol.* **21,** 349–357.
37. Morris, R. (1981) Spatial localization does not require the presence of local cues. *Learn. Motivat.* **12,** 229–260.
38. Hovland Jr., D. N., Machado, A. F., Scott, Jr., W. J., and Collins, M. D. (1999) Differential sensitivity of the SWV and C57BL/6 mouse strains to the teratogenic action of single ad- ministrations of cadmium given throughout the period of anterior neuropore closure. *Tera- tology* **60,** 13–21.
39. Rickard, L. B., et al. (1995) Developmental toxicity of inhaled N-methyformamide in the rat. *Fund. Appl. Tox.* **28,** 167–176.
40. Holson, R. R., Gazzara, R. A., Ferguson, S. A., and Adams, J. (1997) A behavioral and neuroanatomical investigation of the lethality caused by gestational day 11–13 retinoic acid exposure. *Neurotox. Teratol.* **19,** 347–353.
41. Nagao, T., Kuwagata, M., and Saito, Y. (1998) Effects of prenatal exposure to 5-bromo-2'- deoxyuridine on the developing brain and reproductive function in male mouse offspring. *Reprod. Toxicol.* **12,** 477–487.
42. Vancutsem, P. M. and Roessler, M. L. (1997) Neonatal treatment with tamoxifen causes immediate alterations of the sexually dimorphic nucleus of the preoptic area and medial preoptic area in male rats. *Teratology* **56,** 220–228.

3

Developmental Neurotoxicity

What Have We Learned from Guideline Studies?

Gregg D. Cappon and Donald G. Stump

1. INTRODUCTION

The goal of this chapter is to summarize the available developmental neurotoxicology data and to ascertain the value of developmental neurotoxicity as currently
evaluated by the USEPA in the identification of human risk. A whole host of scientific
methodologies have been used to evaluate nervous-system damage and it is beyond the
scope of this chapter to provide a comprehensive overview of the entire body of research in the field of developmental neurotoxicology. Instead, the findings presented
here will focus on developmental neurotoxicology studies executed in general accordance with the most recent US Environmental Protection Agency (EPA) Office of Prevention, Pesticides and Toxic Substances (OPPTS) Guideline 870.6300 (August 1998)
(1). While our discussion revolves around studies executed in agreement with the
OPPTS testing paradigm, the compounds reviewed are not limited to those under EPA
regulatory jurisdiction. The considerable scientific literature available regarding investigation of the potential developmental neurotoxicity of pharmaceuticals and drugs of
abuse *(2)* will also be discussed. However, by focusing on studies performed in general
agreement with regulatory guidelines, we intend to assess the confidence in our ability
to identify potential hazards to the developing nervous system.

2. DESIGN PARADIGMS FOR THE STUDY OF DEVELOPMENTAL NEUROTOXICITY

Myriad behavioral, biochemical, and molecular techniques have been utilized to
ascertain the potential for insult to the developing nervous system *(3–5)*. In combination with a wide variety of exposure regimens, the abundance of information is overwhelming. The current OPPTS guideline requires administration of the test article to
maternal animals from implantation of the embryo through day 10 (LD 10) of lactation,
assuming direct exposure to the offspring *in utero* and indirect exposure by nursing
during lactation. Postnatal behavioral evaluation of the offspring incorporate assessments of physical, sexual, and behavioral development; spontaneous motor activity;
acoustic startle response (ASR); and learning and memory. Recognizing the differen-

From: Handbook of Neurotoxicology, Vol. 2
Edited by: E. J. Massaro © Humana Press Inc., Totowa, NJ

tial sensitivities for tests of cognition, the developmental neurotoxicity guideline allows flexibility for assessment of learning and memory to permit investigation with appropriate methods, taking into consideration reports of sensitive methods for structurally related compounds and the specific expertise of the testing facility. An additional component of the OPPTS-guideline study that has traditionally not been incorporated in behavioral teratogenicity studies is a requirement for neuropathological examination of the offspring.

Given the broad scope of research techniques available for the investigation of developmental neurotoxicity, to focus our discussion it was necessary to establish minimum criteria for the studies incorporated into this review. Prerequisites for inclusion in this discussion are: (1) an exposure regimen covering most of gestation from implantation to parturition, (2) assessment of postnatal growth, (3) evaluation of motor and reflexive behaviors, and (4) an evaluation of cognitive function.

3. EVALUATION OF DEVELOPMENTAL-NEUROTOXICITY STUDIES SUBMITTED FOR OPPTS REVIEW

Given the extensive interest regarding the risk of developmental neurotoxicity from environmental exposure to agricultural and industrial chemicals, we will begin our review by focusing on developmental neurotoxicity studies submitted to the USEPA OPPTS. Because of the proprietary nature of the information, access to most of the study reports is limited, and only several of the submitted studies have been published in the scientific literature. As a result, the primary source for the information summarized in this chapter is a draft manuscript entitled, "A retrospective analysis of twelve developmental neurotoxicity studies submitted to the USEPA Office of Prevention, Pesticides and Toxic Substances" *(6)*. Of the studies reviewed, only those for isopropanol *(7)*, DEET *(8)*, emamectin *(9)*, and chlorpyrifos *(10)* were available for independent review.

3.1. Design of Studies Submitted for OPPTS Review

As would be expected, the studies submitted for OPPTS review are in very close accordance with the specifications outlined in OPPTS guideline 870.6300. The treatment periods generally encompassed from the time of embryonic implantation (gestation day [GD] 6) through at least d 10 of lactation. All studies included assessments of physical and sexual development, motor activity, auditory startle habituation, learning and memory, brain weights and neuropathology of the offspring. An exception to the standard study design is the developmental neurotoxicity evaluation of DEET that was performed as a segment of a multigeneration study. For that study, F_2 offspring of treated F_1 dams were maintained on fortified diet for 9 mo postweaning and then evaluated for functional endpoints *(8)*.

3.2. Evidence of Developmental Neurotoxicity

A summary of the results of the offspring evaluations conducted in the OPPTS review is presented in Table 1. Observations that were strongly indicative of developmental neurotoxicity were noted in 7 of the 12 studies (aldicarb, carbaryl, carbofuran, molinate, emamectin, fipronil, and chlorpyrifos). Aldicarb exposure resulted in decreased pup weight and reduced grip strength. Motor activity in male offspring was

Table 1
Summary of Studies Reviewed by the US EPA

Chemical	Dose levels[b]	Maternally toxic dose	Behavioral indications of neurotoxicity	Neuropathological indications of neurotoxicity
Aldicarb	0.5 0.1 0.3	0.1 0.3	MA MA, ASR	[a] [a] [a]
Carbaryl	0.1 1.0 10	10		Morphometrics
Carbofuran	1.7 6.9 31	6.9 31	Water Y maze Water Y maze	Brain weight Brain weight
Chemical X	40 125 400	125 400	MA	
Chlorpyrifos	0.3 1 5		ASR	Morphometrics, brain weight
Molinate	1.8 6.9 26.1	26.1	ASR ASR MA, ASR, Water Y maze	Morphometrics Morphometrics, brain weight
DEET	22.5 90 225	225	MA	[a] [a] [a]
Emamectin	0.1 0.6 3.6/2.5		MA MA, ASR	Brain weight
Fipronil	0.05 0.9 18.5	18.5	MA, ASR, Water Y maze	Brain weight
Isopropanol	200 700 1200	1200		
TCE	75 250 750			
TGME	300 1650 3000	3000	ASR	

MA, motor activity, ASR, auditory startle response.
[a]Morphometric evaluation not performed.
[b]Dose levels expressed as mg/kg/d or ppm.

decreased when evaluated on postnatal day (PND) 17 and increased when evaluated as adults *(6)*. Maternal carbaryl administration had no effects on offspring development or behavior but demonstrated altered morphometric measurements on both PND 11 and 60 *(6)*. Carbofuran exposure reduced pup survival and weight, delayed physical and sexual maturation, and decreased PND 11 brain weight. Learning was also impaired in a water Y-maze test *(6)*. Molinate exposure resulted in effects on offspring survival and growth, motor activity, startle responsiveness, learning and memory, and brain morphometric measurements *(6)*. Maternal emamectin exposure induced decreases in pup body weights, induced tremors, delayed demonstration of developmental land-marks, altered motor activity and startle responsiveness, and decreased brain weights of adult offspring *(6,9)*. Fipronil administered to pregnant rats reduced pup survival and body weights, altered motor activity and startle responsiveness, impaired learning ability, and reduced brain weights on both PND 11 and 60 *(6)*. Administration of chlorpyrifos to maternal animals impaired offspring growth and survival, modified acoustic startle responsiveness, and altered brain weight and morphometric measure-ments at PND 12 and 62 *(6,10)*.

In three additional studies there was limited evidence of a specific treatment-related neurotoxic effect. These findings consisted of slight changes in motor activity in the studies of DEET *(6,8)*, and Chemical X *(6)*, and altered acoustic startle response in the TGME study *(6)*.

Only two compounds, the solvents 1,1,1-TCE and isopropanol, demonstrated no findings in the offspring *(6)*, even though isopropanol elicited maternal toxicity *(7)*. The findings of the submitted TCE study confirmed an earlier study that also reported that TCE exposure did not induce either maternal toxicity or developmental neurotox-icity *(11)*.

4. STUDIES REPORTED IN SCIENTIFIC LITERATURE

Chemicals were selected for inclusion provided that a single study was performed that was in general compliance with the OPPTS developmental neurotoxicity guideline (Table 2). However, once a chemical was selected for inclusion, findings from devel-opmental neurotoxicity studies that did not fit the criteria for inclusion as guideline studies were used to qualify the findings of the guideline-type study. Therefore, data from several studies of one compound may have been utilized to generate the compre-hensive database for that chemical. Consequently, the studies presented for a particular chemical may have been derived from one or more studies using different rat strains, dosage levels, routes of exposures, and/or different exposure duration and periods.

4.1. Recreational Drugs and Related Compounds

4.1.1. Alcohol (Ethanol)

Evidence from several lines of investigation suggests that the effects in human off-spring following maternal alcohol exposure are expressed as an entire spectrum of disorders ranging from the profound fetal alcohol syndrome (FAS) to less pronounced and more subtle abnormalities of attention and cognitive disorders *(12)*. A comparison of the human and animal literature demonstrated a good deal of congruence with respect to neurobehavioral effects *(13)*. General functional categories, such as deficits in learn-

Table 2
Compounds That Have an OPPTS Guideline Style Developmental Neurotoxicity Study Published in the Scientific Literature

Category

Compound	Exposure period	Reference(s)	Developmental neurotoxicant[a]
Recreational drugs			
Alcohol	Preconception–weaning	(15)	Yes
Methamphetamine	GD 7–20	(24)	Yes
Cocaine	GD 4–20	(30)	Yes
Marijuana	GD 1,2, or 5–weaning	(40-42)	No
Nicotine	GD 4–20	(30)	No
Therapeutic drugs			
Phenytoin	GD 7–18	(53,57)	Yes
Fluoxetine	GD 7–20	(60)	No
Fenfluramine	GD 7–20	(61)	Yes
Chlorpromazine	GD 6–15 or 20	(63,64)	No
Prochlorperazine	GD 7–20	(61)	No
Diazepam	GD 4–19 or GD 7–20	(61,67)	Yes
chlordiazepoxide	GD x–weaning	(73)	Yes
Retinyl palimitate	GD 6 or 7–20	(64,77)	Yes
Propylthiouracil	GD 6–LD 10	(78)	Yes
Methimazole	GD 17–LD 10	(72)	Yes
Naloxone	GD 7–20	(80)	Yes
LAAM	Preconception–birth	(82)	Yes
Propoxyphene	GD 7–20	(61)	Yes
Raloxifene	GD 6–PND 20	(83)	No
MN rgp120/HIV-1	GD 1–20	(84)	No
Metals			
Cadmium	Gestation	(86,87)	Yes
Lead	Preconception–weaning	(91,93)	Yes
Methylmercury	GD 6–15	(98)	No
Aluminum	Gestation	(103,104)	Yes
Tributyltin	GD 6–20	(105)	Yes
Trihexyltin	GD 6–20	(105)	Yes
Manganese	GD 0–PND 30	(108)	Yes
Industrial chemicals			
PCB	GD 6–15 Preconception–weaning	(112,113)	Yes
Methanol	GD 7–19	(122)	No
Styrene	GD 7–20	(123)	Yes
Toluene	GD 7–PND 18	(124)	Yes
Xylene	GD 7–PND 20	(125)	Yes
Ethylene Glycol	GD 7–13 or 14–20	(17,126)	Yes
Dichloromethane	GD x–x	(128)	Yes
Acrylamide	GD 6–LD 10	(6)	Yes

Table 2 *(continued)*

Category

Compound	Exposure period	Reference(s)	Developmental neurotoxicant[a]
Other chemicals			
Aspartame	Preconception–PND 90	*(129)*	Yes
Phenylalanine	Preconception–PND 90	*(129)*	Yes
Brominated vegetable oil	Preconception–weaning	*(130)*	Yes
Hydrogen sulfide	Preconception–GD 19	*(131)*	No
CI-943	GD 15–LD 21	*(132)*	Yes

[a]Based on findings of OPPTS-guideline style evaluations.

ing, inhibition, attention, regulatory behaviors, and motor performance were affected in both humans and laboratory animals *(12,13)*.

In general, rats exposed prenatally to alcohol show deficits in reflex development and tasks that require balance and motor coordination such as righting reflex and negative geotaxis *(14–17)*. Perhaps the most common finding following prenatal alcohol exposure is an increase in the level of activity. This has been demonstrated in open fields, running wheels, and in nose-poke and head-dip tests *(15,18,19)*. While not all studies demonstrate adult learning impairments following gestational alcohol exposure *(14)*, cognitive effects have been reported on numerous tests including operant learning paradigms, multiple avoidance learning tasks, simple discrimination, and Morris water maze *(15,18,20)*.

In a guideline-style study, female rats were exposed to ethanol for approx 1 wk prior to breeding through lactation until weaning *(15)*. Offspring were evaluated for ontogenies of reflexive behaviors, spontaneous motor activity, and cognitive performance in T-maze and shuttle-box paradigms. Exposed offspring demonstrated delayed eye opening and maturation of the air-righting reflex, and elevated spontaneous activity during the first postnatal month. Cognitive impairment was shown by increased escape latencies in both the T-maze and shuttle-box evaluations *(15)*. The findings of this study suggest that an OPPTS developmental-neurotoxicity study is sensitive to the developmental neurotoxicity induced by alcohol.

4.1.2. Amphetamines

Amphetamines are a class of dopaminergic neurostimulants with related pharmacology including amphetamine, methamphetamine, and 3,4-methylene dioxymethamphetamine (MDMA). Amphetamines have high potential for illicit abuse from their neurostimulant effects, and there is considerable concern about the long-term effects resulting from *in utero* exposure. In fact, clinical reports show that *in utero* methamphetamine-exposed offspring exhibit growth retardation, delays in development, impairment in learning, and alterations in brain neurotransmitter levels *(21,22)*.

The developmental neurotoxicity of methamphetamine was evaluated following maternal administration to rats throughout gestation and lactation *(23)*. Methamphetamine-exposed offspring showed a tendency for delayed demonstration of developmental landmarks and increased activity on running wheels. Offspring of maternal animals administered methamphetamine from GD 7–20 demonstrated delays in incisor eruption, eye opening, and testes descent *(24)*. Delayed ontogeny of negative geotaxis and air-righting reflexes and decreased spontaneous activity at weaning were also noted. Adult animals showed cognitive impairment in a conditioned-avoidance test. In a study designed to investigate the critical period for methamphetamine-induced developmental neurotoxicity *(25)*, pregnant rats were treated with methamphetamine from either GD 7–12 or 13–18. Offspring from the early-exposure group demonstrated delayed development of locomotion, and impaired learning in Morris water maze, spontaneous alteration, and passive-avoidance tests. Offspring from the GD 13–18 exposure group showed higher mortality rates, reduced body weights, and neurochemical alterations but did not demonstrate behavior alterations.

Amphetamine is a less potent central nervous system (CNS) stimulant than methamphetamine, but is still of considerable concern regarding illicit use. The results of studies of prenatal amphetamine exposure are not as clearly indicative of developmental neurotoxicity as those for methamphetamine. Findings suggestive of adverse effects include alterations in activity *(26)* and increased ASR *(27)*.

4.1.3. Cocaine

Research examining the effect of prenatal exposure of humans to cocaine has produced an inconsistent pattern of results. Findings from a meta-analysis of studies reported in the scientific literature *(28)* support a general consensus that the reproductive effects of cocaine are minimal. However, a meta-analysis of studies of human infants suggest some long-term functional consequences of *in utero* cocaine exposure *(29)*.

In rats, cocaine administered by continuous infusion from GD 4–20 resulted in reduced maternal weights and offspring birth weights. Cognitive deficits were seen in the Morris water maze and, following propranolol challenge, in the radial-arm maze *(30)*. Based on the findings of this study, cocaine meets the regulatory definition for a developmental neurotoxicant. It should be noted that cocaine-induced behavioral alterations observed in this study were relatively subtle and were only noted following stringent learning evaluations. However, there is substantial literature demonstrating effects of prenatal cocaine exposure on neurotransmitter levels *(31,32)*, receptor binding *(33,34)*, enzyme activity *(35,36)* and sexual behavior *(37)*. This overwhelming evidence clearly indicates that prenatal cocaine exposure induces alteration in offspring CNS function. Therefore, regardless of human findings, the data developed for *in utero* cocaine exposure illustrates how the hazard identification process is intended to function. That is, a potential hazard to the developing nervous system is identified in a screening study and additional highly targeted research provides clearer insight into the underlying biology.

4.1.4. Delta-9-Tetrahydrocannabinol (Marijuana)

Marijuana is the illicit drug most commonly used by pregnant women and delta-9-tetrahydrocannabinol (THC), the principal psychoactive agent in marijuana, readily crosses the placenta *(38)*. Prenatal marijuana exposure has been associated with child behavioral problems at age 10 consisting of increased hyperactivity, impulsivity, inattention, and delinquency *(39)*. Several researchers have evaluated the developmental neurotoxic potential of marijuana in OPPTS-style developmental neurotoxicity studies. The potential developmental neurotoxicity of THC or crude marijuana extract was evaluated following gestational exposure that either incorporated the majority of the gestational period (GD 1, 2, or 5–weaning) *(40–42)* or investigated for possible critical exposure periods (GD 1–7, GD 8–14, and GD 15–22) *(40)*. Exposure during the third week of gestation or throughout the entire gestational period consistently resulted in increased pup mortality and decreased birth weight. *In utero* exposure did not result in neurobehavioral alterations when evaluated for open-field behavior, inclined plane, rotarod performance, or impaired learning when evaluated in spontaneous alteration, two-way shock avoidance, and water-maze learning tasks.

Other studies have shown slight indications of developmental neurotoxicity following gestational marijuana exposure, but in each of these cases the relationship to treatment is uncertain. For example, offspring of maternal animals administered THC from GD 3–parturition were evaluated for behavioral effects using two techniques for measuring social behavior (open-field behavior and push-tube task) and passive-avoidance learning *(43)*. Drug treatment did not affect spontaneous social behavior in the open field, but did demonstrate increased competitiveness in the push-tube task. Passive-avoidance learning demonstrated a transient effect at 21 d of age, however, the limited sample size (n = 5/group) limits the relevance of this finding *(43)*. Exposure to marijuana (cannabis) smoke from GD 1–19 did not affect offspring viability; however, birth weight was reduced and incisor eruption and eye opening were delayed. The maturation of reflex behaviors (surface righting, air-righting cliff avoidance, and visual placing) was not impaired. Motor activity was decreased on PND 7, but recovered by PND 14 *(44)*. This study did not incorporate postnatal behavioral evaluation.

In summary, gestational marijuana exposure clearly induces considerable developmental toxicity, expressed by a reduction in pup survival and body weight. However there is no clear pattern of behavioral alterations following *in utero* marijuana exposure that would suggest insult to the developing CNS.

4.1.5. Nicotine

Levin and Slotkin *(45)* provide an extensive review of the developmental neurotoxicity of nicotine and definitively conclude that nicotine is a developmental neurotoxicant. However, studies designed in accordance with the current OPPTS guidelines do not unequivocally implicate nicotine as a developmental neurotoxicant. Nicotine administered by continuous infusion from GD 4–20 resulted in reduced birth weight but failed to induce learning deficits in the radial-arm maze or the Morris water maze *(30)*. Nicotine exposure from GD 1–LD 19 had no effect on motor activity of adult offspring initially evaluated on PND 90 and then monthly for 36 wk *(23,46)*. In contrast, studies designed to focus on particular aspects of development following gestational exposure have demonstrated altered CNS development and function following gestational exposure. Gestational exposure (GD 6 to term) to nicotine resulted in morphological changes in the hippocampus when examined on PND 40 *(47)*, alterations in 24-h activity patterns *(48)*, and cognitive effects following pharmacological challenge *(49)*.

In summary, the developmental neurotoxicity of nicotine may not be readily apparent in an OPPTS-guideline developmental neurotoxicity study. For example, prenatal nicotine exposure causes alterations in cognitive performance that may not be apparent until the system is challenged either by complicating the behavioral paradigm or by introducing pharmacologic agents that uncover the defects. Therefore, the developmental neurotoxicity of nicotine may only be detectable following thorough cognitive, neurochemical, or neuroanatomical evaluations *(45)*.

4.2. Therapeutic Drugs

4.2.1. Anticonvulsants

The fetal hydantoin syndrome (FHS) in humans consists of craniofacial defects and any two of the following: pre/postnatal growth deficiency, limb defects, major malformations, and mental deficiency *(50,51)*. Animal models of FHS have been developed, and those focusing on developmental neurotoxicity have primary evaluated the effects of phenytoin. Phenytoin produces multiple behavioral dysfunction in rat offspring at subteratogenic and nongrowth-retarding doses *(50,52–56)*. Maternal administration of phenytoin on GD 7–18 resulted in effects on acoustic and tactile startle response (hyperactivity) *(57)*, motor activity *(53,57)*, developmental landmarks (delayed air righting reflex development) *(53,57)*, and impaired learning ability in the Biel maze *(53)*, Y-maze *(53)*, Morris maze *(56,57)* and Cincinnati maze *(55,57)*. Brain neurochemical evaluation of adult offspring demonstrated significant elevations of GABA and smaller increases in other brain amino acids *(54)*. The findings from these studies suggest that intrauterine phenytoin exposure may cause significant effects in offspring even in the absence of malformations or minor dysmorphic features of the fetal hydantoin syndrome. Therefore, not only would phenytoin-induced developmental neurotoxicity be detected in an OPPTS-guideline developmental neurotoxicity study, phenytoin is often considered to be a prototypical developmental neurotoxicant and has been widely used to evaluate developmental neurotoxicity screening batteries.

4.2.2. Antidepressant and Antipsychotic Agents

An estimated 8–20% of all women suffer from depression and many benefit from antidepressant therapy *(58)*. Because half the pregnancies in North America are unplanned, many women take antidepressants drugs during the first few weeks of pregnancy. In addition, there is evidence of impaired cognitive, language, and behavioral skills for children of depressed mothers *(59)*. Therefore, the need to protect the fetus from potential adverse drug effects must be balanced with the benefits of controlling maternal depression. This has spawned a considerable amount research on the potential developmental neurotoxicity of antidepressant agents.

4.2.2.1. SEROTONERGIC AGENTS

Selective serotonin reuptake inhibitors (SSRI) are a class of indirect-acting serotonin agonists therapeutically utilized as antidepressants. Fluoxetine, the first clinically utilized SSRI, was administered to pregnant rats from GD 7–20 and the offspring were evaluated for locomotor activity at three ages (preweaning, juvenile, and adult), ASR, spontaneous alteration, passive avoidance, and complex learning in the Cincinnati maze *(60)*. At the highest dose, fluoxetine caused maternal weight loss during pregnancy, reduced litter size, and increased pup mortality, although offspring growth was not affected. Prenatal fluoxetine exposure produced no treatment-related effects on locomotor activity, acoustic startle, or learning, indicating that fluoxetine does not produce developmental neurotoxicity at doses that are both maternally and developmentally toxic *(60)*.

Fenfluramine is another serotonergic acting compound used as an antidepressant and antiemetic agent. Administration of fenfluramine to pregnant rats from GD 7–20 increased offspring mortality but had little effect on preweaning physical and neuromuscular development *(61)*. Postweaning evaluation of open-field behavior demonstrated increased ambulation and rearing. However, prenatal fenfluramine exposure did not adversely affect cognitive function of the adult offspring.

Although fluoxetine failed to induce developmental neurotoxicity whereas fenfluramine demonstrated slight effects on offspring behavior, the serotonergic-acting agents demonstrate a similar toxic profile following prenatal exposure, i.e., slight effects on neurobehavioral development even at doses resulting in maternal toxicity and impaired offspring viability and growth *(60,61)*. A study designed according to the OPPTS developmental neurotoxicity guideline would be sensitive to the effects induced by *in utero* fenfluramine exposure and would likely result in labeling fenfluramine as a potential developmental neurotoxicant. However, an evaluation of neurobehavioral development of preschool children showed that *in utero* exposure to fluoxetine did not affect global IQ or language and behavioral development *(62)*. The lack of impaired neurodevelopment in humans following *in utero* exposure to a SSRI suggests that the slight effects on neurobehavioral development exhibited in rats may be confounded by the severe general maternal and developmental toxicity observed. Therefore, the characterization of fenfluramine as a potential developmental neurotoxicant based on the results of a developmental neurotoxicity-screening battery may not be appropriate and to fully characterize the developmental neurotoxicologic potential of serotonergic agents will require more exhaustive research.

4.2.2.2. ANTICHOLINERGICS

Chlorpromazine is an anticholinergic compound utilized as an antipsychotic agent. Chlorpromazine administered to pregnant rats from GD 6–15 *(63)* or GD 6–20 *(64)* did not affect preweaning growth or physical and reflexive development of the offspring *(63)*. Postweaning evaluation of offspring exposed from GD 6–15 demonstrated increased open-field activity *(63)* while those exposed from GD 6–20 were not affected *(64)*. Morphometric evaluation of brains collected from adult offspring showed no evidence of neuropathologic alteration *(63)*.

Evaluation of another anticholinergic-acting compound utilized for its antipsychotic properties, prochlorperazine, following maternal exposure from GD 7–20 resulted in increased offspring mortality and impaired growth *(61)*. However, prenatal prochlorperazine did not have an adverse effect on pre- or postweaning neuromuscular development or neurobehavioral function. These findings suggest that the anticholinergic antipsychotics are not developmentally neurotoxic, although there was no lactational exposure. The characterization anticholinergics as not being developmental neurotoxicants is in concordance with a finding that *in utero* exposure to tricyclic (anticholinergic) antidepressants did not affect behavioral development in preschool children *(62)*.

4.2.2.3. BENZODIAZEPINES

Benzodiazepines are versatile compounds used to relieve anxiety (anxiolytic), provide sedation and light anesthesia, for the management of agitation associated with acute alcohol withdrawal, manage skeletal muscle spasticity, and as anticonvulsants; intravenous diazepam is generally considered the drug of choice for termination of status epilepticus. Benzodiazepines readily cross the placenta, however, studies in animals *(65)* and humans *(66)* indicate that prenatal benzodiazapines produce classical teratogenic effects only at doses several orders of magnitude greater than those required for clinical effectiveness. The potential developmental neurotoxicity of diazepam has been investigated following administration to pregnant rats throughout most of gestation (GD 4–19 *[67]* and GD 7–20 *[61]*). Offspring were evaluated for early motor development and coordination, general activity, and learning. Diazepam had only slight effects on pup viability in one study *(61)* and no effect on survival, birth weight, or body-weight gain *(61,67)*. Diazepam had no effect on balance, coordination, or motor activity. However, animals showed a marked impairment in learning acquisition and retention in a discrimination task *(67)* and a slight alteration in a passive-avoidance task *(61)*. Diazepam administered to gravid dams during the last third of gestation (GD 13/14–20) *(68–71)* induced slight reductions in pup body weight gains throughout the preweaning period, potentiation of motor activity in a novel environment, increased ASR and slight cognitive effects *(68,69)*. Administration of diazepam from GD 15 through lactation day (LD) 10 resulted in a deficit in ASR *(72)*, while exposure from LD 1–7 resulted in reduced learning in an active-avoidance task but had no effect in a passive-avoidance task *(70)*.

Administration of the benzodiazepine chlordiazepoxide throughout gestation and lactation resulted in delayed cliff-avoidance development, impaired swimming development, alterations in active-avoidance responses *(73)*, and deficits in a schedule-controlled, food-reinforced responding behavior *(74)*.

These studies implicate benzodiazepines as developmental neurotoxicants that affect an extensive array of neurodevelopmental indices and functional measures. The expansive range of effective gestational exposure paradigms suggest that the susceptible window for diazepam-induced developmental neurotoxicity is quite broad, potentially effecting multiple stages of CNS development. The developmentally neurotoxic effects of diazepam would be readily detected in a guideline developmental neurotoxicity study.

4.2.3. Retinoids

Retinoids, of which vitamin A is the most familiar, have been recognized as teratogenic since the 1950s, but retinoid-induced developmental neurotoxicity was not experimentally demonstrated until the 1970s. Evidence generated from a neuropsychological examination of children exposed prenatally to isotreinoin (Accutane) demonstrated cognitive deficiencies suggestive of developmental neurotoxicity *(75)*. A substantial series of animal studies have conclusively shown that animals exposed to retinoids during organogenesis exhibit a variety of dysfunctions in the absence of malformations *(20,53,64,76,77)*. While a critical period for retinoid-induced developmental neurotoxicity in rats has not been established, several studies have shown that 1–3 d of treatment during midgestation is sufficient to produce developmental delay and cognitive impairment *(20,76)*. In studies that incorporated most measurements required by the current OPPTS developmental neurotoxicity guideline, maternal exposure to retinyl palmitate from GD 7–20 *(77)* or 6–20 *(64)* induced alterations in the ontogeny of developmental reflexes, motor coordination and activity, ASR, and learning ability. These findings indicate that a guideline-like developmental neurotoxicity study would readily detect retinoid-induced developmental neurotoxicity.

4.2.4. Thyroid-Hormone Modulators

In humans, hypothyroidism causes irreversible mental retardation and various neuromotor disabilities. Propylthiouracil administration to pregnant rats is a commonly used experimental model of human congenital hypothyroidism. In a study performed to evaluate the sensitivity of the OPPTS-guideline developmental neurotoxicity screening battery, propylthiouracil was administered from GD 6–LD 10 *(78)*. Offspring were evaluated by use of an observational battery and evaluated for motor activity, ASR, and learning and memory in the Biel water maze. Pup viability and body weights were reduced. Evaluation of offspring with a functional observational battery demonstrated delays in pupillary response, startle reactivity, mobility, and neuromuscular development. ASR was reduced on PND 22. Impaired learning ability of the adult offspring was demonstrated by an increased latency to escape the Biel water maze. Morphometric evaluation of PND 11 pup brains demonstrated statistically significant alterations of the piriform cortex, frontoparietal cortex, and the dentate hilus.

Methimazole is another compound commonly used to induce hypothyroidism in rats. Administration of methimazole by gavage from GD 17 through PND 10 *(79)* resulted in maternal toxicity *(72)*, reduced neonatal body weights *(79)*, and developmental delays *(72,79)*. Behavioral effects included reduced rotorod performance and ASR (neonates), and enhanced motor activity and ASR in young adults *(72)*. Learning and memory, assessed using a shuttle-avoidance paradigm, was not affected *(72)*. Brain weights of pups necropsied on PND 11 were unaffected by treatment and no neuropathological findings were noted *(79)*.

These studies demonstrate that the OPPTS developmental neurotoxicity guideline is sensitive to the developmental neurotoxicity induced by gestational hypothyroidism. However, the differential effects observed between two compounds acting via the same hormonal mechanism when the only appreciable difference in study design is the early prenatal exposure to propylthiouracil, underscores the importance of early gestational exposure in developmental neurotoxicity studies.

4.2.5. Opiate Agonists and Antagonists

Naloxone is an opiate antagonist used for the treatment of opiate-induced depression and acute opiate overdose. Administration of naloxone to pregnant rats on GD 7–20 caused accelerated preweaning development including increased body weight gain, accelerated upper-incisor eruption; facilitated righting, olfactory and startle responses; and impaired learning in the Biel water maze *(80)*. The finding of accelerated preweaning development (righting reflex, negative geotaxis) was also demonstrated following naloxone administration from GD 4–19 *(81)*. Interestingly, in this study neuroanatomical changes in the hippocampal dentate gyrus were demonstrated in brains of pups sacrificed on PND 21 without demonstrable adverse effects on development or learning *(81)*.

The findings of the two developmental-neurotoxicity studies independently support classification of naloxone as a developmental neurotoxicant. However, a weakness of the OPPTS-guideline study is underscored by these data sets; the selective sensitivity of certain learning and memory tests for a particular neurotoxicant insult. Evaluation in a traditional dry maze *(81)* was not able to detect impaired learning ability, while evaluation in a water maze *(80)* was able to uncover a functional deficit. The lack of defined methodologies for the evaluation of learning and memory casts doubt on the reliability of screening for developmental neurotoxicants. However, it should be noted that the demonstration of neuroanatomical alterations following prenatal naloxone exposure *(81)* supports the need for assessing neuropathology as a component of a screening battery.

Levo-Alpha-Acetylmethadol (LAAM) is a clinically effective alternative to methadone for the treatment of heroine addiction. Females rats were administered LAAM via drinking water beginning 1 mo prior to mating and throughout gestation *(82)*. Offspring were fostered to untreated surrogate mothers within 16 h of birth. No effects were noted in preweaning growth and neuromuscular development evaluated by various measures including cliff avoidance, visual placing, negative geotaxis, and grip strength, or in postweaning exploratory activity and learning of a lever-touch response. Indications of impaired cognitive functions were only noted following challenge with a psychotropic drug or when a schedule of reinforcement with strict demands on response output was in effect *(82)*. These data suggest that prenatal LAAM exposure may induce subtle functional alterations that are only demonstrable by rigorous evaluation and likely would not be detected in a guideline type study.

Propoxyphene is a synthetic analgesic that is structurally related to the opiate analgesic methadone. The primary use of propoxyphene is as a mild pain reliever, but it has been used as a supplemental agent for treatment of opiate dependency. Propoxyphene administered to pregnant female rats from GD 7–20 induced a significant delay in the ontogeny of swimming behavior and startle latency *(61)*. Increased activity was demonstrated at both the preweaning (PND 15–17) and postweaning (PND 41–43) open-field evaluations. No impairment in cognitive ability was noted *(61)*. Propoxyphene administered from GD 6–20 corroborated the increase in preweaning activity, but failed to reproduce the developmental delay or increased postweaning activity *(64)*.

4.2.6. Estrogen-Receptor Modulator

Raloxifene is a nonsteroidal selective estrogen receptor modulator (SERM) developed for use as a therapeutic agent for postmenopausal osteoporosis. In a study designed to evaluate both the potential developmental neurotoxicity and evaluations of developmental and reproductive processes that are particularly sensitive to estrogen-modulating compounds (parturition and offspring development), raloxifene was administered to pregnant rats from GD 6 through postpartum d 20 *(83)*. Delayed, extended, and/or disrupted parturition resulted in maternal and fetal mortality. Offspring birth weights were normal but growth was suppressed through lactation. Exposed offspring demonstrated increased negative geotaxis and incisor eruption, but delayed eye opening. Postweaning activity levels, auditory startle, and passive-avoidance performance were not affected. So, even though raloxifene induced considerable developmental toxicity, there was little indication of adverse neurodevelopment.

4.2.7. Recombinant Subunit Vaccine

MN rgp120/HIV-1 is a recombinant subunit vaccine consisting of gp120 prepared from the MN strain of HIV-1 that is currently being developed as a potential AIDS vaccine in pregnant HIV-1 positive females and in children born of HIV positive mothers. The potential for MN rgp120/HIV-1, alone or formulated as a vaccine, to induce developmental neurotoxicity in rats was investigated. Pregnant rats were administered MN rgp120/HIV-1 once every 3 d from GD 1 through parturition. Offspring from the treated and control groups were then administered either the vehicle, MN rgp120/HIV-1 alone, or MN rgp120/HIV-1 formulated as a vaccine from postpartum day 1 through 22 *(84)*. Offspring were evaluated for·neurobehavioral and physical development (preweaning reflex and physical development, sexual maturation, motor activity, acoustic startle, passive-avoidance, functional observational battery, and M-water maze) and brains were weighed and microscopically examined. Administration of MN rgp120/ HIV-1, either alone or formulated as a vaccine, had no effect on behavioral development and neurohistopathological examination did not reveal any pathologic effects.

4.3. Metals

4.3.1. Cadmium

The developmental neurotoxicity of cadmium has been previously reviewed *(85)*. Pregnant rats exposed to cadmium in drinking water throughout gestation *(86,87)* did not result in maternal toxicity and had little effect on litter size, offspring weight, viability, or landmarks of physical development. In one study *(87)*, significant delays were seen in the development of cliff aversion and swimming behavior while other measures of preweaning neurobehavioral development such as surface righting, negative geotaxis, and air righting reflex were normal *(86,87)*. Adult offspring demonstrated reduced motor activity, altered open-field activity, and impaired performance in avoidance acquisition and shuttle-box learning tasks *(86,87)*. Cadmium administered to female rats for 5 wk prior to mating and then daily throughout gestation *(88)* did not result in maternal or developmental toxicity. Offspring of exposed dams demonstrated effects on exploratory motor activity and impaired performance in a rotorod test *(88)*.

In summary, exposure to cadmium during gestation generally resulted in alterations in some aspect of behavior. The most consistent findings were alterations in motor activity and impaired cognitive function and in some instances evidence of developmental neurotoxicity was noted at dosages that did not induce maternal or generalized developmental toxicity. The developmental neurotoxicity of cadmium was detected in OPPTS guideline style studies *(86,87)*, and demonstrations of neurochemical *(85)* and electrophysiological alterations *(89)* following cadmium exposure readily support the findings of the guideline-style studies.

4.3.2. Lead

The effects of lead on CNS development have been extensively investigated in humans as well as laboratory animals *(90–93)* and the neurobehavioral consequences of developmental lead exposure has been thoroughly reviewed *(94)*. Comparison of human and animal findings on the effects of developmental lead exposure suggests that the greatest similarities involve relatively complex behavioral processes such as cognition and learning *(92,94)*. To assess the neurobehavioral effects of early low-lead exposure, female rats were administered lead from 60 d prior to mating through weaning *(93)*. Male offspring were evaluated in an open field, and learning was evaluated using a visual-discrimination task. Exposed offspring were hyperactive in the open field and failed to learn a size-discrimination task *(93)*. This finding parallels the findings of following maternal exposure beginning on PND 22 through breeding, gestation, and lactation until weaning of the F_1 offspring *(91)*. In that study, developmental lead-exposed offspring had more errors, but had significantly shorter acquisition times in both brightness and size-discrimination tasks *(91)*. These studies demonstrate that the developmentally neurotoxic effects of prenatal lead exposure would be readily detected in an OPPTS-guideline study, assuming that the method for evaluating learning and memory is sufficiently challenging.

4.3.3. Methylmercury

Methylmercury is a well-known potent human developmental neurotoxicant *(95–97)*. The potential for prenatal methylmercury exposure to induce developmental neurotoxicity was evaluated in a study designed to evaluate the sensitivity of a standard EPA developmental-neurotoxicity testing battery *(98)*. Maternal animals were treated from GD 6–15 and the offspring were evaluated for acquisition of developmental landmarks, ASR, motor activity, cognitive ability (evaluated at the time of weaning only), and neuropathology. The highest dose of methylmercury resulted in excessive pup mortality, and animals from this dosage were not evaluated in the complete test battery. The mid- and low doses of methylmercury did not affect pup viability or body weight. Preweaning behavioral development (surface righting, pivoting, and negative geotaxis), ASR, and motor activity were not affected by treatment. Cognitive performance of the weanlings, evaluated by olfactory conditioning and T-maze delayed-alteration tasks, was not affected. No differences were noted for regional brain weights, and evaluation of brain tissue from pups euthanized on PND 4 did not reveal any alteration in morphometric measurements or overt pathology. Based on this study, methylmercury does not appear to be a developmental neurotoxicant in rats. However, other studies not designed in strict accordance with the current OPPTS guideline have shown that methylmercury does induce developmental neurotoxicity in rats. For example, the neurotoxicity-test battery used in the collaborative behavioral teratology study (CBTS) *(99)* and the parallel Cincinnati behavioral battery *(100)* study covered most of the behavioral tests listed for the OPPTS study. In these studies, methylmercury exposure from GD 6–9 affected maternal and offspring weight, and the ontogeny of preweaning physical landmarks. Developmental neurotoxicity was demonstrated by alterations in auditory startle habituation, motor activity, response to pharmacological challenge, discrimination learning, and complex water-maze learning *(99,100)*. Interestingly, limited gestational exposure (GD 6–9) in the CBTS and Cincinnati studies *(99,100)* consistently induced the same effect seen following exposure from premating through lactation *(101)*, i.e., alterations in motor activity and impaired learning.

While methylmercury is a well-documented human developmental neurotoxicant *(95)* and substantial scientific literature supports methylmercury as a developmental neurotoxicant in rats *(99–101)*, not all developmental neurotoxicity-study designs were able to demonstrate CNS effects *(98)*. The three primary behavioral methods included in the developmental-neurotoxicity test batteries were motor activity, auditory startle habituation, and learning. In animals, cognitive tests and sensory measures are the most sensitive indicators of methylmercury developmental neurotoxicity *(102)* and the ability to detect methylmercury-induced effects in developmental neurotoxicity studies may be dependent on the learning and memory task. The moderate evidence of developmental toxicity in the CBTS *(99)* and the Cincinnati *(100)* studies, and the failure to detect nervous system-specific insult of a well-known human developmental neurotoxicant in a guideline-style study *(98)*, demonstrates the critical importance of selecting the appropriate cognitive tasks.

4.3.4. Aluminum

Administration of aluminum lactate *(103,104)* or aluminum chloride *(104)* to female rats throughout gestation resulted in increased offspring mortality and a transient delay in growth. Evaluation of preweaning developmental indices demonstrated similar patterns of impaired development of the righting and grasping reflexes, and negative geotaxis response *(103,104)*. Postweaning evaluation of cognitive ability of offspring prenatally exposed to aluminum lactate demonstrated reduced learning ability in an operant-conditioning test *(103)*; animals exposed to aluminum chloride were not evaluated for cognition. These findings suggest that while there may be differing sensitivities based on the salt form, prenatal aluminum exposure induces developmental neurotoxicity in rats.

4.3.5. Organotins

The organotins, tributyltin and trihexyltin, were administered from GD 6–20 to rats at less than maternally toxic dose levels and the offspring were evaluated in a neurotoxicity screening battery *(105)*. No effects were seen on pup viability and growth or in the acquisition of the developmental reflexes, surface righting and negative geotaxis. However, behavioral alterations were noted when the offspring were evaluated as adults. These functional changes consisted of hyperactivity (increased locomotion and rearing), increased activity following amphetamine challenge, and impaired learning in a radial-arm maze task *(105)*. The effects induced by tributyltin were generally more severe than those induced by trihexyltin. However, the behavioral alterations induced by tributyltin and trihexyltin are consistent with findings of impaired radial-arm maze performance for adult rats following neonatal triethyltin exposure *(106)* and alterations in motor activity following prenatal exposure to bis(tri-n-butyltin)oxide *(107)*. These findings indicate that organotins are developmental neurotoxicants in rats and that the most sensitive endpoints for detection are learning ability and locomotion, suggesting that an OPPTS-guideline developmental neurotoxicity study would identify organotins as developmental neurotoxicants.

4.3.6. Manganese

Manganese was administered to pregnant rats in drinking water from conception through PND 30 *(108)*. Manganese-exposed offspring showed reduced body weight gains during most of the postnatal exposure period and hyperactivity on PND 17, but adult offspring demonstrated normal activity in the elevated plus apparatus. Learning was unaffected in the radial-arm maze and the Morris water maze. No neurochemical alterations were noted, but both low- and high-dose manganese offspring demonstrated thinning of the cerebral cortex *(108)*.

4.4. Industrial Chemicals

4.4.1. Polychlorinated Biphenyls (PCBs)

PCBs are stable environmental contaminant mixtures consisting of many individual congeners. A growing body of evidence implicates PCBs as human developmental neurotoxicants *(109,110)*, affecting reflex and motor behavior and cognition with considerable cross-species reliability in demonstration of neurotoxic effects *(111)*.

In an extensive study that provided for an EPA-like postnatal neurobehavioral evaluation, female rats were exposed to Fenclor 42 for 5 d during the 2 wk prior to mating (preconception exposure), from GD 6–15 (*in utero* exposure), or from LD 1–21 (postnatal exposure) *(112)*. PCB exposure did not affect maternal weights or weight of the offspring up to PND 21. Surface righting and negative geotaxis were not affected by treatment. Preconception or *in utero* exposure had no effect on cliff avoidance, while this measure was suppressed in the postnatally exposed group. The development of swimming behavior was affected by all treatment regimens. Rats exposed to PCB prior to conception or postnatally demonstrated reduced open-field activity while offspring exposed *in utero* had normal activity. Learning was evaluated on PND 30 using an active-avoidance task and rats exposed *in utero* and postnatally were impaired in the acquisition of this task *(112)*.

In another series of studies, maternal animals were exposed to PCB 126, a dioxin-like coplanar PCB congener, for 7 wk prior to breeding (Monday through Friday) and then daily throughout gestation and lactation *(113–115)*. In these studies, maternal PCB exposure induced only small effects on scheduled controlled operant behavior *(113)* and low frequency hearing loss *(115)*, but did not cause deficits in attention *(114)*. Perinatal exposure to TCDD (dioxin) *(116,117)* or to the structurally similar coplanar PCBs, PCB 77 or PCB 126, from GD 10–16 resulted in a facilitation of spatial learning in the radial-arm maze for male offspring. No effect was noted when the animals were evaluated in other spatial learning tasks (Morris water maze, T-maze, delayed spatial alternation, and spatial discrimination reversal learning) *(116,117)*. When evaluated in a nonspatial learning task, visual reverse learning, both males and females showed a deficit in learning *(117)*.

Offspring exposed *in utero* (GD 10–16) to the *ortho*-substituted PCBs, PCB 28, PCB 118, or PCB 153, showed no impairment in either working or reference memory tasks on an eight-arm maze. However, when the same animals were later tested in a T-maze delayed spatial alternation task, the high dose of all three PCBs demonstrated impaired acquisition for the females *(118)*.

All together, these studies demonstrate the task-specific effect of PCBs on learning and memory, providing clear evidence of PCB-induced effects on cognition. In addition, these findings suggest that an EPA-style developmental neurotoxicity study would be sensitive to PCB-induced developmental neurotoxicity, assuming that the test for learning and memory was sufficiently rigorous. Finally, the demonstration that *in utero* PCB exposure can induce developmental neurotoxicity in the rat at dosages not affecting pup viability or growth and in the absence of maternal toxicity suggests that PCBs may be selective developmental neurotoxicants.

4.4.2. Solvents

Maternal occupational exposure to aromatic solvents has been strongly linked with congenital anomalies, spontaneous abortion, and fetal death in humans *(119–121)*. The combination of widespread use of organic solvents, risk for occupational exposure, and a potential link between exposure and developmental toxicity, has spawned considerable investigation into the potential for organic solvents to induce developmental neurotoxicity. In this section, developmental neurotoxicity studies of the aromatic solvents methanol, styrene, toluene, xylene, dichloromethane, and ethylene glycol are reviewed.

Methanol is a common organic solvent that has been considered for use as an automobile fuel or fuel additive. Methanol was administered to pregnant rats by wholebody inhalation from GD 7–19 and offspring were evaluated in a neurobehavioral-test battery designed in accordance with the OPPTS developmental neurotoxicity guideline *(122)*. Methanol exposure reduced maternal weight gains and resulted in reduced birth weight and impaired growth of offspring. Behavioral evaluations failed to detect any exposure-related effects on motor activity, olfactory learning, thermoregulation, T-maze learning, ASR, reflex modification, or passive-avoidance learning. Based on the findings of this study, methanol is not considered to be developmentally neurotoxic, although the effect of lactational exposure was not evaluated *(122)*.

Pregnant rats were exposed by inhalation to the organic solvent styrene for 6 h/d from GD 7–20 and the offspring were evaluated for developmental neurotoxicity in a battery designed in accordance with the OPPTS guideline *(123)*. Styrene exposure did not result in maternal toxicity. Birth weights were not affected; however, postnatal growth was slightly inhibited for the high group. Significant delays in acquisition of preweaning developmental landmarks (incisor eruption, eye opening, and vaginal opening) and behavioral development (ASR, and pivoting, bar holding, and surface-righting responses) was noted in the high-dose group. Postweaning evaluation of open field behavior, motor coordination and activity, and learning (operant conditioning) all showed impairment at the high exposure level. Although the behavioral evaluations were performed in accordance with current regulatory guidelines, only a small number of litters were evaluated (5, 2, and 5 litters in the control, mid- and high-dose groups, respectively) *(123)*. So, while the findings of this study clearly raise concern of potential styrene-induced developmental neurotoxicity, due to the small number of litters evaluated, a definitive developmental neurotoxicity study needs to be performed.

Inhalation exposure to toluene, an organic solvent, from GD 7 through LD 18 in rats did not result in maternal toxicity or decreased pup viability *(124)*. Birth weight was slightly reduced and preweaning pup growth was slightly impaired. Litters of exposed dams demonstrated retarded development of simple reflexes (surface righting, auditory startle, and air-righting responses). Exposed offspring demonstrated increased motor activity when evaluated in an open field on PND 28, although evaluation on the rotarod failed to detect alteration in motor coordination. Cognitive impairment was noted when the animals were evaluated as adults for learning using the Morris water maze.

Xylene inhalation exposure from GD 7 through LD 20 to rats did not result in maternal toxicity or adverse effects on offspring viability, birth weight or growth *(125)*. Brain weights of exposed litters were reduced on PND 28. Physical development and ontogeny of simple reflexes were not affected, with the exception of a delay in acquisi-

Table 3
Is There a Developmental Neurotoxicity Solvent Syndrome?[a]

	Developmental landmarks	Reflex development	Activity	Learning and memory	Brain weight and neurochemistry	References
Methanol						*(122)*
Styrene	X	X	X	X		*(123)*
Toluene		X	X	X		*(125)*
Xylene				X	X	*(124)*
Ethylene glycol		X	X		X	*(17,126)*
2-Methoxy ethanol				X		*(127)*
Dichloromethane			X			*(128)*

[a]Not all endpoints were evaluated for each compound.

tion of the air-righting reflex. No effect was noted following evaluation of motor activity or coordination. Slight exposure-related decrements in learning ability were detected in the Morris water maze.

The behavioral teratology of 2-ethoxyethanol (ethylene glycol) was evaluated following inhalation exposure from GD 7–13 or GD 14–20 *(17,126)*. Rats exposed from GD 7–13 demonstrated impaired neuromotor ability (rotarod and ascent test) *(17)* and a slightly better learning in an avoidance task while offspring exposed from GD 14–20 were less active in a running wheel *(126)*. In light of the slight alterations in neurobehavior, it is interesting to note that neurochemical evaluation of brains of offspring from either exposure group demonstrated significant decreases in content of norepinephrine, acetylcholine, and dopamine. The behavioral teratology of a related ethylene glycol, ethylene glycol monomethyl ether (2-methoxy ethanol) was evaluated following maternal administration as liquid diets during organogenesis. No evidence of developmental neurotoxicity was noted except for a slight alteration in the Cincinnati maze learning *(127)*.

Inhalation exposure of pregnant rats to dichloromethane throughout gestation resulted in alterations in motor-activity habituation in a novel environment (habituation). Offspring growth was not affected and no effects were seen in wheel-running activity or avoidance learning *(128)*.

While the results from the methanol study did not indicate developmental neurotoxicity *(122)*, the findings from the evaluation of the organic solvents styrene *(123)*, xylene *(125)*, toluene *(124)*, ethylene glycol *(126)*, ethylene glycol monomethyl ether *(17,127)*, and dichloromethane *(128)* all show evidence of developmental neurotoxicity. The results of these studies lend credence to the claim of a possible "solvent syndrome" that demonstrate similar patterns of positive responses in varied developmental neurotoxicity testing batteries (Table 3).

4.4.3. Acrylamide

Acrylamide is an organic molecule used in production of polyacrylamides, and is primarily a concern for worker exposure. Acrylamide is a well-studied neurotoxicant in animals, inducing behavioral and neuropathological effects associated with peripheral distal axonopathy. The potential for acrylamide to induce developmental neurotoxicity following maternal treatment from GD 6–LD 10 in rats was evaluated in a study that was designed in accordance with the EPA OPPTS guideline *(6)*. Decreased preweaning body weights were noted at all dose levels. Postweaning body-weight gain was decreased only in males of the highest surviving dose group (a higher dose group was terminated early in lactation due to pup mortality). Significant neurobehavioral effects were limited to decreases in horizontal activity and ASR for weanlings of both sexes. The decrease in ASR persisted to adulthood in the females, no other behavioral or neuropathological effects were noted. Because behavior effects were observed only at dosages higher than dosages that induced conventional developmental toxicity (i.e., pup body weights), the authors concluded that while acrylamide may be a developmental neurotoxicant, it is not a selective developmental neurotoxicant.

4.5. Other Chemicals

Aspartame is the generic name for the food sweetener l-methyl *N*-L-α-aspartyl-L-phenylalanine. The potential developmental neurotoxicity of aspartame and one of its components, phenylalanine, was evaluated following continuous dietary exposure from before conception through 90 d of postnatal life in the rat *(129)*. Aspartame and phenylalanine exposures both resulted in increased pup mortality and decreased pup weight. Offspring exposed to aspartame and phenylalanine demonstrated delayed appearance of several developmental reflexes including startle response, forward locomotion, and swimming development. No effects were noted on cognitive performance or adult behavior *(129)*. In general, the effects of aspartame were indistinguishable from those attributable to its phenylalanine content.

The potential of brominated vegetable oils to induce developmental neurotoxicity has been evaluated *(130)*. Adult rats were fed diets containing brominated vegetable oil for 2 wk prior to conception and female exposure continued throughout gestation and lactation. Brominated vegetable oil at dietary dosage levels of up to 2.0% produced severe developmental and reproductive toxicity, including reduced fertility, increased offspring mortality, and impaired physical development. Adverse effects on behavioral development included delays in ontogeny of pivoting behavior, cliff avoidance, negative geotaxis, swimming behavior, and ASR, and decreased activity in an open field. No effects were observed on postweaning open-field activity or learning, however, running-wheel activity was decreased. Brain weights of adult offspring were reduced *(130)*.

The potential developmental neurotoxicity following inhalation exposure of hydrogen sulfide to rats at occupationally relevant exposure concentrations from preconception through GD 19 and then resuming for dams and offspring from LD 5 through 18 was evaluated in a study designed in accordance with the OPPTS developmental neurotoxicity guideline. Exposure to hydrogen sulfide did not affect pup growth, development, or performance in behavioral tests and did not result in any evidence of neuropathology *(131)*.

The developmental neurotoxicity of an antipsychotic with an unknown mechanism of action and identified as CI-943, was evaluated following exposure either from preconception through lactation or from GD 15–LD 21 in rats *(132)*. Offspring were evaluated for developmental neurotoxicity in a behavioral battery that evaluated rotorod performance, spontaneous motor activity, ASR, and learning and memory in a two-way shuttle-avoidance paradigm. Treatment-related effects were evident for each neurobehavioral test. They occurred at both parentally toxic and nontoxic doses and in the absence of effects on offspring growth and vitality. The results indicate that CI–943 is a developmental neurotoxicant regardless of the developmental stage of exposure, although the pattern of response was dependent on the exposure period *(132)*.

5. WHAT HAVE THESE INVESTIGATIONS OF DEVELOPMENTAL NEUROTOXICITY TAUGHT US?

Developmental neurotoxicity is defined as any significant alteration in behavior, neurohistology, neurochemistry, neurophysiology, or gross dysmorphology of the CNS. Chemicals were identified as developmental neurotoxicants if they affected any one of these neurological domains, regardless of the mechanism of action or duration of effect. Based on this definition of developmental neurotoxicity, many of the compounds evaluated were identified as developmental neurotoxicants. It is important to note that positive identification of a compound as a developmental neurotoxicant in the context of a screening battery should not be viewed as a definitive classification. The OPPTS developmental neurotoxicity study design is very complex with a large number of endpoints and is not well-suited for delineating false positives from true developmental neurotoxicants. By design, the screening study incorporates a broad range of functional and neuroanatomical evaluations, and compound-related alterations in any of these domains would be a cause for concern and trigger additional evaluation.

Frequently, neurotoxic effects occurred at dosages that also induced maternal or traditional developmental toxicity (i.e., increased offspring mortality and reduced body weight), and in some cases the developmental effects were severe. Of the studies reviewed by the EPA, in only two (molinate and emamectin) was evidence of developmental neurotoxicity demonstrated at dose levels that did not induce maternal toxicity (Table 1). This raises several issues with regards to interpreting developmental neurotoxicity data: (1) what impact does maternal toxicity have on postnatal development of the offspring, (2) what impact does systemic toxicity have on behavioral evaluations, and (3) if developmental neurotoxicity is expressed only at doses that induced general developmental toxicity, is there reason for heightened concern?

One obvious endpoint that is lacking from the current OPPTS guideline is biochemical evaluations of brain function. While such an evaluation may be difficult to incorporate into a standard screening study, several studies suggest that biochemical alterations may be sensitive indicators of developmental neurotoxicity. For example, alterations in brain neurotransmitter levels occurred following prenatal exposure to methamphetamine *(133)* and 2-ethoxyethanol *(126)* at doses producing little other evidence of developmental neurotoxicity, and prenatal cocaine exposure induced alterations in receptor binding and enzyme activity *(33–35)*. Provisions in the guideline require a traditional neuropathologic examination of neonatal and adult offspring, and a morphometric brain examination on PND 11. Although several of the compounds reviewed by the EPA showed alterations in brain morphometry, the sensitivity of this endpoint has not been established. In addition, it has not been shown that alterations in brain biochemistry, such as those observed following cocaine or 2-ethoxyethanol exposure, have obvious neuroanatomical correlates. Therefore, while perhaps not appropriate for all screening studies, targeted evaluation of biochemical endpoints for chemicals with known neuroactive mechanisms (such as acetylcholinesterase activity for organophosphate pesticides) may provide relevant information for safety assessment.

Myriad behavioral evaluations have been performed in attempts to identify developmental neurotoxicants, including ontogeny of reflexive behaviors, evaluation of sensory functions and spontaneous activity, and cognitive tests. The current OPPTS guideline focuses behavioral evaluations on animal activity, startle responsiveness, and learning and memory, although there is much flexibility around which test of learning and memory is used. In reviewing the developmental neurotoxicity literature, it is often cognitive tests that appear to be the most sensitive for the detection of developmental neurotoxicant exposure. This is especially true of compounds such as ethanol, PCBs, and methylmercury, all of which have been demonstrated to be human developmental neurotoxicants. However, there is great variation in the ability of specific learning and memory tests to detect compound-related alterations. The sensitivity of learning and memory tests to detect alterations appears to be less related to the class of compound and more related to the stringency of the evaluation. In general, complex maze tasks, evaluation of operant behaviors, and tests incorporating pharmacological challenge appear to be the most sensitive. Therefore, raising the standard for learning and memory evaluations in screening studies may increase the probability of detecting developmental neurotoxicants.

Clearly, there is a need to develop more sensitive and relevant methods for the identification of developmental neurotoxicants. Further refinement of the methods used to evaluate potential developmental neurotoxicity and the resultant increased confidence in our ability to detect potential developmental neurotoxicity that will follow may provide an added benefit. In the pharmaceutical industry, pregnant women are not evaluated in premarketing clinical trials due to ethical concerns regarding experimental therapies during pregnancy, and often the default assumption is that pregnant women should not be exposed to drugs. However, the assessment of risk and safety of drugs in pregnancy is complicated by a variety of issues. For example, even when not exposed to medication, infants of mothers with epilepsy have a higher rate of malformation than infants in the general population, and offspring of depressed mothers demonstrate impaired behavioral development *(59)*. Effective treatments for indications such as epilepsy, show considerable variation of impact on neurodevelopment in humans and experimental animals. For example, the anticonvulsant phenytoin has been repeatedly shown to have a negative effect on neurobehavioral development while the anticonvulsant carbamazepine shows no similar effect *(51)*. In this case, a thorough evaluation of the potential for a medication to induce developmental neurotoxicity can increase the confidence in administering the appropriate treatment to alleviate a maternal condition that could potentially have a negative impact on neurodevelopment.

The scientific literature clearly shows that the effects of known human developmental neurotoxicants are readily detected by evaluation using developmental neurotoxicity testing batteries similar to the OPPTS guideline-specified battery. However, due to the inherent difficulty in assessing subtle functional effects in humans, to date only the most potent human developmental neurotoxicants have been identified. To fully optimize hazard identification of potential human developmental neurotoxicants in rodents, further evaluation of the types of endpoints affected (i.e., growth, physical development, innate behaviors, or learning and memory) and methodology is needed.

REFERENCES

1. United States Environmental Protection Agency (1998) Health Effects Test Guidelines OPPTS 870.6300 Developmental Neurotoxicity.
2. Hutchings, D. E. (1990) Issues of risk assessment: lessons from the use and abuse of drugs during pregnancy. *Neurotoxicol. Teratol.* **12**, 183–189.
3. Vorhees, C. V. (1997) Methods for detecting long-term CNS dysfunction after prenatal exposure to neurotoxins. *Drug Chem. Toxicol.* **20**, 387–399.
4. Vorhees, C. V. (1987) Reliability, Sensitivity and validity of behavioral indices of neuro-toxicity. *Neurotoxicol. Teratol.* **9**, 445–464.
5. Rodier, P. M. (1990) Developmental neurotoxicology. *Toxicol. Pathol.* **18**, 89–95.
6. Makris, S., Raffaele, K., Sette, W., and Seed, J. (1998) A retrospective analysis of twelve developmental neurotoxicity studies submitted to the USEPA Office of Prevention, Pesticides, and Toxic Substances (OPPTS). USEPA, Washington, DC.
7. Bates, H. K., McKee, R. H., Bieler, G. S., Gardiner, T. H., Gill, M. W., Strother, D. E., and Masten, L. W. (1994) Developmental neurotoxicity evaluation of orally administered iso-propanol in rats. *Fund. Appl. Toxicol.* **22**, 152–158.
8. Schoenig, G. P., Hartnagel, R. E., Schardein, J. L., and Vorhees, C. V. (1993) Neurotoxic-ity evaluation of *n,n*-Diethyl-*m*-toluamide (DEET) in rats. *Fund. Appl. Toxicol.* **21**, 355–365.
9. Wise, L. D., Allen, H. L., Hoe, C. L., Verbeke, D. R., and Gerson, R.J. (1997) Develop-mental neurotoxicity evaluation of the avermectin pesticide, emamectin benzoate, in Sprague-Dawley rats. *Neurotoxicol. Teratol.* **19**, 315–326.
10. Hoberman, A. M. (1998) Developmental neurotoxicity study of chlorpyrifos administered via oral gavage to Crl:CD BR VAF/Plus presumed pregnant rats. Argus 304–001. Argus Laboratories, Inc., Horsham, PA.
11. Dorfmueller, M. A., Henne, S. P., York, R. G., Bornschein, R. L., and Manson, J. M. (1979) Evaluation of teratogenicity and behavioral toxicity with inhalation exposure of maternal rats to trichloroethylene. *Toxicology* **14**, 153–166.
12. Kaplan-Estrin, M., Jacobson, S. W., and Jacobson, J. L. (1999) Neurobehavioral effects of prenatal alcohol exposure at 26 months. *Neurotoxicol. Teratol.* **21**, 503–511.
13. Driscoll, C. D., Streissguth, A. P., and Riley, E. P. (1990) Prenatal alcohol exposure: Com-parability of effects in humans and animal models. *Neurotoxicol. Teratol.* **12**, 231–237.
14. Lee, M. H., Haddad, R., and Rabe, A. (1980) Developmental impairments in progeny of rats consuming ethanol during pregnancy. *Neurobehav. Toxicol.* **2**, 189–198.
15. Shaywitz, B. A., Griffieth, G. G., and Warshaw, J. B. (1979) Hyperactivity and cognitive deficits in developing rat pups born to alcoholic mothers: an experimental model of the expanded fetal alcohol syndrome (EFAS). *Neurobehav. Toxicol.* **1**, 113–122.
16. Abel, E. L. and Dintcheff, B. A. (1978) Effect of prenatal alcohol exposure on growth and development in rats. *J. Pharmacol. Exp. Therap.* **207**, 916–921.
17. Nelson, B. K., Brightwell, W. S., and Setzer, J. V. (1982) Prenatal interactions between ethanol and the industrial solvent 2-ethoxyethanol in rats: maternal and behavioral terato-genic effects. *Neurobehav. Toxicol. Teratol.* **4**, 387–394.
18. Bond, N. W. (1981) Prenatal alcohol exposure in rodents: a review of its effects on off-spring activity and learning behavior. *Austr. J. Psychol.* **33**, 331–344.
19. Riley, E. P., Shapiro, N. R., and Lochry, E. A. (1979) Nose-poking and head-dipping be-haviors in rats prenatally exposed to alcohol. *Pharmacol. Biochem. Behav.* **11**, 513–519.
20. Vorhees, C. V. (1994) Developmental neurotoxicity induced by therapeutic and illicit drugs. *Environ. Health Perspect.* **102(Suppl. 2),** 145–153.
21. Dixon, S. D. (1989) Effects of transplacental exposure to cocaine and methamphetamine on the neonate. *Wes. J. Med.* **150**, 436–442.
22. Little, B. B., Snell, L. M., and Gilstrap, L. C. (1988) Methamphetamine abuse during preg-nancy: outcome and fetal effects. *Obstet. Gynecol.* **72**, 541–544.

23. Martin, J. C., Martin, D. C., Radow, B., and Sigman, G. (1976) Growth, development and activity in rat offspring following maternal drug exposure. *Exp. Aging Res.* **2,** 235–251.

24. Cho, D., Lyu, H., Lee, H., Kim, P., and Chin, K. (1991) Behavioral teratogenicity of methamphetamine. *J. Toxicol. Sci.* **16,** 37–49.

25. Acuff-Smith, K. D., Schilling, M. S., Fisher, J. E., and Vorhees, C. V. (1996) Stage-specific effects of prenatal D-methamphetamine exposure on eye and behavioral developments in rats. *Neurotoxicol. Teratol.* **18,** 199–215.

26. Hitzemann, B. A., Hitzemann, R. J., Brase, D. A., and Loh, H. H. (1989) Influence of prenatal *d*-amphetamine administration on development and behavior of rats. *Life Sci.* **18,** 605–612.

27. Holson, R. R., Adams, J., Buelke-Sam, J., Gough, B., and Kimmel, C. A. (1976) d-amphetamine as a behavioral teratogen: effects depend on dose, sex, age and task. *Neurobehav. Toxicol. Teratol.* **7,** 753–758.

28. Lutiger, B., Graham, K., Einarson, T. R., and Koren, G. (1991) Relationship between gestational cocaine use and pregnancy outcome: a meta analysis. *Teratology* **44,** 405–414.

29. Held, J. R., Riggs, M. L., and Dorman, C. (1999) The effect of prenatal cocaine exposure on neurobehavioral outcome: a meta-analysis. *Neurotoxicol. Teratol.* **21,** 619–625.

30. Cutler, A. R., Wilkerson, A. E., Gingras, G. L., and Levin, E. D. (1996) Prenatal cocaine and/or nicotine exposure in rats: preliminary findings on long-term cognitive outcome and genital development at birth. *Neurotoxicol. Teratol.* **18,** 635–643.

31. Keller, R. W., Maisonneuve, I. M., Nuccio, D. M., Carlson, J. N., and Glick, S. D. (1994) Effects of prenatal cocaine exposure on the nigrostriatal dopamine system: an in vivo microdialysis study in the rat. *Brain Res.* **634,** 266–274.

32. Henderson, M. G. and McMillen, B. A. (1993) Changes in dopamine, serotonin and their metabolites in discrete brain areas of rat offspring after in utero exposure to cocaine or related drugs. *Teratology* **48,** 421–430.

33. Clow, D. W., Hammer, R. P., Kirstein, C. L., and Spear, L. P. (1991) Gestational cocaine exposure increases opiate receptor binding in weanling offspring. *Dev. Brain Res.* **59,** 179–185.

34. Byrnes, J. J., Pritchard, G. A., Koff, J. M., and Miller, L. G. (1993) Prenatal cocaine exposure: decreased sensitization to cocaine and decreased striatal dopamine transporter binding in offspring. *Neuropharmacology* **32,** 721–723.

35. Akbari, H. M. and Azmitia, E. C. (1992) Increased tyrosine hydroxylase immunoreactivity in the rat cortex following prenatal cocaine exposure. *Dev. Brain Res.* **66,** 277–281.

36. Meyer, J. S. and Dupont, S. A. (1993) Prenatal cocaine administration stimulates fetal brain tyrosine hydroxylase activity. *Brain Res.* **608,** 129–137.

37. Vathy, I., Katay, L., and Mini, K. N. (1993) Sexually dimorphic effects of prenatal cocaine on adult sexual behavior and brain catecholamines in rats. *Dev. Brain Res.* **73,** 115–122.

38. National Institute on Drug Abuse (1996) National Pregnancy and Health Survey. Publication No. 96–3819. National Institutes of Health, Rockville, MD.

39. Goldschmidt, L., Day, N. L., and Richardson, G. A. (2000) Effects of prenatal marijuana exposure on child behavior problems at age 10. *Neurotoxicol. Teratol.* **22,** 325–336.

40. Abel, E. L., Bush, R., Dintcheff, B. A., and Ernst, C. A. S. (1981) Critical periods for marijuana-induced intrauterine growth retardation in the rat. *Neurobehav. Toxicol. Teratol.* **3,** 351–354.

41. Abel, E. L. (1984) Effects of delta-9-tetrahydrocannabinol on pregnancy and offspring in rats. *Neurobehav. Toxicol. Teratol.* **6,** 29–32.

42. Abel, E. L. (1979) Behavioral teratology of marijuana extract in rats. *Neurobehav. Toxicol.* **1,** 285–287.

43. Vardaris, R. M., Weisz, D. J., Fazel, A., and Rawitch, A. B. (1976) Chronic administration of delta–9-tetrahydrocannabinol to pregnant rats: studies of pup behavior and placental transfer. *Pharmacol. Biochem. Behav.* **4,** 249–254.

44. Fried, P. A. (1976) Short and long-term effects of pre-natal cannabis inhalation upon rat offspring. *Psychopharmacology* **50**, 285–289.
45. Levin, E. D. and Slotkin, T. A. (1998) Developmental neurotoxicity of nicotine, in *Handbook of Developmental Neurotoxicology* (Slikker, W. and Chang, L. W., eds.), Academic Press, San Diego, CA, pp. 587–615.
46. Martin, J. C. and Martin, D. C. (1981) Voluntary activity in the aging rat as a function of maternal drug exposure. *Neurobehav. Toxicol. Teratol.* **3**, 261–264.
47. Roy, T. S. and Sabherwal, U. (1998) Effects of gestational nicotine exposure on hippocampal morphology. *Neurotoxicol. Teratol.* **20**, 465–473.
48. Peters, D. A. V., Taub, H., and Tang, S. (1979) Postnatal effects of maternal nicotine exposure. *Neurobehav. Toxicol.* **1**, 221–225.
49. Levin, E. D., Wilkerson, A., Jones, J. P., Christopher, N. C., and Briggs, S. J. (1996) Prenatal nicotine effects on memory in rats: pharmacological and behavioral challenges. *Dev. Brain Res.* **97**, 207–215.
50. Adams, J., Vorhees, C. V., and Middaugh, L. D. (1990) Developmental neurotoxicity of anticonvulsants: Human and animal evidence on phenytoin. *Neurotoxicol. Teratol.* **12**, 203–214.
51. Scolnick, D., Nulman, I., Rovet, J., Gladstone, D., Czuchta, D., Gardner, H. A., et al. (1994) Neurodevelopment of children exposed in utero to phenytoin and carbamazepine monotherapy. *JAMA* **271**, 767–770.
52. Vorhees, C. V. (1983) Fetal anticonvulsant syndrome in rats: dose- and period-response relationships of prenatal diphenylhydantoin, trimethadione and phenobarbital exposure on the structural and functional development of the offspring. *J. Pharmacol. Exp. Ther.* **227**, 274–287.
53. Vorhees, C. V. (1987) Fetal hydantoin syndrome in rats: dose-effect relationships of prenatal phenytoin on postnatal development and behavior. *Teratology* **35**, 287–303.
54. Vorhees, C. V. (1985) Fetal anticonvulsant syndrome in rats: effects on postnatal behavior and brain amino acid content. *Neurobehav. Toxicol. Teratol.* **7**, 471–482.
55. Vorhees, C. V., Acuff-Smith, K. D., Schilling, M. A., and Moran, M. S. (1995) Prenatal exposure to sodium phenytoin in rats induces complex maze learning deficits comparable to those induced by exposure to phenytoin acid at half the dose. *Neurotoxicol. Teratol.* **17**, 627–632.
56. Schilling, M. A., Inman, S. L., Morford, L. L., Moran, M. S., and Vorhees, C. V. (1999) Prenatal phenytoin exposure and spatial navigation in offspring: effects on reference and working memory and on discrimination learning. *Neurotoxicol. Teratol.* **21**, 567–578.
57. Vorhees, C. V. and Minck, D. R. (1989) Long-term effects of prenatal phenytoin exposure on offspring behavior in rats. *Neurotoxicol. Teratol.* **11**, 295–305.
58. Kessler, R. C., McGonagle, K. A., Swartz, M., Blazer, D. G, and Nelson, C. B. (1993) Sex and depression in the national comorbidity survey: lifetime prevelance, chronicity and recurrence. *J. Affect. Disord.* **29**, 85–96.
59. Goodman, S. H. (1992) Understanding the effects of depressed mothers on their children. *Prog. Exp. Pers. Psychopathol. Res.* **15**, 47–109.
60. Vorhees, C. V., Acuff-Smith, K. D., Schilling, M. A., Fisher, J. E., Moran, M. S., and Buelke-Sam, J. (1994) A developmental neurotoxicity evaluation of the effects of prenatal exposure to fluoxetine in rats. *Fund. Appl. Toxicol.* **23**, 194–205.
61. Butcher, R. E. and Vorhees, C. V. (1979) A preliminary test battery for the investigation of behavioral teratology of selected psychotropic drugs. *Neurobehav. Toxicol.* **1(Suppl. 1)**, 207–212.
62. Nulman, I., Rovet, J., Stewart, D. E., Wolpin, J., Gerdner, H.A., Theis, J. G. W., et al. (1997) Neurodevelopment of children exposed in utero to antidepressant drugs. *N. Engl. J. Med.* **336**, 258–262.

63. Robertson, R. T., Majka, J. A., Peter, C. P., and Bokelman, D. L. (1980) Effects of prenatal exposure to chlorpromazine on postnatal development and behavior in rats. *Toxicol. Appl. Pharmacol.* **53,** 541–549.

64. Saillenfait, A. M. and Vannier, B. (1988) Methodological proposal in behavioural teratogenicity testing: assessment of propoxyphene, chlorpromazine, and vitamin A as positive controls. *Teratology* **37,** 185–199.

65. Miller, R. P. and Becker, B. A. (1975) Teratogenicity of oral diazepam and diphenylhydantoin in mice. *Toxicol. Appl. Pharmacol.* **32,** 53–61.

66. Hartz, S. C., Heinonen, O. P., Shapiro, S., Siskind, V., and Slone, D. (1975) Antenatal exposure to meprobamate and chlordiazepoxide in relation to malformations, mental development, and childhood mortality. *N. Engl. J. Med.* **292,** 726–728.

67. Gai, N. and Grimm, V. E. (1982) The effect of prenatal exposure to diazepam on aspects of postnatal development and behavior in rats. *Psychopharmacology* **78,** 225–229.

68. Shore, C. O., Vorhees, C. V., Bornschein, R. L., and Stemmer, K. (1983) Behavioral consequences of prenatal diazepam exposure in rats. *Neurobehav. Toxicol. Teratol.* **5,** 565–570.

69. Kellog, C., Tervo, D., Ison, J., Parisi, T., and Miller, R. K. (1980) Prenatal exposure to diazepam alters behavioral development in rats. *Science* **207,** 205–207.

70. Lauer, J. A., Adams, P. M., and Johnson, K. M. (1987) Perinatal diazepam exposure: Behavioral and neurochemical consequences. *Neurotoxicol. Teratol.* **9,** 213–219.

71. Ryan, C. L. and Pappas, B. A. (1986) Intrauterine diazepam exposure: effects on physical and neurobehavioral development in the rat. *Neurobehav. Toxicol. Teratol.* **8,** 279–286.

72. Henck, J. W., Frahm, D. T., and Anderson, J. A. (1996) Validation of automated behavioral test systems. *Neurotoxicol. Teratol.* **18,** 189–197.

73. Adams, P. M. (1982) Effects of perinatal chlordiazepoxide exposure on rat preweaning and postweaning behavior. *Neurobehav. Toxicol. Teratol.* **4,** 279–282.

74. Harris, R. A. and Case, J. (1979) Effects of maternal consumption of ethanol, barbital, chlordiazepoxide on the behavior of the offspring. *Behav. Neuro. Biol.* **26,** 234–247.

75. Adams, J. and Lammer, J. (1991) Relationship between dysmorphology and neuro-psychological function in children exposed to isotrenoin "in utero," in *Functional Neuroteratology of Short-Term Exposure to Drugs* (Fujii, T. and Boer, G. J., eds.), Teikyo University Press, Tokyo, pp. 159–168.

76. Nolen, G. A. (1986) The effects of prenatal retinoic acid on the viability and behavior of the offspring. *Neurobehav. Toxicol. Teratol.* **8,** 643–654.

77. Vorhees, C. V., Brunner, R. L., and Butcher, R. E. (1979) Psychotropic drugs as behavioral teratogens. *Science* **205,** 1220–1225.

78. Cappon, G. D., Bowen, M., Rhodes, K., Kopp, C., and Radovsky, A. E. (2000) A developmental neurotoxicity study of propylthiouracil in rats. *Toxicol. Sci.* **54,** 293(Abstract).

79. Albee, R. R., Mattsson, J. L., Johnson, K. A., Kirk, H. D., and Breslin, W. J. (1989) Neurological consequences of congenital hypothyroidism in Fischer 344 rats. *Neurotoxicol. Teratol.* **11,** 171–183.

80. Vorhees, C. V. (1981) Effects of prenatal naloxone exposure on postnatal behavioral development of rats. *Neurobehav. Toxicol. Teratol.* **3,** 295–301.

81. Shepanek, N. A., Smith, R. F., Tyer, Z. E., Royall, G. D., and Allen, K. S. (1989) Behavioral and neuroanatomical sequelae of prenatal naloxone administration in the rat. *Neurotoxicol. Teratol.* **11,** 441–446.

82. Lichtblau, L. and Sparber, S. B. (1982) Congenital behavioral effects in mature rats prenatally exposed to Levo-Alpha-Acetylmethadol (LAAM). *Neurobehav. Toxicol. Teratol.* **4,** 557–565.

83. Buelke-Sam, J., Cohen, I. R., Wierda, D., Griffey, K. I., Fisher, L. F., and Francis, P. C. (1998) The selective estrogen receptor modulator, raloxifene: a segment II/III delivery study in rats. *Repro. Tox.* **12,** 271–288.

84. Bussiere, J. L., Hardy, L. M., Peterson, M., Foss, J. A., Garman, R. H., Hoberman, A. M., and Christian, M. S. (1999) Lack of developmental neurtoxicity of MN rgp120/HIV-1 administered subcutaneously to neonatal rats. *Toxicol. Sci.* **48,** 90–99.

85. Hastings, L. L. and Miller, M. L. (1998) Developmental neurotoxicity of cadmium, in *Handbook of Developmental Neurotoxicology* (Slikker, W. and Chang, L. W., eds.), Academic Press, San Diego, CA, pp. 517–538.

86. Baranski, B. (1986) Effects of maternal cadmium exposure on postnatal development and tissue cadmium, copper and zinc concentrations in rats. *Arch. Toxicol.* **58,** 255–260.

87. Ali, M. M., Murthy, R. C., and Chandra, S. V. (1986) Developmental and longterm neurobehavioral toxicity of low level *in-utero* cadmium exposure in rats. *Neurobehav. Toxicol. Teratol.* **8,** 463–468.

88. Baranski, B., Stetkiewicz, I., Sitarek, K., and Szymczak, W. (1983) Effects of oral, subchronic cadmium administration on fertility, prenatal and postnatal progeny development in rats. *Arch. Toxicol.* **54,** 297–302.

89. Desi, I., Nagymajtenyi, L., and Schulz, H. (1998) Behavioral and neurotoxicological changes caused by cadmium treatment of rats during development. *J. Appl. Toxicol.* **18,** 63–70.

90. Bull, R. J., McCauley, P. T., Taylor, D. H., and Crofton, K. M. (1983) The effects of lead on the developing central nervous system of the rat. *Neurotoxicology* **4,** 1–18.

91. Zenick, H., Padich, R., Tokarek, T., and Aragon, P. (1978) Influence of prenatal and postnatal lead exposure on discrimination learning in rats. *Pharmacol. Biochem. Behav.* **8,** 347–350.

92. Davis, J. M., Otto, D. A., Weil, D. E., and Grant, L. D. (1990) The comparative developmental neurotoxicity of lead in humans and animals. *Neurotoxicol. Teratol.* **12,** 215–229.

93. Winneke, G., Brockhaus, A., and Baltissen, R. (1977) Neurobehavioral and systemic effects of long-term blood lead-elevation in rats. *Arch. Toxicol.* **37,** 247–263.

94. Rice, D. C. (1998) Developmental lead exposure: neurobehavioral consequences, in *Handbook of Developmental Neurotoxicology* (Slikker, W. and Chang, L. W., eds.), Academic Press, San Diego, CA, pp. 539–557.

95. Amin-Zaki, L., Elhassani, S., Majeed, M.A., Clarkson, T. W., Doherty, R. A., Greenwood, M. R., and Giovanoli-Jakubczak, T. (1976) Perinatal Methylmercury poisoning in Iraq. *Am. J. Disabl. Child.* **130,** 1070–1076.

96. Harada, Y. (1977) Fetal methylmercury poisoning, in *Minamata Disease* (Tsubak, K. and Inekayama, K., eds.), Elsevier Science, Amsterdam, pp. 38–52.

97. Grandjean, P., Weihe, P., White, R. F., Debes, F., Araki, S., Yokoyama, K., et al. (1997) Cognitive deficit in 7-year-old children with prenatal exposure to methylmercury. *Neurotoxicol. Teratol.* **19,** 417–428.

98. Goldey, E. S., O'Callaghan, J. P., Stanton, M. E., Barone, S., and Crofton, K. M. (1994) Developmental neurotoxicity: evaluation of testing procedures with methylazoxymethanol and methylmercury. *Fund. Appl. Toxicol.* **23,** 447–464.

99. Buelke-Sam, J., Kimmel, C. A., Adams, J., Nelson, C. J., Vorhees, C. V., Wright, D. C., et al. (1985) Collaborative behavioral teratology study: results. *Neurobehav. Toxicol. Teratol.* **7,** 591–624.

100. Vorhees, C. V. (1985) Behavioral effects of methylmercury in rats: a parallel to the collaborative behavioral teratology study. *Neurobehav. Toxicol. Teratol.* **7,** 717–725.

101. Suter, K. E. and Schon, H. (1986) Testing stratagies in behavioral teratology: I. testing battery approach. *Neurobehav. Toxicol. Teratol.* **8,** 561–566.

102. Burbacher, T. M., Rodier, P. M., and Weiss, B. (1990) Methylmercury developmental neurotoxicity: a comparison of the effects in humans and animals. *Neurotoxicol. Teratol.* **12,** 191–202.

103. Muller, G., Bernuzzi, V., Desor, D., Hutin, M., Burnel, D., and Lehr, P. R. (1990) Developmental alterations in offspring of female rats orally intoxicated by aluminum lactate at different gestation periods. *Teratology* **42,** 253–261.

104. Bernuzzi, V., Desor, D., and Lehr, P. R. (1989) Developmental alterations in offspring of female rats orally intoxicated by aluminum chloride or lactate during gestation. *Teratology* **40**, 21–27.

105. Gardlund, A. T., Archer, T., Danielsson, K., Danielsson, B., Fredriksson, A., Lindqvist, N., et al. (1991) Effects of prenatal exposure to tributyltin and trihexyltin on behavior in rats. *Neurotoxicol. Teratol.* **13**, 99–105.

106. Miller, D. B., Eckerman, D. A., Krigman, M. R., and Grant, L. D. (1982) Chronic neonatal organotin exposure alters radial-arm maze performance in adult rats. *Neurobehav. Toxicol. Teratol.* **4**, 185–190.

107. Crofton, K. M., Dean, K. F., Boncek, V. M., Rosen, M. B., Sheets, L. P., Chernoff, N., and Reiter, L. (1989) Prenatal or postnatal exposure to bis(tri-n-butyltin)oxide in the rat: postnatal evaluation of teratology and behavior. *Toxicol Appl Pharmacol* **97**, 113–123.

108. Pappas, B. A., Zhang, D., Davidson, C. M., Crowder, T., Park, G. A. S., and Fortin, T. (1997) Perinatal manganese exposure: behavioral, neurochemical, and histopathological effects in rats. *Neurotoxicol. Teratol.* **19**, 17–25.

109. Winneke, G., Bucholski, A., Heinzow, B., Kramer., U., Schmidt, E., Walkowiak, J., et al. (1998) Developmental neurotoxicity of polychlorinated biphenyls (PCBS): cognitive and psychomotor functions in 7-month old children. *Toxicol. Lett.* **102–103**, 423–428.

110. Stewart, P., Reihman, J., Lonky, E., Darvill, T., and Pagano, J. (2000) Prenatal PCB exposure and neonatal behavioral asessment scale (NBAS) performance. *Neurotoxicol. Teratol.* **22**, 21–29.

111. Tilson, H. A., Jacobson, J. L., and Rogan, W. J. (1990) Polychlorinated biphenyls and the developing nervous system: cross species comparisons. *Neurotoxicol. Teratol.* **12**, 239–248.

112. Pantaleoni, G., Fanini, D., Sponta, A. M., Palumbo, G., Giorgi, R., and Adams, P. M. (1988) Effects of maternal exposure to polychlorobiphenyls (PCBs) on F1 generation behavior in rats. *Fund. Appl. Toxicol.* **11**, 440–449.

113. Rice, D. C. and Hayward, S. (1999) Effects of exposure to 3,3′,4,4′,5-Pentachlorobiphenyl (PCB 126) throughout gestation and lactation on behavior (concurrent random interval-random interval and progressive ratio performance) in rats. *Neurotoxicol. Teratol.* **21**, 679–687.

114. Bushnell, P. J. and Rice, D. C. (1999) Behavioral assessments of learning attention in rats exposed perinatally to 3,3′,4,4′,5-pentachlorobiphenyl (PCB 126). *Neurotoxicol. Teratol.* **21**, 381–392.

115. Crofton, K. M. and Rice, D. C. (1999) Low-frequency hearing loss following perinatal exposure to 3,3′,4,4′,5-pentachlorobiphenyl (PCB 126) in rats. *Neurotoxicol. Teratol.* **21**, 299–301.

116. Schantz, S. L., Seo, B., Moshtaghian, J., Peterson, R. E., and Moore, R. W. (1996) Effects of gestational and lactational exposure to TCDD or coplanar PCBs on spatial learning. *Neurotoxicol. Teratol.* **18**, 305–313.

117. Seo, B., Sparks, A. J., Medora, K., Amin, S., and Schantz, S. L. (1999) Learning and memory in rats gestationally and lactationally exposed to 2,3,7,8-Tetrachlorodibenzo-r-Dioxin (TCDD). *Neurotoxicol. Teratol.* **21**, 231–239.

118. Schantz, S. L., Moshtaghian, J., and Ness, D. K. (1995) Spatial learning deficits in adult rats exposed to *ortho*-substituted PCB congeners during gestation and lactation. *Fund. Appl. Toxicol.* **26**, 117–126.

119. McDonald, J. C., Cote, R., Lavoie, J., and McDonald, A. D. (1987) Chemical exposures at work in early pregnancy and congenital defect: a case-referent study. *Br. J. Ind. Med.* **44**, 527–533.

120. Kristen, K. I., Chu, M., Kopeky, E., Einarson, T. R., and Koren, G. (1998) Pregnancy outcome following maternal organic solvent exposure: a meta-analysis of epidemiologic studies. *Am. J. Industr. Med.* **34**, 288–292.

121. Khattak, S., K-Moghtader, G., Barrera, M., McMartin, K., Kennedy, D., and Koren, G. (1999) Pregnancy outcome following gestational exposure to organic solvents. *JAMA* **281,** 1106–1109.

122. Stanton, M. E., Crofton, K. M., Gray, L. E., Gordon, C. J., Boyes, W. K., et al. (1995) Assessment of offspring development and behavior following gestational exposure to inhaled methanol in the rat. *Fund. Appl. Toxicol.* **28,** 100–110.

123. Kishi, R., Chen, B. K., Katakura, Y., Ikeda, T., and Miyake, H. (1995) Effect of prenatal exposure to styrene on the neurobehavioral development, activity, motor coordination, and learning behavior iof rats. *Neurotoxicol. Teratol.* **17,** 121–130.

124. Hass, U., Lund, S. P., Hougaard, K. S., and Simonsen, L. (1999) Developmental neurotoxicity after toluene inhalation exposure in rats. *Neurotoxicol. Teratol.* **21,** 349–357.

125. Hass, U., Lund, S. P., Simonsen, L., and Fries, A. S. (1995) Effects of prenatal exposure to xylene on postnatal development and behavior in rats. *Neurotoxicol. Teratol.* **17,** 341–349.

126. Nelson, B. K., Brightwell, W. S., Setzer, J. V., Taylor, B. J., Hornung, R. W., and O'Donohue, T. L. (1981) Ethoxyethanol behavioral teratology in rats. *Neurotoxicology* **2,** 231–249.

127. Nelson, B. K., Vorhees, C. V., Scott, W. J., and Hastings, L. L. (1989) Effects of 2-methoxyethanol on fetal development, postnatal behavior, and embryonic intracellular pH of rats. *Neurotoxicol. Teratol.* **11,** 273–284.

128. Bornschein, R. L., Hastings, L. L., and Manson, J. M. (1980) Behavioral toxicity in the offspring of rats following maternal exposure to dichloromethane. *Toxicol. Appl. Pharmacol.* **52,** 29–37.

129. Brunner, R. L., Vorhees, C. V., Kinney, L., and Butcher, R. E. (1979) Aspartame: assessment of developmental psychotoxicity of a new artificial sweetener. *Neurobehav. Toxicol.* **1,** 79–86.

130. Vorhees, C. V., Butcher, R. E., Wootten, V., and Brunner, R. L. (1983) Behavioral and reproductive effects of chronic developmental exposure to brominated vegetable oil in rats. *Teratology* **28,** 309–318.

131. Dorman, D. C., Brenneman, K. A., Struve, M. F., Miller, K. L., James, R. A., Marshall, M. W., and Foster, P. M. D. (2000) Fertility and developmental neurotoxicity effects of inhaled hydrogen sulfide in Sprague-Dawley rats. *Neurotoxicol. Teratol.* **22,** 71–84.

132. Henck, J. W., Petrere, J. A., and Anderson, J. A. (1995) Developmental neurotoxicity of CI–943: a novel antipsychotic. *Neurotoxicol. Teratol.* **17,** 13–24.

133. Acuff-Smith, K. D., George, M., Lorens, S. A., and Vorhees, C. V. (1992) Preliminary evidence for methamphetamine-induced behavioral and occular effect in rat offspring following exposure during early organogenesis. *Psychopharmacology* **109,** 255–263.

4

Risk Assessment of Developmental Neurotoxicants

Hugh A. Tilson

This paper has been reviewed by the National Health and Environmental Effects Research Laboratory, US Environmental Protection Agency, and approved for publication. Mention of trade names or commercial products does not constitute endorsement of recommendation for use.

1. INTRODUCTION

That drugs or chemicals in the environment might affect the development of the nervous system adversely has been a concern of scientists, health officials, and the general public for many years. This concern is based in part on estimates that 70% of developmental defects, which include death, growth retardation, structural alterations, or functional deficits, have no known cause and that exposure to environmental factors during critical periods of development might responsible for some of these defects *(1)*. In addition, the National Academy of Sciences *(2)* has estimated that 12% of the 63 million children under the age of 18 in the United States suffer from one or more mental disorders and identified exposure to toxic substances before or after birth as one of the several risk factors that may make children susceptible to these disorders. It has also been estimated that each day, 1.1 million children between 6 mo and 6 yr of age ingest organophosphate insecticides at levels which exceed the safe daily dose as determined by the Environmental Protection Agency (EPA) *(3)*.

Although it has been noted that the epidemiologic literature on childhood effects of neurotoxicants is difficult to assess due to the complex nature of human brain function and the multiple factors that affect brain development *(4)*, there is ample evidence from the human and animal experimental literature indicating that exposure to chemicals and physical factors during development can have adverse consequences on the developing nervous system. Using behavior as an endpoint, Kimmel *(5)* identified several agents that are strongly suspected to be human developmental neurotoxicants, including several drugs (i.e., ethanol, opiates, cocaine, phenytoin), X-radiation, and environmental agents (lead, methyl mercury, polychlorinated biphenyls [PCBs]). The risk of human developmental neurotoxicity resulting from drug abuse was also reviewed at a New York Academy of Sciences conference in 1989 *(6)*.

Animal research has confirmed the conclusion that exposure to drugs and environmental agents during development can have long-term consequences on nervous sys-

From: Handbook of Neurotoxicology, Vol. 2
Edited by: E. J. Massaro © Humana Press Inc., Totowa, NJ

tem structure or function *(7–9)*. At a workshop sponsored by the EPA in 1989 *(10)*, it was concluded that there was considerable comparability of end-points across species including humans for developmental neurotoxicity; that animal testing methods in developmental neurotoxicity measured qualitatively similar effects in humans; that quantitative differences between animals and humans exist based largely on differing toxicokinetic factors; and that specific effects produced by chemicals including neuropathology in adults, nervous-system teratogenesis, and hormonal activity could be used to trigger more extensive developmental neurotoxicity testing. Concerns were also raised at the workshop about the potential for chemicals to produce adverse effects on the developing nervous system and that regulatory processes needed to be in place to screen chemicals for potential developmental neurotoxicity using animal-test protocols required by regulatory agencies.

Although it is generally accepted that exposure to some chemicals during development can adversely affect the nervous system, there is less consensus concerning efficacy of the current regulatory process to protect infant and children and identify potential developmental neurotoxicants *(11)*. Dews *(12)*, for example, indicated that the developing nervous system appears to be sensitive only to a few agents and that it is quite capable of adapting to insult. This observation might be interpreted as suggesting that neurotoxicological testing in adults may be sufficient to identify potential developmental neurotoxicants. In addition, Lochry *(13)* has noted that screening procedures for developmental neurotoxicity in animals rely heavily on behavioral measures, which may be difficult to interpret, often lack standardization across laboratories, and may not be as sensitive as other indicators of developmental toxicity. Lochry *(13)* also noted that information concerning developmental neurotoxicity could be obtained from routine assessments in other studies on reproductive or developmental toxicity that include measures of embryo/fetal death, fetal malformation, and delayed development. These concerns are important since inappropriate testing could unfairly impede or block the development of useful products *(13)*.

In its report on pesticides in the diets of infants and children, the National Research Council (NRC)*(4)* concluded that current toxicity-testing requirements of the EPA included only a few tests specifically designed to protect infants and children, do not take into account the toxicity and metabolism of chemicals in neonates and adolescent animals, and do not the assess the effects of exposure during early developmental states and effects later in life. The Natural Resources Defense Council (NRDC)*(14)* has also called for the EPA to review and revise, if necessary, its toxicity-testing protocols to ensure they reliably assess the full range of toxic effects most relevant to infants and children, including effects on the developing nervous, immune, endocrine, and reproductive systems.

The purpose of the remainder of this chapter is to address some of the concerns that have been raised about the need to consider the developing animal or human separately from the adult, current testing strategies for developmental neurotoxicity (*see also* Chapter 3 by Cappon and Stump), and salient issues related to the risk assessment of infants and children.

2. BASIS FOR DIFFERENTIAL SENSITIVITY OF DEVELOPING ORGANISMS

The 1993 NRC report on pesticides in the diets of infants and children *(4)* noted that quantitative and qualitative differences in toxicity between children and adults are due in part to age-dependent differences in maturational state, toxicokinetic variables, and differential exposure. Such differences support the requirement to determine the effects of chemicals following exposure during the developing phase and to take into account differential exposure patterns for infants and children in setting pesticide residues.

2.1. Maturational State

The development of the nervous system begins in the fetus and is not complete, at least for humans, until the time of puberty. The integral structure of the nervous system occurs in highly sequenced steps, each dependent on the proper completion of the previous step. Brain development is a complex process starting with specialized structural and biochemical patterns of ontogenesis that proceed in timed multistage processes guided by chemical messengers. During embryogenesis, cells multiply at a rapid rate and are relatively undifferentiated. As organogenesis proceeds, cells become more differentiated and migrate to their appropriate location. Other important steps in nervous-system development include the formation of synapses, myelination of axons, and the development of connections between structural components. Exposure to chemicals prior to conception could cause chromosomal or changes in germ cells that could ultimately affect processes crucial to brain development. Chemical-induced alteration in the temporal or spatial organization of development during gestation and postnatally could directly or indirectly result in dysmorphology or alerted connectivity.

It is now widely accepted that the chief factor in determining the type of developmental neurotoxicity is the ontogenetic stage at the time of chemical perturbation *(15)*. This principle is illustrated by a paper published by Balduini et al. *(16)* who reported that the antimitotic agent methylazoxymethanol (MAMM) produced selective effects on learning and memory in rats depending on the day during gestation that exposure occurred. If exposure occurred on gestational day (GD) 18 or 19, learning deficits were observed, while exposure on any other day during gestation had no effect. Differential sensitivity of the developing nervous system might be related to the fact that rapidly differentiating cells are highly dependent on adequate metabolic support. Chemical-induced alterations in brain metabolism could cause different patterns of dysmorphology dependent on cell types that are differentiating at the time of exposure.

The developing brain is generally dependent on the synthesis of lipids to form new membranes *(9)*. During development, myelination continues for several years after birth and is sensitive to a number of environmental chemicals. An early deficit in myelin is usually persistent. The critical period associated with a permanent hypomyelination is prior to the onset of rapid myelin-membrane synthesis, from 8–14 d postnatal in the rat *(17)*.

Neurons seem to be differentially sensitive to specific signals during their development. Chemical signals that induce neuronal differentiation, growth, migration, and synaptogenesis are all potential sites of attack for environmental agents. Alterations in the timing of these chemical signals could have long-lasting effects on the connectivity of developing neuronal circuits. Differentiating cells are sensitive to alterations in conditions that affect available oxygen and nutrients *(9)*.

The developing nervous system is in a constant state of flux and presents a number of possible sites of attack for chemical perturbation. Since the adult nervous system does not have these sites of attack, it is clear that the developing nervous system will be differentially sensitive to chemical exposure. The point made by Dews *(12)*, however, that the developing nervous system is not always more sensitive than the adult is accurate. For example, acrylamide is a chemical that produces peripheral neuropathy in adult animals, but produces little or no effect following developmental exposure *(18)*. For some pesticides and chemicals, children and infants may be more sensitive than adults; for others less sensitive *(19)*. In addition, for some chemicals, only a subset of children may be uniquely sensitive. For example, acryodynia is a form of mercury poisoning that affects about 1 in 1000 children exposed. These examples illustrate the principle that neurotoxicity observed in adult animals will not be sufficient to predict developmental neurotoxicity.

2.2. Toxicokinetic Variables

The NRC report *(4)* concluded that quantitative differences in pesticide toxicity between children and adults can largely be attributed to differences in toxicokinetic factors, including absorption, metabolism, detoxification, and excretion of xenobiotic compounds. For example, it has also been estimated that the rate of absorption varies with the development of the gastrointestinal system and the volume of distribution depends on the degree of maturity as well as the solubility characteristics of the chemical. This observation is important since it has been estimated that for a well-known developmental neurotoxicant such as lead, adults absorb only about one-tenth of the lead ingested, while children will absorb about half *(4)*. It is also known that human infants have a diminished capacity to metabolize a number of drugs and other chemicals *(4)*. Inefficient metabolism could make the newborn more susceptible to chemicals that are converted to less toxic metabolites. However, there are relatively few studies on age-dependent interspecies differences in toxicokinetic and metabolism of xenobiotics such as pesticides. It is also known that rates of deactivation or activation, number of cell membrane receptors, and rates of excretion vary as a function of age. All of these factors support the conclusion that infants and children can respond differently than adults to chemical exposure and toxicokinetic data may be crucial in estimating risk for infants and children.

Another important feature of adults is that there are protective barriers such as the blood-brain barrier (BBB) that prevent some chemicals in the bloodstream from passing into the brain. It is known that the BBB does not develop fully in children until they are 1–2 yr of age *(19a)*. Therefore, chemicals with structural or other attributes that might prevent them from entering the brain of adults may be active in the developing brain. Furthermore, the placenta may not serve as a barrier to the many chemicals and their metabolites circulating in the bloodstream of the mother. Fetuses also lack full hepatic function until after the middle of gestation and may increase the risk of the fetus to chemicals that are detoxified by metabolism.

It has been suggested that age-dependent changes in body composition may also increase risk for infants and children. For example, the rate at which various bodily constituents increase and their relative proportions in the body change as a function of age. In addition, as the surface area of the infant or child changes, so does the extracellular-fluid volume. A larger extracellular-fluid volume as a function of age would tend to dilute out exposure to a given amount of a chemical. This suggests that for equivalent exposures, target sites in infants and children may be more at risk than in adults.

In terms of toxicity testing using animal models, it has been pointed out that routine studies on metabolism required by the EPA may provide data only on adult animals *(14)*, resulting in a data set that may not be appropriate for determining risk to infants and children. Where toxicokinetic variables appear to be significant in determining a toxic effect, such information in developing animals could prove essential.

2.3. Exposure

The NRC report *(4)* also found that infants and children differ qualitatively and quantitatively from adults in their exposure to pesticide residues in foods. Children tend to consume more calories relative to body weight and fewer types of foods than adults. Infants and children also tend to ingest more of certain types of foods than adults. The NRC report found that infants and children are exposed to pesticides from a variety of sources, including fruits and vegetables, breast milk, drinking water, air, at home and at school. In addition, children and infants exhibit behavioral patterns that could increase exposure to environmental chemicals. For example, it has been shown that pica, i.e., oral ingestion, of paint chips by children living in homes where lead-based paints had been used was a significant source of exposure for this metal. In the aggregate, infants and children are exposed to chemicals from both dietary and nondietary sources that are different from those of adults. In addition, exposure to chemicals having the same or similar mechanism of action frequently occurs, which could lead to cumulative toxicity. To account for these possibilities, the Food Quality Protection Act (FQPA) specifically requires that all route of exposures be part of the risk assessments to establish a pesticide tolerance and that the possibility of cumulative toxicity due to exposure to chemicals having similar mechanisms of action be considered.

In summary, there is clear evidence that the developing nervous system is differentially sensitive to chemical perturbation. Because of the dynamic state of the developing brain, there are many more possible sites of attack for chemicals than the adult brain. Exposure periods used in animals studies should cover the major phases of nervous-system development in order to be provide adequate protection for children and infants. Although not a part of routine assessments in developmental studies, toxicokinetic information in animal studies could provide crucial information relevant to estimating human health risk. Finally, in the exposure-assessment step of the risk-assessment process, age-dependent variations in exposure patterns must be taken into consideration.

3. TESTING STRATEGIES FOR DEVELOPMENTAL NEUROTOXICITY

3.1. Early Test Guidelines

Guidelines for the assessment of developmental neurotoxicity of pharmaceutical agents were introduced in Japan in 1974 and in Great Britain in 1975 *(11,20)*. The

Japanese requirements are for new drugs and include behavioral assessments of off-spring from females during organogenesis (teratology study) and exposure during the last third of gestation and throughout lactation (perinatal study). The regulations state that behavioral observations can be made by a series of procedures that measure motor capabilities, learning sensibility, or emotion. The 1975 British regulations are part of their studies on reproductive guidelines for new drugs and include the requirement that animals be tested for auditory, visual, and behavioral impairment. The guidelines for Great Britain were specified for studies involving exposure prior and after conception (fertility studies), as well as perinatal studies. In both Japan and Great Britain, the choice of the behavioral tests is not specified. Regulations concerning developmental neurotoxicity for food additives, industrial or environmental chemicals have not been promulgated in Japan or Great Britain. In 1983, the European Economic Community (EEC) proposed guidelines for preclinical reproductive and developmental toxicity testing for its member countries. Final guidelines accepted in 1985 call for studies to determine late effects of drugs on the progeny in terms of auditory, visual, and behavioral impairment. General behavioral teratology testing guidelines were proposed by the World Health Organization (WHO) *(21)*. The Organization of Economic Development and Cooperation (OEDC) *(22)* has recently issued a draft guideline for developmental-neurotoxicity testing of drugs chemicals.

The agency responsible for regulation of drugs in the United States, the Food and Drug Administration (FDA), has proposed guidelines on reproduction and developmental toxicity studies that would include developmental neurotoxicity assessments for direct food and color additives *(20)*. Included in these guidelines are a specific histopathological examination of tissue samples representative of all major areas and cellular elements of the brain, spinal cord, and peripheral nervous system (PNS), and a systematic examination of experimental animals inside and outside their cages using a defined battery of functional tests and clinical observations. The objective of the functional assessments is to determine chemical effects on cognitive, sensory, motor, and autonomic function in the mature and developing nervous systems.

3.2. Testing Guidelines for Environmental Agents

The EPA first issued a protocol for developmental neurotoxicity testing of environmental chemicals in 1986. These guidelines were devised to assess in rodents the potential functional and morphological hazards to the nervous system that may arise in the offspring from chemical exposure of the mother during lactation and gestation. The developmental neurotoxicity testing guideline involves a postnatal evaluation of offspring exposed via the mother including observations to detect gross neurological and behavioral abnormalities, tests of motor activity, auditory startle, and learning/memory. These guidelines assume that the nervous system involves a series of anatomical and functional changes over time, which requires assessment at multiple time-points. In addition, it is assumed that one single measure as adequate to identify a chemical-induced change in neural development. Instead, a battery of tests is needed to sample the various developmental steps indicative of changes in anatomical and functional development. Finally, the degree of concordance between anatomical and functional alterations plays an important role in weight of evidence determinations. The developmental neurotoxicity testing guidelines were revised in 1998 *(23)*.

Table 1
EPA's Developmental Neurotoxicity Test Guidelines

Measure	Time of assessment
Observation of dams	Twice during gestational dosing and twice during lactational dosing
Observation of pups	Daily cage side observations-all pups Outside cage observations-subset of pups on PND 4, 11, 21, 35, 45, and 60
Body weights	
Dams	At least weekly and on the day of delivery a PND 11 and 21
Pups	PND 4, 11, 17, 21, and biweekly thereafter
	Developmental milestones
Males	Prepubretal separation
Females	Vaginal opening
Motor activity	PND 13, 17, 21, 58–62
Auditory startle	PND 22, 58–62
Learning and memory	PND 21–24, 58–62
Neuropathology and brain weights	PND 11, end of study

The EPA developmental neurotoxicity testing protocol requires 20 or more litters per dose group and 3 or more dose groups, plus a vehicle control (Table 1). Dams are dosed from GD 6 through postnatal day (PND)10. EPA's protocol is largely based on the results of a Collaborative Teratology Study (CBTS) completed in 1985 *(24)*. The CBTS involved six laboratories that studied the developmental effects of two chemicals, *d*-amphetamine and methyl mercury, using a standard battery of tests for sensory, motor, and learning abilities. The CBTS found that behavioral data were reproducible across laboratories if collected under standardized conditions. In addition, it was found that the detection sensitivities of the tests were acceptable, requiring no more than 5–20% change from control values. It was also determined that replication within study allowed for adequate sample sizes to be tested and that the litter contributed significant amount of variability to behavioral data, supporting the argument that the litter should be the statistical unit. The collaborative study found little evidence that at doses that *d*-amphetamine produced behavioral or physical effects in the offspring at the doses tested. All laboratories found that gestational exposure to methyl mercury affected startle reactivity in the offspring at doses that were not maternally toxic. The generality of these findings was confirmed in two parallel studies *(25,26)* in which another battery of tests (Cincinnati Test Battery) was used to assess the two chemicals. This battery measured many of the same functions as the CBTS protocol, but tended to focus more on measures of neurological and behavioral development. Kutscher et al. *(27)* reported several anatomical changes in methyl mercury-treated animals from the CBTS study. These histopathological data provided support for many of the measures, including morphometric analysis, included in EPA's developmental neurotoxicity screening battery *(23)*. In general, the CBTS indicated that behavioral tests can be sensitive, reliable measures of developmental-neurotoxocity if protocols are standardized and trained personnel are used to conduct the study.

In a subsequent workshop *(8)*, a number of critical issues were addressed for assessing developmental neurotoxicity testing, including the comparability of end-points across species for development neurotoxicity, testing methods in developmental neurotoxicity for use in human risk assessment, weight-of-evidence and quantitative evaluation of data from developmental neurotoxicity studies, and triggers for developmental neurotoxicity testing. In this context, participants of this workshop were asked to review the human and experimental animal data on agents known to cause developmental neurotoxicity in humans, including lead, methyl mercury, phenytoin, drugs of abuse, polychlorinated biphenyls, ethanol, and ionizing radiation. There was a consensus among the chemical experts and participants in various breakout groups that the EPA developmental neurotoxicity testing protocol would have identified each of the agents discussed at the meeting *(28)*. Each agent was shown to have clear effects in rodents that would have been observed in one or more measures used in the EPA protocol. It was also concluded that at the level of functional category (sensory, motivational, cognitive and motor function, and social behavior), there was close agreement across species for all neurotoxic agents reviewed *(29)*.

It was also concluded that animal tests provide an adequate degree of comparability to humans and that quantitative differences between animals and humans are most likely due to differing toxicokinetic variables. There was also agreement that the assessment of developmental neurotoxicity should involve an evaluation of multiple categories of function, which supports the broad behavioral-testing battery described in the current EPA developmental neurotoxicity testing guidelines *(23)*. In fact, many of the tests described by the participants as being sensitive to known human developmental neurotoxicants are included in EPA's developmental neurotoxicity testing guidelines (*see* Chapter 3). It was also noted that for the chemicals discussed, it was frequently the case that behavioral effects were observed at doses below those to produce maternal toxicity, which supports the use of a high dose that should be or just below the threshold for the production of minimal maternal toxicity *(23)*. In addition, there was support for the assessment of various functions at different points in the life-span of the animal model. The latest testing point in most studies tended to be after sexual maturity similar to that used in the developmental neurotoxicity testing guidelines. There was no recommendation or consideration of longitudinal testing of animals beyond 1 or 2 yr of age to determine if early exposure might result in accelerated aging or the early onset of neurodegenerative disease.

As mentioned previously, Lochry *(13)* suggested that end-points used in routine developmental and reproductive toxicity studies could provide the data necessary to determine if a compound has potential developmental neurotoxicity in humans. This observation was followed up in a paper by Faber and O'Donoghue *(30)* who reported that 37 of the 41 developmental neurotoxicants they surveyed could be detected by the Chernoff/Kavlock assay, a battery of tests originally designed as a postnatal screen for developmental toxicity, including teratogenicity and fetotoxicity. This assay includes measures of birth weight, neonatal growth to PND 3, fetal viability, and neonatal survivability, and is much less comprehensive than the developmental neurotoxicity testing guidelines. These authors concluded that the developmental neurotoxicity testing guidelines may not be necessary since such chemicals could be detected in routine developmental toxicity-testing protocols. However, Goldey et al. *(31)* argued that the 41 chemicals selected by Faber and O'Donoghue *(30)* were known teratogens and should have been positive in the Chernoff/Kavlock assay. Goldey et al. *(31)* examined 126 developmental neurotoxicants from several chemical classes, including antiproliferative agents, drugs, food additives, metals, PCBs, pesticides, and solvents. These authors found that only 65% of these chemicals affected measures included in the Chernoff/Kavlock assay. It is interesting to note that the detection rate for pesticides was 50–70% and that there were important agents in each chemical class that were not detected in the Chernoff/Kavlock assay. Goldey et al. *(31)* concluded that reliance on the Chernoff/Kavlock screen could lead to a number of false-negatives for developmental neurotoxicants and that the assay should not be used to replace more comprehensive testing protocols such as the developmental neurotoxicity testing battery.

EPA's developmental neurotoxicity testing battery relies heavily on behavioral measures such as motor activity, startle reactivity, and learning/memory. This is important since it has been pointed out *(13)* that of the tests available for assessing developmental effects of chemicals, behavioral tests appear to be the most problematic. Over reliance on insensitive or highly variable tests could lead to false-negatives or the misidentification of potential human developmental neurotoxicants. To address this issue, Ulbrich and Palmer *(32)* reviewed developmental toxicity data from German regulatory submissions for drugs over a 10-yr period. These studies included measures of fertility, reproduction, embryotoxicity, and behavior. Of 85 drugs that produced behavioral effects, it was observed for 24 that behavioral changes were the only adverse effect detected at any dose, or that occurred at the lowest observable adverse effect level (LOAEL) together with other signs of developmental toxicity. This observation supports the use of behavioral tests for all substances to which the developing human may be exposed *(32)*.

The NRC report *(4)* on pesticides in the diets of infants and children also recommended that the EPA should continue to revise its published guidelines on developmental and functional neurotoxicity testing as new information emerges from the actual conduct of preregistration studies and from on-going research in rodent neurotoxicity. In this regard, Makris et al. *(33)* compared the NOELs of 12 chemicals submitted to the EPA that were tested for adult neurotoxicity, developmental and reproductive toxicity, and developmental neurotoxicity. The data set included nine pesticides (aldicarb, carbaryl, carbofuran, molinate, DEET, emamectin, fipronil, chlorpyrifos, and Chemical X [a nonfood use pesticide]) and three solvents (1,1,1-TCE, TGME, and isopropanol). The survey performed by Makris et al. *(33)* found that there were treatment-related effects on the nervous system for seven of the nine pesticides, while for DEET and Chemical X, findings in the offspring were limited to changes in motor activity at the highest dose tested. For the solvent TGME, alterations in startle reactivity were observed at the highest dose tested, while no findings in the offspring were observed for the other two solvents. Significant decreases in brain weight were noted with five of the nine pesticides, while treatment-related morphometric alterations were noted for three of the six pesticides for which such data were provided.

Table 2
Toxicology Data Requirements for Pesticides

Acute studies–oral, dermal, inhalation
Irritation studies–eye, dermal
Dermal sensitization
90-D feeding studies (rodent and nonrodent)
Chronic feeding studies (rodent and nonrodent)
Oncogenicity studies in two species of rodents
Developmental toxicity studies (rodent and nonrodent)
Two-generation reproduction study (rodents)
Mutagenicity study
General metabolism study (rodents)

Makris et al. *(33)* also found that the no adverse effect level (NOAEL) for developmental neurotoxicity was lower than or about equal to NOELs for acute and/or subchronic neurotoxicity in adult animals for six of the nine chemicals. In eight of nine cases, the NOEL for developmental neurotoxicity was lower than that of the fetal NOEL from prenatal developmental toxicity studies and was equivalent for the remaining chemical. In addition, in two of the nine cases, the NOEL for developmental neurotoxicity was lower than or equal to that for any adult or offspring end-point from prenatal developmental, reproduction, or neurotoxicity studies. These observations indicate that the developmental neurotoxicity test battery is capable of detecting hazards and generating dose-response relationships that could be useful in evaluating chemicals for potential human developmental neurotoxicity (*see* Chapter 3). These results further support the conclusion that the developmental neurotoxicity test battery is as sensitive as or more sensitive than reproductive and developmental toxicity protocols.

Although EPA's developmental neurotoxicity testing battery appears to be relatively sensitive to developmental neurotoxicants and provides data in rodents that evaluates the full range of potential neurotoxic effects in humans (i.e., sensory, motor, learning/ memory, developmental milestones, sexual maturation), there are several issues that remain problematic concerning its use in a screening context. One notable concern is that the developmental neurotoxicity test battery is not currently required for the registration of a food-use chemical (Table 2). For any chemical that is registered for a food use, two developmental toxicity studies (rodent and nonrodent) and a two-generation reproduction study in rats are required. The developmental toxicity protocol exposes mothers only during the prenatal period, while the reproductive study includes some postnatal exposure, but this is only indirect, through breast milk. Offspring of exposed mothers are not evaluated for nervous system structural or functional changes in the reproductive study. A 90-d neurotoxicity study in adult rats may be required, depending on the outcome of the acute-toxicity studies or structure-activity relationship considerations. Acute or subchronic delayed neurotoxicity testing in hens may be required if the substance is an organophosphate or a metabolite or degradation product, which may cause inhibition of acetylcholinesterase, or is structurally related to a chemical that causes delayed neurotoxicity. Under certain circumstances, a developmental neurotoxicity study may also be required. The decision to require such testing is based on criteria or triggers from both adult and developmental toxicity data and a weight-of-evidence review of all available data for each chemical. Triggers for developmental neurotoxicity testing include if the chemical has been shown to cause neuropathy/neurotoxicity in adults, is a hormonally active compound, or causes other types of developmental toxicity. As pointed out by the NRDC *(14)*, this tiered testing strategy has rarely led to the use of the developmental neurotoxicity testing protocol. In fact, the developmental neurotoxicity testing guideline has only been required for the 12 chemicals mentioned in the survey by Makris et al. *(33)*.

EPA's developmental-neurotoxicity testing protocol exposes mothers from GD 6 through PND 10. The development of the brain continues well after birth in both animals and humans and it has been argued that termination of exposure at PND 10 is not adequate *(14)*. Organogenesis and histogenesis are completed prenatally in the rat, while neurogenesis and migration are complete by PND 10 *(11)*. Synaptogenesis, gliogenesis, and myelination also begin prenatally in the rat, but are not complete until maturity. However, brain weight of the rat is more than 80% of maturity at PND 21 or weaning in most strains *(4)* and all postural, locomotor, and related skills have developed by this time as well *(11)*. PND 21 in the rat is approximately similar to 2 yr of age in the human *(4)* and exposure to this time could be sufficient to protect infants and young children. One possibility is to expose pups directly during the postlactational stage to model the extensive postnatal growth and development of the human brain. Unfortunately, there are few studies that have actually compared effects in studies terminated at PND 11 vs at weaning. In the Makris et al. *(33)* survey, studies were conducted with dosing extended to weaning for DDET, emamectin, TGME, and isopropanol, and there were no obvious effects that could be related to late lactation dosing of the offspring via the diet and/or maternal milk. One compelling reason for extending the postnatal dosing period to d 21 is that this protocol would be consistent with other testing protocols. This could alleviate certain logistical problems associated with conducting the developmental neurotoxicity protocol as a stand-alone test. Furthermore, exposure of pups until weaning is consistent with the proposed OCED testing guidelines for developmental neurotoxicity *(22)*.

It has also been argued that the developmental neurotoxicity protocol fails to assess test animals for a long enough period to detect delayed, or latent, effects from toxicity to the developing brain *(14)*. The developmental neurotoxicity testing protocol terminates testing at about PND 60–62, which is well beyond sexual maturity in the rat. It has been suggested that exposure to neurotoxic compounds may be followed years or decades later by clinically evident neurological disease *(34)*. This author points out that the importance of life-long assessment has been repeatedly demonstrated in humans, but such studies are relatively rare in experimental studies of neurotoxicity. Although it may be the case that early exposure to chemicals may increase the risk for neurological diseases that typically develop later in life, such as Alzheimer's or Parkinson's disease (AD/PD), experimental data to support this hypothesis are scarce. Several animal studies have been reported indicating that developmental exposure to chemicals such as triethyl tin or methylmercury can have long-lasting effects on the nervous system. However, in these studies, developmental exposure resulted in functional alterations early in life, which were followed by an appearance of new symptoms or exacerbation of existing symptoms as a function of aging. In the context of screening chemicals for potential developmental neurotoxicity, such effects would have been detected using a battery similar to the developmental-neurotoxicity testing protocol. For example, in the study by Barone et al. *(35)*, rats were dosed with triethyl tin on PND 10 and examined across the life-span for neural damage and functional deficits. In neonatal rats, histological analysis indicated gliosis in the neocortex and loss of neurons in the hippocampus. In addition, there was a significant impairment in a spatial maze test at PND 23. Such effects would most likely have been identified by the developmental neurotoxicity testing protocol. Significant impairments in spatial learning, however, were not observed at 3 or 12 mo of age, although at 2 yr of age, the triethyl tin-treated animals performed more poorly than age-matched controls, suggesting an exacerbation of the triethyl tin effect with aging. Although the possibility of accelerated aging produced by early exposure to an environmental chemical is a crucial finding, it does not suggest that the developmental neurotoxicity testing protocol is insensitive to the developmental neurotoxic effects of triethyl tin. There are few studies showing no anatomical or functional changes as those that would be measured by the developmental neurotoxicity testing protocol up to d 60 of age followed by the appearance of neurotoxicity that resembles neurodegenerative diseases such as AD/PD late in life. Although this remains a fruitful area for future research, required lifetime longitudinal assessments in developmental studies does not seem warranted at this time.

Another concern that has been raised is that EPA's pesticide requirements include no testing for disruption of the endocrine system *(14)*. In addition, the NRC report *(4)* recommended that serum thyroid hormones T3 and T4 and serum thyroid stimulating hormone (TSH) should be routinely added to the EPA chronic/carcinogenicity study protocol or to the subchronic toxicity protocol for the rat so that adverse effects on thyroid function can be determined earlier. The FQPA *(35a)* and amendments to the Safe Drinking Water Act provide the legislative basis for developing and implementing a strategy for screening and testing chemicals for endocrine disruption. EPA's Endocrine Disruptor Screen and Testing Advisory Committee (EDSTAC) has recommended a Tier I screening battery to evaluate the potential for chemicals to act as activators or repressors of the estrogen, androgen, and thyroid receptor using in vitro cell-reporter assays *(35b)*. Other in vivo tests will include a uterotrophic assay to examine effects mediated by the estrogen receptor, an assay to evaluate effects on androgen-receptor function, and a peripubertal test that monitors development of the hypothalamic-pituitary-thyroid gonadal axis. EDSTAC has also recommended additional tests to characterize the nature, likelihood, and dose-response relationship of endocrine disruption of estrogen, androgen, and thyroid activity in humans and wildlife. For purposes of screening, it is anticipated that a two-generation reproduction study will be adequate for this purpose. There is no evidence that chemicals that act on neuroendocrine development would be missed by the proposed two-tier testing strategy or that the developmental-neurotoxicity testing protocol should be required for such chemicals.

In summary, EPA's developmental neurotoxicity testing protocol measures a full range of neurobiological functions in animals. The battery appears to be sensitive to known human developmental neurotoxicants and is relatively sensitive as compared to other measures of developmental and reproductive toxicity. Measures of neurotoxicity in adult animals do not seem sufficient to predict changes in developing animals. It is true that the developmental neurotoxicity testing protocol has been used infrequently and that other measures of developmental and reproductive toxicity are not fully sensitive to developmental neurotoxicity. There is scientific and logistical support for the recommendation to extend the postnatal dosing period to weaning. The possible relationship between early exposure and increased risk of neurodegenerative disease deserves additional research, but there is insufficient data to support introduce lifetime observations into current testing protocols. Finally, proposed in vitro and in vivo tests for endocrine-disruption appear sufficient to detect chemicals that may alter neuroendocrine function during development.

4. RISK ASSESSMENT ISSUES

The purpose of risk assessment is to set acceptable levels exposure. The process typically begins with a determination of a critical adverse effect based on the evaluation of all available human and animal data. An estimate of daily exposure to the human population that is likely to occur without appreciable risk over a lifetime is called the Reference Dose (RfD) or Reference Concentration (RfC) *(36)*. Calculation of the RfD/ RfC is based on determination of a NOAEL or LOAEL from a critical study or studies. The LOAEL is defined as the lowest dose at which there is a statistically or biologically significant increase in the incidence of an adverse effect. The NOAEL is defined as the highest dose at which there is no statistically significant increase in the presence of an adverse effect.

Historically, derivation of the RfD/RfC is based on dividing the NOAEL or LOAEL by safety or uncertainty factors to account for variation in sensitivity among members of the human population, animal-to-human extrapolation, less-than-lifetime exposure, and extrapolating from a LOAEL to the NOAEL in the absence of a NOAEL. In addition, modifying factors may be added to account for scientific uncertainties such as the quality or completeness of the data set. The default value for the uncertainty factors is 10, but may be reduced to another number depending on the availability of other information. Dose-response data from human and animal studies may also be expressed by determining an effective dose (ED) estimated for a given level of response, e.g., the ED10 would be the effective dose that produces a 10% change in response. The lower confidence interval associated with the estimate of the ED is defined as the Benchmark Dose (BMD). Analysis of dose-response data from developmental studies is conducted as part of the overall dose-response evaluation of all available human and animal data. The NOAEL or BMD may also be divided by the estimate of the human exposure to derive a margin of exposure to determine if there are adequate controls on exposure to humans. Although exposure in developmental protocols involves repeated dosing pre- and/or postnatally, it is assumed that adverse developmental effects may be produced by a single exposure occurring during a critical period of development.

In the NRC *(4)* report on pesticides in the diets of infants and children, concerns were raised about the ability of the current risk-assessment process to adequately protect the health of infants and children to pesticide exposure. There are several reports in the literature to support the application of a 10-fold factor to protect 80–95% of the population *(36–39)*. In addition, Sheehan and Gaylor *(40)* reported that the ratios of LD50s of adult to young animals for 238 chemicals were less than 10-fold 86% of the time. Renwick and Lazarus *(41)* also found that the toxicokinetics of infants and children do not differ by an order of magnitude from adults, while Renwick *(42)* concluded from a comparative study of toxicokinetics of young and adult animals and humans that a 10-fold intraspecies factor may provide adequate protection. The NRC report agreed that although the intraspecies uncertainty factor for variation within the human population generally provides adequate protection for infants and children, this population may be uniquely susceptible to chemical exposure at critical states of development. Because of specific periods of vulnerability during development, the NRC report *(4)* recommended an additional uncertainty factor of 10 should be considered when there is evidence of postnatal developmental toxicity and when data from toxicity testing relative to infants and children are incomplete. It should be noted that the NRC report *(4)* indicated that a new, additional uncertainty factor was not necessary. Instead, the NRC committee recommended an extension of an uncertainty factor now routinely applied by agencies related to completeness of the data set. The NRC recommendation is based on the assumption that in absence of data to the contrary infants and children should be considered to be more sensitive to chemicals such as pesticides than adults. In response to the concern about the safety of infants and children, the EPA must take into account that for US threshold effects, an additional 10-fold margin of safety for other chemical residues and other sources of exposure be applied for infants and children to take into account potential pre- and postnatal toxicity and completeness of data with respect to exposure and toxicity to infants and children.

The EPA has on occasion used an uncertainty factor applied to the RfD to account for deficiencies in the available data set. In fact, according to Dourson et al. *(37)*, if data on children's health are not adequate, then an uncertainty factor has been used to account for such deficiencies. For example, a modifying factor of 3 may be applied if either a prenatal toxicity study or a two-generational reproduction study is missing or a factor of 10 may be applied if both are missing. A database uncertainty factor has not been applied in the past for the lack of developmental neurotoxicity data. Inclusion of the developmental-neurotoxicity testing protocol in the core set of required tests (Table 2) should alleviate the need to consider an additional uncertainty or safety factor for the absence of developmental-neurotoxicity data. In general, the size of the uncertainty factor for completeness of the data set will ultimately depend on all available information and how much the missing data may have on estimating the toxicity of the chemical to infants and children.

In summary, concern about adequately protecting infants and children has led to a change in the way regulatory agencies conduct risk assessments. Based largely on recommendations from a NRC report on pesticides in the diets of infants and children, regulatory agencies such as the EPA must consider an additional safety factor would protect infants and children, taking into account their potentially greater vulnerability, as well as their unique patterns of exposure. The application of such an safety factor depends on the completeness of the data base with regard to available information concerning developmental toxicity and exposure data. The EPA has been criticized *(14)* for not using this additional safety factor more frequently in considering pesticide tolerances. In fact, the Agency has applied a 10-fold factor in only about 10% in over 100 decisions. What constitutes a "reliable" or "complete" database to be used in the application of such a safety factor continues to stir debate.

5. SUMMARY AND CONCLUSIONS

The potential vulnerability of infants and children has led to the development of testing guidelines for both pharmaceuticals and environmental chemicals. Recently, the approach taken by regulatory agencies such as the EPA to protect infants and children from overexposure to pesticides and other chemicals has been criticized. One major concern is that although a mechanism is in place to trigger the use developmental-neurotoxicity testing based on results from a core battery of toxicity tests, the developmental-neurotoxicity testing battery has been used only infrequently. Another concern is that the current battery may not include the appropriate tests to evaluate developmental effects in infants and children and may not be sensitive to developmental neurotoxicants. The developmental neurotoxicity testing battery includes measures of sensory, motor, and cognitive development and was validated several years ago by the CBTS. In a workshop held in 1989 *(24)* comparing the effects of several known developmental neurotoxicants in humans and animal models, it was concluded that the developmental neurotoxicity testing battery would have detected all of the chemicals discussed. In addition, it was determined that animal models measure qualitative similarities between animals and humans, although quantitative differences due to toxicokinetic and other factors are apparent. In cases where the developmental neurotoxicity testing protocol has been compared to other measures of reproductive and developmental toxicity, as well as adult neurotoxicity testing, it has been shown to be relatively sensitive and specific.

Although there is evidence that current application of an uncertainty factor for intrapopulation variability may be sufficient to protect most of the population, including infants and children, a report by the NRC *(4)* has raised concern about differential vulnerability of infants and children during critical phases of development This concern led to the passage of the FQPA in 1966, which indicates that, depending on the adequacy of the available data, an additional safety factor must be considered to protect infants and children. The actual application of such a safety factor in the evaluation of over 100 pesticides has not been excessive (about 10%), which has stimulated considerable debate and discussion concerning the definition what constitutes "reliable data" on children's toxicity and exposure to chemicals such as pesticides.

REFERENCES

1. Wilson, J. G. (1977) Embryotoxicity of drugs in man, in *Handbook of Teratology* (Wilson, J. G. and Fraser, F. C., eds.), Plenum Press, New York, pp. 309–355.
2. National Academy of Sciences (NAS) (1988). *Research on Children and Adolescents with Mental, Behavioral, and Developmental Disorders.* National Academy Press, Washington, DC.
3. US Environmental Protection Agency (EPA) (1998) Suggested probabilistic risk assessment methodology for evaluating pesticides with a common mechanism of toxicity: Organophosphate Case Study, US EPA Scientific Advisory Panel.
4. National Research Council (NRC) (1993) *Pesticides in the Diets of Infants and Children.* National Academy Press, Washington, DC.
5. Kimmel, C. A. (1988) Current status of behavioral teratology: Science and regulation. *CRC Crit. Rev. Toxicol.* **19,** 1–10.
6. Hutchings, D. E. (ed.) (1989) *Prenatal Abuse of Licit and Illicit Drugs*, vol 562. New York Academy of Science, New York.
7. Riley, E. P. and Vorhees, C. V. (eds.)(1986) *Handbook of Behavioral Teratology.* Plenum Press, New York.

8. Kimmel, C. A., Rees, D. C., and Francis, E. Z. (1990) Qualitative and quantitative vomparability of human and animal developmental neurotoxicity. *Neurotoxicol Teratol.* **12**, 175–292.

9. Harry, G. J. (ed.) (1994) *Developmental Neurotoxicology.* CRC Press, Boca Raton, FL.

10. Rees, D. C., Francis, E. Z., and Kimmel, C. A. (1990) Scientific and regulatory issues relevant to assessing risk for developmental neurotoxicity: an overview. *Neurotoxicol. Teratol.* **12**, 175–181.

11. Acuff, K. D. and Vorhees, C. V. (1998) Neurobehavioral teratology, in *Introduction to Neurobehavioral Toxicology: Food and Environment* (Niesink, R. J. M., Jaspers, R. M. A., Kornet, L. M. W., van Ree, J. M., and Tilson, H. A., eds.), CRC Press, New York, pp. 27–69.

12. Dews, P. B. (1986) On the assessment of risk, in *Developmental Behavioral Pharmacology* (Krasnegor, N., Gray, J., and Thompson, T., eds.), Lawrence Erlbaum, Hillsdale, NJ, pp. 53–65.

13. Lochry, E. A. (1987) Concurrent use of behavioral/functional testing in existing reproductive and developmental toxicity screens: practical considerations. *J. Am. Coll. Toxicol.* **6**, 433–439.

14. Wallinga, D. (1998) *Putting Children First: Making Pesticide Levels in Food Safer for Infants and Children.* Natural Resources Defense Council.

15. Rodier, P. M. (1976) Critical periods for behavioral anomalies in mice. *Environ. Health Perspect.* **18**, 79–83.

16. Balduini, W., Elsner, J., Lambardelli, G., Peruzzi, G., and Cattabeni, F. (1991) Treatment with methylazoxymethanol at different gestational days: two way shuttle box avoidance and residential maze activity in rat offspring. *Neurotoxicology* **12**, 677–686.

17. Wiggins, R. C. and Fuller, G. N. (1978) Early postnatal starvation causes lasting brain hypomyelination. *J. Neurochem.* **30**, 1231–1238.

18. Edwards, P. M. (1976) The insensitivity of the developing rat foetus to the toxic effects of acrylamide. *Chem. Biol. Interact.* **12**, 13–18.

19. Gaines, T. B. and Linder, R. E. (1986) Acute toxicity of pesticides in adult and weanling rats. *Fund. Appl. Toxicol.* **7**, 299–308.

19a. Lou, H. C. (1982) *Developmental Neurology.* Raven Press, New York.

20. Vorhees, C. V. (1986) Comparison and critique of government regulations for behavioral teratology, in *Handbook of Behavioral Teratology* (Riley, E. P. and Vorhees, C. V., eds.), Plenum Press, New York, pp. 49–66.

21. World Health Organization (WHO) (1986) Draft guidelines for the assessment of drugs and other chemicals for behavioral teratogenicity. WHO Regional Office for Europe, Copenhagen.

22. Organization of Economic Cooperation and Development (OECD) (1998) OECD Guideline for the Testing of Chemicals. Proposal for a New Guideline 426 Developmental Neurotoxicity Study: Draft Document. OECD.

23. US Environmental Protection Agency (EPA) (1998) Health Effects Test Guidelines: Developmental Neurotoxicity Study. OPPTS 870.6300, EPA Document 712-C–98–239, Washington, DC.

24. Kimmel, C. A., Buelke-Sam, J., and Adams, J. (1985) Collaborative behavioral teratology study: implications, current applications and future directions. *Neurobehav. Toxicol. Teratol.* **7**, 669–674.

25. Vorhees, C. V. (1985) Behavioral effects of prenatal d-amphetamine in rats: a parallel trial to the Collaborative Behavioral Teratology Study. *Neurobehav. Toxicol. Teratol.* **7**, 709–716.

26. Vorhees, C. V. (1985) Behavioral effects of prenatal methylmercury in rats: a parallel trial to the Collaborative Behavioral Teratology Study. *Neurobehav. Toxicol. Teratol.* **7**, 717–725.

27. Kutscher, C. L., Sembrat, M, Kutscher, C. S., and Kutscher, N. L. (1985) Effects of the high methylmercury dose used in the Collaborative Behavioral Teratology Study on Brain Anatomy. *Neurobehav. Toxicol. Teratol.* **7**, 775–777.

28. Francis, E. Z., Kimmel, C. A., and Rees, D. C. (1990) Workshop on the qualitative and quantitative comparability of human and animal developmental neurotoxicity: summary and implications. *Neurotoxicol. Teratol.* **12**, 285–292.

29. Stanton, M. E. and Spear, L. P. (1990) Workshop on the qualitative and quantitative comparability of human and animal developmental neurotoxicity, Work Group I Report: comparability of measures of developmental neurotoxicity in humans and laboratory animals. *Neurotoxicol. Teratol.* **12**, 261–267.

30. Faber, W. D. and O'Donoghue, J. L. (1991) Does the Chernoff-Kavlock screening assay for developmental neurotoxicity detect developmental neurotoxicants? *Toxicologist* **11**, 345A.

31. Goldey, E. S., Tilson, H. A., and Crofton, K. M. (1995) Implications of the use of neonatal birth weight, growth, viability, and survival data from predicting developmental neurotoxicity: a survey of the literature. *Neurotoxicol. Teratol.* **17**, 313–332.

32. Ulbrich, B. and Palmer, A. K. (1996) Neurobehavioral aspects of developmental toxicity testing. *Environ. Health Perspect.* **104**, 407–412.

33. Makris, S., Raffale, K., Sette, W., and Seed, J. (1998) A retrospective analysis of twelve developmental neurotoxicity studies submitted to the USEPA Office of Prevention, Pesticides, and Toxic Substances (OPPTS). Presented to the EPA's Science Advisory Panel, December 8–9, 1998.

34. Reuhl, K. R. (1991) Delayed expression of neurotoxicity: the problem of silent damage. *Neurotoxicology* **12**, 341–346.

35. Barone, S., Stanton, M. E., and Mundy, W. R. (1995) Neurotoxic effects of neonatal triethyltin (TET) exposure are exacerbated with aging. *Neurobiol. Aging* **16**, 723–735.

35a. Federal Insecticide, Fungicide and Rodenticide Act, as amended by the Food Quality Protection Act (1996).

35b. Endocrine Disruptor Screening and Testing Advisory Committee (EDSTAC). At http://intranet.epa.gov/opp00002/references/agency.com.htm.

36. Barnes, D. G. and Dourson, D. G. (1998) Reference dose (RfD): description and use in human health risk assessments. *Reg. Toxicol. Pharmacol.* **8**, 471–486.

37. Dourson, M. L. and Stara, J. F. (1983) Regulatory history and experimental support of uncertainty (safety) factors. *Reg. Toxicol. Pharmacol.* **3**, 224–238.

38. Calabrese, E. F. (1985) Uncertainty factors and interindividual variation. *Reg. Toxicol. Pharmacol.* **5**, 190–196.

39. Dourson, M. L., Felter, S. P., and Robinson, D. (1996) Evolution of science-based uncertainty factors in noncancer risk assessment. *Reg. Toxicol. Pharmacol.* **24**, 108–120.

40. Sheehan, D. M. and Gaylor, D. W. (1990) Analysis of the adequacy of safety factors. *Teratology* **41**, 590–591.

41. Renwick, A. G. and Lazarus, N. R. (1998) Human variability and noncancer risk assessment-an analysis of the default uncertainty factor. *Reg. Toxicol. Pharmacol.* **27**, 3–20.

42. Renwick, A. G. (1988) Toxicokinetics in infants and children in relation to the ADI and TDI. *Food Addit. Contam.* **15**, 17–35.

II
DRUGS OF ABUSE

5

Electrophysiologic Evidence of Neural Injury or Adaptation in Cocaine Dependence

Kenneth R. Alper, Leslie S. Prichep,
E. Roy John, Sharon C. Kowalik,
and Mitchell S. Rosenthal

1. INTRODUCTION

The electroencephalogram (EEG) is an emergent phenomenon of neural activity, which suggests that the EEG might reflect the apparently abnormal neurobiology observed in cocaine dependence. The EEG is noninvasive, inexpensive, and quantitative analysis of the EEG (QEEG) is based on information processing technology that is constantly growing with respect to analytic power and accessibility. Clinically, QEEG has been shown to be sensitive to psychiatric conditions, such as depression or attention deficit hyperactivity disorder (ADHD) that are often comorbid with cocaine dependence (1–3). Pretreatment QEEG has been shown to be predictive of subsequent psychotropic drug response in patients with a variety of psychiatric disorders evaluated prospectively (4,5). Neural injury or adaptation in cocaine dependence resulting in changes in the underlying sources of the EEG and reflected quantitatively in the QEEG, could be relevant to "staging" the disorder with respect to the identification of reversible vs irreversible components, and could potentially provide an approach to the development or selection of treatment. This chapter focuses on data obtained from a large population of cocaine-dependent subjects in our ongoing National Institute on Drug Abuse (NIDA) funded work on cocaine dependence. The chapter first provides a brief overview of structural and metabolic imaging studies in cocaine dependence, then reviews studies of EEG power spectral findings in chronic cocaine exposure in animals and humans, and our work on persistence of QEEG abnormality and evidence of electrophysiologic heterogeneity and its clinical correlates in cocaine dependence. Lastly, we attempt an interpretation of our QEEG findings will be considered in the context of hypothetical mechanisms of neural injury or adaptation.

From: Handbook of Neurotoxicology, Vol. 2
Edited by: E. J. Massaro © Humana Press Inc., Totowa, NJ

2. REVIEW OF THE LITERATURE ON COCAINE AND THE EEG POWER SPECTRUM

2.1. Acute Effects in Animals and Humans

Acute administration of cocaine in rats reportedly results in diminished slow EEG power and overall amplitudes, and increased beta frequency power *(6–10)*. These EEG effects appear to be mediated by dopamine (DA) to an important extent, as evidenced by their temporal correspondence to DA levels in the prefrontal cortex and their diminution by D_1 antagonist *(6–9)*. Relative to cocaine-naïve rats, cocaine-sensitized rats also reportedly show a greater relative decrement of EEG power in the delta and theta bands in response to an acutely administered dose of cocaine *(10)*. The possibility that this greater reduction in slow activity reflects increased DA signal transduction is supported by Leung and Yim *(11)* who reported on a delta-frequency rhythm recorded directly from the NAc that they termed "accumbens delta." This delta activation was desynchronized by electrical stimulation of the ventral tegmental area (VTA), suggesting suppression by endogenous DA release. The effect of VTA stimulation on accumbens delta was blocked by haloperidol.

In humans, increased beta power in the EEG following acute cocaine administration, first reported by Berger *(12)* has been well-replicated *(13–15)*. Similar to results reported in animals, the acute effects of cocaine on slow EEG activity may differ as a function of prior exposure to cocaine *(10)*. Relatively inexperienced intranasal cocaine users challenged with intravenous (IV) cocaine have reportedly evidenced a transient delta increase in addition to the expected, and more persistent beta increase in the first 5 min following the injection *(16)*, which coincides with the expected time of peak euphoria *(17)*. However, more experienced intravenous users tested in a later study did not evidence a delta increase *(14)*. The transient enhancement of delta activity in relatively naïve, but not chronic, users could reflect a neuroadaptation due to chronic use, possibly sensitization, resulting in a progressive diminution of activity in global EEG modes (*see* Subheading 2.4.). However, the observation of more beta activity in IV users vs smokers *(18)*, suggests a possible effect of prior route of administration on the EEG.

2.2. Chronic Effects in Animals and Humans

Table 1 summarizes QEEG studies in chronic cocaine-dependent subjects during abstinence as compared to normal controls. Overall, there appears to be significant agreement among these published studies, with respect to reports of slow wave deficit and/or beta excess (in at least a subgroup of subjects). Thus, the chronic QEEG effects of cocaine in animals and humans generally appear to involve some combination of diminished slow activity and/or increased fast activity.

In the studies summarized in Table 1, the EEGs were recorded in the eyes closed resting condition, with the exception of Costa and Bauer *(19)*, who used the eyes open condition. In addition to the comparisons made to a normative database included in the table, Herning et al. *(15)* also reported comparisons to a group of ten controls in the same study, and found that the cocaine users differed only with regard to beta excess. In two studies in which the route of administration was not reported (NR) *(19,20)*, personal communication with the authors suggested a predominance of crack cocaine

Table 1
QEEG in Cocaine Dependence During Drug Abstinence Compared to Normal Controls

Study	N	Length of drug abstinence	Route of administration	EEG power (absolute/relative)			
				Δ	θ	α	β
Alper et al. (21)	7	15.3 d	IN/crack only	↓/↓	0/↓	↑/↑	↑/0 (12.5–25 Hz)
Bauer and Kranzler (90)	18	≤14 d	—	0/0	0/0	0/0	0/0[s];0/0[f]
Noldy et al. (18)	9	2–30 d	IN[7]/IV[2]	NC	NC	NC	↓/↓[β]
Roemer et al. (20)	90	(median 90 d)	NR	↓/↓	↓/↓	0/↑	0/↑ (12.5–25 Hz)
Prichep et al. (132)	52	5–10 d	IN/crack only	↓/↓	↓/↓	0/↑	0/0 (12.5–25 Hz)
Costa and Bauer (19)	21	2.9 mo	NR	0/0	0/0	0/0	↑/0 (13.6–19.0 Hz) ↑/↑ (19.1–13.0 Hz)
Herning et al. (15)	33	10.3 d	"Primarily IV"	NR/↓	NR/↓	NR/↓	NR/↑ (13.6–50.0 Hz)
Prichep et al. (5)	19	5–14 d	IN/crack only	↓/↓	↓/↓	↑/↑	0/0 (12.5–25 Hz)
	16		IN/crack only	↓/↓	↓/↓	0/↑	0/↑ (12.5–25 Hz)

Abbreviations: NR, not reported; IN, intranasal; IV, intravenous.

over IV. Prichep et al. *(5)* reported two QEEG subtypes in the study population at baseline, which differed with respect to treatment outcome.

In four of the studies listed in Table 1, a relative or absolute beta increase was seen *(15,18–20)*. Four studies report decreased delta *(18,20–22)*. These studies in which reduced delta and theta power were noted utilized values derived from normative databases and visual inspection and automatic detection, with exclusion of artifactual epochs to control for EEG artifact. The single study that did not note a slow wave deficit *(19)* relied on a mathematical algorithm to reduce the effect of ocular artifact without the actual exclusion of any artifactual epochs. This is a methodological factor that might have been particularly likely to have affected delta-frequency findings; also the lack of a normative database and inclusion of eyes open data might have limited sensitivity. Excess relative alpha activity was reported in several studies *(14,20–24)*, and was present in one of the two subtypes noted in Prichep et al. *(5)*. The existence of EEG heterogeneity within the cocaine dependent population, which is discussed in Subheading 3.5., is potentially another important factor in the comparability of results reported in the literature.

2.3. QEEG Findings in Other Substances of Abuse

The QEEG findings reported in cocaine-dependent patients appear to have a distinct profile different from those reported in other substance use or other disorders that are frequently comorbid with crack-cocaine dependence. A delta deficit has not generally been reported in alcohol or cannabis dependence, or HIV infection. Reported QEEG characteristics of alcohol dependence include deficit alpha and excess beta and theta *(25–27)*. Cannabis abuse has been shown to be characterized by excess relative power in alpha *(28–30)*, a feature shared with cocaine abuse. There are prominent distinguishing features as well, including the finding of decreased absolute power in slow waves in cocaine but not cannabis dependence.

QEEG data on heroin dependence is scant. However, reported histories of dependence on heroin or intravenous drug abusers (IVDA) were an exclusion criteria mitigating against a potential confound of opiate dependence in our study population. Crack cocaine is a reported risk factor for human immunodeficiency virus (HIV), another confound related to drug abuse *(31)*. Abnormal QEEG has been reported in HIV-seropositive patients *(32)*. The New York City Department of Health has reported an overall seroprevalence of only 7.6% in 1482 Phoenix house clients *(33)*, probably because of the relatively low prevalence of a history of using the IV route of administration. However a reported history of HIV seropositivity, or constitutional signs of HIV, was an exclusion criterion in our study, and the QEEG findings we have reported do not resemble those of early HIV infection in which slow-frequency EEG power is reportedly increased *(32)*.

2.4. Cocaine and Modulation of Cortical EEG Activity

The results in human subjects and animals, chronically or acutely exposed to cocaine appear to share the common general attributes of diminished slow or enhanced fast EEG activity. The effects of such exposure may be viewed as generally consistent with the transition from global to local EEG modes *(25,34,35)*. Global EEG modes tend to originate from sources with a relatively widely dispersed topographic distribution

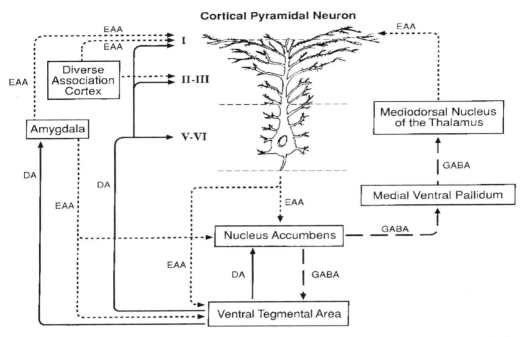

Fig. 1. The cortical pyramidal neuron, the putative generator of delta EEG power, in the frontal cortex, in the context of some major regulatory relationships among structures thought to be relevant to reward and drug abuse. In upper cortical layers, the dendritic arbor of the pyramidal neuron is more widely distributed horizontally than in lower layers. In the sensitized state, increased sensitivity of DA D1 receptors and activity of VTA DA neurons, as well as enhanced inhibition of NAc neurons are predicted to diminish the influence of the more relatively global input to the pyramidal neuron dendritic arbor in the superficial layers, and to potentiate the more relatively local input to somatic dendrites in the deeper layers *(25,119)*. Consequently, cocaine sensitization favors the transition from delta, a frontal cortical global EEG mode, to lower-amplitude, higher-frequency local EEG modes. Solid lines, dopamine (DA); dotted lines, excitatory amino acids (EAA); dashed lines, gamma-aminobutyric acid (GABA).

and have high amplitudes and low frequencies. Functionally, global EEG modes may serve to bind activity of widely distributed neural ensembles, and gate the access of peripheral sensory input to the cortex. Activity in the delta bandwidth in neurologically normal awake humans, and the eyes-closed occipital alpha rhythm are examples of global EEG modes *(36)*. Local EEG modes are higher in frequency, lower in amplitude, and distributed over a more limited topographic area. Functionally, local EEG modes appear to correspond to attending to incoming stimuli or outputting motor action. An example of a local EEG mode is the appearance of beta-frequency activity over visual cortex during a target detection task, or over contralateral motor cortex during a manual movement task *(37)*.

The mesocortical DA projections are an important modulatory influence on the transition between global and local EEG modes in the frontal cortex, a major site of generation of the delta rhythm shown schematically in Fig. 1. The waking delta activity seen in normal adults, and which is reportedly reduced in cocaine users, is distinct from the delta of sleep, or of structural or infectious neurologic illness. There is substantial evidence that delta can appear as a correlate of complex cognitive processes spanning working memory or abstraction such as calculations *(36,38)*, reaction-time tasks *(39)*, abstract thought *(40)*, P300 paradigms *(41,42)* or a delayed match from sample paradigm *(43)*. Delta as a neocortical global mode has been hypothesized to integrate activity across association cortex *(44,45)*. A gating function has been suggested for delta power in the functional disconnection of the cortex from thalamic sensory inputs in order to gate extraneous stimuli from gaining access to global coherent neural assembles during states of "internal concentration" *(36,38)*.

Delta in normal awake humans has been shown to be a correlate of the process of allocating attention, and excluding extraneous stimuli during states in which the cortex is processing its own output. A deficit of delta in cocaine dependence might relate to susceptibility toward preemption of attention by craving and drug-related cues. Local-mode EEG activity, representing the processing of sensory input involving the thalamus, or motor output involving the basal ganglia, could represent a greater relative degree of subcortical determination of cortical processing than global mode activity. Therefore, a bias to local EEG modes might be expected to correspond to a tendency towards a relative reduction in descending cortical regulation of subcortical DA neurotransmission in stimulant sensitization. As noted by Grace *(46)*, the behavioral correlates of relatively diminished neocortical modulatory influence would be expected to include features such as impulsivity, disinhibition, and affective lability that are often evident in the clinical syndrome of cocaine dependence.

3. NEUROMETRIC QEEG STUDIES OF COCAINE DEPENDENCE

3.1. Methodology

The studies conducted in cocaine dependence in this laboratory over the past seven years (NIDA #DA 077070-01-06) use a quantitative EEG methodology known as neurometrics. This section is intended as a general description of this method for the set of studies that follow. It should be noted that in all these studies "baseline" refers to the evaluation done 5–14 d after last reported drug use. Since the studies that follow occurred at different points of data acquisition, the N's vary from study to study.

3.1.1. Cocaine-Dependent Subjects

With the exception of the original pilot study *(21)*, the work from this laboratory reviewed below involves subjects studied during abstinence while in drug-free residential treatment at Phoenix House, a large drug-free therapeutic community (TC) in New York City. Subjects were included who met Diagnostic and Statistical Manual of Mental Disorders-III-R (DSM-III-R) criteria for cocaine dependence for at least 1 yr. The following were criteria for exclusion: a history of ever having met criteria for dependence on any other substance except for alcohol, with alcohol intake limited to non-dependence levels in the year preceding admission; evidence of significant neurologic or medical condition known to affect the EEG; histories of head trauma with loss of consciousness; evidence of HIV infection; a history of ever having used any drug by the IV route; and any history of seizures regardless of association with drug abuse. No history of psychotropic medication treatment within 60 d of intake; IQs within the normal/low normal range. Four subtests of the Wechsler Adult Intelligence Test (WAIS) (vocabulary, arithmetic, block design, and picture arrangement) were used to estimate overall intelligence. This derived IQ (DQ) has been shown to have a significant correlation with fullscale WAIS. All Phoenix House facilities are locked and urine screenings are done randomly throughout treatment, which is an 18-mo program.

Written informed consent (NYU IBRA # H3947) was obtained from all patients meeting inclusion/exclusion criteria prior to entry into the study.

3.1.2. Data Acquisition and Analysis

The EEG evaluation occurred within 24 h of the psychiatric-intake evaluation. Twenty minutes of eyes closed resting EEG data were collected from the 19 monopolar electrode sites of the International 10/20 System, referred to linked earlobes, while the subjects were seated comfortably in a light attenuated room. A differential eye channel was used for the detection of eye movement. All electrode impedances were below 5000 Ohms. The EEG amplifiers had a bandpass from 0.5–70 Hz (3 dB points), with a 60 Hz notch filter. Data were sampled at a rate of 200 Hz with 12 bit resolution.

Artifact contamination is removed in the neurometric methodology by visual examination aided by automatic computer algorithms. Quantitative features are automatically extracted by spectral analysis of the EEG (QEEG), log transformed to obtain normal (Gaussian) distributions, age regressed, and evaluated statistically relative to age-regression equations for every feature in the neurometric database *(27,47)*. All features are transformed to Z scores and expressed in standard deviations (SD) from the age-appropriate normative values. This allows objective assessment of the statistical probability that the measurements obtained from an individual lie outside the normal limits for his or her age.

3.1.3. Use of Normative Database and Age Regression Equations

The neurometric database contains the raw EEG data and quantitative analysis of digital EEG recordings from 550 normally functioning individuals aged 6–90. Details of the norming procedures and construction of the database, including the criteria for inclusion/exclusion can be found in John et al. *(48)* (*see also* refs. *27* and *49*). It is important to note that the number of subjects required for reliability at each age point was statistically determined and were increased until split half replications were satisfactory. This sample requirement was dynamic in that different ages required different N's, for example in the ages from 6–13, where brain maturational changes are rapid, the N's were greater.

Each of the neurometric QEEG features has been expressed as published fourth-order, polynomial age-regression equations *(48)*. For every variable, a specific equation precisely predicts the mean value and SD of the distribution expected from a healthy, normally functioning population of exactly the age of the individual subject whose age has been entered into the equation. Other QEEG norming methods rely upon a reference sample of data obtained from individuals whose ages span one or several decades. In neurometrics, the use of age-regression techniques yields an estimate of the range expected from persons exactly the same age as the subject. Computation of the Z score for the difference between the predicted normative value and the value obtained from the individual then estimates the probability that such a value might be obtained by chance from a healthy peer.

3.1.4. Reliability, Specificity, Gender Effects, and Lack of Ethnic Bias

Significant test retest reliability was demonstrated in short-term (1–2 h), intermediate (wk), and long-term (up to 2 yr) test-retest as reported by John et al. *(50)*. The extremely high reliability found in those retests has recently been confirmed by intensive short- and long-term follow-up studies in a very large sample *(51)*. While expression of general concern about normative databases may sometimes be well-founded, confidence in our normative database derives from the expanding number of references to independent international replications of our normative equations published in the critically peer-reviewed literature by investigators outside of our laboratory. These replications only confirm the high specificity of these norms, but also demonstrate that they are independent of ethnic or cultural bias, accurately evaluating healthy, normally functioning individuals *(49,52–60)*.

3.1.5. Dimensional Source Localization of the EEG

Variable Resolution Electromagnetic Tomography (VARETA) is a recently developed discrete spline-distributed solution *(61)* for estimating the source generators of EEG surface potentials. This tomographic analysis of topographic maps of broad-band EEG spectral parameters has been correlated with lesion volume, location, and volume of surrounding edema indicated by radiological studies in patients with space-occupying lesions *(62–65)*.

Regional sources are co-registered with a Probabilistic Brain Atlas (PBA) developed at the Montreal Neurological Institute (MNI) *(66)*. Use of the PBA was intended to obviate the need for individual magnetic resonance imaging (MRI) scans. In the absence of large space-occupying lesions that grossly distort the brain, the PBA has been shown to closely approximate the MRI obtained from normal individuals. A three concentric-sphere model was fitted to the MNI mean head by a least square procedure. Three-dimensional (3-D) coordinates for the position of each scalp electrode position, defined by the proportional 10/20 International Electrode Placement System, have been published earlier *(67)*. Those coordinates are used to project each electrode position onto the average scalp of the mean head, thus placing the proportional EEG electrode set into spatial registration with the proportional PBA.

Based on this EEG-MRI head model, the problem of the 3-D sources of EEG may be specified in the frequency domain *(68–70)*. Three-dimensional color-coded tomographic images can be generated, with source-generator distributions superimposed upon transaxial, coronal, and sagittal slices of the PBA that correspond to the loci of the inverse solutions. In each case, the frequency at which the maximum significance was found is taken as the frequency of the main source. This must be done taking into consideration the large number of measurements and their intercorrelations. In this work the approach introduced by Worsley et al. *(71)* is taken, and the color codes are selected to only indicate excess or deficit of spectral activity if the appropriate probability level is reached.

3.2. Distinctive QEEG Profile in Crack-Cocaine Dependence

Pilot study findings demonstrated a distinctive QEEG profile in crack cocaine withdrawal *(72)*. These findings were replicated and extended in 52 crack-cocaine subjects (34 males, 18 females) tested at baseline (5–14 d after last use of crack) and after 1 mo of abstinence *(73)*. Previous findings of significant excess of relative alpha power and deficit of absolute and relative delta and theta power were confirmed in this expanded group and persisted after 1 mo of abstinence. Abnormalities greater in anterior than posterior regions, and disturbances in interhemispheric relationships were also observed. Roemer et al. *(20)* replicated these findings as described earlier.

3.3. Persistence of Abnormal EEG Profile in Extended Drug Abstinence

Comparisons between the neurometric profile of the same 17 patients with cocaine dependence at baseline and at 1 and 6 mo of abstinence showed remarkable stability and persistence of abnormal values in the QEEG measure set *(74)*. These results bear an interesting relationship to metabolic studies of abstinent cocaine users indicate a decrease in cortical activity that is persistent and most pronounced in frontal lobes. Using positron emission tomography (PET), Volkow et al. *(75,76)* reported decreased metabolism in the frontal lobes in subjects abstinent for 3 mo. Similarly, subjects evaluated with single photon emission computerized tomography (SPECT), reportedly evidenced frontal perfusion deficits up to 6 mo of drug abstinence *(77–79)*.

Since our database contained QEEG data from periods of abstinence extending to 12 mo, we were able to access the persistence over periods of confirmed abstinence previously unstudied. It was hypothesized that some portion of the QEEG abnormalities might reflect a reversible "state" of neuroadaptation resulting from chronic cocaine exposure. Other more persistent QEEG abnormalities might reflect permanent neurotoxicological injury, or alternatively, might reflect inherent "traits" that might predispose individuals to cocaine addiction or drug-seeking behavior, or that cause differential sensitivity to the effects of cocaine exposure. Preliminary study in a group of 28 male subjects who remained abstinent for at least 9 mo has demonstrated that while certain features remain unchanged during sustained abstinence ("trait" variables), others became more normal ("state" variables) during the same periods of abstinence *(80)*. In addition, the rate of normalization, when it occurs, appears to be different for different QEEG features.

The most consistent, robust (many regions show $p \leq 0.01$), diffuse normalization was seen across the 12-mo period in the mean frequency of the total spectrum. Significant changes toward normal were also reflected in the shift to more normal alpha absolute and relative power. No significant changes in absolute slow-wave power was seen. Frontal coherences in all frequency bands showed normalization in the first 6 mo only. Changes in beta absolute power and frontal slow wave coherence shifted in the abnormal direction.

Probable sources of the scalp recorded EEG data were imaged applying VARETA source-localization algorithms at baseline and after 12 mo of abstinence. Fig. 2 shows the coronal, transaxial, and sagittal views of the VARETA at 1.95 Hz, at the levels indicated by the schematic at the bottom of the figure for a group of 13 of these male subjects. (Note: Following radiological convention, laterality is reversed.) At baseline (top row) deficits of 1.95 Hz activity especially pronounced in the prefrontal, frontal cortex, and anterior cingulate can be seen. After 12 mo of abstinence (bottom row), some normalization was seen posteriorly, while significant deficits remained prominent in the frontal, cingulate, and prefrontal regions. While not shown in this figure, other frequencies, such as 8.97 Hz, showed an overall trend toward normalization across the 12-mo period of abstinence. Further, regionally differentiated rates of change are suggested by the evidence, implying differential regional effects of exposure or vulnerability to the long-term effects of cocaine exposure. These results support our hypoth-

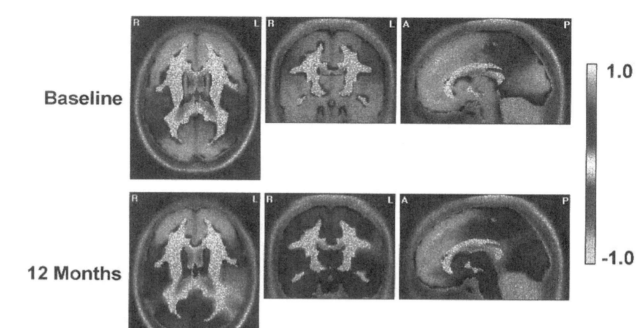

Fig. 2. Group average ($n = 13$) QEEG VARETA 3D images at 1.95 Hz. Images are shown for transaxial, coronal, and sagittal sections at baseline (top row, 5–14 d after last reported use of cocaine) and in the same patients after 12 mo of sustained abstinence (bottom row). Color-coding is in standard deviation units of the distribution of source strengths in each voxel in the normal population, with white representing the center of the scale, shades of red to yellow showing increasing excess, and green showing increasing deficit. The Z scale range is ±1.0, the significance of which is evaluated by multiplying the Z value times the square root of the group size. Note that these images follow radiologic convention, i.e., the nose is up but laterality is reversed so right is left. (*See* color plate 1 appearing in the insert following p. 368.)

esis that certain QEEG features and the corresponding underlying mechanisms demonstrate persistent abnormalities, while others show trend toward normalization with sustained abstinence.

3.4. Effects of Length of Exposure to Cocaine

Correlations between QEEG features and length of exposure (LOE) to cocaine were sought as evidence of a neurobiological effect of cocaine. ANOVAs between length of exposure to crack cocaine and gender were not significant; therefore, genders were combined in these analyses. For 93 subjects evaluated to date (66 males, 27 females), very few significant correlations were found between QEEG variables and LOE to cocaine. It is interesting that all but one of those which were significant ($p > 0.01$, $r > .20$), were QEEG variables quantifying hemispheric relationships, especially in the theta and beta bands between central and posterior regions. Roemer et al. *(20)*, also reported abnormalities of beta interhemispheric asymmetry to be correlated with length of exposure.

Since LOE in this population had a mean of 11.6 yr (± 5.5), it is possible that variance accounted for by length of exposure may asymptote by this point. A potential difficulty in studying humans with histories of chronic cocaine use appears to be a restriction of the dynamic range of the further expression of neuroadaptation in chronic users because of the prior induction of a maximal degree of expression. This effect has been evident, for example in human studies of behavioral sensitization to cocaine or amphetamine. Stimulant-naïve subjects do evidence a sensitized behavioral response to the second of two amphetamine doses *(81,82)*. However, chronic cocaine users reportedly do not clearly evidence a sensitized behavioral response to the second administration of a dose of stimulant relative to the first *(82,83)*. It is apparently difficult to demonstrate the induction of sensitization with an interval change between two stimulant doses in chronic users, because they may already have attained maximal degrees of expression of neuroadaptation to cocaine that no longer increment strongly with successive doses *(84)*.

3.5. Electrophysiologic Heterogeneity in Cocaine Dependence

Given the limited power of behavioral or demographic variables to predict treatment retention *(85)*, there are some reports on the association of baseline electrophysiological features and subsequent treatment outcome. In a study using evoked potentials (EPs) in abstinent cocaine abusers, Bauer *(86)* reported frontal P300 decrements were strongly correlated with presence of anti-social behavior and to have prognostic significance for relapse. Increased beta activity has been reported to correlate with treatment failure in two independent samples of subjects with alcohol dependence *(87,88)*, and as indicated below, is an apparent predictor of treatment failure in our work on cocaine dependence *(89)*. Bauer *(90)* suggests that the enhanced beta found in the relapse-prone alcoholics may reflect the presence of a premorbid trait specific to increased risk for relapse.

3.5.1. Cluster Analysis on Electrophysiologic Features and Differential Treatment Outcome

To assess the presence of electrophysiologic heterogeneity in the cocaine-dependent population, we applied cluster analysis to the QEEG baseline features in 35 males *(91)*. A small subset of selected QEEG baseline variables was submitted to the cluster analysis (BMDP K-Means) and two baseline clusters were obtained. The variables with the highest F ratios (all with $p < 0.0001$) included power gradients between frontal and posterior temporal regions, absolute power in the left lateral and left posterior regions within the right hemisphere, and relative power in the parietal region in the delta band. Cluster 1 was characterized by significant deficits of delta and theta, excess of alpha and more normal amounts of beta and Cluster 2 by deficits of delta, more normal theta, and anterior excess of alpha and beta activity.

No significant relationships were found between subtype membership and length of exposure, any demographic characteristics, or the clinical features of depression and anxiety. However, a significant relationship was found between QEEG subtype membership and length of stay in treatment (LOST), with 81% of the members of Cluster 1 departing from treatment within less than the median LOST of 25 wk, while 84% of the members of Cluster 2 remaining in treatment greater than the median LOST ($p \leq 0.003$). This clustering tended to accurately classify females who left treatment early but not those who remain in treatment longer, suggesting that further heterogeneity might exist among those who stay in treatment longer and implied the need for expansion of the clusters.

We have subsequently expanded the cluster analysis to include both male and female subjects and baseline somatosensory-evoked potential (SEP) features as well as the QEEG measures *(5)*. Fifty-seven cocaine-dependent subjects (16 females, 41 males, mean age 31.2 yr) were included in this cluster analysis. The median length of stay in treatment for this population was 25 wk. Using a small subset of selected QEEG and SEP baseline features were submitted to SAS CLUS and three clusters were constructed. Cluster 2 ($n = 23$) and Cluster 3 ($n = 25$) replicated the subtypes identified in the previous study (described for males only), while Cluster 1 ($n = 9$) had not been previously described. All three clusters contained both male and female subjects. As with the previous results, cluster membership was significantly associated with LOST less than median of 25 wk ($x^2 = 13.789$, $p < 0.001$). Cluster membership was not associated with variables relating to prior exposure to drugs, or any demographic or clinical features. Thus, differential retention was uniquely associated with the electrophysiologically different subtypes, with 78% of Cluster 1 and 65% of Cluster 3 with LOST less than the median of 25 wk, whereas 80% of Cluster 2 remained in treatment for greater than 25 wk *(5)*.

All three clusters shared a common feature of deficit of absolute power in the delta band, suggesting a relationship to cocaine exposure and not subtype membership. Cluster 2, characterized by a significant excess of both absolute and relative alpha power, was electrophysiologically similar to the good prognostic group reported earlier in the two-cluster solution *(5)*, and was likewise associated with greater retention in treatment. Cluster 3, characterized by significant beta-relative power excess, was similar electrophysiologically to the poor prognostic group in the two-cluster solution, and likewise was associated with early departure from treatment. Cluster 1 did not resemble either cluster in the previously described two-cluster solution, and was distinguished by a significant excess relative power in the theta band, maximal in posterior regions. Cluster 1 also featured excess relative beta power in anterior leads, although to a lesser extent than Cluster 3.

Since increased beta power is reported as characteristic of the QEEGs of alcohol dependence *(92,93)* and since the QEEGs of those who drop out of treatment earlier contained more beta, it was important to access the interaction between length of stay in treatment and ethanol (ETOH) use. No significant relationship was found between ETOH use and retention. Increased theta was seen in Cluster 1 and absent in the other two clusters. Given the association of theta with frankly neurological pathology, the presence of theta could reflect a subtype of patients who were more sensitive to the neurotoxic effects of cocaine exposure. In this context it is important to note that the most abnormal somatosensory EP findings were seen in Cluster 1.

3.5.2. Possible Interaction of Psychiatric Comorbidity with QEEG

In order to study the interaction between QEEG and the more frequently reported types of comorbid psychiatric conditions occurring in cocaine dependence, the population was divided into four groups, subjects with: (1) comorbid depression and alcohol abuse, (2) depression but no alcohol abuse, (3) alcohol abuse but no depression, and (4) neither alcohol abuse or depression. QEEG features in these groups showed a predominance of shared features, with all four showing the previously described deficit of delta, excess of alpha, and posterior hypercoherence. Subtle differences could be discerned, e.g., slightly more anterior beta in the group with comorbid alcohol abuse, also reflected in an increased mean frequency in beta. However, analysis of variance (ANOVAs) revealed no significant differences in the QEEG features between the four different comorbidity groups. These results suggest that variance attributable to each of these comorbid factors was small relative to the variance due to cocaine exposure and that the overall QEEG profile shared by these subgroups was relatively invariant *(94)*.

3.6. Prenatal Exposure to Cocaine

In a pilot study of six male children reportedly exposed *in utero* to crack cocaine (but not dependent levels of any other drugs), their QEEGS showed significant deviations from age-expected normal values. This small sample of children also clearly differed from demographically matched controls with ADHD and no apparent intrauterine drug exposure *(95)*. The QEEG profile seen in these children was extremely similar to that we have previously reported in crack cocaine-dependent adults, characterized by significant excess of relative power in the alpha frequency band, and deficits of absolute and relative power in the delta and theta bands. The similarities between the QEEG profiles of those adults with chronic exposure and children with prenatal exposure suggests an alteration that persists in these children at school age. Such differences may suggest an effect of cocaine exposure on brain development, or alternatively, may be evidence of a genetic vulnerability to drug dependence.

3.7. QEEG Differences Between Adult Subjects with or Without Histories of Childhood Abuse

The possible influence of prior exposure to significant stressors such as childhood abuse is a potential confound of interest in evaluating the neurobiological effects of cocaine on the EEG. QEEG was obtained in 15 cocaine-dependent subjects who disclosed a history of abuse in childhood and compared to 14-cocaine dependent subjects matched for gender, age, and reported lifetime cumulative exposure to cocaine *(96)*. The methodology utilized to define sexual and physical abuse is described elsewhere *(97)*. In comparison to subjects who denied a history of abuse, those who disclosed a history of abuse exhibited increased relative theta (3.5–7.5 Hz) power in posterior leads, and increased beta (12.5–25 Hz) mean frequency. While there appears not to have been a prior QEEG study that reported specifically on quantitative differences in the power spectrum in association with abuse histories, the finding reported here regarding increased theta activity in subjects with a history of abuse is consistent with reports of an increased incidence of abnormalities in the conventional, visually evaluated EEG in children with such histories.

The finding of relatively increased theta in association with a prior history of abuse is of interest in view of reports of reduced hippocampal volume measured by MRI in subjects with histories of abuse and/or post-traumatic stress disorder (PTSD) *(98–101)*. The hippocampus is an important generator of theta activity *(102)*. Corticotropin-releasing factor (CRF) is reportedly elevated in the central nervous system (CNS) of victims of trauma and abuse *(103)*, and has anxiogenic behavioral effects. CRF is reported to increase theta activity in animals *(104)*. Theta production is reportedly increased with stress and is augmented with repeated exposure *(105)*, as does the tendency to manifest PTSD with repeated exposure to trauma *(106)*. EEG theta may be a correlate of the persistently elevated CRF and altered response to stress noted in victims of trauma and abuse.

4. HYPOTHETICAL MECHANISMS OF NEURAL INJURY OR ADAPTATION IN COCAINE DEPENDENCE

The existing literature provides support for at least three possible etiologic processes of neuroadaptation or neural injury that could result from chronic exposure to cocaine.

The first possibility is direct neuronal injury. Evidence for this possibility includes an MRI study of cocaine-dependent subjects that showed a significantly increased age-related risk of white matter, but not subcortical gray-matter damage *(107)*. A possible etiologic process mediating direct neuronal injury is suggested by the observation that cocaine-induced vasoconstriction measured by magnetic resonance angiography (MRA) is apparently greater in cocaine dependence, and more pronounced with greater cocaine exposure *(108)*. Studies employing proton magnetic resonance spectroscopy (^{1}H-MRS) *(109)* suggest damage and glial proliferation in the prefrontal and frontal cortices, regions that correspond to the terminal fields of subcortical DA projections. This is possibly consistent with a postmortem study that reported cocaine users have an apparently low number of total DA terminals (although with a high number of dopamine transporter binding sites on dopaminergic neurons) *(110)*.

A second possible mechanism is suggested by neuroendocrine evidence for a functional deficit in serotonin transmission in cocaine-dependent subjects challenged with the serotonin (5-HT) releasers p-chloroamphetamine and d-fenfluramine *(111,112)*.

A third possible mechanism is neuroadaptation involving sensitization, a currently influential hypothesis of the neurobiology of cocaine dependence *(113,114)*. With repeated administration of cocaine or other stimulants, DA neurons in the VTA acquire a pattern of relatively increased or "sensitized" release of DA responsiveness to cocaine and related cues as well as other activating stimuli such as stress, corticosterone, or "priming" doses of rewarding substances *(46,115)*. This would be expected to produce a diminution of cortical activity because the positive feedback of descending cortical excitatory projections would be diminished in the presence of sensitized VTA activity. Diminished cortical activity, consistent with a hypothesis involving either sensitization and/or direct neural injury, has been reported in metabolic imaging studies in cocaine dependence utilizing either PET *(75,76)* or SPECT *(77–79)*. The sensitization model may be pertinent to the persistent nature of the QEEG findings because sensitization appears to persist over a time frame of months to years, unlike other reported changes in DA transmission that resolve within days or weeks of cocaine abstinence *(46)*.

In view of the above, suggested mechanisms underlying the QEEG features which were identified in the ongoing study to distinguish between baseline outcome clusters (increased alpha, theta and beta) and most persistent abnormality identified in the preliminary longitudinal analyses (deficit of delta), are as follows:

4.1. Delta-Power Deficit

There was a significant deficit of delta absolute power in the frontal regions in all three subtypes, described earlier, which appears to persist after months abstinence from cocaine *(74)*. This delta deficit could possibly be accounted for by a neuroadaptation such as sensitization *(25)*, or by direct neuronal injury.

In Fig. 1, the putative generator of the delta rhythm, the pyramidal cell is represented in the context of some of the major modulatory influences considered to be relevant to reward. The figure indicates two pathways by which sensitization can reduce delta EEG power. One involves the DA projections from the VTA. Bursting of VTA DA cells with subsequent enhancement of release from DA terminals *(46,116–118)*, results in increased local-mode activity of cortical pyramidal cells *(119)*. In addition, enhanced signal transduction through DA D1 receptors *(46,120)*, a consistently reported feature of cocaine sensitization, would be expected to enhance cortical local-mode activity as a consequence of the effect of DA D1 receptor stimulation on the response characteristics of pyramidal cells *(119)*. In addition, the context-dependent potentiation of sensitization in response to cocaine-related cues *(116,120)* appears to possibly involve descending excitatory projections from the amygdala, as well as hippocampus and cortex that enhance bursting activity of VTA DA cells.

Another possible pathway suggested in Fig. 1 involves the effect of enhanced inhibition of NAc neurons, a consistently reported correlate of sensitization *(113,122,123)*. Following the general scheme of a striatal-pallidal-thalamic-cortical circuit *(124)*, inhibition of NAc neurons would be expected to cause a net loss of excitatory input to the medial frontal cortex. Reduced NAc inhibitory input to the medial ventral pallidum (VP) would be expected to result in increased activity of VP projections that are inhibitory to the mediodorsal nucleus of the thalamus (MDT). The projections from the MDT to the cortex are mainly excitatory *(125)* and directed to superficial cortical layers, which feature a wide horizontal distribution of dendrites favoring global-mode EEG activity. Diminished excitatory input to the superficial cortical layers due to increased inhibition of the MDT would theoretically favor a local-mode response of pyramidal cells *(119)*.

4.2. Theta Power Excess

Excess theta was a distinguishing characteristic of one of the QEEG subtypes we identified, the members of which did not remain abstinent. Evidence exists that theta is generated within the septal-hippocampal pathway. The septal nucleus and the nucleus accumbens receive inhibitory modulation through dopaminergic innervation from the ventral tegmental area, via D_2 receptors *(126,127)*. Cholinergic efferents modulate hippocampal and cingulate cortex with these hippocampal pathways acting to slow down the septal nucleus. Thus, a theta excess can occur with an overactivation of the septal-hippocampal pathway or, as most likely in the case of cocaine dependence, via disinhibition from diminished inhibitory DA input *(128)*.

4.3. Alpha Power Excess

There was a diffuse and very significant excess of both absolute and relative alpha power in the QEEG subtype we identified, the members of which were found to remain abstinent. Alpha activity arises from thalamo-cortico-thalamic reverberations generated initially by oscillating pacemaker neurons in the thalamus *(26)*. This thalamic-cortical resonance receives excitatory modulation from the ascending reticular activating system (ARAS) via acetylcholine and inhibitory regulation through nucleus reticularis of the thalamus via GABA. In turn the ARAS receives further modulation via the dopaminergic striatal/nigral system. Disregulation of this system can lead to alpha excess by hyperactivation of the thalamus that may be secondary to over-stimulation of the midbrain reticular formation, because of decreased inhibition via the dopaminergic nigral system, or hypoactivation of the prefrontal cortex and a resulting disinhibition from nucleus reticularis. Thus, both a theta and/or alpha excess might result from a functional deficit of DA in cocaine dependence suggested by the neuroimaging and the postmortem studies described earlier.

The alpha findings are possibly also consistent with a functional deficit of serotonergic transmission, as suggested by neuroendocrine studies in cocaine-dependent subjects *(111,112)*. Alpha is reportedly decreased by treatment with multiple varieties of antidepressants, including the specific serotonin reuptake inhibitors (SSRI) and tricyclics *(4)*, which share the common pharmacologic effect of enhancing functional serotonin transmission *(129)*. The finding of asymmetry of alpha that normalizes with time in cocaine withdrawal is also possibly consistent with a hypothesis of a functional deficit of serotonergic transmission, given the reported asymmetric cortical distribution of serotonergic terminals in humans *(130)* and the positive association of baseline alpha with relatively favorable treatment outcome *(5)*.

4.4. Beta-Power Excess

As discussed earlier, excess beta absolute power was associated with failure to remain in treatment in our work on cocaine dependence, and has been correlated with negative treatment outcome in alcohol dependence *(87,88)*. The observation that VTA stimulation in animals enhances beta power and diminishes delta power *(11,131)* is possibly consistent with a hypotheses attributing excess beta EEG activity to neural sensitization in the mesotelencephalic DA system *(25)*.

5. CONCLUSIONS

The persistently abnormal QEEG pattern we have described in cocaine dependence may be acquired from cocaine exposure, and may reflect neuronal injury and persistent neuroadaptation such as stimulant sensitization. EEG studies in humans cannot directly measure direct neuronal injury or neuroadaptation, although as suggested earlier, such possible cocaine-related alterations of the CNS could be expected to have correlates reflected in the EEG. The possibility of direct neuronal injury might be addressed by evaluating the same subjects with structural imaging techniques and the EEG. The possibility of a neuroadaptation such as cocaine sensitization could be tested in animal models by correlating the EEG with signs of sensitization over the time interval corresponding to the initiation and maintenance of cocaine self-administration. Observations of EEG or unit activity in animals self-administering cocaine recorded from the cortex, anterior striatum, ventral pallidum, and VTA might also be informative regarding possible relationships between drug self-administration, the expression of neuronal injury or neurodaptations such as sensitization, and the EEG. The apparent similarity of QEEG abnormality in a small series of children with a history of *in utero* cocaine exposure to adults with cocaine dependence *(132)* suggests the possibility of a general pattern of neurotoxicological injury. The hypothesis that this pattern is an acquired abnormality as opposed to an inherited trait can be confirmed by evaluating non-drug exposed family members of cocaine-dependent subjects.

The finding of an apparent relationship of baseline QEEG profile and subsequent retention in treatment *(5)* suggests the possibility that the EEG may indeed access determinants of human behavior that are pre-attentive and not available to conscious introspection. If substantiated, this finding is significant validating evidence, as it would correlate the EEG with the cardinal clinical feature of cocaine dependence, the tendency to repeatedly resume use. On the basis of the evidence reviewed earlier, it is also possible that the neurotoxicological consequences of chronic cocaine exposure may be reflected in the EEG. To the extent that the EEG can be correlated with underlying processes of neuroadaptation or neuronal injury, it could potentially provide a noninvasive and clinically feasible means of assessing neurotoxicological consequences and identifying prognostic and differentially treatment-responsive subtypes in cocaine dependence.

ACKNOWLEDGMENT

This work was supported in part by the National Institute on Drug Abuse grant #RO1 DA07707. The authors wish to express their appreciation for the cooperation and support of this project by the staff of the Phoenix House Foundation Induction Facility. The contribution of MeeLee Tom, Bryant Howard, Henry Merkin, and Nestor Lagares to the data acquisition and analyses is also gratefully acknowledged.

REFERENCES

1. Alper, K. (1995) Quantitative EEG and Evoked Potentials in Adult Psychiatry, in *Advances in Biological Psychiatry*, vol. 1 (Pankseep, J., ed.), JAI Press, Greenwich, CT, pp. 65–112.
2. Chabot, R. J., Merkin, H., Wood, L. M., Davenport, T. L., and Serfontein, G. (1996) Sensitivity and specificity of qeeg in children with attention deficit or specific developmental learning disorders. *Clin. EEG* **27**, 26–34.
3. Hughes, J. R. and John, E. R. (1999) Conventional and quantitative electroencephalography in psychiatry. *J. Neuropsychiatry Clin. Neurosci.* **11**, 190–208.
4. Prichep, L. S., Mas, F., Hollander, E., Liebowitz, M., John, E. R., Almas, M., et al. (1993) Quantitative EEG (QEEG) subtyping of obsessive compulsive disorder. *Psychiat. Res.* **50(1)**, 25–32.
5. Prichep, L. S., Alper, K. R., Kowalik, S., Vaysblat, L., Merkin, H. A., Tom, M., et al. (1999) Prediction of treatment outcome in cocaine dependent males using quantitative EEG. *Drug Alcohol Depend.* **54**, 35–43.
6. Luoh, H. F., Kuo, T. B., Chan, A. H., and Pan, W. T. (1994) Power spectral analysis of electroencephalographic desynchronization induced by cocaine in rats: correlation with microdialysis evaluation of dopaminergic neurotransmission at the medial prefrontal cortex. *Synapse* **16**, 29–35.
7. Chang, A. W., Kuo, T. J., Chen, C. F., and Chan, S. H. (1995) Power spectral analysis of electroencephalographic desynchronization induced by cocaine in rats: correlation with evaluation of noradrenergic neurotransmission at the medial prefrontal cortex. *Synapse* **21**, 149–157.
8. Kropf, W. and Kuschinsky, K. (1993) Effects of stimulation of Dopamine D1 receptors on the cortical EEG in rats: different influences by a blockade D2 receptors and by an activation of putative Dopamine autoreceptors. *Neuropharmacology* **32**, 493–500.
9. Ferger, B., Kropf, W., and Kuschinsky, K. (1994) Studies on electroencephalogram (EEG) in rats suggest that moderate doses of cocaine or d-amphetamine activate D1 rather than D2 receptors. *Psychopharmacology* **114**, 297–308.
10. Ferger, B., Stahl, D., and Kuschinsky, K. (1996) Effects of cocaine on the EEG power spectrum of rats are significantly altered after its repeated administration: do they reflect sensitization phenomena? *Naunyn Schmiedebergs Arch. Pharmacol.* **353**, 545–551.
11. Leung, L. S. and Yim, C. Y. (1993) Rythmic delta-frequency activities in the nucleus accumbens of anesthetized and freely moving rats. *Can. J. Physiol. Pharmacol.* **71**, 311–320.

12. Berger, H. A. (1937) Electroencephalogram of man. *Arch. Psychiar. Nervenkr* **106,** 577–584.
13. Herning, R. I., Hooker, W. D., and Jones, R. T. (1987) Cocaine effects on electroencephalographic cognitive event-related potentials and performance. *EEG Clin. Neurophysiol.* **66,** 34–42.
14. Herning, R. I., Glover, B. J., Koeppl, B., Phillips, R. L., and London, E. D. (1994) Cocaine-induced increases in EEG alpha and beta: evidence for reduced cortical processing. *Neuropsychopharmacology* **11,** 1–9.
15. Herning, R. I., Guo, X., Better, W. E., Weinhold, L. L., Lange, W. R., Cadet, J. L., and Gorelick, D. A. (1997) Neurophysiological signs of cocaine dependence: increased electroencephalogram beta during withdrawal. *Biol. Psychiat.* **41,** 1087–1094.
16. Herning, R. I., Jones, R. T., Hooker, W. D., Mendelson, J., and Blackwell, L. (1985) Cocaine increases EEG beta: a replication and extension of Hans Berger's historic experiments. *EEG Clin. Neurophysiol.* **60,** 470–477.
17. Lukas, S. E. (1991) Topographic brain mapping during cocaine-induced intoxication and self-administration, in *Biological Psychiatry*, vol. 2 (Racagni, G., Brunello, N., and Fukuda, T., eds.), Elsevier Science, Amsterdam, pp. 25–29.
18. Noldy, N. E., Santos, C. V., Politzer, N., Blair, G. R. D., and Carlen, P. L. (1994) Quantitative EEG changes in cocaine withdrawal: evidence for long-term CNS effects. *Neuropsychobiology* **30,** 189–196.
19. Costa, L. and Bauer, L. (1997) Quantitative electroencephalographic differences associated with alcohol, cocaine, heroin and dual-substance dependence. *Drug and Alcohol Depend.* **46,** 87–93.
20. Roemer, R. A., Cornwall, A., Dewart, D., Jackson, P., and Ercegovac, D. V. (1995) Quantitative electroencephalographic analysis in cocaine-preferring polysubstance abusers during abstinence. *Psychiatry Res.* **58,** 247–257.
21. Alper, K. R., Chabot, R. J., Kim, A. H., Prichep, L. S., and John, E. R. (1990) Quantitative EEG correlates of crack cocaine dependence. *Psychiatry Res.* **35,** 95–106.
22. Prichep, L. S., Kowalik, S. C., Alper, K. R., and Chabot, R. J. (1997) Distinctive quantitative EEG (QEEG) abnormalities in children exposed to cocaine in utero, in *Problems of Drug Dependence* (Harris, L. S., ed.), Proceedings of the 59th Annual Scientific Meeting, NIDA Research Monograph 178. NIDA, Bethesda, MD.
23. Lukas, S. E., Mendelson, J. H., Woods, B T., Mello, N. K., and Seoh, S. K. (1989) Topographic distribution of EEG alpha activity during ethanol-induced intoxication in women. *J. Studies Alcohol* **50,** 176–184.
24. Lukas, S. E. (1993) Advanced electrophysiological imaging techniques for studying drug effects, in *Imaging Drug Action in the Brain* (London, E. D., ed.), CRC Press, Boca Raton, FL, pp. 389–404.
25. Alper, K. R. (1999) The EEG and cocaine sensitization: a hypothesis. *J. Neuropsychiat. Clin. Neurosci.* **11,** 209–221.
26. Hughes, J. R. and John, E. R. (1999) Conventional and quantitative electroencephalography in psychiatry. *J. Neuropsychiatry Clin. Neurosci.* **11,** 190–208.
27. John, E. R., Prichep, L. S., Friedman, J., and Easton, P. (1988) Neurometrics: computer assisted differential diagnosis of brain dysfunctions. *Science* **293,** 162–169.
28. Struve, F. A., Straumanis, J. J., Patrick, G., and Price, L. (1989) Topographic mapping of quantitative EEG variables in chronic heavy marijuana users: empirical findings with psychiatric patients. *Clin. EEG* **20,** 6–23.
29. Struve, F. A., Straumanis, J. J., and Patrick, G. (1994) Persistent topographic quantitative EEG sequelae of chronic marijuana use: a replication study and initial discriminant function analysis. *Clin. EEG* **25,** 63–75.
30. Struve, F. A., Straumanis, J. J., Patrick, G., Leavitt, J., Manno, J. E., and Manno, B. R. (1999) Topographic quantitative EEG sequelae of chronic marihuana use: a replication

using medically and psychiatrically screened normal subjects. *Drug Alcohol Depend.* **56,** 167–179.

31. Booth, R. E., Watters, J. K., and Chitwood, D. D. (1993) HIV risk-related sex behaviors among injection drug crack smokers, and injection drug users who smoke. *Am. J. Public Health* **83,** 1144–1148

32. Riedel, R-R., Alper, K. R., Bulau, P., Niese, D., Schieck, U., and Gunther, W. (1995) QEEG in hemophiliacs infected with HIV. *Clin. EEG* **26,** 84–91.

33. Lehner, T., Torian, L., Alper, K., Geringer, W., Horton, T., Gonzalez, I., and Weisfuse, I. (1995) HIV infection among non-injecting drug users entering drug treatment facility in New York City. Abstracts, 35th Interscience Conference Antimicrobial Agents and Chemotherapy, San Francisco, CA.

34. Nunez, P. L. (1995) Experimental connections between EEG data and the global wave theory, in *Neocortical Dynamics and Human EEG Rhythms* (Nunez, P. L., ed.), Oxford University Press, New York, pp. 534–590.

35. Miller, E. N., Satz, P., and Visscher, B. (1991) Computerized and conventional neuropsychological assessment of HIV–1-infected homosexual men. *Neurology* **41,** 1608–1616.

36. Harmony, T., Fernández, T., Silva, J., Bernal, J., Diaz-Comas, L., Reyes, A., Marosi, E., and Rodriquez, M. (1996) EEG delta activity: an indicator of attention to internal processing during performance of mental tasks. *Int. J. Psychophysiol.* **24,** 161–171.

37. Pulvermuller, F., Birbaumer, N., Lutzenberger, W., and Mohr, B. (1997) High-frequency brain activity: it's possible role in attention, perception and language processing. *Prog. Neurobiol.* **52,** 427–445.

38. Fernandez, T., Harmony, T., Rodriguez, M., Bernal, J., Silva, J., Reyes, A., and Marosi, E. (1995) EEG activation patterns during the performance of tasks involving different components of mental calculation. *EEG Clin. Neurophysiol.* **94,** 175–182.

39. Van Dijk, J. G., Caekebeke, V. J. F., and Zwinderman, A. H. (1992) Background EEG reactivity in auditory event-related potentials. *EEG Clin. Neurophysiol.* **83,** 44–51.

40. Michel, C. M., Henggeler, B., Brandeis, D., and Lehmann, D. (1993) Localization of sources of brain alpha\theta\delta activity and the influence of the mode of spontaneous mentation. *Physiol. Meas.* **14,** 21–26.

41. Basar-Eroglu, C., Basar, E., Demiralp, T., and Schurmann, M. (1992) P300-response: Possible psychophysiological correlates in delta and theta frequency channels: a review. *Intl. J. Psychophysiol.* **13,** 161–179.

42. Roschke, J. and Fell, J. (1997) Spectral analysis of P300 generation in depression schizophrenia. *Neuropsychobiology* **35,** 108–114.

43. John, E. R., Easton, P., Isenhart, R., Allen, P., and Gulyashar, A. (1996) Electrophysiological analysis of the registration, storage and retrieval of information in delayed match from samples. *Intl. J. Psychophysiol.* **24,** 127–144.

44. Freeman, W. J. and Barrie, J. M. (1994) Chaotic oscillations and the genesis of the meaning in cerebral cortex, in *Temporal Coding in the Brain* (Buzsaki, G. L., Llinas, R., Singer, W., Bertroz, A., and Christen, Y., eds.), Springer Verlag, Berlin, pp. 13–38.

45. Bullock, T. H. (1992) Introduction to induced rhythms: a widespread, heterogeneous of oscillations, in *Induced Rhythms in the Brain* (Basar, E. and Bullock, T. H., eds.), Birkhauser, Boston, pp. 1–26.

46. Grace, A. A. (1995) The tonic/phasic model of dopamine system regulation: its relevance for understanding how stimulant abuse can alter basal ganglia function. *Drug Alcohol Depend.* **37,** 111–129.

47. John, E. R. and Prichep, L. S. (1993) Principles of neurometrics and neurometric analysis of EEG and evoked potentials, in *EEG: Basic Principles, Clinical Applications and Related Fields* (Niedermeyer, E. and Lopes Da Silva, F., eds.), Williams and Wilkins, pp. 989–1003.

48. John, E. R., Prichep, L. S., and Easton, P. (1987) Normative data banks and neurometrics: basic concepts, methods and results of norm construction, in *Handbook of*

Electroencephalography and Clinical Neurophysiology, vol. I (Gevins, A. S. and Remond, A., eds.), Elsevier, Amsterdam, pp. 449–495.

49. Ahn, H., Prichep, L. S., John, E. R., Baird, H., Trepetin, M., and Kaye, H. (1980) Developmental equations reflect brain dysfunction. *Science* **210**, 1259–1262.

50. John, E. R., Prichep, L. S., Ahn, H., Easton, P., Fridman, J., and Kaye, H. (1983) Neurometric evaluation of cognitive dysfunctions and neurological disorders in children. *Prog. Neurobiol.* **21**, 239–290.

51. Kondacs, A. and Szabo, M. (1999) Long-term intra-individual variability of the background EEG in normals. *Clin. Neurophysiol.* **110**, 1708–1716.

52. Verleger, R., Gasser, T., and Mocks, J. (1982) Corrections of EOG artifacts in event-related potentials of the EEG: aspects of reliability and validity. *Psychophysiology* **19**, 472–480.

53. Jonkman, E. J., Poortvliet, D. C. J., Veering, M. M., DeWeerd, A. W., and John, E. R. (1985) The use of neurometrics in the study of patients with cerebral ischemia. *EEG Clin. Neurophys.* **61**, 333–341.

54. Yingling, C. D., Galin, D., Fein, G., Peltzman, D., and Davenport, L. (1986) Neurometrics does not detect 'pure' dyslexics. *EEG Clin. Neurophysiol.* **63**, 426–430.

55. Alvarez, A., Pascual, R., and Valdes, P. (1987) U.S. EEG development equations confirmed for Cuban school children. *EEG Clin. Neurophysiol.* **67**, 330–332.

56. Diaz de Leon, A. E., Harmony, T., Marosi, E., Becker, J., and Alvarez, A. (1988) Effect of different factors on EEG spectral parameters. *Intl. J. Neurosci.* **43**, 123–131.

57. Duffy, F. H., Albert, M. S., and McAnulty, G. B. (1993) The pattern of age-related differences in electrophysiological activity of healthy subjects. *Neurobiol. Aging* **14**, 73–74.

58. Matsuura, M., Okubo, Y., Toru, M., Kojima, T., He, Y., Hou, Y., Shen, Y., and Lee, C. (1993) A cross-national study of children with emotional behavioral problems: a WHO collaborative study in the Pacific Region. *Biol. Psychiatry* **34**, 59–65.

59. Veldhuizen, R. J., Jonkman, E. J., and Poortvliet, J. D. C. (1993) Sex differences in age regression parameters of adults-normative data. *EEG Clin. Neurophysiol.* **86**, 377–384.

60. Duffy, F. H., Jones, K., McAnulty, G. B., and Albert, M. (1995) Spectral coherence in normal adults: unrestricted principal components analysis. *Clin. EEG* **26**, 30–46.

61. Bosch-Bayard, P., Valdes-Sosa, P., Virues-Alba, T., Aubert-Wazquez, E., John, E. R. et al. (2001) 3D statistical parametric mapping of EEG source spectra by means of Variable Resolution Electromagnetic Tomography (VARETA). *Clin. EEG* **32**, 47–61.

62. Harmony, T., Fernandez-Bouzas, A., and Marosi, E. (1993) Correlation between computed tomography and voltage and current source density spectral EEG parameters in patients with brain lesions. *EEG Clin. Neurophysiol.* 87, 196–205.

63. Harmony, T., Fernandez-Bouzas, A., Marosi, E., Fernandez, T., Valdes, P., Bosch, J., et al. (1995) Frequency source analysis in patients with brain lesions. *Brain Topogr.* **8**, 109–117.

64. Fernandez-Bouzas, A., Casanova, R., Harmony, T., Valdes, P., Aubert, E., Silva, J., et al. (1997) EEG frequency domain distributed inverse solutions in lesions. *EEG Clin. Neurophysiol.* **103**, 195.

65. Fernandez-Bouzas, A., Harmony, T., Bosch, J. A. E., Fernandez, T., Valdes, P., Silva, J., et al. (1999) Sources of abnormal EEG activity in the presence of brain lesions. *Clin. EEG* **30**, 1–7.

66. Evans, A. C., Collins, D. L., Mills, S. R., Brown, E. D., Kelly, R. L., and Peters, T. M. (1993) 3D statistical neuroanatomical models from 305 MRI volumes. Proceedings of IEEE-Nuclear Science Symposium and Medical Imaging Conference 95: 1813–1817

67. Scherg, M. and Von Crainon, D. (1985) Two bilateral sources of the late AEP as identified by a spatio-temporal dipole model. *EEG Clin. Neurophysiol.* **62**, 32–44.

68. Valdes-Sosa, P., Bosch, J., Gray, F., Hernandez, J., Riera, J., Pascual, R., and Biscay, R. (1992) Frequency domain models of the EEG. *Brain Topogr.* **4**, 309–319.

69. Casanova, R., Valdes-Sosa, P., Garcia, F. M., Aubert, E., Riera, J., Korin, J., and Lins, O. (1996) Frequency domain distributed inverse solution. Proceedings of the 10th International Conference on Biomagnetism, Santa Fe, New Mexico.

70. Valdes-Sosa, P., Riera, J., and Casanova, R. (1996) Spatio temporal distributed inverse solutions. Santa Fe, New Mexico.

71. Worsley, K. J., Marrett, S., Neelin, P., Vandal, A. C., Friston, K. J., and Evans, A. C. (1995) A unified approach for determining significant signals in images of cerebral activation. *Human Brain Mapping* **4,** 58–73.

72. Alper, K. R., Chabot, R. J., Kim, A. H., Prichep, L. S., and John, E. R. (1990) Quantitative EEG correlates of crack cocaine dependence. *Psychiatry Res.* **35,** 95–106.

73. Prichep, L. S., Alper, K. R., Kowalik, S. C., John, E. R., Merkin, H. A., Tom, M., and Rosenthal, M. S. (1996) Quantitative electroencephalographic characteristics of crack cocaine dependence. *Biol. Psychiatry* **40,** 986–993.

74. Alper, K. R., Prichep, L. S., Kowalik, S. C., and Rosenthal, M. S. (1998) Persistent qEEG abnormality in crack cocaine users at 6 months of drug abstinence. *Neuropsychopharmacology* **19,** 1–9.

75. Volkow, N. D., Hitzemann, R., Wang, G., Fowler, J. S., Wolf, A. P., Dewey, S. L., and Handleman, L. (1992) Long-term frontal brain metabolic changes in cocaine abusers. *Synapse* **11,** 184–190.

76. Volkow, N. D., Wang, G. J., Fowler, J. S., Logan, J., Hitzeman, R., Gatley, S. J., MacGregor, R. R., and Wolf, A. P. (1996) Cocaine uptake is decreased in the brain of detoxified cocaine abusers. *Neuropsychopharmacology* **14,** 159–168.

77. Strickland, T. L., Villanueva-Meyer, J., Miller, B. L., Cummings, J., Mehringer, C. M., Satz, P., and Myers, H. (1993) Cerebral perfusion and neuropsychological consequences of chronic cocaine use. *J. Neuropsychiatry Clin. Neurosci.* **5,** 4419–4427.

78. Levin, J. M., Holman, B. L., and Mendelson, J. H. (1994) Gender differences in cerebral perfusion in cocaine abuse. *J. Nucl. Med.* **35,** 1902–1909.

79. Gatley, S. J. and Volkow, N. D. (1998) Addiction and imaging of the living human brain. *Drug Alcohol Depend.* **51,** 97–108.

80. Prichep, L. S., Alper, K. R., Rausch, L., Vaysblat, L., Merkin, H., Tom, M., et al. (1999) Normalization of the QEEG with long-term abstinence in cocaine dependence. Problems of Drug Dependence: Proceedings of the 61st Annual Scientific Meeting. NIDA, Acapulco, Mexico.

81. Strakowski, S. M., Sax, K. W., Setters, M. J., and Keck, P. E., Jr. (1996) Enhanced response to repeated d-amphetamine challenge: evidence behavioral sensitization in humans. *Biol. Psychiatry* **40,** 872–880.

82. Gorelick, D. A. and Rothman, D. B. (1997) Stimulant sensitization in humans. *Biol. Psychiatry* **40,** 230–231.

83. Rothman, R. B., Gorelick, D. A., Guo, X. Y., Herning, R. I., Rickworth, W. B., and Gendon, T. M. (1994) Lack of evidence for context specific cocaine induced sensitization in humans: preliminary studies. *Pharmacol. Biochem. Behav.* **49,** 583–588.

84. Phillips, T. J. (1997) Behavioral genetics of drug sensitization. *Crit. Rev. Neurobiol.* **11,** 21–33.

85. DeLeon, G. (1991) Retention in drug-free therapeutic communities, in *Improving Drug Abuse Treatment* (Pickens, R., Leukfeld, C., and Schuster, C. R., eds.), Research monograph No. 106, NIDA, Bethesda, MD, pp. 218–244.

86. Bauer, L. O. (1997) Frontal P300 decrements, childhood conduct disorder, family and the prediction of relapse among abstinent abusers. *Drug Alcohol Depend.* **44,** 1–10.

87. Bauer, L. O. (1994) Photic driving of EEG alpha activity in recovering cocaine-dependent and alcohol-dependent patients. *Am. J. Addictions* **3,** 49–57.

88. Herrmann, W. M. and Winterer, G. (1996) Electroencephalography in psychiatry: a review of literature. *Nerenarzt* **67,** 349–359.

89. Prichep, L. S., Alper, K., Kowalik, S. C., and Rosenthal, M. S. (1996) Neurometric QEEG studies of crack cocaine dependence and treatment outcome. *J. Addictive Dis.* **15,** 39–53.

90. Bauer, L. O. and Kranzler, H. R. (1994) Electroencephalographic activity and mood in cocaine-dependent outpatients: effects of cocaine cue exposure. *Biol. Psychiatry* **36,** 189–197.

91. Prichep, L. S., Alper, K. R., Kowalik, S. C., John, E. R., Merkin, H. A., Tom, M., and Rosenthal, M. S. (1996) Quantitative electroencephalographic characteristics of crack cocaine dependence. *Biol. Psychiatry* **40,** 986–993.

92. Pollock, V. E., Gabrielli, W. F., Mednick, S. A., and Goodwin, D. W. (1988) EEG identification of subgroups of men at risk for alcoholism. *Psychiatry Res.* **26,** 101–114.

93. Alper, K. R., Prichep, L. S., Kowalik, S., Rosenthal, M. S., John, E. R., Tom, M., and Merkin, H. A. (1995) Persistence of QEEG abnormality in crack cocaine withdrawal. Problems of Drug Dependence: Proceedings of the 57th Annual Scientific Meeting. NIDA, Scottsdale, AZ.

94. Prichep, L. S., Alper, K. R., Kowalik, S. C., and John, E. R. (2000) Invariant QEEG features independent of comorbidity in cocaine dependence. *J. Neuropsychiat.*, in review.

95. Prichep, L. S., Kowalik, S. C., Alper, K. R., and De Jesus, C. (1995) Quantitative EEG characteristics of children exposed in utero to crack cocaine. *Clin. EEG* **26,** 166–172.

96. Alper, K. A., Prichep, L. S., Kowalik, S. C., and Rosenthal, M. S. (1999) College of Problems of Drug Dependence 61st Annual Scientific Meeting, Acapulco, Mexico (Abstract).

97. Alper, K., Devinsky, O., Perrine, K., and Luciano, D. (1993) Nonepileptic seizures: childhood sexual and physical abuse. *Neurology* **43,** 1950–1953.

98. Bremner, J. D., Randal, P., Vermetten, E., Staib, L., Bronen, R. A., Mazure, C., et al. (1997) Magnetic resonance imaging-based measurement of hippocampal volume in post-traumatic stress disorder related to childhood physical and sexual abuse: a preliminary report. *Biol. Psychiatry* **41,** 23–32.

99. Stein, M. B., Koverola, C., Hanna, C., Torchia, M. G., and McClarty, B. (1997) Hippocampal volume in women victimized by childhood sexual abuse. *Psychol. Med.* **27,** 951–959.

100. Bremner, J. D., Vermetten, E., Southwick, S. M., Krystal, J. H., and Charney, D. S. (1998) Trauma, memory and dissociation: an integrative formulation, in *Trauma, Memory and Dissociation* (Bremner, J. D. and Marmar, C., eds.), APA Press, Washington, DC, pp. 365–402.

101. Gurvits, T. G., Shenton, M. R., Hokama, H., et al. (1996) Magnetic resonance imaging study of hippocampal volume in chronic combat-related post-traumatic stress disorder. *Biol. Psychiatry* **40,** 192–199.

102. Steriade, M., Gloor, P., Llinas, R. R., Lopes Da Silva, F., and Mesulam, M. M. (1990) Basic mechanisms of cerebral rhythmic activities. *EEG Clin. Neurophysiol.* **76,** 481–508.

103. Arborelius, L., Owens, M. J., Plotsky, P. M., and Nemeroff, C. B. (1999) The role of corticotropin-releasing factor in depression and anxiety disorders. *J. Endocrinol.* **160,** 1–12.

104. Mazziotta, J. C., Pelizzari, C. C., Chen, G. T., Bookstein, F. L., and Valentino, D. (1991) Region-of-interest issues: the relationship between structure and function in the brain. *J. Cereb. Blood Flow Metab.* 11, A51–A56.

105. Shors, T. J., Gallegos, R. A., and Breindl, A. (1997) Transient and persistent consequences of Acute Stress on long-term potentiation (LTP), synaptic efficacy, theta rhythms and in area CA1 of the hippocampus. *Synapse* **26,** 209–217.

106. Breslau, N., Chilcoat, H. D., Kessler, R. C., and Davis, G. C. (1999) Previous exposure to trauma and PTSD effects of subsequent trauma: results from the Detroit Area Survey of Trauma. *Am. J. Psychiatry* **156,** 902–907.

107. Bartzokis, G., Goldstein, I. B., Hance, D. B., Beckson, M., Shapiro, D., Lu, P. H., et al. (1999) The incidence of T2-weighted MR imaging signal abnormalities in the brain of cocaine-dependent patients is age-related and region-specific. *Am. J. Neuroradiol.* **20,** 1628–1635.

108. Kaufman, M. J., Levin, J. M., Ross, M. H., Lange, N., Rose, S. L., Kukes, T. J., Mendelson, J. H., Lukas, S. E., Cohen, B. M., and Renshaw, P. F. (1998) Cocaine-induced cerebral vasoconstriction detected in humans with magnetic resonance angiography. *JAMA* **275**, 376–380.

109. Chang, L., Ernst, T., Strickland, T., and Mehringer, C. M. (1999) Gender effects on persistent cerebral metabolite changes in the frontal lobes of abstinent cociane users. *Am. J. Psychiatry* **156**, 5716–5722.

110. Little, K. Y., Zhang, L., Desmond, T., Frey, K. A., Dalack, G. W., and Cassin, B. J. (1999) Striatal dopaminergic abnormalities in human cocaine users. *Am. J. Psychiatry* **156**, 238–245.

111. Levy, A. D., Baumann, M. H., and Van de Kar, L. D. (1994) Monoaminergic regulation of neuroendocrine function and its modification by cocaine. *Front Neuroendocrinol.* **15**, 85–156.

112. Buydens-Branchey, L., Branchey, M., Fergeson, P., Hudson, J., and McKernin, C. (1997) The metachlorophenylpiperazine challenge test in cocaine addicts: hormonal and psychological responses. *Biol. Psychiatry* **41**, 1071–1086.

113. White, F. J. and Kalivas, P. W. (1998) Neuroadaptations involved in amphetamine and cocaine addiction. *Drug Alcohol Depend.* **51**, 141–153.

114. Robinson, T. E. and Berridge, K. C. (1993) The neural basis of drug craving: an incentive-sensitization theory of addiction. *Brain Res.Revs.* **18**, 247–291.

115. Kiyatkin, E. A. (1995) Functional significance of mesolimbic dopamine. *Neurosci. Biobehav. Revs.* **19**, 578–598.

116. Karreman, M. and Moghaddam, B. (1996) The prefrontal cortex regulates the basal release of dopamine in in the limbic striatum: an effect mediated by ventral tegmental area. *J. Neurochem.* **66**, 589–598.

117. Brudzynski, S. M. and Gibson, C. J. (1997) Release of dopamine in the nucleus accumbens caused by stimulation of the subiculum in freely moving rats. *Brain Res. Bull.* **42**, 303–308.

118. Taber, M. T. and Fibiger, H. C. (1997) Feeding-evoked dopamine release in the nucleus accumbens: regulation by glutamatergic mechanisms. *Neuroscience* **76**, 1105–1112.

119. Yang, C. R. and Seamans, J. K. (1996) Dopamine D1 receptor actions in layers V-VI rat prefrontal cortex neurons in vitro: modulation of dendritic-somatic signal integration. *J. Neurosci.* **16**, 1922–1935.

120. Henry, D. J. and White, F. J. (1995) The persistence of behavioral sensitization to cocaine enhanced inhibition of nucleus accumbens neurons. *J. Neurosci.* **15**, 6287–6299.

121. Anagnostaras, S. G. and Robinson, T. E. (1996) Sensitization to the psychomotor stimulant effects of amphetamine: Modulation by associative learning. *Behav. Neurosci.* **110**, 1397–1414.

122. Kiyatkin, E. A. and Rebec, G. V. (1996) Dopaminergic modulation of glutamate-induced excitations of neurons the neostriatum and nucleus accumbens of awake unrestrained rats. *J. Neurophysiol.* **75**, 142–153.

123. O'Donnell, P. and Grace, A. A. (1996) Dopaminergic reduction of excitability in nucleus accumbens neurons recorded in vitro. *Neuropsychopharmacology* **15**, 87–97.

124. Mogenson, G. J., Brudzynski, S. M., Wu, M., Yang, C. R., and Yim, C. Y. (1993) From motivation to action: a review of dopaminergic regulation of limbic—nucleus—accumbens—ventral pallidum—pendunculopontine nucleus circuitries involved in limbic-motor integration. *Limbic Motor Circuits Neuropsychiatry* 193–236.

125. Jones, M. W., Kilpatrick, I. C., and Phillipson, O. T. (1987) Regulation of dopamine function in the prefrontal cortex of the rat by the thalamic mediodorsal nucleus. *Brain Res. Bull.* **19**, 9–17.

126. DeBoer, P. and Abercrombie, E. (1996) Physiological release of striatal acetylcholine in vivo: modulation of d1 and d2 dopamine receptor subtypes. *J. Pharmacol. Exp. Ther.* **277**, 775–783.

127. Icarashi, Y., Takahashi, H., Aral, T., and Maruyama, Y. (1997) Suppression of cholinergic activity via the dopamine d2 receptor in the rat stratum. *Neurochem. Intl.* **30,** 191–197.

128. Russel, V., de Villiers, A., Sagvolden, T., et al. (1995) Altered dopaminergic function in the prefrontal cortex, nucleus accumbens and caudate-putamen of an animal model of attention deficit hyperactivity disorder. *Brain Res.* **676,** 343–351.

129. Markou, A., Kosten, T. R., and Koob, G. F. (1998) Neurobiological similarities in depression and drug dependence: a self-medication hypothesis. *Neuropsychopharmacology* **18,** 135–174.

130. Arato, M., Frecska, E., Tekes, K., and Crimmon, D. J. (1991) Serotonergic interhemispheric asymmetry: gender difference in the orbital cortex. *Acta Psychiatry Scand.* **84,** 110–111.

131. Rougeul-Buser, A. (1994) Electrocortical rhythms in the 40 Hz band in cat: in search of their behavioral correlates, in *Temporal Coding in the Brain* (Buzsaki, G., Llinas, R., Singer, W., Berthoz, A., Christen, Y., eds.), Springer-Verlag, Berlin, pp. 103–114.

132. Prichep, L. S., Alper, K. R., and Kowalik, S. C. (1995) Persistent QEEG abnormalities in abstinent cocaine dependent patient. 6th International Congress of the International Society Brain Electromagnetic Topography (ISBET) (Abstract).

6

Addictive Basis of Marijuana and Cannabinoids

Eliot L. Gardner

1. BRAIN REWARD SUBSTRATES

The brain's reward circuitry consists of synaptically interconnected neurons that link the ventral tegmental area (VTA), nucleus accumbens (Acb), ventral pallidum (VP), and medial prefrontal cortex (MPFC). Laboratory animals avidly self-administer mild electrical stimulation to these loci, and to the medial forebrain bundle (MFB), which interconnects the VTA, Acb, and MPFC. Mild electrical stimulation of this circuit produces an intense subjective experience of pleasure in humans. This circuit is strongly implicated in the neural substrates of drug abuse, and in such phenomena as withdrawal dysphoria and craving. Not surprisingly, natural rewards (e.g., food, sex) also activate these same brain substrates. Cannabinoids are euphorigenic in humans and have abuse liability, but were long considered to be devoid of pharmacological action on these brain-reward substrates. Work with cannabinoids over the last decade, however, make it clear that they activate these brain substrates and influence reward-related mechanisms in a manner strikingly similar to that of other drugs of abuse.

1.1. Neuroanatomy, Neurophysiology, and Neurochemistry of Brain Reward

The neuroanatomy, neurophysiology, and neurochemistry of brain-reward mechanisms is known to involve a series of neural links located primarily in the ventral limbic forebrain and associated with the MFB (1). Neuroanatomically, this system appears to consist of "first-stage," "second-stage," and "third-stage" reward-related neurons "in series" with one another (1). On the basis of anatomical-tracing studies and electrophysiological studies from which one can infer direction of neuronal conduction (2), the first-stage neurons appear to originate diffusely from a group of ventral limbic-forebrain loci termed by some neuroanatomists as "the anterior bed nuclei of the medial forebrain bundle" (horizontal limb of the diagonal band of Broca, olfactory tubercle, magnocellular preoptic nucleus, lateral preoptic area, interstitial nucleus of the stria medullaris, VP, substantia innominata, and anterior lateral hypothalamus). These first-stage neurons are myelinated and moderately fast-conducting, and they project posteriorly through the MFB to synapse on VTA dopamine (DA) cells. The second-stage neurons are DA in nature, and project anteriorly within the MFB to synapse in the Acb. Only a small subset of these DA neurons appear specialized for carrying reward-rel-

From: Handbook of Neurotoxicology, Vol. 2
Edited by: E. J. Massaro © Humana Press Inc., Totowa, NJ

evant information *(1)*. From Acb, third-stage enkephalinergic reward-relevant neurons carry the neural signal to VP. This third-stage pathway appears critical for expression of reward-related and incentive-related behaviors *(3–5)*. The VTA, Acb, and VP are mutually interconnected by reciprocal anatomic pathways. These interconnections appear to regulate reward functions and reward-driven behaviors. The medium spiny Acb projection neurons (which use γ-aminobutyric acid [GABA] as their neurotransmitter) may constitute another brain-reward output path *(6)*. Additional neural elements synapse onto the first-stage, second-stage, or third-stage components of this brain reward system, presumably to regulate aspects of hedonic tone *(1)*. These regulatory inputs include opioid peptidergic, serotonergic, glutamatergic, and GABAergic neural elements *(1)*. On the basis of studies in which single-neuron electrophysiological recordings have been coupled with reward-related behavioral contingencies, it appears that the neurons in these pathways are exceedingly heterogeneous in terms of their reward-related functions. Some neurons seem to encode reward itself while others seem to encode expectancy of reward, errors in reward-prediction, prioritized reward, and other more complex aspects of reward-driven learning and reward-related incentive motivation *(7–14)*. There also appears to be significant functional plasticity within these systems with respect to the encoding of reward-related events *(9,11)*. Even taking into account the significant functional heterogeneity and plasticity found in these systems, one of the primary functions of these reward substrates is to compute hedonic tone and neural "payoffs" *(15–18)*. It appears that these brain substrates evolved to subserve natural, biologically significant rewards *(19)*.

1.2. Actions of Drugs of Abuse on Brain-Reward Substrates

Drugs of abuse activate the brain-reward substrates delineated earlier. Specifically, they appear to activate the second-stage DA neurons of the VTA-Acb axis, thus producing the pleasurable/euphoric effects that constitute the "high" sought by drug abusers. For some drugs of abuse (e.g., amphetamines, cocaine), the action on the VTA-Acb DA neurons appears to be direct. For other drugs of abuse (e.g., opiates, nicotine), the action on the VTA-Acb DA neurons appears to be indirect and even transsynaptic *(1)*. The DA component appears to be a crucial common substrate upon which drugs of abuse (regardless of chemical structure or pharmacological category) act to enhance brain reward substrates, and thus the subjective experience of reward and reward-related behaviors. Drug reward by itself and drug potentiation of electrical brain-stimulation reward (BSR) appear to have common actions within these reward substrates *(20)*. BSR and the pharmacological reward produced by drugs of abuse are both more powerful than the reward produced by natural, biologically essential reinforcers *(19)*. Drugs of abuse appear to gain this power by "hijacking" the reward substrates that originally evolved to subserve natural rewards *(19)*.

1.3. Hedonic Dysregulation of Brain-Reward Substrates as an Underlying Cause of Drug Abuse

That drugs of abuse activate the aforementioned brain-reward substrates appears clear, as does the inference that the high that drug users seek derives therefrom. What is not clear is why some human users of these drugs can use them on an occasional recreational basis, while other users of these same drugs deteriorate into an obsessional, compulsive, addictive use pattern that is patently self-destructive. Genetic factors may well play a role *(21)*. At the animal level, genetic factors are also known to play a role in proclivity to self-administer drugs of abuse, and in the degree of ease with which initially neutral environmental cues can acquire positive incentive salience as a result of being paired with exposure to drugs of abuse *(22–25)*. At the cellular and molecular level, these genetic vulnerabilities to drugs of abuse appear to correlate with a decreased neurofilamentary transport system for tyrosine hydroxylase (the rate-limiting enzyme in DA synthesis) in mesolimbic DA neurons of the VTA-Acb neural axis *(26,27)*. This, in turn, produces a DA deficiency in these brain-reward substrates, which has been hypothesized to underlie the observed behavioral vulnerability to drugs of abuse *(28,29)*. A more complex explanatory scheme of the cellular neurobiological mechanisms underlying vulnerability to drug abuse and relapse to drug abuse—involving a cascade of homeostatic dysregulations within both the brain's VTA-Acb reward substrates and in circuits interconnecting with these reward substrates—has also been advanced *(30,31)*. In this conception, the increased vulnerability to drug abuse conferred by genetic factors, drug use, or withdrawal dysphoria is conceived to involve decreased VTA-Acb reward function coupled with increases in the brain-stress neurotransmitter corticotropin-releasing factor (CRF) in the central nucleus of the amygdala. In this view, it is the combination of decreased positive drug-induced reward, increased opponent neural processes within the reward substrates, and recruitment of brain-stress neural systems within the extended amygdala that provides the allostatic change in overall hedonic set-point that leads to the compulsive drug-seeking and drug-taking that characterizes drug abuse *(30–32)*.

2. CANNABINOID ACTIONS ON BRAIN-REWARD SUBSTRATES

Even though cannabinoids have clear abuse potential at the human level *(33–39)*, some workers in the field have considered them to be "anomalous," i.e., lacking interaction with brain-reward substrates (e.g., *40*). However, it has become clear over the last decade that marijuana and other cannabinoids act on the aforementioned brain-reward substrates in strikingly similar fashion to noncannabinoid drugs of abuse.

2.1. Acute Cannabinoid Exposure

2.1.1. Cannabinoid Effects on Electrical BSR

Δ^9-Tetrahydrocannabinol (THC), the psychoactive and addictive constituent of marijuana and hashish, enhances electrical BSR (i.e., lowers brain-reward thresholds) in the VTA-Acb neural reward axis in laboratory animals *(41–45)*, as demonstrated using both an auto-titration quantitative electrophysiological reward-threshold measurement technique and the so-called "rate-frequency curve-shift" quantitative electrophysiological reward-threshold measurement technique. In the former technique *(41)*, animals are studied in test chambers containing two response levers. Each response by an animal on the primary or "stimulation" lever delivers BSR, the initial intensity of which is optimized for each animal at a clearly supra-threshold reward level (in µA), and decreases by a fixed amount at every third press of the primary lever. The animal can reset the current back to the initial intensity maximum at any time by pressing a "reset" lever (which does not deliver BSR; it only resets the system back to initial stimulus

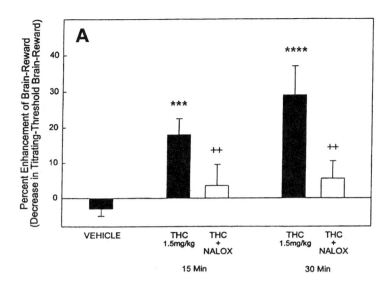

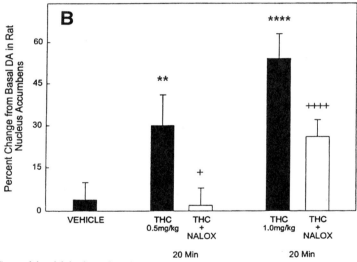

Fig. 1. Cannabinoid-induced enhancement of electrical brain-stimulation reward (**A**; top panel) and extracellular dopamine overflow in the nucleus accumbens (**B**; bottom panel). A: Enhancement of electrical brain-stimulation reward produced by acute low-dose administration of Δ^9-tetrahydrocannabinol (THC), and attenuation of THC-induced enhancement by acute low-dose naloxone (NALOX). Enhancement of electrical brain-stimulation reward was measured as decreases in brain-reward threshold using an auto-titration quantitative electrophysiological reward measurement technique with stimulation electrodes implanted in the medial forebrain bundle. Significantly different from vehicle control: ***$p < .005$, ****$p < .001$. Significantly different from THC alone: ++$p < .01$. (B) Enhancement of extracellular dopamine overflow in nucleus accumbens produced by acute low-dose administration of THC, and attenuation of THC-induced enhancement by acute low-dose naloxone (NALOX). Enhancement of extracellular dopamine overflow was measured by in vivo brain microdialysis in the nucleus accumbens, using 20-min sampling periods. Significantly different from vehicle control: **$p < .01$, ****$p < .001$. Significantly different from THC alone: +$p < .05$, ++++$p < .001$.

strength). The mean self-determined reset level is taken to be the animal's self-chosen reward threshold (below which the animal feels no subjective reward). In the latter technique *(44,45)*, animals are trained to lever-press for a series of 16 different reward-ing electrical-pulse frequencies, ranging from 25–141 Hz, presented in descending order. The initial frequency is optimized for each animal at a clearly supra-threshold reward level. At each pulse frequency, animals are given the opportunity to lever-press for rewarding electrical BSR for two 30-s time periods ("bins"), following which the pulse frequency decreases by 0.05 log units. Two measures of reward threshold are taken: M_{50}, the pulse frequency at which the animal lever-presses at half-maximum speed; and θ_0, the frequency at which the animal ceases to respond for rewarding elec-trical BSR. Both are reliable indices of reward efficacy. Using either technique, THC at low doses (e.g., 1.0 mg/kg) is clearly observed to reliably and significantly lower brain-reward thresholds, i.e., to enhance brain-reward substrates (e.g., *see* Fig. 1, top panel) *(41–45)*.

2.1.2. Cannabinoid Effects on Brain-Reward Neurochemical Substrates

2.1.2.1. In Vitro Studies

THC appears to enhance the synthesis of DA, as studied by in vitro assay systems *(46,47)*. 9-Nor-9beta-hydroxyhexahydrocannabinol, a cannabinoid with potent antinociceptive activity, appears to share this feature *(48)*. With respect to effects on DA uptake mechanisms, several laboratories have reported that THC inhibits DA neu-ronal uptake, as studied by in vitro assay systems *(49–52)*. With respect to DA release in in vitro assay systems, the picture is much less clear. Cannabinoid enhancement of DA release has been reported *(52,53)*. But other studies report either no effect *(54)* or cannabinoid-induced inhibition of electrically stimulated DA release *(55)*.

2.1.2.2. In Vivo Studies

Beginning more than a decade ago, the technique of in vivo brain microdialysis began to be used to measure THC effects on extracellular DA overflow in reward-relevant brain loci of awake behaving animals *(56)*. These early studies found that THC acutely enhances extracellular DA overflow in reward-related forebrain loci, including the Acb. Subsequent work, both from the Gardner laboratory in New York *(57–60)* and from other research groups *(61–63)*, confirms these findings. The DA-enhancing effect is tetrodotoxin-sensitive, calcium-dependent, and naloxone-blockable *(42,43,60,62)*, and is also blocked by the selective cannabinoid antagonist SR141716A *(62)*. The effect is also seen with the synthetic cannabinoid agonist WIN–55212–2 *(62)*. Cannabinoid-induced DA enhancement is seen not only in Acb *(60)* but also in other reward-relevant forebrain DA terminal projection loci, including medial prefron-tal cortex (59) and neostriatum *(56,57,61,63)*. Within the Acb, THC's DA-enhancing effect occurs selectively within the Acb shell *(62)*. This latter finding is congruent with a large literature implicating the shell as the anatomic domain within Acb most special-ized for mediating drug-enhanced brain reward *(1,64–67)*. Also beginning more than a decade ago, the technique of in vivo brain voltammetric electrochemistry was used to measure THC effects on extracellular DA overflow in reward-relevant brain loci, and showed robust THC-induced synaptic DA enhancement in reward-relevant forebrain loci *(57)*. Thus, despite one negative report *(69)*, the overwhelming evidence from several different labs and using two different in vivo neurochemical techniques is that cannabinoids enhance extracellular DA in the reward-relevant forebrain (e.g., *see* Fig. 1, bottom panel).

2.1.3. Cannabinoid Effects on DA Neuronal Firing in Brain-Reward Substrates

Drugs of abuse enhance DA functions in reward-relevant brain loci in a wide variety of ways *(1)*. Some, such as cocaine and amphetamines, accomplish this by enhancing DA release or inhibiting DA reuptake *(1)*. Others, such as nicotine and opioids, accomplish this by stimulating the firing rate of the second-stage reward-relevant DA neurons *(1,70,71)*. To assess whether cannabinoids augment DA function in the DA reward system by influencing DA release/reuptake or by influencing DA neuronal firing, a number of laboratories have employed in vivo single-neuron electrophysiological recording techniques in conjunction with cannabinoid administration in living laboratory animals *(72–76)*. With one exception *(72)*, the findings are that THC and the potent synthetic cannabinoids WIN-55,212-2, and CP-55,940 enhance neuronal firing of DA neurons in forebrain reward substrates *(73–76)*. The effect is seen in VTA-Acb DA neurons, and also in the adjacent nigro-striatal and meso-prefrontal DA neurons *(73–76)*. The enhanced DA firing is more pronounced in the VTA-Acb DA axis than in other forebrain DA loci *(74)*, which is congruent with the known preferential action of other drugs of abuse on DA neurons of the VTA-Acb axis *(1,8,65,77)*. The effect is blocked by the selective CB1 cannabinoid receptor antagonist SR141716A *(73,75,76)*, although not by the opiate antagonist naloxone *(73)*. In a small number of meso-prefrontal DA neurons, cannabinoid administration did not increase firing rate, but rather produced an increase in bursting activity of those neurons *(76)*. This latter finding is provocative, as it is known that the burst-firing state of mesotelencephalic DA neurons produces dramatically increased (supra-additive) DA release at axon terminals *(78)*.

2.2. Chronic Cannabinoid Exposure

Studies of the effects of chronic cannabinoid exposure are mixed. Furthermore, this is primarily an older literature using in vitro assay techniques performed on tissue dissected from the brains of chronically treated animals. Some studies report that chronic THC produces increased DA in the mediobasal hypothalamus (through which runs the VTA-Acb DA reward axis) *(79,80)*. Others report no effects of chronic cannabinoids on DA in dissected brain tissue *(81,82)*. One study reports that chronic THC produces no effects on DA indices in striatum or Acb, while decreasing DA metabolism (as assessed by DOPAC:DA ratios) in medial prefrontal cortex *(83)*. Yet another study indicates that chronic THC administration produces tolerance to the enhanced DA reuptake produced by acute THC *(84)*. A very recent report *(85)* indicates that chronic THC administration produces sensitization to the psychomotor-stimulant effects of amphetamine, a behavioral measure usually taken to indicate increased DA tone within the VTA-Acb neural axis.

2.3. Cannabinoid Withdrawal

As delineated earlier, drugs of abuse enhance BSR and augment DA in brain-reward substrates. Conversely, withdrawal from drugs of abuse produces inhibition of BSR and depletion of DA in brain reward substrates *(86–92)*. The question thus arises as to whether cannabinoid withdrawal mimics withdrawal from other addicting drugs, either in regards to BSR thresholds or DA function in the VTA-Acb reward axis. With respect to BSR, withdrawal from as little as a single 1.0 mg/kg dose of THC produces significant elevation in brain reward threshold *(93)*, identical to that seen in withdrawal from other drugs of abuse. With respect to DA function within the VTA-Acb neural reward axis, withdrawal from chronic THC—precipitated either by abrupt THC discontinuance or by the selective CB1 cannabinoid receptor antagonist SR141716A—produces a reduction in VTA-Acb DA cell activity (reversed by the administration of THC in the case of the discontinuance-precipitated withdrawal) *(94)* and a reduction in in vivo microdialysate-measured DA in the Acb shell *(95)*. These findings indicate that cannabinoid withdrawal is characterized by reduced DA transmission in the VTA-Acb reward system, similar to that observed with other drugs of abuse. Recently, it has been proposed that another common feature of withdrawal from drugs of abuse is elevation of CRF in the central nucleus of the amygdala *(32,96,97)*. This is provocative, as the amygdala has been implicated in mediating neural substrates of an emotional memory system that facilitates drug-seeking behavior *(98–102)*. The question thus arises as to whether cannabinoid withdrawal mimics withdrawal from other drugs of abuse, with respect to amygdaloid CRF. Recent reports suggest strongly that it does: cannabinoid withdrawal is accompanied by marked elevation in extracellular amygdaloid CRF similar to that seen in withdrawal from other drugs of abuse *(103)*. Thus, it may be stated that cannabinoid withdrawal mimics withdrawal from other drugs of abuse with respect to effects seen in the two main brain systems believed to subserve initial drug-taking behavior and relapse *(31)*.

2.4. Endocannabinoid Function and DA Brain-Reward Substrates

The advances in knowledge of the brain mechanisms subserving cannabinoid action on the brain during the past decade have been stunning *(104–111)*. Specific brain receptors for cannabinoids have been discovered, cloned, and sequenced. Their neuroanatomical distribution has been mapped. Endogenous brain agonists for these receptors have been identified, and the signal-transduction cascades that these receptors activate have been delineated. Evidence has accumulated that these endogenous cannabinoid agonists serve neurotransmitter and/or neuromodulatory functions in the brain. Recent studies have attempted to explore the relationship between these endogenous cannabinoid ("endocannabinoid") systems and DA brain substrates. This research is new, and comparatively few clear-cut findings have emerged.

2.4.1. Endocannabinoid Regulation of DA Substrates

The selective cannabinoid CB1 receptor antagonist SR141716A increases the neural population response of nigrostriatal DA neurons without altering their spontaneous firing rates or apomorphine-induced rate inhibition *(112)*. SR141716A also prevents amphetamine-induced inhibition of nigrostriatal DA neurons *(112)*. These findings are interpreted to indicate that an endocannabinoid endogenous neural tone modulates nigrostriatal DA function. Similar effects were not seen in the VTA-Acb DA neural axis *(112)*.

2.4.2. DA Regulation of Endocannabinoid Substrates

Repeated DA D_1 receptor stimulation enhances cannabinoid-induced catalepsy produced by the potent synthetic cannabinoid receptor agonist HU–210 *(113)*. DA D_2

receptor stimulation, but not DA D_1 receptor stimulation, induces endogenous release of the endocannabinoid neurotransmitter/neuromodulator anandamide *(114)*. Chronic L-DOPA treatment increases cannabinoid CB1 receptor mRNA expression in 6-hydroxydopamine-lesioned rats *(115)*. All of these findings were observed in the nigrostriatal DA system, and it is not known to what extent similar findings may obtain in the mesoaccumbens VTA-Acb axis.

3. GENETIC VARIATIONS IN CANNABINOID ACTIONS ON BRAIN-REWARD SUBSTRATES

Genetic differences exist in preference for specific drugs of abuse and in propensity to self-administer such drugs *(22,23,25,26,116–118)*. Some animal strains that show high ethanol preference and self-administration generalize this drug-seeking behavior to other drugs of abuse such as nicotine and opiates *(22,117,119,120)*, suggesting that generalized vulnerability to the rewarding effects of drugs of abuse may be genetically influenced. The Lewis rat strain is particularly intriguing. Lewis rats appear to be inherently drug-seeking and drug-preferring: they work harder for opiate and cocaine self-administration, cue-condition more readily to opiates and cocaine, and voluntarily drink ethanol more readily, than other rat strains *(22,23,25,26,121)*. The question arises as to whether cannabinoid effects on brain-reward show similar genetic variation. To this end, cannabinoid effects have been studied on brain reward substrates in various rat strains. Using quantitative electrophysiological brain-stimulation techniques, it has been determined that THC produces robust enhancement of BSR in drug-preferring Lewis rats, moderate enhancement in drug-neutral Sprague-Dawley rats, and no change in drug-resistant Fischer 344 rats *(44,45,122,123)*. Using in vivo brain microdialysis, it has been determined that THC produces robust enhancement of Acb DA in drug-preferring Lewis rats, moderate enhancement in drug-neutral Sprague-Dawley rats, and no change in drug-resistant Fischer 344 rats *(124,125)*.

4. ENDOGENOUS OPIOID INVOLVEMENT IN CANNABINOID ACTIONS ON BRAIN-REWARD SUBSTRATES

It has been known for almost a decade that cannabinoid and opioid receptors are both coupled to similar postsynaptic intracellular-signaling mechanisms, involving activation of G_i proteins and consequent inhibition of adenylyl cyclase and decreased cAMP production *(126)*. In fact, it has been suggested that cannabinoids and opioids may interact at the level of their signal transduction mechanisms *(127)*. Also, CB1 cannabinoid receptors are co-localized with μ opioid receptors in the Acb *(128)*. The question arises as to functional cannabinoid-opioid interactions that may be relevant to drug abuse.

4.1. Cannabinoid Effects on Endogenous Brain-Opioid Systems

Adult rats exposed to chronic THC administration show increased methionine-enkephalin- and β-endorphin-like immunoreactivity in the preoptic area and mediobasal hypothalamus *(79)*. Newborn rat pups given THC daily for 4 d show significantly elevated methionine-enkephalin and β-endorphin levels in anterior hypothalamus/preoptic area and mediobasal hypothalamus *(129)*. Rats given subchronic THC show increased mRNA levels for pro-opiomelanocortin, the precursor for the opioid neurotransmitter β-endorphin *(130)*, and for pro-enkephalin and pro-dynorphin, the precursors for the opioid enkephalins and dynorphins, respectively *(131)*, although none of these findings was in reward-relevant brain areas. More germane to reward-related substrates, Acb pro-enkephalin mRNA levels are elevated in animals given subchronic administration of the powerful synthetic cannabinoid CP-55,940 *(132)*, although Acb pro-enkephalin mRNA was unchanged following subchronic THC or R-methanandamide (although the latter two cannabinoids did increase pro-enkephalin mRNA in other brain areas) *(132)*. Morphine's reinforcing properties and its ability to enhance Acb DA are both markedly reduced in knockout mice lacking the CB1 cannabinoid receptor *(133,134)*.

4.2. Endogenous Opioid Mediation of Cannabinoid Actions on Brain-Reward Substrates

DA brain-reward substrates are anatomically and functionally interconnected with endogenous brain-opioid peptide neural systems in the VTA, Acb, and VP *(1)*. These endogenous opioid peptide systems appear importantly involved in the set-point of hedonic tone, and in the expression of reward-related and incentive-related behaviors *(1)*. Provocatively, the enhanced brain reward produced by all well-studied drugs of abuse (including nonopiates such as ethanol, barbiturates, benzodiazepines, phencyclidine, amphetamines, and cocaine) is blocked or attenuated by opiate antagonists *(1)*, implicating endogenous opioid mechanisms in mediating the rewarding actions of such drugs. The question thus arises as to the possible role of endogenous opioid mechanisms in cannabinoid effects on brain-reward systems. This question has been addressed using BSR and in vivo microdialysis techniques. With respect to BSR, the opiate antagonist naloxone attenuates THC-induced BSR enhancement (e.g., *see* Fig. 1, top panel) *(42,43,135)*. Naloxone also attenuates THC-induced enhancement of Acb DA (e.g., *see* Fig. 1, bottom panel) *(42,43,58,60,62,136)*. The selective μ_1 opiate antagonist naloxonazine duplicates the naloxone effect, implicating the μ_1 opiate receptor subtype in mediating cannabinoid effects on brain reward *(62)*. These findings using in vivo microdialysis are congruent with an older report that naloxone attenuates THC-enhanced DA synthesis in brain, as measured by in vitro biochemistry *(137)*.

5. NEURAL AND SYNAPTIC MODELS OF CANNABINOID ACTIONS ON BRAIN-REWARD SUBSTRATES

From the evidence presented earlier, and from additional reports, hypotheses may be hazarded concerning *where* in the brain and *how* in the brain cannabinoids act to alter brain reward substrates.

5.1. Neural Sites of Action of Cannabinoid Effects on Brain-Reward Substrates

Different drugs of abuse enhance brain reward by acting at different sites within the brain's reward substrates. Nicotine, ethanol, benzodiazepines, and barbiturates appear to act (primarily transsynaptically) in VTA; cocaine, amphetamines, and dissociative anesthetics appear to act primarily in Acb *(1)*. Opiates act on reward substrates in VTA, Acb, and VP *(1)*. The question arises as to the sites of action in the brain where cannabinoids act to alter brain reward. This has been addressed in several ways, both direct

and inferential. One of the direct ways has been to study the effects of local cannabinoid microinjection on DA overflow in brain-reward substrates *(138)*. THC
microinfusions into Acb dose-dependently enhance Acb DA *(138)*. THC microinjections into VTA dose-dependently enhance VTA DA, but do not enhance Acb DA *(138)*.
This suggests that local VTA THC does not alter local DA neuronal firing, and further
suggests that the elevated Acb DA and augmented BSR produced by systemic THC
result from local actions by THC at or near the reward-relevant Acb DA axon terminals
(138). However, as noted earlier, systemic THC administration does enhance VTA-
Acb DA neuronal firing *(73–75)*, and local microinjections of the μ_1 opioid antagonist
naloxonazine into VTA attenuate cannabinoid-enhanced Acb DA *(62)*. Critically, however, systemic naloxone (at doses generally considered high enough to block endogenous opioid mechanisms) does not inhibit THC's enhancement of VTA-Acb neuronal
firing *(73)*. This combination of findings is frankly puzzling, as it is by no means clear
why local brain microinjections of an opioid antagonist should attenuate the cannabinoid effects, while systemic administration of an opioid antagonist fails to do so. Thus,
it may be hypothesized that cannabinoids enhance Acb DA by acting at a combination
of brain loci: (1) within the Acb, acting on mechanisms closely linked to axon terminal
DA release; (2) within the VTA, acting on endogenous opioid mechanisms not linked
to activation of neuronal firing, but rather linked to mechanisms of DA synthesis, transport, and/or release; and (3) within the VTA, acting on non-endogenous-opioid mechanisms linked to activation of neuronal firing.

5.2. Neural Mechanisms of Action of Cannabinoid Effects on Brain-Reward Substrates

As noted earlier, different drugs of abuse enhance brain reward by acting through
different mechanisms within the brain's reward substrates. Amphetamines (and probably some phencyclidine-like dissociative anesthetics) act as presynaptic DA releasers,
cocaine as a presynaptic DA reuptake blocker, opiates and nicotine as transsynaptic
enhancers of DA neuronal firing, and other addictive drugs by yet other mechanisms
(1). The question arises as to the mechanisms of action in the brain through which
cannabinoids act to alter brain reward, a question obviously related to the issues raised
in the previous section on brain sites of cannabinoid action. As noted in Subheading
5.1., studies using local intracerebral THC microinjections have led to the hypothesis
that one of THC's sites of action is in the vicinity of the reward-relevant Acb DA axon
terminals *(138)*. As also noted earlier, THC-induced Acb DA augmentation is calcium-
dependent and tetrodotoxin-sensitive *(42,43,60)*, implicating an action-potential-
dependent mechanism. Additional studies—using in vivo voltammetric
electrochemistry to study THC-induced synaptic DA overflow in forebrain DA terminal projection fields—indicate that the THC-induced electrochemical "signature"
resembles that of a DA reuptake blocker rather than that of a presynaptic DA releaser
(57). Further explorations of this hypothesis have taken place. First, studies of the
effects of various combinations of THC and the DA antagonist haloperidol on Acb DA
using in vivo brain microdialysis have been carried out *(139)*. The rationale for this is
that impulse-induced facilitation of DA release underlies a synergistic effect between
DA antagonists and DA-reuptake inhibitors *(140)*. The findings were provocative: pretreatment with the DA antagonist haloperidol has a synergistic effect on THC's

enhancement of Acb DA, and THC pretreatment before haloperidol has a similar synergistic effect on haloperidol's enhancement of Acb DA *(139)*. Tetrodotoxin perfused locally into the Acb abolished the synergism between THC and haloperidol *(139)*. Since this type of synergistic effect on DA is highly characteristic of the effect seen with co-administration of a DA antagonist such as haloperidol and a DA reuptake blocker such as GBR12909 *(140,141)*, this suggests that the synergistic enhancement of haloperidol-induced increase in Acb DA by THC is consistent with the hypothesis that THC's enhancing action on Acb DA results from DA reuptake blockade (possibly indirect or transsynaptically-mediated) at Acb DA terminals *(42,43,139)*. This hypothesis has also been explored using in vivo microdialysis of the DA metabolite 3-methoxytyramine (3-MT) *(142)*. While only a small portion of released DA is metabolized to it, 3-MT is believed to be a sensitive index of enhanced extracellular DA *(143)* and, most importantly, a sensitive marker for distinguishing DA releasing agents from DA reuptake blockers, since DA releasers such as amphetamine and methamphetamine increase 3-MT levels while DA reuptake blockers such as bupropion and nomifensine do not *(144)*. Studies were therefore undertaken on the effects of amphetamine, cocaine, nomifensine, and THC on extracellular Acb 3-MT levels using in vivo microdialysis. It was found that the DA releaser amphetamine significantly increased both DA and 3-MT in Acb, while the DA reuptake blockers cocaine and nomifensine increased only DA *(142)*. THC increased only DA, resembling the DA reuptake blockers *(142)*. These in vivo findings are congruent with older in vitro studies showing that cannabinoids have DA reuptake blockade actions in brain tissue, as previously noted *(49,52,84)*. It is tempting to speculate that such a mechanism may underlie cannabinoid action on DA reward substrates locally within the Acb. Cannabinoid action within the VTA—acting on endogenous opioid mechanisms not linked to activation of neuronal firing, but rather linked to mechanisms of DA synthesis, transport, and/or release—may be mediated by a cannabinoid-receptor inhibition of an inhibitory endogenous opioid peptidergic synaptic link to VTA DA neurons that regulates their synthesis, transport, and/or release of DA rather than cell firing. Cannabinoid action within the VTA—acting on nonendogenous-opioid mechanisms linked to activation of neuronal firing—could conceivably be mediated by a cannabinoid-receptor inhibition of feedback Acb-VTA projection neurons that normally exert inhibitory synaptic tone on VTA DA cells. This suggestion would be congruent with the known co-localization of cannabinoid receptors with DA D_1 receptors on striatonigral inhibitory projection neurons *(145)*.

6. INTEGRATION AND SUMMARY

On the basis of more than a decade of electrophysiological and biochemical evidence, cannabinoids appear to enhance brain-reward substrates in similar fashion to other drugs of abuse. Also on the basis of electrophysiological and biochemical evidence, cannabinoid withdrawal appears to activate the same withdrawal substrates in brain as activated by other drugs of abuse. Cannabinoids are euphorigenic in humans and have addictive liability in vulnerable persons, but were long considered "anomalous" drugs of abuse, lacking pharmacological action on brain-reward substrates or on the anhedonic substrates activated in withdrawal. This position is no longer tenable. Rather, cannabinoids appear to share a common final neural action as other drugs of abuse in activating the VTA-Acb DA system and in inhibiting it (as well as activating amygdaloid CRF systems) during withdrawal.

REFERENCES

1. Gardner, E. L. (1997) Brain reward mechanisms, in *Substance Abuse: A Comprehensive Textbook,* 3rd ed. (Lowinson, J. H., Ruiz, P., Millman, R. B., and Langrod, J. G., eds.), Williams & Wilkins, Baltimore, pp. 51–85.
2. Gallistel, C. R., Shizgal, P., and Yeomans J. S. (1981) A portrait of the substrate for self-stimulation. *Psychol. Rev.* **88,** 228–273.
3. Bardo, M. T. (1998) Neuropharmacological mechanisms of drug reward: beyond dopamine in the nucleus accumbens. *Crit. Rev. Neurobiol.* **12,** 37–67.
4. Napier, T. C. and Mitrovic I. (1999) Opioid modulation of ventral pallidal inputs. *Ann. NY Acad. Sci.* **877,** 176–201.
5. McBride, W. J., Murphy, J. M., and Ikemoto S. (1999) Localization of brain reinforcement mechanisms: intracranial self-administration and intracranial place-conditioning studies. *Behav. Brain Rev.* **101,** 129–152.
6. Carlezon, W. A. Jr. and Wise, R. A. Rewarding actions of phencyclidine and related drugs in nucleus accumbens shell and frontal cortex. *J. Neurosci.* **16,** 3112–3122.
7. Gardner, E. L. and Lowinson, J. H. (1993) Drug craving and positive/negative hedonic brain substrates activated by addicting drugs. *Sem. Neurosci.* **5,** 359–368.
8. Di Chiara, G. (1995) The role of dopamine in drug abuse viewed from the perspective of its role in motivation. *Drug Alcohol Depend.* **38,** 95–137.
9. Schultz, W., Dayan, P., and Montague, P. R. (1997) A neural substrate of prediction and reward. *Science* **275,** 1593–1599.
10. Wickelgren, I. (1997) Getting the brain's attention. *Science* **278,** 35–37.
11. Woodward, D. J., Chang, J. Y., Janak, P., Azarov, A., and Anstrom, K. (1999) Mesolimbic neuronal activity across behavioral states. *Ann. NY Acad. Sci.* **877,** 91–112.
12. Redgrave, P., Prescott, T. J., and Gurney, K. (1999) Is the short-latency dopamine response too short to signal reward error? *Trends Neurosci.* **22,** 146–151.
13. Everitt, B. J., Parkinson, J. A., Olmstead, M. C., Arroyo, M., Robledo, P., and Robbins, T. W. (1999) Associative processes in addiction and reward: the role of amygdala-ventral striatal subsystems. *Ann. NY Acad. Sci.* **877,** 412–438.
14. Berridge, K. C. and Robinson, T. E. (1998) What is the role of dopamine in reward: hedonic impact, reward learning, or incentive salience? *Brain Res. Rev.* **28,** 309–369.
15. Kornetsky, C. and Bain, G. (1992) Brain-stimulation reward: a model for the study of the rewarding effects of abused drugs. *Natl. Inst. Drug Abuse Res. Monogr. Ser.* **124,** 73–93.
16. Kornetsky, C. and Duvauchelle, C. (1994) Dopamine, a common substrate for the rewarding effects of brain stimulation reward, cocaine, and morphine. *Natl. Inst. Drug Abuse Res. Monogr. Ser.* **145,** 19–39.
17. Shizgal, P. (1997) Neural basis of utility estimation. *Curr. Opinion Neurobiol.* **7,** 198–208.
18. Peoples, L. L., Uzwiak, A. J., Gee, F., Fabbricatore, A. T., Muccino, K. J., Mohta, B. D., and West, M. O. (1999) Phasic accumbal firing may contribute to the regulation of drug taking during intravenous cocaine self-administration. *Ann. NY Acad. Sci.* **877,** 781–787.
19. Goldstein, A. (1994) *Addiction: From Biology to Drug Policy.* W.H. Freeman, New York.
20. Wise, R. A. (1996) Addictive drugs and brain stimulation reward. *Annu. Rev. Neurosci.* **19,** 319–340.
21. Uhl, G., Blum, K., Noble, E., and Smith, S. (1993) Substance abuse vulnerability and D2 receptor genes. *Trends Neurosci.* **16,** 83–88.
22. George, F. R. and Goldberg, S. R. (1989) Genetic approaches to the analysis of addiction processes. *Trends Pharmacol. Sci.* **10,** 78–83.
23. Suzuki, T., George, F. R., and Meisch, R. A. (1989) Differential establishment and maintenance of oral ethanol reinforced behavior in Lewis and Fischer 344 inbred rat strains. *J. Pharmacol. Exp. Ther.* **245,** 164–170.

24. Kosten, T. A., Miserendino, M. J., Haile, C. N., DeCaprio, J. L., Jatlow, P. I., and Nestler, E. J. (1997) Acquisition and maintenance of intravenous cocaine self-administration in Lewis and Fischer inbred rat strains. *Brain Res.* **778**, 418–429.

25. Guitart, X., Beitner-Johnson, D., and Nestler, E. J. (1992) Fischer and Lewis rat strains differ in basal levels of neurofilament proteins and in their regulation by chronic morphine. *Synapse* **12**, 242–253.

26. Nestler, E. J. (1993) Molecular mechanisms of drug addiction in the mesolimbic dopamine pathway. *Sem. Neurosci.* **5**, 369–376.

27. Self, D. W. and Nestler, E. J. (1995) Molecular mechanisms of drug reinforcement and addiction. *Annu. Rev. Neurosci.* **18**, 463–495.

28. Gardner, E. L. (1999) The neurobiology and genetics of addiction: implications of the "reward deficiency syndrome" for therapeutic strategies in chemical dependency, in *Addiction: Entries and Exits* (Elster, J., ed.), Russell Sage, New York, pp. 57–119.

29. Blum, K., Cull, J. G., Braverman, E. R., and Comings, D. E. (1996) Reward deficiency syndrome. *Amer. Scientist* **84**, 132–145.

30. Koob, G. F. and Le Moal, M. (1997) Drug abuse: hedonic homeostatic dysregulation. *Science* **278**, 52–58.

31. Koob, G. F. (1999) The role of the striatopallidal and extended amygdala systems in drug addiction. *Ann. NY Acad. Sci.* **877**, 445–460.

32. Koob, G. F., Markou, A., Weiss, F., and Schulteis, G. (1993) Opponent process and drug dependence: neurobiological mechanisms. *Sem. Neurosci.* **5**, 351–358.

33. Kozel, N. J. and Adams, E. H. (1986) Epidemiology of drug abuse: an overview. *Science* **234**, 970–974.

34. Goldstein, A. and Kalant, H. (1990) Drug policy: striking the right balance. *Science* **249**, 1513–1521.

35. MacCoun, R. and Reuter, P. (1997) Interpreting Dutch cannabis policy: reasoning by analogy in the legalization debate. *Science* **278**, 47–52.

36. Kleber, H. D. (1988) Introduction —cocaine abuse: historical, epidemiological, and psychological perspectives. *J. Clin. Psychiat.* **49(2)[Suppl.]**, 3–6.

37. Crowley, T. J., Macdonald, M. J., Whitmore, E. A., and Mikulich, S. K. (1998) Cannabis dependence, withdrawal, and reinforcing effects among adolescents with conduct symptoms and substance use disorders. *Drug Alcohol Depend.* **50**, 27–37.

38. Anthony, J. C., Warner, L. A., and Kessler, R. C. (1994) Comparative epidemiology of dependence on tobacco, alcohol, controlled substances and inhalants: basic findings from National Comorbidity Study. *Exp. Clin. Psychopharmacol.* **2**, 244–268.

39. Hall, W., Solowij, N., and Lemon, J. (1994) The Health and Psychological Consequences of Cannabis Use (National Drug Strategy Monograph Series No. 25). Australian Government Publishing Service, Canberra.

40. Felder, C. C. and Glass, M. (1998) Cannabinoid receptors and their endogenous agonists. *Annu. Rev. Pharmacol Toxicol.* **38**, 179–200.

41. Gardner, E. L., Paredes, W., Smith, D., Donner, A., Milling, C., Cohen, D., and Morrison, D. (1988) Facilitation of brain stimulation reward by Δ^9-tetrahydrocannabinol. *Psychopharmacology* **96**, 142–144.

42. Gardner, E. L. and Lowinson, J. H. (1991) Marijuana's interaction with brain reward systems: update 1991. *Pharmacol. Biochem. Behav.* **40**, 571–580.

43. Gardner, E. L. (1992) Cannabinoid interaction with brain reward systems: the neurobiological basis of cannabinoid abuse, in *Marijuana/Cannabinoids: Neurobiology and Neurophysiology* (Murphy, L. L. and Bartke, A., eds.), CRC Press, New York, pp. 275–335.

44. Gardner, E. L., Liu, X., Paredes, W., Savage, V., Lowinson, J., and Lepore, M. (1995) Strain-specific differences in Δ^9-tetrahydrocannabinol (THC)-induced facilitation of electrical brain stimulation reward (BSR). *Soc. Neurosci. Abstr.* **21**, 177.

45. Lepore, M., Liu, X., Savage, V., Matalon, D., and Gardner, E. L. (1996) Genetic differences in Δ^9-tetrahydrocannabinol-induced facilitation of brain stimulation reward as mea-

sured by a rate-frequency curve-shift electrical brain stimulation paradigm in three different rat strains. *Life Sci. (Pharmacol. Lett.)* **58**, PL365–PL372.

46. Bloom, A. S. (1982) The effect of Δ^9-tetrahydrocannabinol on the synthesis of dopamine
    and norepinephrine in mouse brain synaptosomes. *J. Pharmacol. Exp. Ther.* **221**, 97–103.

47. Navarro, M., Fernández-Ruiz, J. J., de Miguel, R., Hernández, M. L., Cebeira, M., and
    Ramos, J. A. (1993) An acute dose of Δ^9-tetrahydrocannabinol affects behavioral and neu-
    rochemical indices of mesolimbic dopaminergic activity. *Behav. Brain Res.* **57**, 37–46.

48. Bloom, A. S., Dewey, W. L., Harris, L. S., and Brosius, K. K. (1977) 9-Nor-9beta-hydroxy-
    hexahydrocannabinol, a cannabinoid with potent antinociceptive activity: comparisons
    with morphine. *J. Pharmacol. Exp. Ther.* **200**, 263–270.

49. Banerjee, S. P., Snyder, S. H., and Mechoulam, R. (1975) Cannabinoids: influence on
    neurotransmitter uptake in rat brain synaptosomes. *J. Pharmacol. Exp. Ther.* **194**, 74–81.

50. Johnson, K. M., Dewey, W. L., and Harris, L. S. (1976) Some structural requirements for
    inhibition of high-affinity synaptosomal serotonin uptake by cannabinoids. *Mol.
    Pharmacol.* **12**, 345–352.

51. Hershkowitz, M., Goldman, R., and Raz, A. (1977) Effect of cannabinoids on neurotrans-
    mitter uptake, ATPase activity and morphology of mouse brain synaptosomes. *Biochem.
    Pharmacol.* **26**, 1327–1331.

52. Poddar, M. K. and Dewey, W. L. (1980) Effects of cannabinoids on catecholamine uptake
    and release in hypothalamus and striatal synaptosomes. *J. Pharmacol. Exp. Ther.* **214**,
    63–67.

53. Jentsch, J. D., Wise, A., Katz, Z., and Roth, R. H. (1998) Alpha-noradrenergic receptor
    modulation of the phencyclidine- and Δ^9-tetrahydrocannabinol-induced increases in
    dopamine utilization in rat prefrontal cortex. *Synapse* **28**, 21–26.

54. Szabo, B., Muller, T., and Koch, H. (1999) Effects of cannabinoids on dopamine release in
    the corpus striatum and the nucleus accumbens in vitro. *J. Neurochem.* **73**, 1084–1089.

55. Cadogan, A. K., Alexander, S. P., Boyd, E. A., and Kendall, D. A. (1997) Influence of
    cannabinoids on electrically evoked dopamine release and cyclic AMP generation in the
    rat striatum. *J. Neurochem.* **69**, 1131–1137.

56. Ng Cheong Ton, J.M. and Gardner, E.L. (1986) Effects of delta-9-tetrahydrocannabinol on
    dopamine release in the brain: intracranial dialysis experiments. *Soc. Neurosci. Abstr.*
    12, 135.

57. Ng Cheong Ton, J. M., Gerhardt, G. A., Friedemann, M., Etgen, A. M., Rose, G. M.,
    Sharpless, N. S., and Gardner, E. L. (1988) The effects of Δ^9-tetrahydrocannabinol on
    potassium-evoked release of dopamine in the rat caudate nucleus: an in vivo electrochemi-
    cal and in vivo microdialysis study. *Brain Res.* **451**, 59–68.

58. Chen, J., Paredes, W., Li, J., Smith, D., and Gardner, E. L. (1989) In vivo brain
    microdialysis studies of Δ^9-tetrahydrocannabinol on presynaptic dopamine efflux in
    nucleus accumbens of the Lewis rat. *Soc. Neurosci. Abstr.* **15**, 1096.

59. Chen, J., Paredes, W., Lowinson, J. H., and Gardner, E. L. (1990) Δ^9-Tetrahydrocannab-
    inol enhances presynaptic dopamine efflux in medial prefrontal cortex. *Eur. J. Pharmacol.*
    190, 259–262.

60. Chen, J., Paredes, W., Li, J., Smith, D., Lowinson, J., and Gardner, E. L. (1990) Δ^9-
    Tetrahydrocannabinol produces naloxone-blockable enhancement of presynaptic basal
    dopamine efflux in nucleus accumbens of conscious, freely-moving rats as measured by
    intracerebral microdialysis. *Psychopharmacology* **102**, 156–162.

61. Taylor, D. A., Sitaram, B. R., and Elliot-Baker, S. (1988) Effect of Δ-9-tetrahydrocannab-
    inol on release of dopamine in the corpus striatum of the rat, in *Marijuana: An Interna-
    tional Research Report* (Chesher, G., Consroe, P., and Musty, R., eds.), Australian
    Government Publishing Service, Canberra, pp. 405–408.

62. Tanda, G., Pontieri, F. E., and Di Chiara, G. (1997) Cannabinoid and heroin activation of
    mesolimbic dopamine transmission by a common μ_1 opioid receptor mechanism. *Science*
    276, 2048–2050.

63. Malone, D. T. and Taylor, D. A. (1999) Modulation by fluoxetine of striatal dopamine release following Δ^9-tetrahydrocannabinol: a microdialysis study in conscious rats. *Br. J. Pharmacol.* **128,** 21–26.

64. McBride, W. J., Murphy, J. M., and Ikemoto, S. (1999) Localization of brain reinforcement mechanisms: intracranial self-administration and intracranial place-conditioning studies. *Behav. Brain Res.* **101,**129–152.

65. Pontieri, F. E., Tanda, G., and Di Chiara, G. (1995) Intravenous cocaine, morphine, and amphetamine preferentially increase extracellular dopamine in the "shell" as compared with the "core" of the rat nucleus accumbens. *Proc. Natl. Acad. Sci. USA* **92,** 12,304–12,308.

66. Johnson, P. I., Goodman, J. B., Condon, R., and Stellar, J. R. (1995) Reward shifts and motor responses following microinjections of opiate-specific agonists into either the core or shell of the nucleus accumbens. *Psychopharmacology* **120,** 195–202.

67. Carlezon, W. A. Jr. and Wise, R. A. (1996) Rewarding actions of phencyclidine and related drugs in nucleus accumbens shell and frontal cortex. *J. Neurosci.* **16,** 3112–3122.

68. Carlezon, W. A. Jr. and Wise, R. A. (1996) Microinjections of phencyclidine (PCP) and related drugs into nucleus accumbens shell potentiate medial forebrain bundle brain stimulation reward. *Psychopharmacology* **128,** 413–420.

69. Castañeda, E., Moss, D. E., Oddie, S. D., and Whishaw, I. Q. (1991) THC does not affect striatal dopamine release: microdialysis in freely moving rats. *Pharmacol. Biochem. Behav.* **40,** 587–591.

70. Gysling, K. and Wang, R. Y. (1983) Morphine-induced activation of A10 dopamine neurons in the rat. *Brain Res.* **277,** 119–127.

71. Grenhoff, J., Aston-Jones, G., and Svensson, T. H. (1986) Nicotinic effects on the firing pattern of midbrain dopamine neurons. *Acta Physiol. Scand.* **128,** 351–358.

72. Gifford, A. N., Gardner, E. L., and Ashby, C. R. Jr. (1997) The effect of intravenous administration of delta–9-tetrahydrocannabinol on the activity of A10 dopamine neurons recorded in vivo in anesthetized rats. *Neuropsychobiology* **36,** 96–99.

73. French, E. D. (1997) Δ^9-Tetrahydrocannabinol excites rat VTA dopamine neurons through activation of cannabinoid CB1 but not opioid receptors. *Neurosci. Lett.* **226,** 159–162.

74. French, E. D., Dillon, K., and Wu, X. (1997) Cannabinoids excite dopamine neurons in the ventral tegmentum and substantia nigra. *Neuroreport* **8,** 649–652.

75. Gessa, G. L., Melis, M., Muntoni, A. L., and Diana, M. (1998) Cannabinoids activate mesolimbic dopamine neurons by an action on cannabinoid CB1 receptors. *Eur. J. Pharmacol.* **341,** 39–44.

76. Diana, M., Melis, M., and Gessa, G. L. (1998) Increase in meso-prefrontal dopaminergic activity after stimulation of CB1 receptors by cannabinoids. *Eur. J. Neurosci.* **10,** 2825–2830.

77. Di Chiara, G. and Imperato, A. (1986) Preferential stimulation of dopamine release in the nucleus accumbens by opiates, alcohol, and barbiturates: studies with transcerebral dialysis in freely moving rats. *Ann. NY Acad. Sci.* **473,** 367–381.

78. Overton, P. G. and Clark, D. (1997) Burst firing in midbrain dopaminergic neurons. *Brain Res. Rev.* **25,** 312–334.

79. Kumar, M. S., Patel, V., and Millard, W. J. (1984) Effects of chronic administration of Δ^9-tetrahydrocannabinol on the endogenous opioid peptide and catecholamine levels in the diencephalon and plasma of the rat. *Substance Alcohol Actions/Misuse* **5,** 201–210.

80. Patel, V., Borysenko, M., and Kumar, M. S. (1985) Effect of Δ^9-THC on brain and plasma catecholamine levels as measured by HPLC. *Brain Res. Bull.* **14,** 85–90.

81. Taylor, D. A. and Fennessy, M. R. (1982) Time-course of the effects of chronic Δ^9-tetrahydrocannabinol on behaviour, body temperature, brain amines and withdrawal-like behaviour in the rat. *J. Pharm Pharmacol.* **34,** 240–245.

82. Ali, S. F., Newport, G. D., Scallet, A. C., Gee, K. W., Paule, M. G., Brown, R .M., and Slikker, W. Jr. (1989) Effects of chronic Δ^9-tetrahydrocannabinol (THC) administration on neurotransmitter concentrations and receptor binding in the rat brain. *Neurotoxicology* **10,** 491–500.

83. Jentsch, J. D., Verrico, C. D., Le, D., and Roth, R. H. (1998) Repeated exposure to Δ^9-tetrahydrocannabinol reduces prefrontal cortical dopamine metabolism in the rat. *Neurosci. Lett.* **246,** 169–172.

84. Hershkowitz, M. and Szechtman, H. (1979) Pretreatment with Δ^1-tetrahydrocannabinol and psychoactive drugs: effects on uptake of biogenic amines and on behavior. *Eur. J. Pharmacol.* **59,** 267–276.

85. Gorriti, M. A., Rodríguez de Fonseca, F., Navarro, M., and Palomo, T. (1999). Chronic (-)-Δ^9-tetrahydrocannabinol treatment induces sensitization to the psychomotor effects of amphetamine in rats. *Eur. J. Pharmacol.* **365,** 133–142.

86. Schaefer, G. J. and Michael, R. P. (1986) Changes in response rates and reinforcement thresholds for intracranial self-stimulation during morphine withdrawal. *Pharmacol. Biochem. Behav.* **25,** 1263–1269.

87. Frank, R. A., Martz, S., and Pommering, T. (1988) The effect of chronic cocaine on self-stimulation train-duration thresholds. *Pharmacol. Biochem. Behav.* **29,** 755–758.

88. Schulteis, G., Markou, A., Gold, L. H., Stinus, L., and Koob, G. F. (1994) Relative sensitivity of multiple indices of opiate withdrawal: a quantitative dose-response analysis. *J. Pharmacol. Exp. Ther.* **271,** 1391–1398.

89. Wise, R. A. and Munn, E. (1995) Withdrawal from chronic amphetamine elevates baseline intracranial self-stimulation thresholds. *Psychopharmacology* **117,** 130–136.

90. Parsons, L. H., Smith, A. D., and Justice, J. B. Jr. (1991) Basal extracellular dopamine is decreased in the rat nucleus accumbens during abstinence from chronic cocaine. *Synapse* **9,** 60–65.

91. Pothos, E., Rada, P., Mark, G. P., and Hoebel, B. G. (1991) Dopamine microdialysis in the nucleus accumbens during acute and chronic morphine, naloxone-precipitated withdrawal and clonidine treatment. *Brain Res.* **566,** 348–350.

92. Rossetti, Z. L., Hmaidan, Y., and Gessa, G. L. (1992) Marked inhibition of mesolimbic dopamine release: a common feature of ethanol, morphine, cocaine and amphetamine abstinence in rats. *Eur. J. Pharmacol.* **221,** 227–234.

93. Gardner, E. L. and Lepore, M. (1996) Withdrawal from a single dose of marijuana elevates baseline brain-stimulation reward thresholds in rats. Paper presented at meetings of the Winter Conference on Brain Research, Aspen, CO, USA, January 1996.

94. Diana, M., Melis, M., Muntoni, A. L., and Gessa, G. L. (1998) Mesolimbic dopaminergic decline after cannabinoid withdrawal. *Proc. Natl. Acad. Sci. USA* **95,** 10,269–10,273.

95. Tanda, G., Loddo, P., and Di Chiara, G. (1999) Dependence of mesolimbic dopamine transmission on Δ^9-tetrahydrocannabinol. *Eur. J. Pharmacol.* **376,** 23–26.

96. Merlo Pich, E., Lorang, M., Yeganeh, M., Rodríguez de Fonseca, F., Raber, J., Koob, G. F., and Weiss, F. (1995) Increase in extracellular corticotropin-releasing factor-like immunoreactivity levels in the amygdala of awake rats during restraint stress and ethanol withdrawal as measured by microdialysis. *J. Neurosci.* **15,** 5439–5447.

97. Koob, G. F. (1996) Drug addiction: the yin and yang of hedonic homeostasis. *Neuron* **16,** 893–896.

98. Cador, M., Robbins, T. W., and Everitt, B. J. (1989) Involvement of the amygdala in stimulus-reward associations: interaction with the ventral striatum. *Neuroscience* **30,** 77–86.

99. Everitt, B. J., Cador, M., and Robbins, T. W. (1989) Interactions between the amygdala and ventral striatum in stimulus-reward associations: studies using a second-order schedule of sexual reinforcement. *Neuroscience* **30,** 63–75.

100. Gaffan, D. (1992) Amygdala and the memory of reward, in *The Amygdala: Neurobiological Aspects of Emotion* (Aggleton, J. P., ed.), Wiley, New York, pp. 471–483.
101. Hiroi, N. and White, N. M. (1991) The lateral nucleus of the amygdala mediates expression of the amphetamine conditioned place preference. *J. Neurosci.* **11,** 2107–2116.
102. White, N. M. and Hiroi, N. (1993) Amphetamine conditioned cue preference and the neurobiology of drug-seeking. *Sem. Neurosci.* **5,** 329–336.
103. Rodríguez de Fonseca, F., Carrera, M. R. A., Navarro, M., Koob, G. F., and Weiss, F. (1997) Activation of corticotropin-releasing factor in the limbic system during cannabinoid withdrawal. *Science* **276,** 2050–2054.
104. Matsuda, L. A. (1997) Molecular aspects of cannabinoid receptors. *Crit. Rev. Neurobiol.* **11,** 143–166.
105. Pertwee, R. G. (1998) Pharmacological, physiological and clinical implications of the discovery of cannabinoid receptors. *Biochem. Soc. Trans.* **26,** 267–272.
106. Di Marza, V., Melck, D., Bisogno, T., and De Petrocellis. (1998) Endocannabinoids: endogenous cannabinoid receptor ligands with neuromodulatory action. *Trends Neurosci.* **21,** 521–528.
107. Felder, C. C. and Glass, M. (1998) Cannabinoid receptors and their endogenous agonists. *Annu. Rev. Pharmacol. Toxicol.* **38,** 179–200.
108. Axelrod, J. and Felder, C. C. (1998) Cannabinoid receptors and their endogenous agonist, anandamide. *Neurochem. Res.* **23,** 575–581.
109. Martin, B. R., Mechoulam, R., and Razdan, R. K. (1999) Discovery and characterization of endogenous cannabinoids. *Life Sci.* **65,** 573–595.
110. Khanolkar, A. D. and Makriyannis, A. (1999) Structure-activity relationships of anandamide, an endogenous cannabinoid ligand. *Life Sci.* **65,** 607–616.
111. Shire, D., Calandra, B., Bouaboula, M., Barth, F., Rinaldi-Carmona, M., Casellas, P., and Ferrara, P. (1999) Cannabinoid receptor interactions with the antagonists SR 141716A and SR 144528. *Life Sci.* **65,** 627–635.
112. Gueudet, C., Santucci, V., Rinaldi-Carmona, M., Soubrie, P., and Le Fur, G. (1995) The CB1 cannabinoid receptor antagonist SR 141716A affects A9 dopamine neuronal activity in the rat. *Neuroreport* **6,** 1421–1425.
113. Rodríguez de Fonseca, F., Martin Calderon, J. L., Mechoulam, R., and Navarro, M. (1994) Repeated stimulation of D1 dopamine receptors enhances (-)–11-hydroxy-Δ^8-tetrahydrocannabinol-dimethyl-heptyl-induced catalepsy in male rats. *Neuroreport* **5,** 761–765.
114. Giuffrida, A., Parsons, L. H., Kerr, T. M., Rodríguez de Fonseca, F., Navarro, M., and Piomelli, D. (1999) Dopamine activation of endogenous cannabinoid signaling in dorsal striatum. *Nature Neurosci.* **2,** 358–363.
115. Zeng, B. Y., Dass, B., Owen, A., Rose, S., Cannizzaro, C., Tel, B. C., and Jenner, P. (1999) Chronic L-DOPA treatment increases striatal cannabinoid CB1 receptor mRNA expression in 6-hydroxydopamine-lesioned rats. *Neurosci. Lett.* **276,** 71–74.
116. Cannon, D. S. and Carrell, L. E. (1987) Rat strain differences in ethanol self-administration and taste aversion. *Pharmacol. Biochem. Behav.* **28,** 57–63.
117. George, F. R. (1987) Genetic and environmental factors in ethanol self-administration. *Pharmacol. Biochem. Behav.* **27,** 379–384.
118. Kosten, T. A., Miserendino, M. J., Chi, S., and Nestler, E. J. (1994) Fischer and Lewis rat strains show differential cocaine effects in conditioned place preference and behavioral sensitization but not in locomotor activity or conditioned taste aversion. *J. Pharmacol. Exp. Ther.* **269,** 137–144.
119. George F. R. and Meisch, R. A. (1984) Oral narcotic intake as a reinforcer: genotype x environment interaction. *Behav. Genet.* **14,** 603.
120. Khodzhagel'diev, T. (1986) Formirovanie vlecheniia k nikotinu u myshei linii C57Bl/6 i CBA [Development of nicotine preference in C57Bl/6 and CBA mice]. *Biull. Eksp. Biol. Med.* **101,** 48–50.

121. Misenrendino, M. J. D., Kosten, T. A., Guitart, X., Chi, S., and Nestler, E. J. (1992) Individual differences in vulnerability to drug addiction: behavioral and biochemical correlates. *Soc. Neurosci. Abstr.* **18,** 1078.

122. Gardner, E. L., Paredes, W., Smith, D., Seeger, T., Donner, A., Milling, C., Cohen, D., and Morrison, D. (1988) Strain-specific sensitization of brain stimulation reward by Δ^9-tetrahydrocannabinol in laboratory rats. *Psychopharmacology* **96(Suppl.),** 365.

123. Gardner, E. L., Chen, J., Paredes, W., Li, J., and Smith, D. (1989) Strain-specific facilitation of brain stimulation reward by Δ^9-tetrahydrocannabinol in laboratory rats is mirrored by strain-specific facilitation of presynaptic dopamine efflux in nucleus accumbens. *Soc. Neurosci. Abstr.* **15,** 638.

124. Gardner, E. L., Chen, J., Paredes, W., Li, J., and Smith, D. (1989) Strain-specific facilitation of brain stimulation reward by Δ^9-tetrahydrocannabinol in laboratory rats is mirrored by strain-specific facilitation of presynaptic dopamine efflux in nucleus accumbens. *Soc. Neurosci. Abstr.* **15,** 638.

125. Chen, J., Paredes, W., Lowinson, J. H., and Gardner, E. L. (1991) Strain-specific facilitation of dopamine efflux by Δ^9-tetrahydrocannabinol in the nucleus accumbens of rat: an in vivo microdialysis study. *Neurosci. Lett.* **129,** 136–140.

126. Childers, S. R., Fleming, L., Konkoy, C., Marckel, D., Pacheco, M., Sexton, T., and Ward, S. (1992) Opioid and cannabinoid receptor inhibition of adenylyl cyclase in brain. *Ann. NY Acad. Sci.* **654,** 33–51.

127. Thorat, S. N. and Bhargava, H. N. (1994) Evidence for a bidirectional cross-tolerance between morphine and Δ^9-tetrahydrocannabinol in mice. *Europ. J. Pharmacol.* **260,** 5–13.

128. Navarro, M., Chowen, J., Carrera, M. R. A., del Arco, I., Villanúa, M. A., Martin, Y., et al. (1998) CB$_1$ cannabinoid receptor antagonist-induced opiate withdrawal in morphine-dependent rats. *NeuroReport* **9,** 3397–3402.

129. Kumar, A. M., Haney, M., Becker, T., Thompson, M.L., Kream, R. M., and Miczek, K. (1990) Effects of early exposure to δ–9-tetrahydrocannabinol on the levels of opioid peptides, gonadotropin-releasing hormone and substance P in the adult male rat brain. *Brain Res.* **525,** 78–83.

130. Corchero, J., Fuentes, J. A., and Manzanares, J. (1997) Δ^9-Tetrahydrocannabinol increases proopiomelanocortin gene expression in the arcuate nucleus of the rat hypothalamus. *Eur. J. Pharmacol.* **323,** 193–195.

131. Corchero, J., Avila, M. A., Fuentes, J. A., and Manzanares, J. (1997) Δ^9-Tetrahydrocannabinol increases prodynorphin and proenkephalin gene expression in the spinal cord of the rat. *Life Sci. [Pharmacol. Lett.]* **61,** PL39–PL43.

132. Manzanares, J., Corchero, J., Romero, J., Fernandez-Ruiz, J. J., Ramos, J. A., and Fuentes, J. A. (1998) Chronic administration of cannabinoids regulates proenkephalin mRNA levels in selected regions of the rat brain. *Mol. Brain Res.* **55,** 126–132.

133. Ledent, C., Valverde, O., Cossu, G., Petitet, F., Aubert, J.F., Beslot, F., et al. (1999) Unresponsiveness to cannabinoids and reduced addictive effects of opiates in CB1 receptor knockout mice. *Science* **283,** 401–404.

134. Mascia, M. S., Obinu, M. C., Ledent, C., Parmentier, M., Böhme, G. A., Imperato, A., and Fratta, W. (1999) Lack of morphine-induced dopamine release in the nucleus accumbens of cannabinoid CB$_1$ receptor knockout mice. *Eur. J. Pharmacol.* **383,** R1–R2.

135. Gardner, E. L., Paredes, W., Smith, D., and Zukin, R. S. (1989) Facilitation of brain stimulation reward by Δ^9-tetrahydrocannabinol is mediated by an endogenous opioid mechanism. *Adv. Biosci.* **75,** 671–674.

136. Gardner, E. L., Chen, J., Paredes, W., Smith, D., Li, J., and Lowinson, J. (1990) Enhancement of presynaptic dopamine efflux in brain by Δ^9-tetrahydrocannabinol is mediated by an endogenous opioid mechanism, in *New Leads in Opioid Research* (van Ree, J. M., Mulder, A. H., Wiegant, V. M., and van Wimersma Greidanus, T. B., eds.), Elsevier Science Publishers, Amsterdam, pp. 243–245.

137. Bloom, A. S. and Dewey, W. L. (1978) A comparison of some pharmacological actions of morphine and Δ^9-tetrahydrocannabinol in the mouse. *Psychopharmacology* **57,** 243–248.

138. Chen, J., Marmur, R., Pulles, A., Paredes, W., and Gardner, E. L. (1993) Ventral tegmental microinjection of Δ^9-tetrahydrocannabinol enhances ventral tegmental somatodendritic dopamine levels but not forebrain dopamine levels: evidence for local neural action by marijuana's psychoactive ingredient. *Brain Res.* **621,** 65–70.

139. Gardner, E. L., Paredes, W., and Chen, J. (1990) Further evidence for Δ^9-tetrahydrocannabinol as a dopamine reuptake blocker: brain microdialysis studies. *Soc. Neurosci. Abstr.* **16,** 1100.

140. Westerink B. H., Tuntler, J., Damsma, G., Rollema, H., and de Vries, J. B. (1987) The use of tetrodotoxin for the characterization of drug-enhanced dopamine release in conscious rats studied by brain dialysis. *Naunyn Schmiedeberg's Arch. Pharmacol.* **336,** 502–507.

141. Shore, P. A., McMillen, B. A., Miller, H. H., Sanghera, M. K., Kiserand, R. S., and German, D. C. (1979) The dopamine neuronal storage system and non-amphetamine psychotogenic stimulants: a model for psychosis, in *Catecholamines: Basic and Clinical Frontiers* (Usdin, E., Kopin, I. J., and Barchas, J., eds.), Pergamon Press, New York, pp. 722–735.

142. Chen, J., Paredes, W., and Gardner, E. L. (1994) Δ^9-Tetrahydrocannabinol's enhancement of nucleus accumbens dopamine resembles that of reuptake blockers rather than releasers: evidence from in vivo microdialysis experiments with 3-methoxytyramine. *Natl. Inst. Drug Abuse Res. Monogr. Ser.* **141,** 312.

143. Wood, P. L. and Altar, C. A. (1988) Dopamine release in vivo from nigrostriatal, mesolimbic, and mesocortical neurons: utility of 3-methoxytyramine measurements. *Pharmacol. Rev.* **40,** 163–187.

144. Heal, D. J., Frankland, A. T. J., and Buckett, W. R. (1990) A new and highly sensitive method for measuring 3-methoxytyramine using HPLC with electrochemical detection: studies with drugs which alter dopamine metabolism in the brain. *Neuropharmacology* **29,** 1141–1150.

145. Herkenham, M., Lynn, A. B., de Costa, B. R., and Richfield, E. K. (1991) Neuronal localization of cannabinoid receptors in the basal ganglia of the rat. *Brain Res.* **547,** 267–274.

7

Dopamine and Its Modulation of Drug-Induced Neuronal Damage

Donald M. Kuhn

1. INTRODUCTION

Dopamine (DA), or 3-hydroxytyramine, is a chemical species that has immense importance for the proper functioning of a number of the body's organ systems. Perhaps DA exerts its most profound influence in its role as a neurotransmitter. DA is distributed in a rather discrete manner throughout the central nervous system (CNS), with its cell bodies originating in the mesencephalon. Its axonal processes ramify from here to many distant sites where DA participates in the process of neuronal communication. As a neurotransmitter, DA is known to mediate a wide-variety of physiological processes and behaviors including locomotor activity, modulation of the cardiovascular system, food-intake, regulation of body temperature, and neuroendocrine function, to mention but a few. DA also mediates the reinforcing effects of a number of psychostimulant drugs of abuse such as cocaine and the amphetamines. In a broader sense, DA is actually considered the neurotransmitter in the brain's pleasure center (i.e., the nucleus accumbens) where it decodes the reinforcing effects of diverse stimuli. When the DA neuronal system does not function properly, it is possible that the ensuing disruption in higher-cognitive processes can lead to psychiatric illness. Furthermore, if the nigrostriatal DA system damaged or destroyed, the effects can manifest themselves as a neurological disorder, and Parkinson's disease (PD) is the best known example of this. Therefore, the DA neuronal system is extremely important to brain function and it maintains a delicate balance between normal function and dysfunction.

Alterations in the function of the DA neuronal system can occur at many biological sites. Two elements of the DA neuronal phenotype are particularly important in ensuring that DA function remains within normal limits. First, tyrosine hydroxylase (TH) is the initial and rate-limiting enzyme in the biosynthesis of DA. It is generally assumed that any neuron that contains TH is a DA neuron, and changes in the activity of TH can lead to corresponding changes in the amount of DA that is synthesized and released into the synapse. Second, the DA neuronal transporter (DAT) is an integral membrane protein that transports released (i.e., synaptic) DA back into the presynaptic nerve ending. The DAT therefore serves to terminate the synaptic action of DA. The DAT, like TH, is thought to be a phenotypic marker for DA neurons. Other elements of the DA

From: Handbook of Neurotoxicology, Vol. 2
Edited by: E. J. Massaro © Humana Press Inc., Totowa, NJ

neuronal phenotype are equally important in transducing the neurotransmitter functions of DA (e.g., the family of receptors for DA and their second-messenger systems), but TH and the DAT are particularly relevent when one considers drugs of abuse, psychiatric disorders, and neurologic disorders that are mediated by DA.

The purpose of this chapter is to focus on the role of DA in conditions that are associated with damage to the CNS. To do this, it is necessary to include discussions of TH and the DAT because these important proteins appear to be targeted for damage by various neurotoxicants. Reductions in their function will therefore be predicted to have severe consequences on neurochemical function, and, at the same time, their modification by certain neurotoxicants could serve as an early indication that more serious effects will ensue. Losses in TH or DAT function do not necessarily follow loss of neuronal integrity, but may actually serve as an index of the mechanisms of action by which DA neurons are being damaged. The remaining discussion will focus on the hypothesis that DA actually participates in the process by which DA neurons are damaged by drugs and other toxins. It may sound anthropomorphic to discuss a neurotransmitter in this manner, but the participation by DA in a neurotoxic process is unwitting, and may well represent an unfortunate combination of events that lead to a very selective form of neurotoxicity. Before this hypothesis can be delineated, it must be established how an important neurotransmitter like DA can participate in toxicity.

2. ROLES FOR DA IN NEUROTOXICITY

DA itself, and many other catechol compounds including L-DOPA, can be quite toxic to cells and neurons under the appropriate conditions. Certain aspects of DA chemistry make it a strong candidate for an endogenous neurotoxicant. DA readily oxidizes nonenzymatically to the corresponding quinone *(1,2)* and it is well-known that quinones can modify cellular proteins and enzymatic processes *(1,3–6)* and DNA *(7)*. The metabolism of DA by monoamine oxidase (MAO) also produces H_2O_2 *(8,9)*, and the generation of reactive oxygen species (ROS) downstream of the peroxide, such as superoxide or hydroxyl radicals *(10)*, could also underlie the damaging effects of DA in neural tissue. High concentrations of DA can inhibit DA *(11,12)* and glutamate transporter function in vitro *(12)* and cause toxic effects in brain or cultured neurons *(13–17)*. Studies of DA cellular toxicity have not yet identified a specific target protein or nucleotide in brain tissue, but it is evident that DOPA and DA can be quite toxic to neurons in situ and in vivo. Are these toxic effects restricted to in vitro and cell culture situations, or is it possible that DA can participate in the process of neurotoxicity in vivo?

The amphetamine derivatives methamphetamine and 3,4-methylenedioxymethamphetamine (MDMA) are well-known drugs of abuse. These drugs are now known to have persistent, if not permanent effects on the DA and serotonin neuronal systems *(18–20)*. The spectrum of their toxic effects includes significant reductions in function of TH and the DAT. It has been known for some time now that the toxic effects of methamphetamine, and to some extent MDMA, are dependent on endogenous DA. If animals are depleted of DA prior to treatment with methamphetamine, the reductions in TH (and DA levels) and DAT function caused by the substituted amphetamine are largely prevented. When depleted brain levels of DA are restored to near normal with L-DOPA treatment, the toxic effects of methamphetamine (i.e., reductions in TH, DA levels, and DAT function) are restored *(21–24)*. Finally, if endogenous DA is elevated to supra-normal levels with L-DOPA treatment, the toxic effects of methamphetamine on the DA neuronal phenotype are heightened *(25,26)*. Vesicular monoamine transporter knockout mice have much higher levels of cytoplasmic DA and show enhanced methamphetamine-induced toxicity *(27)*. Direct-acting DA receptor agonists do not apparently share this effect with DA, so it appears to be associated with the DA molecular itself and not with a receptor-transduced process. Enzymatic and nonenzymatic breakdown of DA can lead to the generation of various downstream reactants, particularly in the cellular cytoplasm *(3,9,18,28)*. Therefore, it is significant that the neurotoxic amphetamines cause the redistribution of DA from synaptic vesicles (a protective, chemically reductive environment) into the cytoplasm (an oxidative environment), probably through a weak-base action and collapse of the pH gradient across the vesicle membrane *(29–33)*. While certain DA receptor antagonists protect the brain from methamphetamine, it is not thought that the toxicity of the amphetamines is transduced by receptor mediated events, and most evidence points directly at DA itself. By comparison, the excitatory amino acid neurotransmitter glutamate does transduce its toxic effects through receptor-mediated events. Taken together, these results paint a rather interesting image of DA being positively linked to the toxic effects of methamphetamine: higher levels of DA resulting in more extensive damage to DA nerve endings, and lower levels of DA resulting in protection against methamphetamine-induced toxicity.

Apart from amphetamine-induced damage to DA nerve endings, it has also been suggested that DA could play a role in the neurodegeneration associated with PD. As mentioned earlier, a confluence of events related to altered metabolism of intraneuronal (i.e., cytoplasmic) DA could establish conditions allowing for the creation of a DA-derived species that results in neurodegeneration. Obviously, one source of increased intraneuronal DA in PD could be L-DOPA itself, the preferred and most effective therapy for DA-replacement in this neurological disorder. DOPA, like DA, can also be very toxic to cells in culture *(34–38)*, but the evidence relating DOPA itself to worsening of Parkinson's symptomology, or to causing Parkinson's-like pathology in treated animals, is inconclusive and remains a matter of some debate *(39)*. Another approach to the therapy of PD that focused on modifying the production of a DA-derived substance involved monoamine oxidase inhibitors (MAOI). If it is assumed that the DA itself is not the actual toxin, but that MAO-mediated generation of hydrogen peroxide was, then it should be possible to prevent damage or slow its progression by MAOI therapy. This approach was bolstered with the observation that the known DA neurotoxin MPTP was prevented from damaging DA neurons by MAOIs *(40)*. The large Datatop clinical study that assessed the protective effects of MAOI therapy on the progression of PD was not able to detect a DA-derived product from MAO action on the neurotransmitter as the DA neuronal toxin *(41)*, but DA remains as a viable source of toxicity. The neurochemical consequences of increased DA on the toxicity associated with MPTP, or with the progression of PD, does not seem as clear as the situation with methamphetamine, but it is generally acknowledged that intraneuronal DA could also play an integral role in the neurodegenerative processes that are operative in PD. Is it possible that a monoamine neurotransmitter can be neurotoxic itself or contribute to neurotoxicity?

3. REACTIVE OXYGEN SPECIES AND REACTIVE NITROGEN SPECIES ARE PROBABLE MEDIATORS OF DA NEUROTOXICITY

The entry of methamphetamine into DA nerve ending seems necessary but is not sufficient for damage to occur. Therefore, something must "transduce" the damaging properties of the amphetamines. Oxidative stress, in its broadest definition, refers to the deleterious and damaging effects that reactive oxygen species (ROS) and reactive nitrogen species (RNS) have on cellular proteins and organelles. Species like nitric oxide (NO), superoxide radical, hydroxyl radical, and hydrogen peroxide, to list but a few, are extremely reactive and need not be radicals (i.e., possessing an unpaired electron) to cause neuronal damage. A rapidly growing body of evidence is linking amphetamine toxicity to oxidative stress, and it has been shown that methamphetamine causes the production in vivo of hydroxyl radical (*42–44*), heightened expression of the neuronal form of NOS (45)*,* and increases NO production *(46)*. Oxidative stress is a heuristically appealing and testable mechanism to explain amphetamine-induced neuronal deficits. Most, if not all, known in vivo effects of the amphetamines on their identified targets (e.g., DAT, serotonin transporter, TH, and tryptophan hydroxylase) can be mimicked in in vitro studies when these same target proteins are exposed to ROS/RNS. Furthermore, drugs that scavenge ROS and RNS, or that bolster cellular antioxidant capability *(47,48)*, protect against amphetamine-induced damage. Many ROS/RNS are known to react kinetically with cellular proteins and organelles at rates that are faster than their reaction with glutathione. Therefore, drug-induced oxidative stress can readily override cellular defenses, and presents an important mechanism mediating the effects of the substituted amphetamines.

The extreme complexity of oxidative stress makes it clear why the toxic mechanisms of action of drugs like methamphetamine are so difficult to understand. Reactions of individual ROS and RNS with each other and with their cellular targets are among the fastest known in biological systems. Therefore, studies of individual ROS or RNS as mediators of amphetamine-induced damage could easily be predicted to be futile, but instead, they have been quite productive. For instance, targeted disruption of the gene for nitric oxide synthase (NOS), the enzyme responsible for synthesis of NO, protects mice from methamphetamine toxicity *(49,50)*. Compounds that inhibit NOS also protect animals from methamphetamine (METH) and MDMA *(51–54)*. Transgenic mice overexpressing superoxide dismutase (SOD), the enzyme responsible for discharging the superoxide radical in vivo, are resistant to amphetamine-induced damage *(55–62)* and SOD inhibitors enhance methamphetamine toxicity *(63)*. Taken together, roles for NO and superoxide radical in substituted amphetamine toxicity have been substantiated, but are these reactive species the active, toxic agents?

NO and superoxide are almost certainly involved in the damaging effects of the amphetamines, establishing conditions for production of another reactive chemical species-peroxynitrite (ONOO⁻). ONOO⁻ is formed by the near diffusion-limited reaction of NO with superoxide *(64–67)*. Because the rate of this reaction is $> 10^9 \ M^{-1} \ s^{-1}$, it is highly likely that the production of ONOO⁻ will occur in any cellular location where NO is generated *(64,68)*. ONOO⁻ is a powerful oxidant *(69)* and it also nitrates free tyrosine and tyrosine residues in proteins *(70–72)*. Very recent evidence has established that ONOO⁻ is probably more cytotoxic than either of its precursors NO and superoxide, and it can damage proteins and DNA, cause lipid peroxidation, and diminish mitochondrial function *(64,67,68,73–75)*, effects associated with many drugs that damage DA neurons (i.e., methamphetamine and N-methyl-4-phenyl-1,2,3,6-tetrahydropyridine [MPTP]). By searching for tyrosine nitration in conditions associated with cytotoxicity *(72)*, emerging evidence is pointing to a role for $ONOO^-$ in apoptosis, Alzheimers disease (AD), Parkinson's disease, and Huntington's disease (HD) *(76)*. The DA-selective neurotoxin MPTP has also been linked to $ONOO^-$-induced tyrosine nitration in proteins *(77)*. Protection of animals from substituted amphetamine toxicity by blocking NO or superoxide production could point to these agents as the damaging species, but it could indicate that $ONOO^-$ is active because removal of either NO or superoxide from the equation would also prevent $ONOO^-$ production. The participation of $ONOO^-$ in amphetamine-induced toxicity has been investigated in only one study to date, and the preliminary data in this paper indicated a METH-induced increase in free nitrotyrosine formation *(78)*. Evidence for $ONOO^-$ participation in amphetamine-induced damage to DA and serotonin nerve endings is compelling (although insufficiently studied at present), but is $ONOO^-$ the active, toxic species?

Using MPTP and/or its active metabolite MPP^+ to model the DA neuronal toxicity of PD in animals and cell culture, strong mechanistic evidence exists supporting roles for these ROS and RNS as mediators of cell damage *(79–82)*. While any one of these reactive species, or combinations of them, could potentially cause damage to DA neurons, evidence for the participation of superoxide and NO has been the most convincing when considering MPTP-induced neurotoxicity. For instance, the autooxidation of MPTP and some of its intermediary metabolites involves the production of superoxide radical *(83–85)*. Transgenic mice expressing increased levels of SODs are also resistant to MPTP-induced neurotoxicity *(58,86–88)*. Perhaps the strongest evidence that NO is involved in MPTP-induced damage to DA neurons, and in PD by extension, are the results showing that animals lacking the gene for NOS are resistant to the damaging effects of MPTP *(89,90)*. It has been demonstrated very recently that MPTP causes extensive gliosis and a robust upregulation of the inducible form of NOS (iNOS;*91*), and mice lacking the gene for iNOS are resistant to MPTP-induced neurotoxicity *(91)*. Inhibitors of NOS also protect DA neurons from MPTP-induced damage *(89,90,92,93)*. Therefore, an emerging picture implicates both superoxide radical and NO in the early events leading to DA neuronal damage and cell death in PD, as modeled by MPTP. While MPTP and methamphetamine share some elements and pathways of neurotoxicity, they differ in the extent to which they damage the nigrostriatal system. MPTP eventually damages the entire DA neuronal systems, from nerve endings to cell bodies, whereas the damaging effects of methamphetamine appear to be restricted to nerve endings.

Recent evidence from analyses of the incidence of PD in identical twins has diminished the role of genetic factors in the development of PD and this, in turn, has shifted emphasis to environmental and endogenous neurochemical factors as contributing elements in this neurodegenerative disorder. These studies are only mentioned because they establish a rather significant and interesting departure from the foregoing discussion with regard to methamphetamine and MPTP. Among a long list of potential environmental risk factors, epidemiological studies have identified pesticide exposure as a solid candidate *(94–97)*. Postmortem studies of PD brains have revealed a strong association between the presence of the organochlorine insecticide dieldrin and a diagnosis of PD *(98)*. Well-water consumption and a rural-life setting, both of which could possibly expose individuals to environmental contaminants like agricultural pesticides and herbicides, increase the risk of developing PD *(94,96,99,100)*. It was recognized some time ago that paraquat (PQ)-treated frogs showed Parkinson's-like behavioral and neurochemical changes *(101)*. The strong structural resemblance between PQ and 1-methyl-4-phenylpyridium (MPP^+), the active DA neurotoxin derived from MPTP, aroused suspicion that DA neurons may be selectively targeted by this agent. Indeed, Brooks et al. *(102)* have established recently that PQ treatment of rats causes extensive losses of DA containing cells of the nigrostriatal system, resulting in a behavioral syndrome very similar to that caused by MPTP (and as seen in PD).

Dieldrin is also known to cause extensive loss of neuronal DA in various species *(103,104)*, and this effect could underlie the hypokinesia and tremor seen in exposed animals. Dieldrin is very toxic to DA neurons in mesencephalic cultures *(105)* and one basis for its ability to damage DA neurons could be inhibition of mitochondrial oxidative phosphorylation *(106)*. Miller et al. *(107)* recently extended DA neurotoxic potential to the organochlorine insecticide heptachlor by showing that its active metabolite, heptachlor epoxide, significantly inhibited vesicular DA uptake. In fact, the vesicular DA transporter has been implicated as a target for a wide variety of herbicides and pesticides *(108)*. It is generally believed that the cytotoxicity of DA is enhanced by increasing its cytoplasmic levels, and the heptachlor-induced reduction in vesicular DA uptake adds weight to the suggestion that pesticides and herbicides are interacting with endogenous neurochemical systems (i.e., DA) and causing neurotoxicity via oxidative stress, DNA damage, mitochondrial dysfunction, and apoptosis (*see* below).

The herbicidal activity of PQ is actually based on its ability to generate superoxide in chloroplasts, subjecting plants to severe oxidative stress. PQ toxicity in mammals is thought to involve oxidative stress and it has been shown that mice lacking the genes for various forms of SOD are extremely sensitive to PQ lethality *(109,110)*. Although PQ is a structural analog of MPP^+ and might be expected to have many effects with in common with it, studies of the neurotoxic mechanisms of action of PQ lag far behind those of MPTP. Nevertheless, it seems likely that PQ, dieldrin, and heptachlor, share with MPTP and methamphetamine the ability to generate ROS and RNS *(111,112)*, and their spectrum of effects on DA cells includes DNA fragmentation, increased AP-1 binding, and apoptotic cell death *(113)*. Only recently has it been realized that pesticides and herbicides may share much in common with MPTP, and the escalating search for their participation in DA neurotoxicity has uncovered some very interesting parallels between MPTP and PQ. However, important mechanistic differences exist between these agents. Perhaps the most striking distinction is the ability of PQ to interact directly with NOS, the enzyme that produces NO. It appears that NOS can function as a PQ diaphorase. Day et al. *(114)* have established that PQ actually uses NOS as an electron source to generate superoxide, and this interaction decreases the production of NO. The PQ-NOS interaction reduces the generation of $ONOO^-$ by increasing superoxide production at the expense of NO *(114)*. Therefore, MPTP and PQ diverge mechanistically at the point of NO involvement—MPTP appears to cause DA neuronal damage in a manner dependent on increased production of both NO and superoxide, to create

ONOO⁻, whereas PQ appears to reduce NO production and increase superoxide production, minimizing a role for ONO.

4. INTERACTIONS OF DA WITH ROS AND RNS CAN GENERATE ENDOGENOUS TOXINS: DA-QUINONES

At the risk of appearing naive or overly simple, it must be emphasized that DA neurons contain a substance that is not found in other neurochemical cell types: namely DA. This places DA neurons in a unique position to influence their reaction to ROS/RNS and to determine the consequences of oxidative stress therein. Although not fully appreciated, ONOO⁻ reacts almost instantaneously with DA to form the o-quinone of DA, and this reaction occurs at the expense of the tyrosine nitrating properties of ONOO⁻ *(115,116)*. It is reasonably inferred that ONOO⁻ production will cause cytotoxicity via tyrosine nitration *(76)*, yet DA-quinones are highly reactive in their own right and can have detrimental effects on cells. For instance, cysteinyl-DA, an indirect index of quinone formation, is detected under in vivo conditions favoring DA-induced striatal damage *(4,14,117,118)*, including METH administration *(119)*. Catechol-quinones may be involved in the damage to DA neurons seen in PD *(120,121)*, and it has been shown recently that antiserum from patients with PD react with quinoproteins in vitro *(122)*. Like ONOO⁻-induced tyrosine nitration, posttranslational modification of proteins (including TH, tryptophan hydroxylase, DAT, and the serotonin transporter) by DA-quinone could serve as a "footprint" of an ONOO⁻-DA reaction following administration of MPTP or methamphetamine. A quinone of DA could help explain how DA participates in methamphetamine-induced damage, and the chemical properties of the DA-quinone are sufficiently distinct from those of DA itself that it may enter serotonin cells or damage them from the synaptic side. In the classic paper on catechol-quinone formation, Graham *(2)* showed that DA-quinones readily cyclize into species that have indole ring structures and could conceivably serve as substrates for uptake into serotonin neurons. Mayer has suggested that ONOO⁻ would not likely nitrate tyrosine residues under conditions of physiological pH *(123)*, yet Ischiropoulos *(76)* has reviewed impressive evidence that tyrosine nitration (presumably via ONOO⁻ action) occurs in dozens of animal and human diseases. A reaction between ONOO⁻ and DA, in DA nerve endings, to create o-quinones, certainly falls somewhere between these two extreme positions. Therein could lie a mechanism by which the neurotoxic amphetamines damage both DA and serotonin nerve endings.

It is not well-appreciated, but superoxide interacts directly with DA to produce the o-quinone *(124–126)*, much like ONOO⁻ oxidizes DA to its o-quinone. In fact, Fridovich originally used the ability of SOD to block catechol-quinone formation caused by superoxide as an early assay of SOD activity *(127,128)*. PQ, viewed as an intracellular generator of superoxide, appears not to utilize NO in its cytotoxic properties, but can result in the production of DA-quinones via the reaction of superoxide with DA. Catechol-quinones could exert many of the same effects attributed to NO, superoxide, and ONOO⁻ including modification of proteins, mitochondria, and DNA, and evidence of quinone involvement in DA neuronal death and in PD is emerging. Therefore, if DA is viewed as more than a neurotransmitter, to include consideration as an active participant in the process that damages or destroys DA neurons (as heretical as this may seem), it becomes important to study DA-quinones for their role in DA neuronal damage.

PQ is a significant environmental risk factor for PD. It is not considered a risk factor for any other neurodegenerative condition at this point in time. Administration of PQ to animals does not cause nonspecific neurodegeneration, but a Parkinson's (and MPTP)-like destruction of DA neurons. The single, endogenous neurochemical factor that can impart selectivity to the neurotoxic actions of PQ is DA. In fact, as discussed earlier, the most viable point of overlap among methamphetamine, MPTP, and PQ lies in their ability to lead to DA-quinone formation via the interaction of ONOO⁻ or superoxide with DA.

5. DA-QUINONES MODIFY PROTEINS IMPORTANT FOR DA NEURONAL FUNCTION

The proposal that DA-quinones could be involved in a variety of conditions associated with DA neurotoxicity is plausible, and several general elements relating to the toxicity of DA-quinones have emerged recently. For instance, DA-quinones have been shown to cause a reduction in the mitochondrial complex I enzyme activity and to provoke an opening of the mitochondrial transition pore *(129)*. Relating specifically to the DA neuronal system, it has also been shown that the function of the DAT is also compromised under conditions promoting the formation of quinones from DA *(11,12)*. In an attempt to assign potential in vivo relevance to the actions of DA-quinone, we have studied their effects on the activity and function of TH *(130)*. The quinones of DA and DOPA each cause concentration-dependent decreases in the activity of TH. Figure 1 shows that quinones synthesized enzymatically (by tyrosinase) or chemically (via reaction with $NaIO_4$) cause significant inactivation of TH. The $NaIO_4$-generated quinone of N-acetyl-DA also caused extensive inactivation of TH. Therefore, it appears to be a general property of catechol-quinones to mediate reductions in TH activity. Various antioxidants and reducing agents were tested for the ability to protect TH from quinone-induced inactivation and these results are presented in Table 1. Glutathione, dithiothreitol, and cysteine each protected TH from quinone inactivation. These reagents are known to reduce (i.e., chemically) catechol-quinones back to the catechol moiety *(1,2)* and each could also provide protection by forming thiol-catechol derivatives as well *(120)*. These same reagents that prevented inactivation of TH could not reverse the inhibition if added to the enzyme after exposure to the catechol-quinones, confirming the irreversible nature of enzyme inhibition. The quinone-induced inactivation of TH could not be prevented by catalase, SOD, or dimethylsulfoxide (DMSO), suggesting that hydrogen peroxide, superoxide, or hydroxyl radicals, respectively, were not playing roles in the inactivation process. These data show that the inactivating species were indeed the catechol-quinones and not another downstream reactant. Therefore, various catechol-quinones share in common the ability to cause extensive inhibition of TH, implying that the in vivo formation of these substances within DA nerve endings could also function in a similar regard.

6. MECHANISM OF INACTIVATION OF TH BY DA-QUINONES

It has been suggested that the inhibition of TH seen in animals treated with MPTP is related to the eventual nitration of the enzyme by ONOO⁻ *(77)*. Studies from our labo-

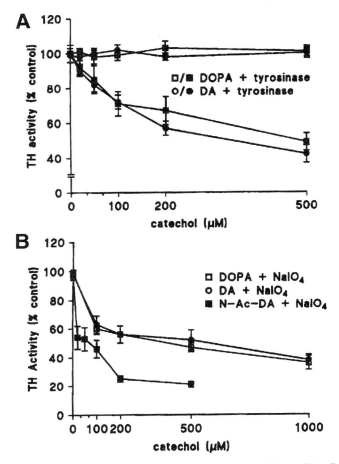

Fig. 1. Inactivation of TH by the quinones of DOPA, DA, and N-Ac-DA. Recombinant TH was expressed as a glutathione S-transferase (GST)-fusion protein and purified by affinity chromatography on GSH-agarose beads. **(A)** Immobilized TH (15–18 μg protein/tube) was exposed to increasing concentrations of DOPA (□/■) or DA (○/●) in the absence (open symbols) or presence (closed symbols) of tyrosinase (50 U/mL) for 15 min at 30°C. **(B)** The o-quinones of DOPA (□), DA (○), and Na-Ac-DA (■) were synthesized by reacting increasing concentrations of the catechols with sodium periodate (NaIO$_4$). Samples were then washed 3× with 100 vol of 0.05 M potassium phosphate buffer, pH 6.0, at 4°C and residual TH activity was determined as described previously. Results represent means ± SEM of four separate experiments run in duplicate. The concentration effects of all catechol-quinones on TH were statistically significant ($p < 0.001$, ANOVA).

ratory have confirmed that ONOO$^-$ causes the coincident nitration of TH and its inhibition, but we concluded that the oxidation of cysteine-sulfhydryls caused by ONOO$^-$ was the actual mechanism by which TH was inhibited *(131)*. Quinones are also highly reactive species and they are known to modify cysteine sulfhydryls. Therefore, it becomes evident that DA-quinones might inactivate TH via sulfhydryl oxidation, so we tested the effects of catechol-quinones on TH sulfhydryl status. Titration of TH sulfhydryl groups revealed that catechol-quinones caused varying amounts of sulfhydryl modification, measured as losses of DTNB reactivity. These data are shown in Table 2

Table 1

Protection of TH Against Inhibition by Catechol-Quinones with Reducing Agents and Antioxidants[a]

Conditions	DOPA + tyrosinase	DA + tyrosinase	N-Ac-DA + NaIO$_4$	DOPA + NaIO$_4$	DA + NaIO$_4$
Catechol-quinone	60.0 ± 4[*]	47.0 ± 5[*]	22.9 ± 3[*]	54.3 ± 3[*]	56.2 ± 3[*]
+ GSH (1 mM)	92.8 ± 6[**]	83.6 ± 4[**]	90.2 ± 9[**]	82.9 ± 7[**]	85.4 ± 6[**]
+ DTT (1 mM)	90.1 ± 4[**]	83.1 ± 4[**]	95.7 ± 6[**]	74.9 ± 6[**]	88.4 ± 5[**]
+ Cysteine (1 mM)	96.8 ± 2[**]	88.6 ± 2[**]	99.5 ± 6[**]	84.7 ± 4[**]	87.7 ± 6[**]
+ SOD (125 U/mL)	45.0 ± 4	42.0 ± 6	20.0 ± 2	57.5 ± 5	59.0 ± 4
+ DMSO (25 mM)	40.7 ± 7	46.2 ± 3	18.6 ± 2	58.2 ± 3	56.4 ± 4
+ Catalase (0.13 U/mL)	53.4 ± 4	47.4 ± 5	24.5 ± 3	50.2 ± 4	55.5 ± 3

[a]TH-GST immobilized on GSH-affinity beads was incubated with the indicated catechol-quinones at 30°C for 15 min. All catechols were used at a concentration of 500 μM and tyrosinase was used at a concentration of 50 U/mL. One equivalent of NaIO$_4$ (500 μM) was reacted with N-Ac-DA, and two equivalents of NaIO$_4$ (1 mM) were reacted with DOPA and DA to synthesize the respective o-quinones of the catechols. Agents tested for the ability to protect the enzyme from inactivation were added 5 min prior to the catechol-quinones. Results are expressed as % control TH activity (DOPA or DA omitted) and are the mean ± SEM for three independent experiments carried out in duplicate. The effects of all catechol-quinones on TH activity were statistically significant by comparison to untreated controls ([*]$p < 0.05$ for each, Bonferroni test). The effects of GSH, dithiothreitol (DTT), and cysteine were significantly different from the catechol-quinone values ([**]$p < 0.05$ for each, Bonferroni test).

and indicate that untreated TH contains a total of 7 cysteine residues, as expected from its deduced amino acid composition *(132)*. Equimolar concentrations of the catechol-quinones (200 μM) caused the modification of 4–5 sulfhydryl groups, out of the total of 7. In general, the extent of sulfhydryl modification by any quinone was related to the loss of enzyme activity. For comparison, TH was also reacted with pCMB or IBZ, both of which selectively oxidize sulfhydryl groups in proteins, and the results in Table 2 show that these reagents also caused extensive inactivation of TH activity. These results suggest that catechol-quinones are targeting cysteinyl residues in TH and imply that quinone-induced modification of these residues underlies the modification of catalytic activity.

Catechol compounds are Fe(III) chelators and are capable of binding to TH and inhibiting its catalytic activity. In fact, DA can bind to TH so tightly in vivo that it can be detected in TH preparations after exhaustive purification of the protein from adrenal tissue *(133)*. TH-bound DA is proposed to exert a variety of regulatory influences over TH *(134–138)*, and it could be possible that the catechol-quinones are altering TH via Fe(III) binding. The effects of catechol-quinones on TH do not appear to be related to iron-chelation for several reasons. First, the recombinant form of TH expressed in bacteria has little iron to serve as a target for catechol-quinone binding. Second, the binding of catechols to TH-bound iron is reversible, and the effects of the catechol-quinones are not. Third, bacterial hosts for TH expression do not contain catecholamines. Fourth, catechol binding to Fe(III) results in the appearance of a blue-green chromophore with an absorption max between 660–700 nm and quinone-modified TH does not display evidence of this catechol-Fe(III) chromophore (data not shown). Thus, the effects of

Table 2
Effects of Catechol-Quinones on Sulfhydryl Group Reactivity and TH Enzyme Activity[a]

Treatment	Sulfhydryl/TH monomer	Activity (% control)
None	7.07 ± 0.3	100
DOPA + tyrosinase	3.75 ± 0.5	64.6 ± 8
DA + tyrosinase	2.40 ± 0.2	52.7 ± 6
DOPA + NaIO$_4$	3.55 ± 0.4	62.6 ± 7
DA + NaIO$_4$	3.35 ± 0.3	54.3 ± 4
N-Ac-DA + NaIO$_4$	2.44 ± 0.3	23.6 ± 4
pCMB	0.72 ± 0.1	2.4 ± 0.1
IBZ	1.03 ± 0.2	37.3 ± 2

[a]TH was cleaved from the GST fusion tag with thrombin and treated with the indicated catechol (200 μ*M* for all) plus tyrosinase (50 U/mL) or plus NaIO$_4$ (one molar equivalent with N-Ac-DA and two molar equivalents with DOPA and DA) for 15 min at 30°C. In some experiments, TH was incubated with the sulfhydryl oxidants para-chloromercuribenzoic acid (pCMB) (100 μ*M*) or iodosobenzoic acid (IBZ) (1 m*M*) for 15 min at 30°C. Samples were dialyzed against 50 m*M* potassium phosphate buffer, pH 7.4, for 60 min at room temperature and then a small aliquot of enzyme was assayed for catalytic activity and the remainder (approx 3–4 μ*M* TH) was reacted with 200 μ*M* 5,5'-dithio-bis(2-nitrobenzoic acid) (DTNB) under denaturing conditions for 60 min at room temperature. The number of sulfhydryl groups remaining in TPH after quinone treatment was determined by the molar extinction coefficient $E_{412} = 13,600$ $M^{-1}cm^{-1}$. Results are the mean ± SEM from 3–4 experiments run in duplicate.

catechol-quinones on TH activity probably reflect a covalent modification of cysteinyl residues, not a reversible binding of the catechol moieties to enzyme-bound Fe(III).

7. COVALENT MODIFICATION OF TH BY DA-QUINONES

As an additional test of cysteinyl alteration of TH by catechol-quinones, attempts were made to document the presence of catechol-modified cysteinyls within TH. Purified TH was treated with DOPA + tyrosinase as a representative catechol-quinone and the data in Fig. 2 presents the results. Under the present high performance liquid chromatography (HPLC)-EC conditions, standards of DOPA and cysteinyl-DOPA eluted at 5.3 and 7.1 min, respectively (Fig. 2A). It can be seen that DOPA-quinone-modified TH contained an electrochemically active peak eluting from the HPLC column with a retention time and 7.1 min, in addition to the internal standard of DOPA eluting with a retention time of 5.3 min (Fig. 2B). These results substantiate that DOPA-quinones modify cysteinyl residues in TH. Treatment of TH with DOPA + NaIO$_4$ or with DA-quinones resulted in chromatograms showing the presence of the respective cysteinyl-catechol (data not shown). These chromatographic results are consistent with previous studies investigating catechol-modified cysteinyl residues in proteins *(4,139,140)*.

The mechanism by which catechol-quinones modify protein cysteinyls *(3,14)* suggests that a protein-bound quinone moiety may undergo redox-cycling. Therefore, we examined the ability of the catechol-quinones to convert TH to a redox-cycling quinoprotein. The data in Fig. 3A demonstrate that treatment of TH with the tyrosinase-generated quinones of DOPA or DA resulted in concentration-dependent increases in redox-cycling of nitro blue tetrazolium (NBT) in the presence of glycinate buffer at pH 10.0. Neither DOPA nor DA alone (without tyrosinase) caused this change in TH.

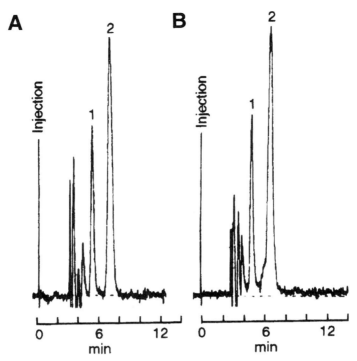

Fig. 2. HPLC-EC analysis of DOPA-quinone modified TH. TH (4.2 mg) was treated with DOPA (200 μ*M*) + tyrosinase (50 U/mL) and exposed to acid hydrolysis and HPLC-EC analysis as described previously. Chromatographs represent standards of enzymatically generated cysteinyl-DOPA **(A)** and dopa-quinone modified TH **(B)**. The peaks in A and B are identified as follows: peak 1, DOPA, retention time = 5.3 min added to each sample as an internal standard; and peak 2, cysteinyl-DOPA, retention time = 7.1 min.

When DOPA- or DA-quinone-modified TH was exposed to sodium dodecyl sulfate polyacrylamide gel electrophoresis (SDS-PAGE) and electroblotted to nitrocellulose, quinolated TH retained its redox-cycling properties (Fig. 3A inset). Treatment of TH with the NaIO$_4$-generated quinones of DOPA, DA, or N-acetyl-DA produced similar effects on TH as shown in Fig. 3B.

8. QUINONE-MODIFIED TH COULD EXERT EFFECTS ON OTHER PROTEINS AND CELLULAR COMPONENTS

The catechol-quinone-induced modification of TH is very interesting because protein-bound quinones retain the ability to alter their redox status. Catechol-quinones caused a concentration-dependent increase in redox cycling by modified TH, shown by the ability of quino-TH to mediate the oxidation/reduction of NBT in the presence of glycinate *(141)*. Exposure of quinone modified TH to denaturing gel electrophoresis and blotting revealed that the redox-active species was associated with the TH monomer (MW = 60 kDa). Dean and colleagues have shown that the presence of reducing moieties on proteins *(142–146)* can result in a transfer of chemical reactivity from the modified protein to other proteins. The ability of catechol-quinone-modified TH to influence other proteins was assessed by measuring its ability to reduce the heme-iron

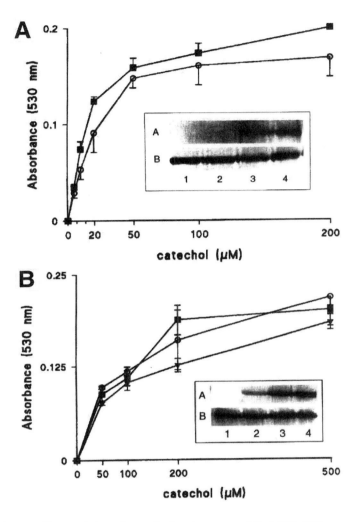

Fig. 3. Redox-cycling activity of catechol-quinone modified TH. TH was cleaved from its GST-fusion tag with thrombin and the isolated protein was treated **(A)** with the indicated concentrations of DOPA (■) or DA (○) in the presence of tyrosinase (50 U/mL) or **(B)** with the indicated concentrations of DOPA (■), DA (○), or N-Ac-DA (▼) plus $NaIO_4$ as described previously. Unreacted quinones were removed by dialysis against 50 mM potassium phosphate buffer, pH 7.4, and the modified proteins were tested for redox cycling. The results are the means ± SEM of three experiments carried out in duplicate. The concentration effects of catechol-quinones on the generation of formazan were statistically significant for both DOPA and DA ($p < 0.001$, ANOVA). *Insets*: TH modified by the respective catechol-quinones (200 µM for each) in (A) or (B) were exposed to SDS-PAGE and electroblotted to nitrocellulose for redox-cycling analysis. Row A in each inset represents redox-cycling staining whereas row B in each inset is Ponceau S staining of recombinant TH proteins. Lanes in the inset to panel A represent: *lane 1* (in both panels), untreated TH; *lane 2*, TH treated with tyrosinase alone; *lane 3*, TH treated with DOPA + tyrosinase; and *lane 4*, TH treated with DA + tyrosinase. Lanes in the inset to panel B represent: *lane 1*, untreated TH; *lane 2*, TH treated with DOPA + $NaIO_4$, *lane 3*, TH treated with DA + $NaIO_4$; and *lane 4*, TH treated with N-Ac-DA + $NaIO_4$.

in cytochrome c. The results of these experiments (data not shown) indicate that TH-bound quinones are capable of causing more than stoichiometric reduction of cyto-chrome c. The quinones of DOPA and DA were capable of reducing 4–5 moles of iron per mole of TH subunit, reflecting its redox-cycling property. This result is entirely consistent with estimates of the number of sulfhydryl groups in TH that are modified by the catechol-quinones. Thus, TH is modified at 4–5 sulfhydryls sites and each site appears capable of iron-reductive capacity. The generality of the reductive properties of quino-TH on transition metals was extended from iron to copper (data not shown), and is consistent with findings of Dean and colleagues *(142–146)*.

9. CONCLUSIONS

The covalent modification of TH by DA-quinones to form a redox-cycling quinoprotein represents a novel finding for this important brain enzyme and provokes interesting speculation with regard to DA neurotoxicity. As a quinoprotein, TH could undergo continuous redox-cycling that could contribute to depletion of cellular-energy stores and endogenous reductants. Indeed, redox-cycling proteins have been implicated in several forms of neurotoxicity *(147,148)* and redox cycling is likely to be more pronounced with protein-bound quinones than with free quinones in solution *(141)*. Cellular defense mechanisms that might be expected to protect against oxidative stress (e.g., GSH or ascorbate) could actually contribute to redox-cycling of a quinoprotein *(5,141,148)*. Quinoproteins could also have longer lived effects than those of ROS, DA, or DA-quinones in solution *(3,14,149,150)*. TH represents just one of few identi-fied targets for DA-quinone attack, and as a phenotypic marker for DA neurons, it would be in a position to have detrimental cellular effects in vivo through its redox-cycling properties.

A role for a TH-quinoprotein in amphetamine-, MPTP, or PQ-induced neurotoxicity is certainly plausible, as discussed earlier, but the specificity of DA-quinone modifica-tion of proteins is an important issue to address in order to define the scope of any role played by quinoproteins. TH has 7 cysteinyl residues in its primary structure, or 28 per tetramer *(132)*, and would appear to be a good substrate for cysteinyl-based quinone attack. Very few proteins have been identified heretofore as catechol-induced quinoproteins. Exposure of crude brain extracts to high concentrations of DA results in the formation of just two redox-cycling quinoproteins *(148,151)*. The identity of these proteins has not been established beyond the characterization of their molecular weights of 45 kDa and 56 kDa. These proteins were originally referred to as a serotonin-bind-ing proteins *(152)* and the 56 kDa protein is close to the molecular weight of TH (60 kDa). Studies of a very limited set of other catechol-quinone labeled proteins indicates that they vary widely in the extent to which they are labeled *(140)*. Therefore, it does not appear that catechol-quinones nonspecifically label large numbers of proteins. The rather selective modification of proteins by DA-quinones would be consistent with the highly delineated neuronal toxicity caused by DA neurotoxins. While TH and TPH are certainly not specific targets for attack by DA-quinones, the collective effects of cat-echol-quinone modification of numerous proteins within DA neurons could extend the breadth of its impact to the point of cell damage. We agree with Smythies and Galzinga *(153)* who have asserted that the oxidation of catecholamines to quinones in brain occurs to a much greater extent than previously appreciated and the potential of catechol-quinones to modify DA neuronal function has probably been underestimated.

ACKNOWLEDGMENTS

The research presented in this chapter was generously supported by NIDA grant DA–10756, by a Department of Veteran's Affairs Merit Award, and by the Parkinson's Disease Foundation.

REFERENCES

1. Graham, D. G., Tiffany, S. M., Bell, W. R., Jr., and Gutknecht, W. F. (1978) Autoxidation versus covalent binding of quinones as the mechanism of toxicity of dopamine, 6-hydroxydopamine, and related compounds toward C1300 neuroblastoma cells in vitro. *Mol. Pharmacol.* **14,** 644–653.
2. Graham, D. G. (1978) Oxidative pathways for catecholamines in the genesis of neuromelanin and cytotoxic quinones. *Mol. Pharmacol.* **14,** 633–643.
3. Hastings, T. G., Lewis, D. A., and Zigmond, M. J. (1996) Reactive dopamine metabolites and neurotoxicity: implications for Parkinson's disease. *Adv. Exp. Med. Biol.* **387,** 97–106.
4. Hastings, T. G. and Zigmond, M. J. (1994) Identification of catechol-protein conjugates in neostriatal slices incubated with [^{3}H]dopamine: impact of ascorbic acid and glutathione. *J. Neurochem.* **63,** 1126–1132.
5. Gieseg, S. P., Simpson, J. A., Charlton, T. S., Duncan, M. W., and Dean, R. T. (1993) Protein-bound 3,4-dihydroxyphenylalanine is a major reductant formed during hydroxyl radical damage to proteins. *Biochemistry* **32,** 4780–4786.
6. Terland, O., Flatmark, T., Tangeras, A., and Gronberg, M. (1997) Dopamine oxidation generates an oxidative stress mediated by dopamine semiquinone and unrelated to reactive oxygen species. *J. Mol. Cell. Cardiol.* **29,** 1731–1738.
7. Stokes, A. H., Brown, B. G., Lee, C. K., Doolittle, D. J., and Vrana, K. E. (1996) Tyrosinase enhances the covalent modification of DNA by dopamine. *Brain Res. Mol. Brain Res.* **42,** 167–170.
8. Maker, H. S., Weiss, C., Silides, D. J., and Cohen, G. (1981) Coupling of dopamine oxidation (monoamine oxidase activity) to glutathione oxidation via the generation of hydrogen peroxide in rat brain homogenates. *J. Neurochem.* **36,** 589–593.
9. Cohen, G., Farooqui, R., and Kesler, N. (1997) Parkinson disease: a new link between monoamine oxidase and mitochondrial electron flow. *Proc. Natl. Acad. Sci. USA* **94,** 4890–4894.
10. Halliwell, B. (1992) Reactive oxygen species and the central nervous system. *J. Neurochem.* **59,** 1609–1623.
11. Berman, S. B., Zigmond, M. J., and Hastings, T. G. (1996) Modification of dopamine transporter function: effect of reactive oxygen species and dopamine. *J. Neurochem.* **67,** 593–600.
12. Berman, S. B. and Hastings, T. G. (1997) Inhibition of glutamate transport in synaptosomes by dopamine oxidation and reactive oxygen species. *J. Neurochem.* **69,** 1185–1195.
13. Filloux, F. and Townsend, J. J. (1993) Pre- and postsynaptic neurotoxic effects of dopamine demonstrated by intrastriatal injection. *Exp. Neurol.* **119,** 79–88.
14. Hastings, T. G., Lewis, D. A., and Zigmond, M. J. (1996) Role of oxidation in the neurotoxic effects of intrastriatal dopamine injections. *Proc. Natl. Acad. Sci. USA* **93,** 1956–1961.
15. Hoyt, K. R., Reynolds, I. J., and Hastings, T. G. (1997) Mechanisms of dopamine-induced cell death in cultured rat forebrain neurons: interactions with and differences from glutamate-induced cell death. *Exp. Neurol.* **143,** 269–281.
16. Lai, C. T. and Yu, P. H. (1997) Dopamine- and L-beta-3,4-dihydroxyphenylalanine hydrochloride (L-Dopa)-induced cytotoxicity towards catecholaminergic neuroblastoma

SH-SY5Y cells. Effects of oxidative stress and antioxidative factors. *Biochem. Pharmacol.* **53**, 363–372.

17. Rosenberg, P. A. (1988) Catecholamine toxicity in cerebral cortex in dissociated cell culture. *J. Neurosci.* **8**, 2887–2894.

18. Cadet, J. L. and Brannock, C. (1998) Free radicals and the pathobiology of brain dopamine systems. *Neurochem. Int.* **32**, 117–131.

19. McCann, U. D., Wong, D. F., Yokoi, F., Villemagne, V., Dannals, R. F., and Ricaurte, G. A. (1998) Reduced striatal dopamine transporter density in abstinent methamphetamine and methcathinone users: evidence from positron emission tomography studies with [11C]WIN–35,428. *J. Neurosci.* **18**, 8417–8422.

20. McCann, U. D., Szabo, Z., Scheffel, U., Dannals, R. F., and Ricaurte, G. A. (1998) Positron emission tomographic evidence of toxic effect of MDMA ("Ecstasy") on brain serotonin neurons in human beings [see comments]. *Lancet* **352**, 1433–1437.

21. Gibb, J. W., Johnson, M., Elayan, I., Lim, H. K., Matsuda, L., and Hanson, G. R. (1997) Neurotoxicity of amphetamines and their metabolites. *NIDA Res. Monogr.* **173**, 128–145.

22. Schmidt, C. J., Ritter, J. K., Sonsalla, P. K., Hanson, G. R., and Gibb, J. W. (1985) Role of dopamine in the neurotoxic effects of methamphetamine. *J. Pharmacol. Exp. Ther.* **233**, 539–544.

23. Stone, D. M., Johnson, M., Hanson, G. R., and Gibb, J. W. (1988) Role of endogenous dopamine in the central serotonergic deficits induced by 3,4-methylenedioxymethamphetamine. *J. Pharmacol. Exp. Ther.* **247**, 79–87.

24. Gibb, J. W., Stone, D. M., Johnson, M., and Hanson, G. R. (1989) Role of dopamine in the neurotoxicity induced by amphetamines and related designer drugs, *NIDA Res. Monogr.* **94**, 161–178.

25. Schmidt, C. J., Black, C. K., and Taylor, V. L. (1991) L-DOPA potentiation of the serotonergic deficits due to a single administration of 3,4-methylenedioxymethamphetamine, p-chloroamphetamine or methamphetamine to rats. *Eur. J. Pharmacol.* **203**, 41–49.

26. Aguirre, N., Barrionuevo, M., Lasheras, B., and Del Rio, J. (1998) The role of dopaminergic systems in the perinatal sensitivity to 3, 4-methylenedioxymethamphetamine-induced neurotoxicity in rats. *J. Pharmacol. Exp. Ther.* 286, 1159–1165.

27. Fumagalli, F., Gainetdinov, R. R., Wang, Y. M., Valenzano, K. J., Miller, G. W., and Caron, M. G. (1999) Increased methamphetamine neurotoxicity in heterozygous vesicular monoamine transporter 2 knock-out mice. *J. Neurosci.* **19**, 2424–2431.

28. Cohen, G. (1994) Enzymatic/nonenzymatic sources of oxyradicals and regulation of antioxidant defenses. *Ann. NY Acad. Sci.* **738**, 8–14.

29. Cubells, J. F., Rayport, S., Rajendran, G., and Sulzer, D. (1994) Methamphetamine neurotoxicity involves vacuolation of endocytic organelles and dopamine-dependent intracellular oxidative stress. *J. Neurosci.* **14**, 2260–2271.

30. Sulzer, D., Chen, T. K., Lau, Y. Y., Kristensen, H., Rayport, S., and Ewing, A. (1995) Amphetamine redistributes dopamine from synaptic vesicles to the cytosol and promotes reverse transport. *J. Neurosci.* **15**, 4102–4108.

31. Fon, E. A., Pothos, E. N., Sun, B. C., Killeen, N., Sulzer, D., and Edwards, R. H. (1997) Vesicular transport regulates monoamine storage and release but is not essential for amphetamine action. *Neuron* **19**, 1271–1283.

32. Rudnick, G. and Wall, S. C. (1992) The molecular mechanism of "ecstasy" [3,4-methylenedioxy-methamphetamine (MDMA)]: serotonin transporters are targets for MDMA-induced serotonin release. *Proc. Natl. Acad. Sci. USA* **89**, 1817–1821.

33. Schuldiner, S., Steiner-Mordoch, S., Yelin, R., Wall, S. C., and Rudnick, G. (1993) Amphetamine derivatives interact with both plasma membrane and secretory vesicle biogenic amine transporters. *Mol. Pharmacol.* **44**, 1227–1231.

34. Pardo, B., Mena, M. A., Casarejos, M. J., Paino, C. L., and De Yebenes, J. G. (1995) Toxic

effects of L-DOPA on mesencephalic cell cultures: protection with antioxidants. *Brain Res.* **682,** 133–143.

35. Newcomer, T. A., Rosenberg, P. A., and Aizenman, E. (1995) Iron-mediated oxidation of 3,4-dihydroxyphenylalanine to an excitotoxin. *J. Neurochem.* **64,** 1742–1748.

36. Cheng, N., Maeda, T., Kume, T., Kaneko, S., Kochiyama, H., Akaike, A., Goshima, Y., and Misu, Y. (1996) Differential neurotoxicity induced by L-DOPA and dopamine in cultured striatal neurons. *Brain Res.* **743,** 278–283.

37. Basma, A. N., Morris, E. J., Nicklas, W. J., and Geller, H. M. (1995) L-dopa cytotoxicity to PC12 cells in culture is via its autoxidation. *J. Neurochem.* **64,** 825–832.

38. Alexander, T., Sortwell, C. E., Sladek, C. D., Roth, R. H., and Steece-Collier, K. (1997) Comparison of neurotoxicity following repeated administration of l-dopa, d-dopa and dopamine to embryonic mesencephalic dopamine neurons in cultures derived from Fisher 344 and Sprague-Dawley donors. *Cell Transplant* **6,** 309–315.

39. Fahn, S. (1998) Welcome news about levodopa, but uncertainty remains [editorial] [see comments]. *Ann. Neurol.* **43,** 551–444.

40. Heikkila, R. E., Manzino, L., Cabbat, F. S., and Duvoisin, R. C. (1985) Studies on the oxidation of the dopaminergic neurotoxin 1-methyl-4-phenyl-1,2,5,6-tetrahydropyridine by monoamine oxidase B. *J. Neurochem.* **45,** 1049–1054.

41. Shoulson, I. (1998) DATATOP: a decade of neuroprotective inquiry. Parkinson Study Group. Deprenyl and tocopherol antioxidative therapy of Parkinsonism. *Ann. Neurol.* **44,** S160–S166.

42. Giovanni, A., Liang, L. P., Hastings, T. G., and Zigmond, M. J. (1995) Estimating hydroxyl radical content in rat brain using systemic and intraventricular salicylate: impact of methamphetamine. *J. Neurochem.* **64,** 1819–1825.

43. Shankaran, M., Yamamoto, B. K., and Gudelsky, G. A. (1999) Mazindol attenuates the 3,4-methylenedioxymethamphetamine-induced formation of hydroxyl radicals and long-term depletion of serotonin in the striatum. *J. Neurochem.* **72,** 2516–2522.

44. Yamamoto, B. K. and Zhu, W. (1998) The effects of methamphetamine on the production of free radicals and oxidative stress. *J. Pharmacol. Exp. Ther.* **287,** 107–114.

45. Deng, X. and Cadet, J. L. (1999) Methamphetamine administration causes overexpression of nNOS in the mouse striatum [In Process Citation]. *Brain Res.* **851,** 254–257.

46. Zheng, Y. and Laverty, R. (1998) Role of brain nitric oxide in (+/-)3,4-methylene-dioxymethamphetamine (MDMA)-induced neurotoxicity in rats. *Brain Res.* **795,** 257–263.

47. Gudelsky, G. A. (1996) Effect of ascorbate and cysteine on the 3,4-methylenedioxy-methamphetamine-induced depletion of brain serotonin. *J. Neural. Transm.* **103,** 1397–1404.

48. Hom, D. G., Jiang, D., Hong, E. J., Mo, J. Q., and Andersen, J. K. (1997) Elevated expression of glutathione peroxidase in PC12 cells results in protection against methamphetamine but not MPTP toxicity. *Brain Res. Mol. Brain Res.* **46,** 154–160.

49. Sheng, P., Cerruti, C., Ali, S., and Cadet, J. L. (1996) Nitric oxide is a mediator of methamphetamine (METH)-induced neurotoxicity. In vitro evidence from primary cultures of mesencephalic cells. *Ann. NY Acad. Sci.* **801,** 174–186.

50. Itzhak, Y., Martin, J. L., and Ali, S. F. (1999) Methamphetamine- and 1-methyl-4-phenyl–1,2,3,6-tetrahydropyridine-induced dopaminergic neurotoxicity in inducible nitric oxide synthase-deficient mice, *Synapse* **34,** 305–312.

51. Itzhak, Y. and Ali, S. F. (1996) The neuronal nitric oxide synthase inhibitor, 7-nitroindazole, protects against methamphetamine-induced neurotoxicity in vivo. *J. Neurochem.* **67,** 1770–1773.

52. Ali, S. F. and Itzhak, Y. (1998) Effects of 7-nitroindazole, an NOS inhibitor on methamphetamine-induced dopaminergic and serotonergic neurotoxicity in mice. *Ann. NY Acad. Sci.* **844,** 122–130.

53. Callahan, B. T. and Ricaurte, G. A. (1998) Effect of 7-nitroindazole on body temperature and methamphetamine-induced dopamine toxicity. *NeuroReport* **9**, 2691–2695.

54. Di Monte, D. A., Royland, J. E., Jakowec, M. W., and Langston, J. W. (1996) Role of nitric oxide in methamphetamine neurotoxicity: protection by 7-nitroindazole, an inhibitor of neuronal nitric oxide synthase. *J. Neurochem.* **67**, 2443–2450.

55. Jayanthi, S., Ladenheim, B., Andrews, A. M., and Cadet, J. L. (1999) Overexpression of human copper/zinc superoxide dismutase in transgenic mice attenuates oxidative stress caused by methylenedioxymethamphetamine (Ecstasy). *Neuroscience* **91**, 1379–1387.

56. Jayanthi, S., Ladenheim, B., and Cadet, J. L. (1998) Methamphetamine-induced changes in antioxidant enzymes and lipid peroxidation in copper/zinc-superoxide dismutase transgenic mice. *Ann. NY Acad. Sci.* **844**, 92–102.

57. Hirata, H., Asanuma, M., and Cadet, J. L. (1998) Superoxide radicals are mediators of the effects of methamphetamine on Zif268 (Egr-1, NGFI-A) in the brain: evidence from using CuZn superoxide dismutase transgenic mice. *Brain Res. Mol. Brain Res.* **58**, 209–216.

58. Cadet, J. L., Ali, S. F., Rothman, R. B., and Epstein, C. J. (1995) Neurotoxicity, drugs and abuse, and the CuZn-superoxide dismutase transgenic mice. *Mol. Neurobiol.* **11**, 155–163.

59. Cadet, J. L., Ladenheim, B., Hirata, H., Rothman, R. B., Ali, S., Carlson, E., Epstein, C., and Moran, T. H. (1995) Superoxide radicals mediate the biochemical effects of methylenedioxymethamphetamine (MDMA): evidence from using CuZn-superoxide dismutase transgenic mice. *Synapse* **21**, 169–176.

60. Hirata, H., Ladenheim, B., Rothman, R. B., Epstein, C., and Cadet, J. L. (1995) Methamphetamine-induced serotonin neurotoxicity is mediated by superoxide radicals. *Brain Res.* **677**, 345–347.

61. Cadet, J. L., Ladenheim, B., Baum, I., Carlson, E., and Epstein, C. (1994) CuZn-superoxide dismutase (CuZnSOD) transgenic mice show resistance to the lethal effects of methylenedioxyamphetamine (MDA) and of methylenedioxymethamphetamine (MDMA). *Brain Res.* **655**, 259–262.

62. Cadet, J. L., Ali, S., and Epstein, C. (1994) Involvement of oxygen-based radicals in methamphetamine-induced neurotoxicity: evidence from the use of CuZnSOD transgenic mice. *Ann. NY Acad. Sci.* **738**, 388–391.

63. Kita, T., Paku, S., Takahashi, M., Kubo, K., Wagner, G. C., and Nakashima, T. (1998) Methamphetamine-induced neurotoxicity in BALB/c, DBA/2N and C57BL/6N mice. *Neuropharmacology* **37**, 1177–1184.

64. Beckman, J. S. and Koppenol, W. H. (1996) Nitric oxide, superoxide, and peroxynitrite: the good, the bad, and the ugly. *Am. J. Physiol.* **271**, C1424–C1437.

65. Crow, J. P. and Beckman, J. S. (1995) The role of peroxynitrite in nitric oxide-mediated toxicity. *Curr. Top. Microbiol. Immunol.* **196**, 57–73.

66. Crow, J. P. and Beckman, J. S. (1995) Reactions between nitric oxide, superoxide, and peroxynitrite: footprints of peroxynitrite in vivo. *Adv. Pharmacol.* **34**, 17–43.

67. Koppenol, W. H., Moreno, J. J., Pryor, W. A., Ischiropoulos, H., and Beckman, J. S. (1992) Peroxynitrite, a cloaked oxidant formed by nitric oxide and superoxide. *Chem. Res. Toxicol.* **5**, 834–842.

68. Beckman, J. S., Chen, J., Ischiropoulos, H., and Crow, J. P. (1994) Oxidative chemistry of peroxynitrite. *Methods Enzymol.* **233**, 229–240.

69. Radi, R., Beckman, J. S., Bush, K. M., and Freeman, B. A. (1991) Peroxynitrite oxidation of sulfhydryls. The cytotoxic potential of superoxide and nitric oxide. *J. Biol. Chem.* **266**, 4244–4250.

70. Crow, J. P. and Ischiropoulos, H. (1996) Detection and quantitation of nitrotyrosine residues in proteins: in vivo marker of peroxynitrite. *Methods Enzymol.* **269**, 185–194.

71. Souza, J. M., Daikhin, E., Yudkoff, M., Raman, C. S., and Ischiropoulos, H. (1999) Factors determining the selectivity of protein tyrosine nitration. *Arch. Biochem. Biophys.* **371**, 169–178.

72. van der Vliet, A., Eiserich, J. P., Kaur, H., Cross, C. E., and Halliwell, B. (1996) Nitrotyrosine as biomarker for reactive nitrogen species. *Methods Enzymol.* **269,** 175–184.

73. Ischiropoulos, H. and al-Mehdi, A. B. (1995) Peroxynitrite-mediated oxidative protein modifications. *FEBS Lett.* **364,** 279–282.

74. Smith, M. A., Richey Harris, P. L., Sayre, L. M., Beckman, J. S., and Perry, G. (1997) Widespread peroxynitrite-mediated damage in Alzheimer's disease. *J. Neurosci.* **17,** 2653–2657.

75. Crow, J. P. and Beckman, J. S. (1996) The importance of superoxide in nitric oxide-dependent toxicity: evidence for peroxynitrite-mediated injury. *Adv. Exp. Med. Biol.* **387,** 147–161.

76. Ischiropoulos, H. (1998) Biological tyrosine nitration: a pathophysiological function of nitric oxide and reactive oxygen species. *Arch. Biochem. Biophys.* **356,** 1–11.

77. Ara, J., Przedborski, S., Naini, A. B., Jackson-Lewis, V., Trifiletti, R. R., Horwitz, J., and Ischiropoulos, H. (1998) Inactivation of tyrosine hydroxylase by nitration following exposure to peroxynitrite and 1-methyl-4-phenyl-1,2,3,6-tetrahydropyridine (MPTP). *Proc. Natl. Acad. Sci. USA* **95,** 7659–7663.

78. Imam, S. Z., Crow, J. P., Newport, G. D., Islam, F., Slikker, W., Jr., and Ali, S. F. (1999) Methamphetamine generates peroxynitrite and produces dopaminergic neurotoxicity in mice: protective effects of peroxynitrite decomposition catalyst. *Brain Res.* **837,** 15–21.

79. Simonian, N. A. and Coyle, J. T. (1996) Oxidative stress in neurodegenerative diseases. *Annu. Rev. Pharmacol. Toxicol.* **36,** 83–106.

80. Fahn, S. and Cohen, G. (1992) The oxidant stress hypothesis in Parkinson's disease: evidence supporting it. *Ann. Neurol.* **32,** 804–812.

81. Tatton, W. G. and Olanow, C. W. (1999) Apoptosis in neurodegenerative diseases: the role of mitochondria [see comments]. *Biochim. Biophys. Acta* **1410,** 195–213.

82. Gutteridge, J. M. (1994) Hydroxyl radicals, iron, oxidative stress, and neurodegeneration. *Ann. NY Acad. Sci.* **738,** 201–213.

83. Zang, L. Y. and Misra, H. P. (1993) Generation of reactive oxygen species during the monoamine oxidase-catalyzed oxidation of the neurotoxicant, 1-methyl-4-phenyl-1,2,3,6-tetrahydropyridine. *J. Biol. Chem.* **268,** 16,504–16,512.

84. Zang, L. Y. and Misra, H. P. (1992) EPR kinetic studies of superoxide radicals generated during the autoxidation of 1-methyl-4-phenyl-2,3-dihydropyridinium, a bioactivated intermediate of parkinsonian-inducing neurotoxin 1-methyl-4-phenyl-1,2,3,6-tetrahydropyridine. *J. Biol. Chem.* **267,** 23,601–23,608.

85. Zang, L. Y. and Misra, H. P. (1992) Superoxide radical production during the autoxidation of 1-methyl-4-phenyl-2,3-dihydropyridinium perchlorate. *J. Biol. Chem.* **267,** 17,547–17,552.

86. Klivenyi, P., St. Clair, D., Wermer, M., Yen, H. C., Oberley, T., Yang, L., and Flint Beal, M. (1998) Manganese superoxide dismutase overexpression attenuates MPTP toxicity. *Neurobiol. Dis.* **5,** 253–258.

87. Andrews, A. M., Ladenheim, B., Epstein, C. J., Cadet, J. L., and Murphy, D. L. (1996) Transgenic mice with high levels of superoxide dismutase activity are protected from the neurotoxic effects of 2'-NH2-MPTP on serotonergic and noradrenergic nerve terminals. *Mol. Pharmacol.* **50,** 1511–1519.

88. Przedborski, S., Kostic, V., Jackson-Lewis, V., Naini, A. B., Simonetti, S., Fahn, S., et al. (1992) Transgenic mice with increased Cu/Zn-superoxide dismutase activity are resistant to N-methyl-4-phenyl-1,2,3,6-tetrahydropyridine-induced neurotoxicity. *J. Neurosci.* **12,** 1658–1667.

89. Matthews, R. T., Beal, M. F., Fallon, J., Fedorchak, K., Huang, P. L., Fishman, M. C., and Hyman, B. T. (1997) MPP$^+$ induced substantia nigra degeneration is attenuated in nNOS knockout mice. *Neurobiol. Dis.* **4,** 114–121.

90. Przedborski, S., Jackson-Lewis, V., Yokoyama, R., Shibata, T., Dawson, V. L., and Dawson, T. M. (1996) Role of neuronal nitric oxide in 1-methyl-4-phenyl-1,2,3,6-tetrahydropyridine (MPTP)-induced dopaminergic neurotoxicity. *Proc. Natl. Acad. Sci. USA* **93,** 4565–4571.

91. Liberatore, G. T., Jackson-Lewis, V., Vukosavic, S., Mandir, A. S., Vila, M., McAuliffe, W. G., et al. (1999) Inducible nitric oxide synthase stimulates dopaminergic neurodegeneration in the MPTP model of Parkinson disease. *Nature Med.* **5,** 1403–1409.

92. Hantraye, P., Brouillet, E., Ferrante, R., Palfi, S., Dolan, R., Matthews, R. T., and Beal, M. F. (1996) Inhibition of neuronal nitric oxide synthase prevents MPTP-induced parkinsonism in baboons [see comments], *Nature Med.* **2,** 1017–1021.

93. Schulz, J. B., Matthews, R. T., Muqit, M. M., Browne, S. E., and Beal, M. F. (1995) Inhibition of neuronal nitric oxide synthase by 7-nitroindazole protects against MPTP-induced neurotoxicity in mice. *J. Neurochem.* **64,** 936–939.

94. Golbe, L. I. (1993) Risk factors in young-onset Parkinson's disease [editorial; comment]. *Neurology* **43,** 1641–1643.

95. Hubble, J. P., Cao, T., Hassanein, R. E., Neuberger, J. S., and Koller, W. C. (1993) Risk factors for Parkinson's disease [see comments]. *Neurology* **43,** 1693–1697.

96. Semchuk, K. M., Love, E. J., and Lee, R. G. (1991) Parkinson's disease and exposure t o rural environmental factors: a population based case-control study. *Can. J. Neurol. Sci.* **18,** 279–286.

97. Seidler, A., Hellenbrand, W., Robra, B. P., Vieregge, P., Nischan, P., Joerg, J., et al. (1996) Possible environmental, occupational, and other etiologic factors for Parkinson's disease: a case-control study in Germany. *Neurology* **46,** 1275–1284.

98. Fleming, L., Mann, J. B., Bean, J., Briggle, T., and Sanchez-Ramos, J. R. (1994) Parkinson's disease and brain levels of organochlorine pesticides. *Ann. Neurol.* **36,** 100–103.

99. Semchuk, K. M., Love, E. J., and Lee, R. G. (1992) Parkinson's disease and exposure to agricultural work and pesticide chemicals. *Neurology* **42,** 1328–1335.

100. Koller, W., Vetere-Overfield, B., Gray, C., Alexander, C., Chin, T., Dolezal, J., et al. (1990) Environmental risk factors in Parkinson's disease. *Neurology* **40,** 1218–1221.

101. Barbeau, A., Dallaire, L., Buu, N. T., Poirier, J., and Rucinska, E. (1985) Comparative behavioral, biochemical and pigmentary effects of MPTP, MPP$^+$ and paraquat in Rana pipiens. *Life Sci.* **37,** 1529–1538.

102. Brooks, A. I., Chadwick, C. A., Gelbard, H. A., Cory-Slechta, D. A., and Federoff, H. J. (1999) Paraquat elicited neurobehavioral syndrome caused by dopaminergic neuron loss. *Brain Res.* **823,** 1–10.

103. Wagner, S. R. and Greene, F. E. (1978) Dieldrin-induced alterations in biogenic amine content of rat brain. *Toxicol. Appl. Pharmacol.* **43,** 45–55.

104. Heinz, G. H., Hill, E. F., and Contrera, J. F. (1980) Dopamine and norepinephrine depletion in ring doves fed DDE, dieldrin, and Aroclor 1254. *Toxicol. Appl. Pharmacol.* **53,** 75–82.

105. Sanchez-Ramos, J., Facca, A., Basit, A., and Song, S. (1998) Toxicity of dieldrin for dopaminergic neurons in mesencephalic cultures. *Exp. Neurol.* **150,** 263–271.

106. Bergen, W. G. (1971) The in vitro effect of dieldrin on respiration of rat liver mitochondria. *Proc. Soc. Exp. Biol. Med.* **136,** 732–735.

107. Miller, G. W., Kirby, M. L., Levey, A. I., and Bloomquist, J. R. (1999) Heptachlor alters expression and function of dopamine transporters [In Process Citation]. *Neurotoxicology* **20,** 631–637.

108. Vaccari, A. and Saba, P. (1995) The tyramine-labelled vesicular transporter for dopamine: a putative target of pesticides and neurotoxins. *Eur. J. Pharmacol.* **292,** 309–314.

109. Ho, Y. S., Gargano, M., Cao, J., Bronson, R. T., Heimler, I., and Hutz, R. J. (1998) Reduced fertility in female mice lacking copper-zinc superoxide dismutase. *J. Biol. Chem.* **273,** 7765–7769.

110. Huang, T. T., Yasunami, M., Carlson, E. J., Gillespie, A. M., Reaume, A. G., Hoffman, E. K., et al. (1997) Superoxide-mediated cytotoxicity in superoxide dismutase-deficient fetal fibroblasts. *Arch. Biochem. Biophys.* **344,** 424–432.

111. Yang, W. and Sun, A. Y. (1998) Paraquat-induced free radical reaction in mouse brain microsomes. *Neurochem. Res.* **23,** 47–53.

112. Yang, W. L. and Sun, A. Y. (1998) Paraquat-induced cell death in PC12 cells. *Neurochem. Res.* **23,** 1387–1394.

113. Li, X. and Sun, A. Y. (1999) Paraquat induced activation of transcription factor AP-1 and apoptosis in PC12 cells. *J. Neural. Transm.* **106,** 1–21.

114. Day, B. J., Patel, M., Calavetta, L., Chang, L. Y., and Stamler, J. S. (1999) A mechanism of paraquat toxicity involving nitric oxide synthase. *Proc. Natl. Acad. Sci. USA* **96,** 12,760–12,765.

115. Kerry, N. and Rice-Evans, C. (1998) Peroxynitrite oxidises catechols to o-quinones. *FEBS Lett.* **437,** 167–171.

116. Pannala, A. S., Razaq, R., Halliwell, B., Singh, S., and Rice-Evans, C. A. (1998) Inhibition of peroxynitrite dependent tyrosine nitration by hydroxycinnamates: nitration or electron donation? *Free Radic. Biol. Med.* **24,** 594–606.

117. Hastings, T. G. and Zigmond, M. J. (1997) Loss of dopaminergic neurons in parkinsonism: possible role of reactive dopamine metabolites. *J. Neural. Transm.* (Suppl.)**49,** 103–110.

118. Stokes, A. H., Hastings, T. G., and Vrana, K. E. (1999) Cytotoxic and genotoxic potential of dopamine. *J. Neurosci. Res.* **55,** 659–665.

119. LaVoie, M. J. and Hastings, T. G. (1999) Dopamine quinone formation and protein modification associated with the striatal neurotoxicity of methamphetamine: evidence against a role for extracellular dopamine. *J. Neurosci.* **19,** 1484–1491.

120. Spencer, J. P., Jenner, P., Daniel, S. E., Lees, A. J., Marsden, D. C., and Halliwell, B. (1998) Conjugates of catecholamines with cysteine and GSH in Parkinson's disease: possible mechanisms of formation involving reactive oxygen species. *J. Neurochem.* **71,** 2112–2122.

121. Montine, T. J., Picklo, M. J., Amarnath, V., Whetsell, W. O., Jr., and Graham, D. G. (1997) Neurotoxicity of endogenous cysteinylcatechols. *Exp. Neurol.* **148,** 26–33.

122. Rowe, D. B., Le, W., Smith, R. G., and Appel, S. H. (1998) Antibodies from patients with Parkinson's disease react with protein modified by dopamine oxidation. *J. Neurosci. Res.* **53,** 551–558.

123. Pfeiffer, S. and Mayer, B. (1998) Lack of tyrosine nitration by peroxynitrite generated at physiological pH. *J. Biol. Chem.* **273,** 27,280–27,285.

124. Ohnishi, T., Yamazaki, H., Iyanagi, T., Nakamura, T., and Yamazaki, I. (1969) One-electron-transfer reactions in biochemical systems. II. The reaction of free radicals formed in the enzymic oxidation. *Biochim. Biophys. Acta* **172,** 357–369.

125. Iyanagi, T. and Yamazaki, I. (1969) One-electron-transfer reactions in biochemical systems. 3. One-electron reduction of quinones by microsomal flavin enzymes. *Biochim. Biophys. Acta* **172,** 370–381.

126. Iyanagi, T. and Yamazaki, I. (1970) One-electron-transfer reactions in biochemical systems. V. Difference in the mechanism of quinone reduction by the NADH dehydrogenase and the NAD(P)H dehydrogenase (DT-diaphorase). *Biochim. Biophys. Acta* **216,** 282–294.

127. McCord, J. M. and Fridovich, I. (1969) Superoxide dismutase. An enzymic function for erythrocuprein (hemocuprein). *J. Biol. Chem.* **244,** 6049–6055.

128. Misra, H. P. and Fridovich, I. (1972) The role of superoxide anion in the autoxidation of epinephrine and a simple assay for superoxide dismutase. *J. Biol. Chem.* **247,** 3170–3175.

129. Berman, S. B. and Hastings, T. G. (1999) Dopamine oxidation alters mitochondrial respiration and induces permeability transition in brain mitochondria: implications for Parkinson's disease. *J. Neurochem.* **73,** 1127–1137.

130. Kuhn, D. M., Arthur, R. E., Jr., Thomas, D. M., and Elferink, L. A. (1999) Tyrosine hydroxylase is inactivated by catechol-quinones and converted to a redox-cycling quinoprotein: possible relevance to Parkinson's disease. *J. Neurochem.* **73,** 1309–1317.

131. Kuhn, D. M., Aretha, C. W., and Geddes, T. J. (1999) Peroxynitrite inactivation of tyrosine hydroxylase: mediation by sulfhydryl oxidation, not tyrosine nitration. *J. Neurosci.* **19,** 10,289–10,294.

132. Grima, B., Lamouroux, A., Blanot, F., Biguet, N. F., and Mallet, J. (1985) Complete coding sequence of rat tyrosine hydroxylase mRNA. *Proc. Natl. Acad. Sci. USA* **82,** 617–621.

133. Andersson, K. K., Vassort, C., Brennan, B. A., Que, L., Jr., Haavik, J., Flatmark, T., et al. (1992) Purification and characterization of the blue-green rat phaeochromocytoma (PC12) tyrosine hydroxylase with a dopamine-Fe(III) complex. Reversal of the endogenous feedback inhibition by phosphorylation of serine-40. *Biochem. J.* **284,** 687–695.

134. Almas, B., Le Bourdelles, B., Flatmark, T., Mallet, J., and Haavik, J. (1992) Regulation of recombinant human tyrosine hydroxylase isozymes by catecholamine binding and phosphorylation. Structure/activity studies and mechanistic implications. *Eur. J. Biochem.* **209,** 249–255.

135. Haavik, J., Martinez, A. and Flatmark, T. (1990) pH-dependent release of catecholamines from tyrosine hydroxylase and the effect of phosphorylation of Ser–40. *FEBS Lett.* **262,** 363–365.

136. Haavik, J., Le Bourdelles, B., Martinez, A., Flatmark, T., and Mallet, J. (1991) Recombinant human tyrosine hydroxylase isozymes. Reconstitution with iron and inhibitory effect of other metal ions. *Eur. J. Biochem.* **199,** 371–378.

137. Ramsey, A. J., Daubner, S. C., Ehrlich, J. I., and Fitzpatrick, P. F. (1995) Identification of iron ligands in tyrosine hydroxylase by mutagenesis of conserved histidinyl residues. *Protein Sci.* **4,** 2082–2086.

138. Ribeiro, P., Wang, Y., Citron, B. A., and Kaufman, S. (1992) Regulation of recombinant rat tyrosine hydroxylase by dopamine. *Proc. Natl. Acad. Sci. USA* **89,** 9593–9597.

139. Kuhn, D. M. and Arthur, R., Jr. (1998) Dopamine inactivates tryptophan hydroxylase and forms a redox-cycling quinoprotein: possible endogenous toxin to serotonin neurons. *J. Neurosci.* **18,** 7111–7117.

140. Kato, T., Ito, S., and Fujita, K. (1986) Tyrosinase-catalyzed binding of 3,4-dihydroxyphenylalanine with proteins through the sulfhydryl group. *Biochim. Biophys. Acta* **881,** 415–421.

141. Paz, M. A., Fluckiger, R., Boak, A., Kagan, H. M., and Gallop, P. M. (1991) Specific detection of quinoproteins by redox-cycling staining. *J. Biol. Chem.* **266,** 689–692.

142. Simpson, J. A., Narita, S., Gieseg, S., Gebicki, S., Gebicki, J. M., and Dean, R. T. (1992) Long-lived reactive species on free-radical-damaged proteins. *Biochem. J.* **282,** 621–624.

143. Simpson, J. A., Gieseg, S. P., and Dean, R. T. (1993) Free radical and enzymatic mechanisms for the generation of protein bound reducing moieties. *Biochim. Biophys. Acta* **1156,** 190–196.

144. Dean, R. T., Fu, S., Stocker, R., and Davies, M. J. (1997) Biochemistry and pathology of radical-mediated protein oxidation. *Biochem. J.* **324,** 1–18.

145. Dean, R. T., Gebicki, J., Gieseg, S., Grant, A. J., and Simpson, J. A. (1992) Hypothesis: a damaging role in aging for reactive protein oxidation products? *Mutat. Res.* **275,** 387–393.

146. Davies, M. J., Fu, S., Wang, H., and Dean, R. T. (1999) Stable mlarkers of oxidant dam-

age to proteins and their application in the study of human disease *Free Rad. Biol. Med.* **27,** 1151–1163.

147. Brunmark, A. and Cadenas, E. (1989) Redox and addition chemistry of quinoid compounds and its biological implications. *Free Rad. Biol. Med.* **7,** 435–477.

148. Velez-Pardo, C., Jimenez Del Rio, M., Ebinger, G., and Vauquelin, G. (1996) Redox cycling activity of monoamine-serotonin binding protein conjugates. *Biochem. Pharmacol.* **51,** 1521–1525.

149. Shen, X. M. and Dryhurst, G. (1996) Oxidation chemistry of (-)-norepinephrine in the presence of L-cysteine. *J. Med. Chem.* **39,** 2018–2029.

150. Shen, X. M., Zhang, F. and Dryhurst, G. (1997) Oxidation of dopamine in the presence of cysteine: characterization of new toxic products. *Chem. Res. Toxicol.* **10,** 147–155.

151. Liu, K. P., Gershon, M. D., and Tamir, H. (1985) Identification, purification, and characterization of two forms of serotonin binding protein from rat brain. *J. Neurochem.* **44,** 1289–1301.

152. Tamir, H. and Liu, K. P. (1982) On the nature of the interaction between serotonin and serotonin binding protein: effect of nucleotides, ions, and sulfhydryl reagents. *J. Neurochem.* **38,** 135–141.

153. Smythies, J. and Galzigna, L. (1998) The oxidative metabolism of catecholamines in the brain: a review. *Biochim. Biophys. Acta* **1380,** 159–162.

8

NMDA Antagonist-Induced Neurotoxicity and Psychosis

The Dissociative Stimulation Hypothesis

Kevin Noguchi

1. INTRODUCTION

1.1. History

There has been much research on N-methyl-D-aspartate (NMDA) antagonists since they were first discovered in mid-part of the 20th century. Initially, it was hoped that that some noncompetitive NMDA antagonists (the most common being ketamine, phencyclidine [PCP], and, more recently, MK-801) could be utilized as a new class of anesthetics with quick onset, short duration, and surprisingly good preservation of brainstem reflexes *(1)*. Unfortunately, while these drugs induced an anesthetic state, they concomitantly induced certain aspects of arousal and even seizures *(2–4)*. This finding correlated quite well with these drug's ability to selectively depress neocortical areas while stimulating limbic areas as measured by the electroencephalogram (EEG) *(3,4)*. To reflect this paradoxical ability to both inhibit and excite, these types of drugs were placed in their own drug class named dissociative anesthetics *(4,5)*. Another unfortunate property of NMDA antagonists included the ability to induce a model psychosis almost indistinguishable from schizophrenia (for an excellent review, *see* Jentsch and Roth *[6]*). As ketamine and PCP developed as drugs of abuse, this psychosis became familiar in emergency rooms across the country *(7)*. After further research, it became apparent that this class of drugs possessed the ability to produce both positive and negative symptoms of schizophrenia, which has made it one of the most widely accepted animal models for this disease *(6)*. This made NMDA antagonists a more complete animal model than dopamine agonists, the only other class of psychotomimetic drugs that induce only the positive symptoms of schizophrenia.

1.2. Glutamate Pharmacology

With the application of new technologies in receptor pharmacology, it was discovered that dissociative anesthetics all have the ability to antagonize the NMDA receptor. Additionally, this antagonism was curious in that these drug ligands did not directly

From: Handbook of Neurotoxicology, Vol. 2
Edited by: E. J. Massaro © Humana Press Inc., Totowa, NJ

Box 1
The NMDA Receptor Complex

The glutamatergic NMDA receptor is currently the focus of intense research due to it being a receptor subtype for the most common excitatory neurotransmitter and its role in neural mechanisms of synaptic plasticity. One unique aspect of this receptor is the multiple regulatory sites located within its structure (Fig. 1). Several of these are absolute requirements that need to be fulfilled in order for it to open and allow the influx of calcium ions. These requirements include: (1) depolarization of the postsynaptic membrane which removes the magnesium ion block from within the receptor ionophore, (2) the binding of glutamate and glycine to its receptor, and (3) the absence of binding to the PCP receptor (Fig. 1). This allows the receptor to act as a coincident detector whereby presynaptic (glutamate release) and postsynaptic (depolarization) activation are necessary for the ion channel to open. Additionally, the purpose of the glycine and PCP channel are currently unknown. Under normal physiological conditions, there should always be enough synaptic glycine available for binding. Moreover, an endogenous ligand that actually binds to the PCP receptor has yet to be found. Finally, although this review does not list all the modulatory sites for the NMDA receptor, it does illustrate the complexity of this structure. This use of such a multitude of regulatory sites may impart a vulnerability in that each additional one may allow another mechanism for NMDA antagonism and dissociative stimulation.

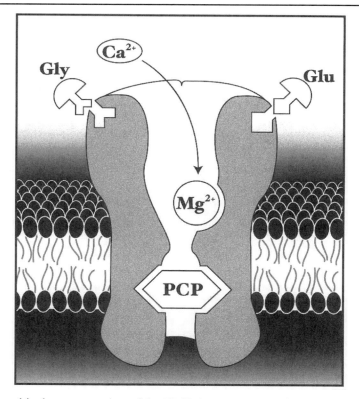

Fig. 1. A graphical representation of the NMDA receptor complex, which includes the glycine (Gly), glutamate (Glu), and PCP ligands along with the calcium (Ca^{2+}) and magnesium (Mg^{2+}) divalent cations.

compete at the NMDA receptor to mediate their effect but instead blocked the NMDA receptor ion channel by binding to a PCP receptor located within it (Box 1). Because of this attribute, the term "noncompetitive" NMDA antagonist was used to describe these drugs. It is interesting to note that no endogenous ligand has been found that binds to the PCP receptor although a name has already been suggested if its found; angeldustin (obviously from the term "angel dust," the street name for PCP). In fact, it may actually be possible that no ligand exists and that the shape of noncompetitive NMDA antagonists somehow fits and blocks the conformation of the NMDA ionophore serendipitously.

At this point, it might be helpful to review the receptor pharmacology of the glutamate receptor. Glutamate is the most common excitatory neurotransmitter in the brain and has three known receptor subtypes to which it can bind. The first glutamate receptor is the ionotropic NMDA receptor, which is unique in that, in general, its ion channel is the only one able to gate calcium (Fig. 1). The second sub-type is the ionotropic alpha-amino-3-hydroxy-5-methyl-4-isoxazolepropionic acid (AMPA)/ kainate receptor, which can gate monovalent cations such as sodium and mediates a majority of glutamatergic synaptic transmission. The final glutamate receptor subtype is the metabotropic glutamate receptor that is composed of several other subclassifications.

1.3. Excitotoxicity

In addition to glutamate's importance in neurotransmission, studies by John Olney discovered that too much extracellular amounts of this neurotransmitter could induce excitotoxicity; literally the overstimulation of a neuron to death by glutamate *(8,9)*. Since then, excitotoxicity has been implicated as a common route for inducing neurodegeneration in several different types of insults including seizures and ischemia *(10,11)*. This discovery led to the possible novel use of NMDA antagonists as neuroprotectants. It was thought that by blocking the entry of calcium (known to be essential for inducing any excitotoxicity) through the NMDA ion channel, one might be able to block the excitotoxic process. In practice, while NMDA antagonists were found to be neuroprotective, paradoxically they were also found to actually induce degeneration in a specific subset of structures *(12)*. Therefore, based on NMDA antagonists' ability to be a neuroprotectant, a neuroexcitant, an anesthetic, and an animal model for schizophrenia, there has been intense research on the possible mechanisms for NMDA antagonist-induced neurodegeneration (NAN) in recent years.

2. A POSSIBLE MECHANISM FOR NAN: THE DISSOCIATIVE STIMULATION HYPOTHESIS

In this chapter, a novel mechanism for NAN and psychosis will be hypothesized. In this model, the administration of NMDA antagonists leads to a reciprocal increase in glutamate/aspartate release. While the protected NMDA receptor remains unaffected, this glutamate/aspartate release can still stimulate the unprotected non-NMDA glutamate receptors leading to certain characteristic abnormalities. This theory would be able to explain how these dissociative anesthetics may be able to induce inhibition (through NMDA antagonism) and excitation (through non-NMDA agonism) during drug exposure. Moreover, by correlating this pattern of stimulation with previous re-

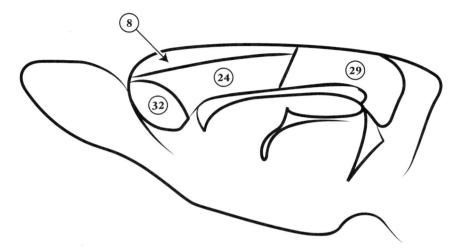

Fig. 2. Diagram of the midsagittal view of the surface of the rat brain with numbers indicating Brodmann areas. Areas 24 and 29 represent the anterior and posterior cingulate cortices respectively.

search with limbic epilepsy (*see* below; *34*), one can provide a possible mechanism for NMDA antagonist induced psychosis. Finally, the non-NMDA receptor stimulation may be able to explain how NMDA antagonists could induce degeneration through the previously mentioned excitotoxicity and explain several other characteristics of NAN.

One of the most essential questions of this theory is whether or not NMDA antagonists can increase glutamate/aspartate release. Using microdialysis, research has found that this is indeed possible with glutamate/aspartate elevations seen with ketamine *(13)*, PCP *(14)*, MK-801 *(15,16)*, and even the competitive NMDA antagonist AP5 *(17)*. Unfortunately, much of these studies used probes in areas that do not necessarily degenerate with NAN, although the hippocampus *(17)* and retrosplenial cortex *(16)* are exceptions to this. The importance of this research is that it illustrates the ability of NMDA antagonists to increase glutamate/aspartate release. Because of this fact, it would be hard to imagine how this would not result in increased non-NMDA receptor stimulation. Whether or not this stimulation would result in NAN would be dependent on the amount of stimulation and the ability of the neurons to protect themselves from toxicity. Fortunately, by looking at correlates between the characteristics of NAN and non-NMDA induced excitotoxicity, one might be able to gain insight into this possibility.

3. CHARACTERISTICS OF NAN AND THE DISSOCIATIVE STIMULATION HYPOTHESIS

3.1. Pattern of Degenerated Structures

Research in NAN has revealed a very characteristic pattern of degeneration dependent on the drug regimen given. At lower acute dosages of NMDA antagonist exposure, degeneration is isolated primarily to layers III and IV of the retrosplenial cortex (Fig. 2). It should be noted that this structure is synonymous with the posterior cingulate cortex in rats *(18)* but differs in humans (Box 2). As the drug regimen is given at

---

Box 2
Cingulate Cortex Connections and Homology

Unfortunately, while the cingulate cortex is one of the main neuroanatomical structures of this chapter, its relative inaccessibility has limited its research *(108)*. In fact, novel research on the cytoarchitecture of this brain region is still ongoing *(113,114)*. Nevertheless, it is known that layer IV (where most of the degeneration occurs) of the posterior cingulate is the convergence point for several important afferents. These include: (1) subicular inputs from the hippocampal formation to layers III and IV *(32,33,115)*; (2) anterior thalamic (limbic thalamus) afferents to layer I, III, and IV *(32,116,117)*; and (3) cholinergic inputs from the ventral globus pallidus/substantia innominata to layer IV *(118)*.

It should also be noted that there are considerable differences in homology between the rat and human cingulate cortices. Nevertheless, it is useful to divide this area into anterior and posterior portions regardless of the species examined. The anterior cingulate (Brodmann area 24) is agranular due to a absence of a layer IV, whereas the posterior cingulate (*see* below for Brodmann areas) has either a dense granular layer II–IV or a thin (dysgranular) granular layer IV *(119)*. The differences between the rat (Fig. 2) and human (Figs. 3 and 4) is far more pronounced in the posterior cingulate. In the rat, the posterior cingulate (area 29) is synonymous with the retrosplenial cortex, which is named due to its spatial relationship with the splenium (the posterior fifth of the corpus callosum) (Fig. 1). As one progresses to primates, the posterior cingulate includes Brodmann areas 23, 29, and 30 with the retrosplenial cortex including only areas 29 and 30 (Fig. 2). Area 23, which some have described as transitional cortex between area 24 and 29 in the rat *(32)*, comprises the largest part of the posterior cingulate cortex in humans. Due to the expansion of this area, the retrosplenial cortex is located more ventrally and buried into the depths of the callosal sulcus (Fig. 3).

---

higher or more chronic doses, this degeneration pattern spreads to other limbic regions including: (1) the hippocampal formation, particularly the dentate gyrus granule cells, scattered pyramidal cells in CA1 and CA3, and cells in the subiculum; (2) the entorhinal cortex; (3) the piriform cortex; and (4) other olfactory-related areas *(19–21)*.

It is suggested here that some degeneration in NAN is caused by excitotoxic stimulation of non-NMDA glutamate receptors. Fortunately, there has been much research on the stimulation of the non-NMDA kainate receptor through exposure to kainic acid. This has been done in animals to mimic limbic seizures in humans, which can lead to excitotoxicity mediated through excess glutamatergic stimulation. This research has found that kainic acid can induce a very specific pattern of degeneration showing some strong correlations to NAN. The major areas that show degeneration in kainic acid induced seizures and NAN include: (1) the hippocampal formation, including (in order of vulnerability) pyramidal CA1 cells, pyramidal CA3 cells, and dentate granule cells *(22,23)*; (2) the entorhinal cortex *(22,23)*; (3) the piriform cortex *(23,24)*; and (4) other olfactory-related areas including the tenia tecta *(23,24)*. While the retrosplenial cortex (the most sensitive area to NAN) is generally not considered a major area that degenerates in kainic acid toxicity, it has been reported in the literature *(22,25)*. One reason for this may be that excitotoxic degeneration of this area has been hard to detect by some researchers without more sensitive histological techniques *(26)*.

While there is a strong correspondence between the areas that degenerate in both these types of insults, it should be noted that several areas do not, with the most conspicuous being the amygdala proper and thalamus. This may mean these structures are either not as strongly stimulated, are able to protect themselves from neurotoxicity, or both. The amygdala is much more strongly connected with the anterior cingulate while the posterior cingulate is more intimately connected with the hippocampus *(79)*. Therefore the amygdala may not be receiving as much stimulation due to poor interconnections with the areas that degenerate during NMDA-antagonist administration. It is interesting to note that the posterolateral amygdala is one of the more sensitive areas to degenerate in NAN *(27)* although the amygdala proper seems to be fairly resistant to toxicity. As far as the thalamus is concerned, because it does not degenerate does not mean it is not involved in the degeneration. Excellent research has found that MK-801 injected directly into the anterior thalamus can injure retrosplenial neurons *(28)*. Similarly, GABA injected into the same area can be neuroprotective to retrosplenial neurons during NMDA antagonists' exposure *(28)*. This may mean that the thalamus is sending powerful efferent stimulation to the retrosplenial cortex. Regardless, even not considering the amygdala and thalamus, kainic acid exposure does induce a more extensive pattern of degeneration than NMDA antagonists in general.

One reason why there may be less toxicity in NAN could be due to the substantial NMDA receptor-mediated toxicity seen with kainic acid induced degeneration. This effect is thought to be caused by the presynaptic release of glutamate/aspartate leading to NMDA receptor-mediated excitotoxicity during kainic acid exposure *(23,29)*. Since NAN happens in the complete absence of ion gating through the NMDA receptor, one may predict a less pronounced pattern of toxicity. In support of this, research has shown that NMDA antagonism can be neuroprotective against excitotoxicity induced from kainic acid administration independent of its anti-seizure effects *(23)*.

Finally, degeneration caused by the metabotropic glutamate receptor should not be overlooked. Stimulation of this receptor may contribute to excitotoxicity through the release of calcium through intracellular stores *(31)*. In fact, research with the glutamatergic metabotropic agonist DCG-IV has revealed that high doses can produce degeneration in the cingulate cortex (although whether or not this was the retrosplenial cortex or not was not revealed) and the subiculum *(31)*. This may suggest that the afferents from the subiculum to layers III and IV of the retrosplenial cortex *(32,33)* are being stimulated to the point of degeneration.

Therefore, using this information, it seems obvious that there are strong correlations with the degeneration seen in NAN and neurodegeneration induced by non-NMDA receptor stimulation. It is suggested here that at least some of the degeneration produced by NMDA antagonists is caused by non-NMDA mediated excitotoxicity and the seizures they can cause (*see* below). In later sections of this chapter, the possibility that this stimulation may lead to limbic seizures will be talked about in more depth and the possibility that this type of stimulation pattern may be responsible for psychosis will be explored.

3.2. NAN and Ultrastructural Morphology

Ultrastructural examination has shown that neurons that degenerate during NAN show a characteristic vacuolization isolated primarily to the mitochondria and endoplasmic reticulum *(35)* in addition to a swelling of the dendrites in the area of toxicity *(19,21)*. As will be outlined later, these two observations strongly suggest excitotoxicity as the mechanism for degeneration.

In order to explain these electron microscopic findings, it is important to look at the excitotoxic process and how neurons protect themselves from it. First, it is known that high amounts of free intracellular calcium are produced by any excitotoxic mechanism *(9)*. When neurons are exposed to this, they protect themselves initially by using calcium-binding proteins that can inactivate some of the intracellular calcium. If this is unsuccessful, the neuron then sequesters the calcium in two types of organelles: the mitochondria and endoplasmic reticulum *(38)*. Therefore, it is suggested that the vacuolization caused by NMDA antagonists may be because of the ability of these two organelles, and only these two organelles, to sequester free intracellular-calcium concentrations *(38)*. As further evidence for this, electron microscopy following kainic acid induced excitotoxicity has shown this same vacuolization in the mitochondria and endoplasmic reticulum *(36,37)*. It should be noted that efforts have been made to detect intracellular-calcium changes during NAN which have been unsuccessful *(39,40)*. This may not be surprising though because others have tried to detect the same calcium changes during well-known excitotoxic processes without success. The authors suggested that this may be because of the inability of the technique to catch the full spatial or temporal profile of calcium changes *(9,41)*.

Dendritic swelling is another feature of NAN that is seen following examination with electron microscopy *(19,21)*. This fits research showing that one of the hallmark characteristics of kainic acid induced excitotoxicity is dendritic swelling *(42,43)*, probably due to the stress and ionic gating occurring during insult.

Therefore, the two main ultrastructural characteristics seen with NAN can simply be explained by relating them to the excitotoxic process. Similar parallels will be drawn in the next sections with regard to the effects of age on NAN.

3.3. Effects of Age on NAN

The age of the rat has an extremely pronounced effect in NAN with a complete resistance to NAN (this does not include apoptotic degeneration) at ages less than 1 mo and increasing susceptibility as the animal ages *(41,44)*. This seems to correlate well with the vulnerability of rats to kainic acid induced toxicity as a function of age. Research has found that animals 21 d and younger are extremely resistant to kainic acid-induced toxicity *(45)* but, as the animals age, they become more and more vulnerable to this type of degeneration *(46)*. Therefore, both kainic acid and NAN show a resistance to degeneration in the immature rat but, as the rat ages, they become more susceptible to insult. This may suggest a common mechanism of degeneration through non-NMDA mediated excitotoxicity. Finally, it should be noted that not all patterns of degeneration show this general trend of increased susceptibility based on age. NMDA-mediated excitotoxicity shows an exact opposite relationship to degeneration, with a decreasing vulnerability to toxicity as the animal ages *(45)*. This would also suggest the age dependency seen with kainic acid degeneration is due to non-NMDA glutamatergic stimulation.

3.4. Effects of Gender on NAN

There are other factors besides age that can dramatically effect the susceptibility to NAN. The toxicity of NAN is known to be sexually dimorphic with females being much more susceptible than males *(40)*. While one might look at the effects of sex hormones on degeneration, it turns out that the hormonal effects on pharmacokinetics may be much more important.

Looking at the effects of sex hormones on seizure-induced excitotoxicity does not lead to a clear prediction as to their effects. For instance, estradiol is known to potentiate seizures, progesterone is thought to decrease them *(47)*, and the effects of testosterone is uncertain *(47,48)*. Confusing the matter further, testosterone can be converted into estradiol in males, which may have effects on seizures *(47)*. Finally, even though estrogens can potentiate seizures, they are also known to be neuroprotective against excitotoxicity *(49)*. The most revealing study would look at sex differences on seizure-induced excitotoxicity but no literature on this could be found.

The effects of sex hormones on pharmacokinetics seem to play a much more important role in this dimorphism. It has been known for quite awhile that the plasma half-life of PCP is much longer in females than males *(50)*. In fact, the clearance rate for PCP has been shown to be up to 45% lower in females than in males *(51)*. Interestingly, the sex dependent sensitivity (as measured behaviorally and through hepatic metabolic indicators) can be reversed between the sexes by removing the gonads and administrating the sex hormones of the opposite sex at 4 wk of age *(52)*. Based on this information, the sexual dimorphism (at least with PCP) seen in NAN may be from the influence of sex hormones on pharmacokinetics. Whether this effect applies for other types of NMDA antagonists is unknown as research on this subject could not be found.

4. SEIZURES: A POSSIBLE MECHANISM FOR TOXICITY AND PSYCHOSIS

4.1. Introduction

In this chapter, it is proposed that NMDA antagonists lead to a reciprocal release of glutamate/aspartate leading to stimulation of non-NMDA glutamatergic receptors, and, eventually excitotoxicity. Surprisingly, this proposal would be the exact opposite of what many experts in the field would predict. In fact, when MK-801 was first introduced, it was thought that this glutamate antagonist would prevent the formation of seizures. This was due to the general feeling in the field that glutamatergic agonism plays a central role in seizures. The thought that these glutamatergic antagonists would lead to excess stimulation caused by glutamate/aspartate release is not what one would predict. In this section, research will be introduced suggesting that NMDA antagonists can induce a specific pattern of stimulation that closely mimics the functional anatomy of limbic seizures *(34)*, the seizure subtype most closely associated with a psychosis very similar to schizophrenia *(53–56)*. This idea can explain the ability of NMDA antagonists to cause psychosis and induce a specific pattern of degeneration.

4.2. NMDA Antagonists and the Measurement of Seizures

In evaluating whether NMDA antagonists lead to a dissociative stimulation pattern whereby neocortical areas are depressed and areas in the phylogenetically older limbic cortex are stimulated, one needs to be careful to use the correct dependent variables. This would suggest that many of the more traditional and less invasive measures of seizures such as scalp EEGs and some behavioral measures (such as convulsions, which depend on spread of the seizure to the motor cortex *[57]*) may not give us the complete picture. This later point is not to say there are no behavioral correlates to this type of dissociative stimulation. In fact, it is suggested that this type of stimulation may be the mechanism for NMDA antagonist-induced psychosis.

4.3. The Effect of NMDA Antagonists on Animal Models of Limbic Epilepsy

One of the paradoxical effects seen with NMDA antagonists in different animal models of epilepsy is the dissociation between inhibition of convulsions (probably from neocortical inhibition of the motor cortex) while concomitantly exacerbating EEG depth electrode measures of seizures *(58–62)*. These studies include a wide variety of epilepsy models including kindling *(58)*, pilocarpine *(59)*, and kainic acid *(60)*. This dissociation has probably led to some fallacious conclusions regarding the anti-epileptic effects of NMDA antagonists on seizures, particularly when using only scalp EEGs or behavioral scales (i.e., Racine behavioral scale) of evaluation. Therefore, this research dramatically replicates previous work *(3,4)* showing that NMDA antagonists can produce dissociative stimulation, with the convulsion inducing *(57)* motor cortex (including the surrounding neocortex) being inhibited and limbic areas being stimulated. Others have come to somewhat different conclusions, suggesting that limbic areas are stimulated and NMDA antagonists prevent the spread to neocortical regions *(59,63)*. Nevertheless, inhibition of certain regions of the brain may not be surprising, because this drug does lead to antagonism of the NMDA receptor and, therefore, hypofunction might be expected. Additionally, this inhibition may provide a mechanism for the ability of NMDA antagonists to induce hypofrontality that can be seen during prolonged exposure *(6)*.

It should be mentioned that at higher doses, NMDA antagonists have even been shown to induce convulsions in animal models of limbic epilepsy *(65,66)*. This may be because of non-NMDA glutamatergic stimulation dominating the NMDA-mediated inhibition and ultimately leading to seizure spread to the motor cortex.

Finally, it is of interest that there are different seizure types caused by different mechanisms. Therefore, NMDA antagonists may have different effects on seizures dependent on their etiology. As an example of this, Turski gave three glutamate agonists for each glutamate receptor subtype at seizure causing doses: NMDA, kainic acid, and quisqualate (a metabotropic glutamate-receptor agonist) *(66)*. He found that MK-801 only inhibited the NMDA-mediated seizures but exacerbated kainic- and quisqualate-induced seizures.

In summary, research in this section has looked at the ability of NMDA antagonists to potentiate seizures in different animal models of epilepsy. One criticism of this research is that the manipulations of the animal models may cloud the true effects of the NMDA antagonist. Therefore, the next sections will look at the ability of NMDA antagonists to induce seizures when given alone.

4.4. The Ability of NMDA Antagonists Alone to Induce Seizures

The ability of NMDA antagonists to worsen seizures seen in animal models of limbic epilepsy may be from the interaction of several factors. In order to gain a more direct idea of the effects of NMDA antagonists on the brain by themselves, this section will look at the effects of NMDA antagonists alone on seizures.

Although not commonly mentioned, the ability of NMDA antagonists to induce seizures has been known since they were first discovered. Because ketamine and PCP were thought of as a possible new class of anesthetic, several studies were done in order to test their safety. These revealed ketamine and PCP could induce seizures in animals and humans in limbic structures *(3,4,68–71)* with the largest effect and point of origin being in the hippocampus *(3,4)*. These effects were so dramatic that some even suggested that the anesthetic effect of NMDA antagonists could be mediated through the same mechanisms that petit mal seizures cause a loss of consciousness *(4,68)*. Additionally, just like in animal models of limbic epilepsy, they could depress neocortical areas while stimulating limbic structures *(3,4)* and induce seizures in the absence of convulsions when given alone *(4,71)*. More recent research has found that the noncompetitive NMDA antagonist MK-801 has shown similar results, with seizures induced in the hippocampus at doses as low as 0.3 mg/kg i.p. *(72)*. Therefore, based on these studies there is incontrovertible evidence that NMDA antagonists can cause enough stimulation when given alone to induce seizures in both animals and humans. It will be seen later in this chapter that schizophrenics may show this same type of excitation as measured by depth EEGs even though no abnormalities can be seen in scalp EEGs.

4.5. NMDA Antagonists and Seizure-Induced Neurodegeneration

The fact that NMDA antagonists can induce seizures does not necessarily mean they are the cause of NAN. In fact, specific neuronal populations have different abilities to protect themselves from excitotoxic attack *(23,74)*. Therefore, seizure-induced degeneration is a function of both stimulation and the ability to protect against insult. Fortunately, research has shown that limbic seizures of more than 1 h (which can be classified as status epilepticus *[23]*) consistently lead to neurodegeneration *(24)*. Pilot data from this lab has found that high doses of phencyclidine result in seizures that can happen over multiple-hour time periods in areas that degenerate including the dentate gyrus, retrosplenial cortex, and the piriform cortex *(75)*. Based on this, it may be no surprise that this higher dose of PCP is known to induce degeneration in many of the areas classically known to degenerate in limbic seizures such as the piriform cortex, entorhinal cortex, and hippocampal formation *(19)*. Therefore, it is suggested here that the ability of high doses of NMDA antagonists to induce NAN is caused, at least in part, by its ability to induce limbic status epilepticus. In fact, it would be hard to imagine how this tremendous amount of stimulation could not contribute in some way to NAN. Based on the previously mentioned research, one surprising prediction may be that limbic seizures are caused more by non-NMDA receptor stimulation. This might explain why convulsions are easily controlled with traditional anticonvulsants but limbic seizures are extremely resistant to treatment *(64)*.

In retrospect, considering the strong interconnectedness of the areas that degenerate in NAN, seizures seem a natural mechanism for degeneration. As these seizures spread throughout the limbic system, it is easy to imagine they could lead to excitotoxicity, the primary mechanism for seizure-induced degeneration *(24,73)*.

4.6. NMDA Antagonist-Induced Seizures and Psychosis

Limbic seizures are the seizure subtype most closely associated with a psychosis very similar to schizophrenia *(53–56)*. Due to the ability of NMDA antagonists to induce both seizures and psychosis, it is suggested here that NMDA antagonists cause a stimulation pattern that mimics limbic seizures which can eventually lead to psychosis in man.

It is of interest that one of the most important limbic seizure subtypes, the temporobasal seizure subtype *(34)*, seems to be very similar to NMDA antagonist induced seizures. The temperobasal seizure subtype is the most distinct of the limbic-seizure subtypes starting in the hippocampus and spreading primarily to two areas, the posterior cingulate and the retrosplenial cortex *(34)* (*see* Box 2). These seizures rarely spread to the anterior cingulate (which is fairly resistant to NAN) but frequently spread to the amygdala *(34)*. From this we can see that the functional anatomy of temporobasal seizures resemble the areas that degenerate in NAN. The primary areas that receive temporobasal stimulation are the most sensitive areas to degenerate in NAN. In addition to this, temperobasal seizures *(3,4)*, just like NMDA antagonist-induced seizures, begin in the hippocampus *(34)*.

What about the dissociative stimulation sometimes seen with NMDA antagonists? A similar phenomena can be seen in epileptics who develop a type of psychosis called "forced normalization." During this phenomena, epileptics undergoing seizures will sometimes develop psychosis at the same time seizure discharge, as measured by scalp EEG, is depressed *(76,77)*. This effect is most frequently seen following anti-epileptic drug treatment *(80)*. It should be pointed out that forced normalization is somewhat of a misnomer probably due to problems in German translation *(76)*. When it was first reported by Landolt *(78)*, it was used to describe an excess inhibition in the scalp EEG but not necessarily a normal scalp EEG *(76)*. Additionally, psychosis and seizures are not necessarily inversely related in this phenomena. Even if the scalp EEG was normal, this may not reflect what was happening subcortically. Just as in the previously mentioned studies *(58,60)*, the scalp EEG can be a horrible, misleading measure of seizures subcortically due to their inability to measure areas deep in the cerebral hemisphere. Such areas include the posterior cingulate and retrosplenial cortices that are tucked deep in the longitudinal fissure (Figs. 3 and 4) in addition to the rhinencephalic structures (hippocampal formation, entorhinal cortex, and piriform cortex) that are located just off midline at the base of the brain. Therefore, the scalp EEG may just be recording the dissociative depression in the neocortex during strong limbic stimulation.

Fortunately, research has been done using depth electrodes during forced normalization. This research has revealed that during what appears to be forced normalization (as measured by scalp EEG), focal subcortical seizures (as measured by depth electrodes) can actually be found *(76,80–82)*. Therefore, during anti-epileptic exposure, these drugs may be inhibiting the neocortex while limbic structures continue to seize leading to forced normalization. This idea is also consistent with the finding that the most susceptible people to anti-epileptic drug-induced forced normalization are epileptics with regular seizures that are focal in origin in the limbic system *(83)*. In other words, it is suggested that forced normalization may be seizure-induced psychosis where the seizures go undetected from the inability of the scalp EEG to record limbic

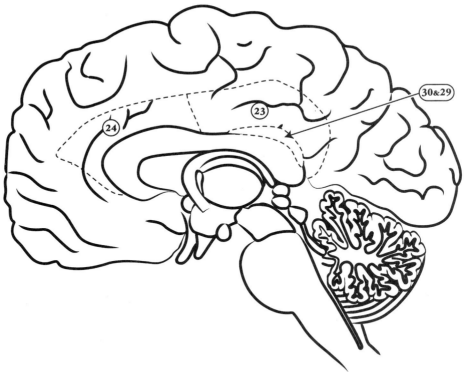

Fig. 3. Diagram of the midsagittal view of the surface of the human brain with numbers indicating Brodmann areas. Area 24 represents the anterior cingulate whereas areas 23, 29, and 30 represent the posterior cingulate cortex. Note the callosal sulcus is exposed in order to visualize the retrosplenial cortex (areas 29 and 30) located within it.

seizures *(84,85)*. It is of interest that even when seizures are detected, psychosis is thought to be caused by activation and inhibition of different parts of the brain *(86)* and it may be possible that forced normalization may be an extreme form of this abnormality. Using this information, it is suggested that this strong limbic stimulation combined with the inhibition of the higher neocortical areas may lead to the full spectrum of the symptoms seen in psychosis. It should be noted that research has shown that seizure-induced psychosis more closely mimics the positive symptoms of schizophrenia *(86)*. Therefore, the negative symptoms induced by NMDA antagonists may be more related to the hypofrontality *(6)* and/or neocortical inhibition *(3,4)* these drugs can cause concurrently.

It should additionally be mentioned that there is still much controversy regarding the relationship between seizures and psychosis. Interestingly, it was initially believed that seizures and psychosis were inversely related to each other *(88,89)* but subsequent research has refuted such claims *(85,87)* (*see* below). One other controversy involves the causal relationship between these two phenomena *(85)*. It is currently unknown whether: (1) seizures cause psychosis directly, (2) seizures induce physiological changes that result in psychosis, (3) there is a common phenomena that induces both seizures and psychosis, or (4) psychoses leads to seizures. Confusing matters even more, psychosis can occur ictally (during seizure detection), post-ictally (following

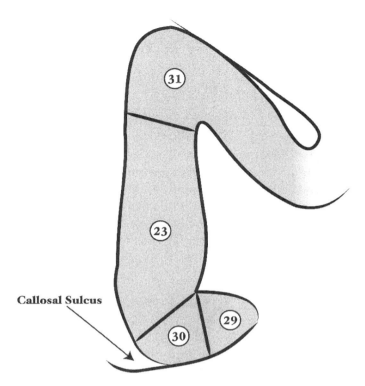

Fig. 4. Diagram of a coronal section through the posterior cingulate cortex in the human brain. Note how, compared to the rat brain, the retrosplenial cortex (areas 29 and 30) is ventralized and tucked into the callosal sulcus.

detection of seizures), or inter-ictally (both seizure detection and psychosis present but no temporal relationship can be found) *(85,86)*. The second possibility, that seizures can induce physiological changes, is worth elaboration. Some have suggested that seizures may produce psychosis through the process of kindling *(90)*. In this phenomena, a specific pattern of stimulation (such as that seen in seizures) can lead to a relatively permanent change in synaptic strength specific to the areas stimulated. If this pattern of stimulation behaviorally manifests itself as psychosis, a chronic condition can result whereby these same synaptic connections can more easily be stimulated. The result is an individual with a low threshold for displaying this psychotic pattern of stimulation which can happen, possibly, at subseizure levels of stimulation. Therefore, the ability of seizures to induce psychosis may be produced by insult to specific areas in the brain or may be caused by changes in synaptic strength in the complete absence of neurodegeneration *(91)*. This also leaves open the possibility that the psychosis NMDA antagonist cause may be due to sub-seizure amounts of stimulation.

In summary, it is suggested here that the ability of NMDA antagonists to cause psychosis may be due to the same mechanisms involved in psychosis associated with temporobasal seizures. Since seizures associated with psychosis usually leads to the positive symptoms of schizophrenia, the negative symptoms NMDA antagonists can invoke may be related more to the inhibition these drug can cause. Finally, while a full discussion of the relationship between seizures and psychosis is beyond the scope of this text, it is sufficient to say that psychosis and seizures can be correlated with each other and that NMDA antagonists can show an amazing similarity to both of these phenomena during drug exposure.

5. IMPLICATIONS FOR SCHIZOPHRENIA

5.1. Introduction

There are two predominant animal models of schizophrenia that are based on the drugs that, when given in a certain drug regimen to humans, are known to cause a psychosis that closely mimics the disease. The first type is primarily composed of two stimulants, cocaine and amphetamine, while the other type is composed of drugs that are noncompetitive NMDA antagonists. While these two animal models are both psychotomimetic, they induce their effects primarily through different neurotransmitter systems and cause different types of symptoms. The stimulants are thought to exert their effects through dopamine agonism and are known to only cause positive symptoms of schizophrenia *(6)*. Alternatively, the NMDA antagonists are known to exert their effects through the blockade of the NMDA ion channel and are known to cause both positive and negative symptoms of schizophrenia *(6)*. Because of this, the NMDA antagonist-induced psychosis is thought to be a more representative animal model of schizophrenia.

Further research with NMDA antagonists revealed other amazing similarities to schizophrenia. This includes the ability of NMDA antagonists to induce degeneration (as mentioned earlier) in many of the same limbic structures known to show abnormalities in schizophrenics *(92)*. In addition to this, the rat is extremely resistant to NAN until early adulthood *(41,44)*, which mirrors the susceptibility of humans to schizophrenia. While these similarities are notable, an important question to be discussed is whether schizophrenics show the same type of dissociative stimulation seen with NMDA antagonists.

5.2. Dissociative Stimulation and Schizophrenia: Functional Neuroimaging

It has previously been suggested that dissociative stimulation may be responsible for the full psychosis induced by NMDA antagonists. This information is based on research showing that NMDA antagonists can induce both inhibition of the neocortex (including the prefrontal cortex) and stimulation in limbic structures *(3,4,6)*. One question that remains is: Can this same idea be applied to what is seen in schizophrenia? One way to look at this possibility is through functional neuroimaging in schizophrenics. One of the most established findings using this method is hypofunction of the prefrontal cortex *(94,95)* in schizophrenics, which is known to be positively correlated with the negative symptoms of schizophrenia *(95)*. On the other hand, the positive symptoms of schizophrenia have been shown to be correlated to increases in cerebral blood-flow measures in subcortical limbic areas *(96)*. These structures include, but are not limited to, the hippocampus, posterior cingulate gyrus, and the parahippocampal gyrus (which includes the entorhinal and piriform cortices) *(96)*. Additionally, functional-imaging studies of the cingulate cortex have found that the anterior cingulate has lower metabolic rates and the posterior cingulate has higher metabolic rates relative to normals *(97)*. Therefore, there may even be a dissociation of stimulation within the cingulate cortex that mirrors the degeneration seen in NAN. This increase in the metabolic rates in the posterior cingulate coincides nicely with a similar study that has found increased metabolic rates in the retrosplenial cortex *(98)*. Therefore, looking at functional neuroimaging, there does seem to be some evidence for a dissociation between cortical and subcortical areas. It should be noted that while functional neuroimaging allows one the tremendous advantage of looking in vivo at changes in humans, the results from these studies are sometimes controvertible *(99)*. In fact, at least one study has found a negative correlation between the positive symptoms of schizophrenia and posterior cingulate function *(95)*, which is inconsistent with the previously mentioned results *(96)*. Due to these and other shortcomings, there is not yet a clear picture as to what functional imaging tells us about schizophrenics. For a more direct measure of this cerebral activity, the next section will describe research using depth electrodes in schizophrenics previously thought to be seizure free.

5.3. Dissociative Stimulation and Schizophrenia: Depth Electrode Studies

What about the possibility that schizophrenics may have strong stimulation in sub-cortical areas possibly to the point of seizures? It is interesting to note that the first person to suggests such a relationship between schizophrenia and epilepsy was Kraepelin *(100)*, the first person to classify schizophrenia (dementia preacox) into its major symptoms, and the first to develop a widely accepted classification of mental disorders. As mentioned earlier, functional neuroimaging data is somewhat consistent with this idea but a much more direct way to measure this would be to use depth electrodes. While the invasiveness of such a procedure on pure schizophrenics has limited this type of research, it is probably necessary in order to get a representative look at the whole brain due to the limitations of the scalp EEG. As evidence for this, one study looking at temporal-lobe seizures with depth and scalp electrodes has found that 72.2% of seizures found with depth electrodes showed no changes in scalp EEGs during auras *(101)*. When considering seizures that showed no obvious behavioral correlate, this finding increased to 90%. Therefore, in the following section, research will be described looking at depth electrode studies on schizophrenic patients with no prior history of seizures. It should be noted that, out of necessity, all of these studies were done during or before the 1960s, with much of the research during this period inspired by Meduna's findings that schizophrenics had a much lower rate of epilepsy than the general population *(88,89)*. This erroneous finding was due in part to the fact any schizophrenic who has seizures was automatically classified as an epileptic with psychosis *(102)*. Therefore, because of the methods for classification at the time, all schizophrenics as a rule are supposed to be seizure-free.

One of the first researchers to look at depth electrodes in schizophrenic patients was Sem-Jacobsen. He looked at a patient population of chronic schizophrenics that had been hospitalized for an average of nine years with no prior history of seizures *(103)*. His research found that over half (34 out of 60) of the schizophrenics he looked at showed intermittent, high-voltage, paroxysmal seizures in depth electrodes even though the scalp EEG appeared normal throughout *(103)*. These seizures were highly focal and oftentimes located in the parietal lobe and the medial ventral portion of the temporal and frontal lobes *(103,104)*. Additionally, several cases where seizures were highly correlated with hallucinations were described *(104)*. Although the exact brain structures where the electrodes were placed were not given, the medial ventral portion of the temporal and frontal lobes are located in the general area where several of the rhinencephalic structures in which we are interested are located. Other studies have revealed similar results. Kendrick and Gibbs wanted to use depth EEGs to look at temporal-lobe epileptics with psychosis *(105)*. As a control group, they wanted a group of individuals with psychosis but no seizures and decided to use chronic schizophrenics ($n = 62$). Their serendipitous finding was that a comparison between the groups was impossible because of the fact that around 50% of the schizophrenics showed focal seizures in the medial ventral portion of the temporal and frontal lobes. As in the previous study, these seizure discharges frequently appeared in the complete absence of scalp EEG abnormalities. The final study mentioned in this section was done by Heath using depth EEGs on schizophrenics ($n = 40$), epileptics ($n = 8$), and a control group ($n = 6$) *(106)*. One advantage of this study was the addition of the control group of patients with other disorders (intractable pain, narcolepsy, or Parkinson's disease [PD]) which found no abnormalities in the depth EEGs. The major finding of the study was seizures in the schizophrenic group primarily located in the septal region (located in the ventral medial frontal lobe) and to a lesser extent in the hippocampus and amygdala (located in the ventral medial temporal lobe) during psychosis. This same group showed recordings that were essentially the same as the control group when not psychotic. Unlike the Kendrick and Gibbs study *(105)*, the authors concluded that the epileptic group and the schizophrenic group displayed different depth EEG patterns *(106)*, with epileptics showing a higher concentration of seizures in the hippocampus and amygdala. Based on this information, there is a highly conserved finding that around 50% of chronic schizophrenics with no history of seizures can display seizures as detected by depth EEGs in the ventral medial portion of the temporal and frontal lobes that usually can not be detected by scalp EEGs. It should be mentioned that in the normal brain, seizure-like patterns can appear that are unrelated to the epileptic processes *(107)*. Fortunately, the fact that a control group showed no such seizures *(106)* suggests that these seizures are abnormal discharges. Finally, it should not be forgotten that up to 50% of schizophrenics showed no seizures. This may imply that abnormalities as a result of seizures or strong subseizure like stimulation (abnormal synaptic connectivity) may play a role in psychosis. Regardless, the presence of focal seizures in a highly conserved region with such a high percentage of seemingly seizure-free schizophrenics suggests that abnormally strong amounts of stimulation may play a role in schizophrenia. This idea is bolstered by the positive correlation of these aberrant patterns that can be seen during the psychosis *(104,106)*. While there is no mention of these seizures spreading to the posterior cingulate or retrosplenial cortex, it is unsure that depth electrodes were placed in this area to detect such stimulation. It is known that access to this area is difficult (Figs. 3 and 4), which has hindered functional and neurological research in the past *(108)*. Another possibility is that depth electrode placement was not proximal enough to the seizures for detection.

Taken as a whole, these studies do confirm that there is strong stimulation in some schizophrenics in rhinencephalic areas. This, as well as functional-neuroimaging studies provide evidence that schizophrenics may display a very similar type of dissociative stimulation that NMDA antagonists and seizures can cause.

6. DISCUSSION

6.1. Summary

In this chapter, a theory has been proposed to explain how NMDA antagonists can induce both neurodegeneration and a psychosis indistinguishable from schizophrenia. This has been done by showing exposure to NMDA antagonists can induce a dissociative stimulation whereby limbic structures are stimulated and higher neocortical areas are inhibited. It is suggested that this strong stimulation in limbic structures leads to degeneration, at least in part, via non-NMDA induced excitotoxicity. As evidence for this, depth EEGs have shown limbic status epilepticus during NMDA antagonist administration in many of the areas that degenerate for periods known to consistently induce degeneration. Moreover, these seizures may provide a mechanism for NMDA antagonists induced psychosis. This is because the seizures induced by NMDA antagonists are neuroanatomically similar to limbic seizures, the seizure subtype most closely correlated with the positive symptoms of schizophrenia. Because seizures associated with psychosis are known to cause more of the positive symptoms of schizophrenia *(86)*, the negative symptoms may be a result of the concurrent inhibition that NMDA antagonists can produce *(3,4,6)*. It should be mentioned that while this chapter mostly focuses on seizures and psychosis, there is a strong possibility that sub-seizure dissociative stimulation may be the cause of psychosis. In fact, Flor-Henry *(100)* described abnormal sub-seizure amounts of stimulation in the hippocampal-amygdaliod-cingular projections as a possible cause for psychosis seen in epileptics. Finally, evidence was presented illustrating how schizophrenia can produce a similar type of dissociative stimulation using modern techniques such as functional neuroimaging and more established approaches such as depth EEGs. This may suggest that similar mechanisms are involved in both schizophrenia and NMDA antagonist-induced psychosis.

6.2. Concluding Remarks

It is hoped that through the presentation of the ideas mentioned in this chapter that researchers will gain a different perspective on the ability of NMDA antagonists to induce degeneration and psychosis. This includes the ability of NMDA antagonists to induce limbic status epilepticus, which may suggest a surprising mechanism for some limbic seizures. Such an etiology may explain why this disorder is so resistant to traditional drug treatments *(64)* and may provide new ideas for anti-epileptic drug therapies, which might include non-NMDA antagonists and possibly even NMDA agonists. In addition to this, the dissociative stimulation hypothesis provides a different framework from which to view the effects of NMDA antagonists on the brain. For example, it would suggest that NMDA antagonists may not be the best drug class to protect neurons from excitotoxic insults such as ischemia and seizures. Previous research on seizures has, in general, supported this view *(109)*.

Finally, based on the similarities of schizophrenia and NMDA antagonist's effects on the brain, it is hoped that research on NAN may provide insights into the etiology of this disease. It would suggest that the NMDA receptor, while providing the framework for higher cognitive thought, may produce a liability through which psychosis can be invoked through dissociative stimulation. This would include an abnormal amount of stimulation in the phylogenetically older limbic structures (possibly through non-

NMDA receptor stimulation) and inhibition of higher neocortical areas (possibly through NMDA receptor inhibition). Finally, although dissociative stimulation is hardly mentioned in the current literature, this idea has been around since the 1960s *(5)*. The fact that researchers of the time called these drugs "dissociative anesthetics" *(4)* exhibits how characteristic they felt this type stimulation was to this drug class. More recently, the re-conceptualization of dopamine hypothesis has proposed that excitation and inhibition of mesolimbic and mesocortical neurotransmission, respectively, may lead to a similar dissociation seen in schizophrenia *(93)*. In this, hypofrontality caused by low mesocortical dopamine activity leads to a reciprocal increase in mesolimbic dopamine activity. While this theory has some similarities to the dissociative stimulation hypothesis, there are significant differences. Research by this lab has shown that NMDA antagonists can cause an increase in limbic stimulation minutes following exposure *(75)*, whereas others have found that hypofrontality only appears after long term exposure *(6,110)*. Because of the temporal order of these phenomena, the limbic stimulation probably is not a result of hypofrontality (at least when using NMDA antagonists as an animal model of schizophrenia). A more likely mechanism may be the ability of the strong connections from the medial temporal lobe structures to influence the prefrontal cortex *(92)* when the former is abnormally stimulated. The fact that abnormalities in the medial temporal lobe to occur first may explain why there is only hypofrontality following long-term exposure to NMDA antagonists *(6)*. The hypofrontality seen with NMDA antagonists may also simply be due to the direct inhibition of the NMDA receptor in prefrontal areas. One final possibility for hypofrontality may be the interaction of NMDA antagonism with dopamine release leading to decreased mesocortical neurotransmission (*111*, but *see* ref. *112*). This illustrates that the effects of NMDA antagonists are not isolated to glutamate/aspartate neurotransmission and probably leads to a complex interaction of several neurotransmitter systems.

In evaluating NMDA antagonists as a model of schizophrenia, some reservation is needed. It is important to realize one is causing in a short time what takes decades to develop in a schizophrenic. Moreover, the cingulate cortex of rats and humans show significant differences in homology (Box 2), therefore, research in one species may not apply to the other. Finally, the symptomatology of schizophrenia is not unitary and neurological abnormalities may be as diverse as the symptoms of this disease. Nevertheless, good theories gain support by looking at the same problem from disparate sources which all come to a common sound conclusion. It is believed that the dissociative stimulation hypothesis does this by explaining several different characteristics of NAN and psychosis at the ultrastructural, cellular, neuroanatomical, functional, and behavioral level in both animals and humans. It is hoped that these ideas will help researchers gain new perspectives and stimulate research in both neurodegeneration and therapies for disease.

ACKNOWLEDGMENTS

The author would like to acknowledge gratefully the excellent work of Incognito Advertising and Design (incognito@vel.net) for the production of all figures in this text and Janice Carlson for help and advice throughout the writing of this chapter.

REFERENCES

1. Corssen, G., Groves, E., and Gomez, S. (1969) Ketamine: its place in anesthesia for neurosurgical diagnostic procedures. *Anesth. Analg.* **48,** 181–188.
2. Bennett, D., Madsen, J., Jordan, W., and Wiser, W. (1973) Ketamine anesthesia in brain-damaged epileptics: Electroencephalographic and clinical observations. *Neurology* **23(5),** 449–460.
3. Corssen, G., Miyasaka, M., and Domino, E. (1968) Changing concepts in pain control during surgery: dissociative anesthesia with CI–581. a progress report. *Anesth. Analg.* **47,** 746–759.
4. Kayama, Y. and Iwama, K. (1972) The EEG, evoked potentials, and single unit activity during ketamine anesthesia in the cat. *Anesthesiology* **36,** 316–328.
5. Myasaka, M. and Domino, E. (1968) Neuronal mechanisms of ketamine induced anesthesia. *Int. J. Neuropharmacol.* **7,** 557–573.
6. Jentsch, J. D. and Roth, R. H. (1999) The neuropsychopharmacology of phencyclidine: from NMDA receptor hypofunction to the dopamine hypothesis of schizophrenia. *Neuropsychopharmacology* **20(3),** 201–225.
7. Siegel, R. (1978) Phencyclidine and ketamine intoxication: a study of four populations of recreational users. *NIDA Res. Monograph* **21,** 119–147.
8. Olney, J. (1971) Glutamate-induced neuronal necrosis in the infant mouse hypothalamus. An electron microscopic study. *J. Neuropathol. Exp. Neurol.* **30,** 75–90.
9. Choi, D. (1992) Excitotoxic cell death. *J. Neurobiol.* **23(9),** 1261–1276.
10. Olney, J. (1985) Excitatory transmitters and epilepsy-related brain damage. *Int. Rev. Neurobiol.* **27,** 337–362.
11. Olney, J. (1993) Role of excitotoxins in developmental neuropathology. *APMIS* **40(Suppl. 1),** 103–112.
12. Olney, J., Labruyere, J., and Price, M. (1989) Pathological changes induced in cerebrocortical neurons by phencyclidine and related drugs. *Science* **244(4910),** 1360–1362.
13. Moghaddam, B., Adams, B., Verma, A., and Daly, D. (1997) Activation of glutamatergic neurotransmission by ketamine: a novel step in the pathway from NMDA receptor blockade to dopaminergic and cognitive disruptions associated with the prefrontal cortex. *J. Neurosci.* **17(8),** 2921–2927.
14. Adams, B. and Moghaddam, B. (1998) Corticolimbic dopamine neurotransmission is temporally dissociated from the cognitive and locomotor effects of phencyclidine. *J. Neurosci.* **18(14),** 5545–5554.
15. Bustos, G., Abarca, J., Forray, M., Gysling, K., Bradberry, C., and Roth, R. (1992) Regulation of excitatory amino acid release by N-methyl-D-asparate receptors in rat striatum: in vivo microdialysis studies. *Brain Res.* **585,** 105–115.
16. Noguchi, K. and Ellison, G. unpublished results
17. Liu, J. and Moghaddam, B. (1995) Regulation of glutamate efflux by excitatory amino acid receptors: evidence for tonic inhibitory and phasic excitatory regulation. *J. Pharmacol. Exp. Ther.* **274(3),** 1209–1215.
18. Domesick, V. (1969) Projections from the cingulate cortex in the rat. *Brain Res.* **12,** 296–320.
19. Corso, T., Sesma, M., Tenkova, T., Der, T., Wozniak, D., Farber, N., and Olney, J. (1997) Multifocal brain damage induced by phencyclidine is augmented by pilocarpine. *Brain Res.* **752,** 1–14.
20. Ellison, G. (1995) The N-methyl-D-aspartate antagonists phencyclidine, ketamine, and dizocilpine as both behavioral and anatomical models of the dementias. *Brain Res. Brain Res. Rev.* **20,** 250–267.
21. Wozniak, D. F., Dikranian, K., Ishimaru, M. J., Nardi, A., Corso, T., Tenkova, T., Olney, J. W., and Fix, A. S. (1998) Disseminated corticolimbic neuronal degeneration induced in rat brain by MK–801: potential relevance to Alzheimer's Disease. *Neurobiol. Diss.* **5,** 305–322.

22. Gass, P., Prior, P., and Kiessling, M. (1995) Correlation between seizure intensity and stress protien expression after limbic epilepsy in the rat brain. *Neuroscience* **65(1)**, 27–36.

23. Wasterlain, C., Fujikawa, D., LaRoy, P., and Sankar, R. (1993) Pathophysiological mechanisms of brain damage from status epilepticus. *Epilepsia* **34(Suppl. 1)**, S37–S53.

24. Olney, J., Collins, R., and Sloviter, R. (1986) Excitotoxic mechanisms of epileptic brain damage. *Adv. Neurol.* **44**, 857–877.

25. O'Shaughnessy, D. and Gerber, G. (1986) Damage induced by systemic kainic acid in rats is dependent upon seizure activity—A behavioral and morphological study. *Neurotoxicology* **7(3)**, 187–202.

26. Nunn, J. and Jarrard, L. (1994) Silver impregnation reveals neuronal damage in cingulate cortex following 4 VO ischaemia in the rat. *NeuroReport* **5**, 2363–2366.

27. Horvath, Z. C., Czopf, J., and Buzsaki, G. (1997) MK-801-induced neuronal damage in rats. *Brain Res.* **753(2)**, 181–195.

28. Tomitaka, S., Tomitaka, M., Tolliver, B., and Sharp, F. (2000) Bilateral blockade of NMDA receptors in anterior thalamus by dizocilpine (MK-801) injures pyramidal neurons in the rat retrosplenial cortex. *Eur. J. Neurosci.* **12**, 1420–1430.

29. Brown, J. and Nijjar, M. (1995) The release of glutamate and aspartate from rat brain synaptosomes in response to domoic acid (amnesic shellfish toxin) and kainic acid. *Mol. Cell Biochem.* **151**, 49–54.

30. Frandsen, A. and Schousboe, A. (1993) Excitatory amino acid-mediated cytotoxicity and calcium homeostasis in cultured neurons. *J. Neurochem.* **60(4)**, 1202–1211.

31. Shinozaki, H. (1994) Neuron damage induced by some potent kainoids and neuroprotective action of new agonists for metabotropic glutamate receptors. *Eur. Neurol.* **34 (Suppl. 3)**, 2–9.

32. Finch, D. M., Derian, E., and Babb, T. (1984) Afferent fibers to rat cingulate cortex. *Exp. Neurol.* **83**, 468–485.

33. Wyss, J. and Van Groen, T. (1992) Connections between the retrosplenial cortex and the hippocampal formation in the rat: a review. *Hippocampus* **2(1)**, 1–11.

34. Wieser, H. (1983) *Electroclinical Features of the Psychomotor Seizure: A Stereoelectroencephalographic Study of Ictal Symptoms and Chronotopographical Seizure Patterns Including Clinical Effects of Intracerebral Stimulation.* Gustav Fischer Verlag: New York, pp. 193–196.

35. Auer, R. (1994) Assessing structural changes in the brain to evaluate neurotoxicological effects of NMDA receptor antagonists. *Psychopharmacol. Bull.* **30**, 585–591.

36. Lassmann, H., Petsche, U., Kitz, K., Baran, H., Sperk, G., Seitelberger, F., and Hornykiewicz, O. (1984) The role of brain edema in epileptic brain damage induced by systemic kainic acid injection. *Neuroscience* **13(3)**, 691–704.

37. Sperk, G., Lassman, H., Baran, H., Kish, S., Seitelberger, F., and Hornykiewicz, O. (1983) Kainic acid induced seizures: neurochemical and histopathological changes. *Neuroscience* **10(4)**, 1301–1315.

38. Frandsen, A. and Schousboe, A. (1993) Excitatory amino acid-mediated cytotoxicity and calcium homeostasis in cultured neurons. *J. Neurochem.* **60(4)**, 1202–1211.

39. Auer, R. and Coulter, K. (1994) The nature and time course of neuronal vacuolation induced by the NMDA antagonist MK-801. *Acta Neuropathol. (Berl.)* **87(1)**, 1–7.

40. Auer, R. (1996) Effect of age and sex on N-methyl-D-aspartate antagonist-induced neuronal necrosis in rats. *Stroke* **27(4)**, 743–746.

41. Randall, R. D. and Thayer, S. A. (1992) Glutamate-induced calcium transient triggers delayed calcium overload and neurotoxicity in rat hippocampal neurons. *J. Neurosci.* **12(5)**, 1882–1895.

42. Sperk, G. (1994) Kainic acid seizures in the rat. *Prog. Neurobiol.* **42**, 1–32.

43. Coyle, J. (1983) Neurotoxic action of kainic acid. *J. Neurochem.* **4**, 1–11.

44. Farber, N., Wozniak, D., Price, M., Labruyere, J., Huss, J., Peter, H., and Olney, J. (1995)

Age-specific neurotoxicity in the rat associated with NMDA receptor blockade: potential relevance to schizophrenia. *Biol. Psychiatry* **38**, 788–796.

45. MacDonald, J. and Johnston, M. (1990) Physiological and pathophysiological roles of excitatory amino acids during central nervous system developement. *Brain Res. Brain Res. Rev.* **15**, 41–70.

46. Wozniak, D., Stewart, G., Miller, P., and Olney, J. (1991) Age-related sensitivity to kainate neurotoxicity. *Exp. Neurol.* **114**, 250–253.

47. Herzog, A. and Eisenberg, C. (1997) Hormonal treatment, in *Epilepsy: A Comprehensive Textbook* (Engel, J. and Pedley, T., ed.), Lippincott-Raven, Philadelphia, pp. 1345–1351.

48. Backstrom, T. and Rosciszewska, D. (1997) Effect of hormones on seizure expression, in *Epilepsy: A Comprehensive Textbook* (Engel, J. and Pedley, T., ed.), Lippincott-Raven, Philadelphia, pp. 1345–1351.

49. Regan, R. and Guo, Y. (1997) Estrogens attenuate neuronal injury due to hemoglobin, chemical hypoxia, and excitatory amino acids in murine cortical cultures. *Brain Res.* **764**, 133–140.

50. Nabeshima, T., Yamaguchi, K., Yamada, K., Hiramatsu, M., Kuwabara, Y., Furukawa, H., and Kameyama, T. (1984) Sex-dependent differences in the pharmacological actions and pharmacokinetics of phencyclidine in rats. *Eur. J. Pharmacol.* **97(3–4)**, 217–227.

51. Shelnutt, S., Gunnell, M., and Owens, S. (1999) Sexual dimorphism in phencyclidine in vitro metabolism and pharmacokinetics in rats. *J. Pharmacol. Exp. Ther.* **290(3)**, 1292–1298.

52. Nabeshima, T., Yamaguchi, K., Furukawa, H., and Kameyama, T. (1984a) Role of sex hormones in sex-dependent differences in phencyclidine-induced stereotyped behaviors in rats. *Eur. J. Pharmacol.* **105(3–4)**, 197–206.

53. Adachi, N., Onuma, T., Nishiwaki, S., Murauchi, S., Akanuma, N., Ishida, S., and Takei, N. (2000) Inter-ictal and post-ictal psychoses in frontal lobe epilepsy: a retrospective comparison with psychoses in temporal lobe epilepsy. *Seizure* **9**, 328–335.

54. Reynolds, E. H. and Trimble, M. R. (eds.) (1981) *Epilepsy and Psychiatry*. Churchill Livingstone, Edinburgh.

55. Sindrup, E. H. and Kristensen, O. (1980) Psychosis and temporal lobe epilepsy, in *Epilepsy and Behavior '79* (Kulig, B., Meinardi, H., and Stores, G. eds.), Swets and Zeitlinger B.V., Lisse, pp. 133–139.

56. Wieser, H. (1983) Depth recorded limbic seizures and psychopathology. *Neurosci. Biobehav. Rev.* **7**, 427–440.

57. Hughes, P., Young, D., and Dragunow, M. (1993) MK–801 sensitizes rats to pilocarpine induced limbic seizures and status epilepticus. *NeuroReport* **4**, 314–316.

58. Gilbert, M. (1994) The NMDA antagonist MK–801 suppresses behavioral seizures, augments afterdischarges, but does not block development of perforant path kindling. *Epilepsy Res.* **17**, 145–156.

59. Lee, M., Chou, J., Lee, K., Choi, B., Kim, S., and Kim, C. (1997) MK–801 augments pilocarpine-induced electrographic seizure but protects against brain damage in rats. *Prog. Neuropsychopharmacol. Biol. Psychiatry* **21**, 331–344.

60. Fariello, R., Golden, G., Smith, G., and Reyes, P. (1989) Potentiation of kainic acid epileptogenicity and sparing from neuronal damage by an NMDA receptor antagonist. *Epilepsy Res.* **3**, 206–213.

61. Wada, Y., Hasegawa, H., Nakamura, M., and Yamaguchi, N. (1992) The NMDA receptor antagonist MK–801 has a dissociative effect on seizure activity of hippocampal cats. *Pharmacol., Biochem. Behavior* **43**, 1269–1272.

62. Sagratella, S. (1995) NMDA antagonists: Antiepileptic-neuroprotective drugs with diversified neuropharmacological profiles. *Pharmacolog. Res.* **32(1)**, 1–13.

63. Young, D. and Dragunow, M. (1993) Non-NMDA glutamate receptors are involved in the maintenance of status epilepticus. *NeuroReport* **5**, 81–83.

64. Lothman, E., Bertram, E., and Stringer, J. (1991) Functional anatomy of hippocampal seizures. *Prog. Neurobiol.* **37**, 1–82.
65. Starr, M. and Starr, B. (1993) Paradoxical facilitation of pilocarpine-induced seizures in the mouse by MK–801 and the nitric oxide synthesis inhibitor L-NMDA. *Pharmacol., Biochem. Behavior* **45**, 321–325.
66. Turski, L., Niemann, W., and Stephans, D. (1990) Differential effects of antiepileptic drugs and beta-carbolines on seizures induced by excitatory amino acids. *Neuroscience* **39(3)**, 799–807.
67. Corssen, G. and Domino, E. (1966) Dissociative anesthesia: Further pharmacologic studies and first clinical experience with the phencyclidine derivitive CI–581. *Anesth. Analg.* **45(1)**, 29–39.
68. Corssen, G., Litle, S., and Tavakoli, M. (1974) Ketamine and epilepsy. *Anesth. Analg.* **53(2)**, 319–333.
69. Mori, K., Kawamata, M., Mitani, H., Yamazaki, Y., and Fujita, M. (1971) A neurophysiologic study of ketamine anesthesia in the cat. *Anesthesiology* **35**, 373–383.
70. Greifenstein, F., DeVault, M., Yoshitake, J., and Gajewski, J. (1958) 1-Aryl cyclo hexyl amine for anesthesia. *Anesthesiology* **37(5)**, 283–294.
71. Contreras, C., Guzman-Flores, C., Mexicano, G., Ervin, F., and Palmour, R. (1984) Spike and wave complexes produced by four hallucinogenic compounds in the cat. *Physiol. Behav.* **33(6)**, 981–984.
72. Feinberg, I., Campbell, I., and Marrs, J. (1995) Intraperitoneal dizocilpine induces cortical spike-wave seizure discharges in rat. *Neurosci. Lett.* **196(3)**, 157–160.
73. Meldrum, B. (1993) Excitotoxicity and selective neuronal loss in epilepsy. *Brain Pathol.* **3**, 405–412.
74. Meldrum, B. (1993) Excitotoxicity and selective neuronal loss in epilepsy. *Brain Pathol.* **3**, 405–412.
75. Noguchi, K. and Ellison, G. unpublished results.
76. Wolf, P. (1991) Acute behavioral symptomatology at disappearance of epileptiform EEG abnormality: paradoxical or forced normilazation. *Adv. Neurol.* **55**, 127–142.
77. Pakalnis, A., Drake, M., John, K., and Kellum, J. (1987) Forced Normalization: Acute psychosis after seizure control in seven patients. *Arch. Neurol.* **44**, 289–292.
78. Landolt, H. (1953) Some clinical electroencephalographical correlations in epileptic psychoses (twilight states). *Electroencephalogr. Clin. Neurophysiol.* **5**, 121.
79. Mega, M., Cummings, J., Salloway, S., and Malloy, P. (1997) The limbic system: An anatomic, phylogenetic, and clinical perspective. *J. Neuropsychiatry Clin. Neurosci.* **9**, 315–330.
80. Krishnamoorthy, E. and Trimble, M. (1999) Forced normalization: clinical and therapeutic relevance. *Epilepsia* **40(Suppl. 10)**, S57–S64.
81. Wieser, H. (1979) 'Psychische Anfalle' und deren stereo-electroenzephpalographisches Korrelat. *Z EEG-EMG* **10**, 197–206.
82. Pacia, S. and Ebersole, J. (1997) Intracranial EEG substrates of scalp ictal patterns from temporal lobe foci. *Epilepsia* **38(6)**, 642–654.
83. Trimble, M. (ed.) (1991) *The Psychosis of Epilepsy*. Raven Press, New York.
84. Engel, J., Caldecott-Hazard, S., and Bandler, R. (1986) Neurobiology of behavior: anatomic and physiological implications related to epilepsy. *Epilepsia* **27(Suppl. 2)**, S3–s13.
85. Sachdev, P. (1998) Schizophrenia-like psychosis and epilepsy: the status of the association. *Am. J. Psychiatry* **155**, 325–336.
86. Lancman, M. (1999) Psychosis and peri-ictal confusional states. *Neurology* **53**(Suppl. 2), S33–S38.
87. Slater, E. and Beard, A. W. (1963) The schizophrenia-like psychoses of epilepsy, V: Discussion and conclusions. *J. Neuropsychiatry Clin. Neurosci.* **7(3)**, 372–378.
88. Meduna, L. (1934) Uber experimentelle Campherepilepsie *Arch. fur Psychiatrie* **102**, 333–339.

89. Yde, A., Lohse, E., and Faurbye, A. (1940) On the relation between schizophrenia, epilepsy, and induced convulsions. *Acta Psychiatry Scand.* **15,** 325–388.
90. Smith, P. and Darlington, C. (1996) The development of psychosis in epilepsy: a reexamination of the kindling hypothesis. *Behav. Brain Res.* **75(1–2),** 59–66.
91. Harrison, P. (1999) The neuropathology of schizophrenia: A critical review of the data and their interpretation. *Brain* **122,** 593–624.
92. Bogerts, B. (1999) The neuropathology of schizophrenic diseases: historical aspects and present knowledge. *Eur. Arch. Psychiatry Clin. Neurosci.* **249(Suppl. 4),** IV/2–IV/13.
93. Davis, K., Kahn, R., Ko, G., and Davidson, M. (1991) Dopamine in schizophrenia: a review and reconceptualization. *Am. J. Psychiatry* **148(11),** 1474–1486.
94. Ingvar, D. and Franzen, G. (1974) Distribution of cerebral activity in chronic schizophrenia. *Lancet* **2,** 1484–1486.
95. Liddle, P. Friston, K., Frith, C., Hirsch, S. Jones, T., and Frackowiak, R. (1992) Patterns of cerebral blood flow in schizophrenia. *Br. J. Psychiatry* **160,** 179–186.
96. Silbersweig, D., Stern, E., Frith, C., Cahill, C., Holmes, A., Grootoonk, S., et al. (1995) A functonal neuroanatomy of hallucinations in schizophrenia. *Nature* **378,** 176–179.
97. Haznedar, M., Buchsbaum, M., Luu, C., Hazlett, E., Siegel, B., Lohr, J., et al. (1997) Decreased anterior cingulate gyrus metabolic rate in schizophrenia. *Am. J. Psychiatry* **154,** 682–684.
98. Andreasen, N., O'Leary, D., Flaum, M., Nopoulos, P., Watkins,G., Boles Ponto, L., and Hichwa, R. (1997) Hypofrontality in schizophrenia: distributed dysfunctional circuits in neuroleptic-naive patients. *Lancet* **349,** 1730–1734.
99. Fu, C. and McGuire, P. K. (1999) Functional neuroimaging in psychiatry. *Philos. Trans. R. Soc. Lond.* **354,** 1359–1370.
100. Flor-Henry, P. (1969) Psychosis and temporal lobe epilepsy. *Epilepsia* **10,** 363–395.
101. Lieb, J., Walsh, G., Babb, T., Walter, R., and Crandell, P. (1976) A comparison of EEG seizure patterns recorded with surface and depth electrodes in patients with temporal lobe epilepsy. *Epilepsia* **17,** 137–160.
102. Gibbs, F., Gibbs, E., and Lennox, W. (1938) The likeness of the cortical dysrhythmias of schizophrenia and psychomotor epilepsy. *Am. J. Psychiatry* **95,** 255–269.
103. Sem Jacobsen, C., Petersen, M., Lazarte, J., Dodge, H., and Holman, C. (1955) Electroencephalographic rhythms from the depths of the frontal lobe in 60 psychotic patients. *Electroencephalogr. Clin. Neurophysiol.* **7,** 193–210.
104. Sem Jacobsen, C., Petersen, M., Lazarte, J., Dodge, H., and Holman, C. (1955) Intracerebral electrographic recordings from psychotic patients during hallucinations and agitation. *Am. J. Psychiatry* **112,** 278–288.
105. Kendrick, J. and Gibbs, F. (1957) Origin, spread and neurosurgical treatment of the psychomotor type of seizure discharge. *J. Neurosurg.* **14,** 270–284.
106. Heath, R. (1962) Common characteristics of epilepsy and schizophrenia: clinical observation and depth electrode studies. *Am. J. Psychiatry* **118,** 1013–1026.
107. Klass, D. and Westmoreland, B. (1985) Nonepileptogenic epileptiform electroencephalographic activity. *Ann. Neurol.* **18,** 627–635.
108. Vogt, B. (1993) Structural organization of the cingulate cortex: areas, neurons, and somatodendritic transmitter receptors, in *Neurobiology of the Cingulate Cortex and Limbic Thalamus* (Vogt, B. and Gabriel, M., eds.), Birkhauser, Boston, MA, pp. 19–69.
109. Loscher, W. (1998) Pharmacology of glutamate receptor antagonists in the kindling model of epilepsy. *Prog. Neurobiol.* **54,** 721–741.
110. Hertzman, M., Reba, R., and Kotlyarove, E. (1990) Single photon emission computerized tomography in phencyclidine and related drug abuse. *Am. J. Psychiatry* **147,** 255–256.
111. Kalivas, P., Duffy, P., and Barrow, J. (1989) Regulation of the mesocorticolimbic dopamine system by glutamic acid receptor subtypes. *J. Pharmacol. Exp. Ther.* **251(1),** 378–387.

112. Hondo, H., Yonezawa, Y., Nakahara, T., Nakamura, K., Hirano, M., Uchimura, H., and Tashiro, N. (1994) Effects of phencyclidine on dopamine release in the rat prefrontal cortex: an in vivo microdialysis study. *Brain Res.* **633,** 337–342.

113. Morris, R., Patrides, M., and Pandya, D. (1999) Architecture and connection of the retrosplenial area 30 in the rhesus monkey (macaca mulatta). *Eur. J. Neuroscience* **11,** 2506–2518.

114. Morris, R., Patrides, M., and Pandya, D. (2000) Architectonic analysis of the human retrosplenial cortex. *J. Comp. Neurol.* **421,** 14–28.

115. Meibach, R. C. and Siegel, A. (1977) Subicular projections to the posterior cingulate cortex in rats. *Exp. Neurol.* **57,** 264–274.

116. Sripanidkulchai, K. and Wyss, J. M. (1987) The laminar organization of efferent neuronal cell bodies in the retrosplenial granular cortex. *Brain Res.* **406,** 255–269.

117. Van Groen, T. and Wyss, J. (1990) Connections of the retrosplenial granular a cortex in the rat. *J. Comp. Neurol.* **300,** 593–606.

118. Stewart, D. J., MacFabe, D. F., and Leung, L. W. (1985) Topographical projection of cholinergic neurons in the basal forebrain to the cingulate cortex in the rat. *Brain Res.* **358(1–2),** 404–407.

119. Krieg, W. (1946) Connections of the cerebral cortex. I. The albino rat. B. Structure of the cortical areas. *J. Comp. Neurol.* **84,** 277–323.

9

Emerging Drugs of Abuse

Use Patterns and Clinical Toxicity

Katherine R. Bonson and Matthew Baggott

1. INTRODUCTION

The desire to change one's consciousness through the use of drugs is thought to be as old as humanity. Given the limitations of our biology, there are restrictions on what responses are possible as the result of self-administering exogenous compounds. Historically, scientists have generally categorized drugs of abuse into one of the following broad classes: depressants/anxiolytics (opioids, alcohol, benzodiazepines), stimulants (cocaine, amphetamines, caffeine), hallucinogenic drugs (LSD, mescaline, THC), and nicotine. In many ways, though, these categories are insufficient to adequately characterize the experiences produced by many of the drugs that are used illicitly.

As our knowledge of the neurochemistry of the brain has expanded, there has been a concomitant increase in our understanding of how drugs with reinforcing properties can have multiple actions in various neurotransmitter systems. Identification of novel pharmacological agents or mechanisms has often been accompanied by explorations of the potential of these compounds for reinforcing effects, both in the laboratory and among illicit drug users. Drugs that were previously thought to affect only peripheral sites are now recognized as having centrally acting properties. Interactions between drugs of different classes have been exploited by drug users for their reinforcing effects. The present chapter presents a summary of compounds that are somewhat outside of the typical classifications used for drugs of abuse. This includes discussions on N-methyl-D-aspartate (NMDA) antagonists such as dextromethorphan and ketamine, gamma hydroxybutyrate (GHB), the potentiation of hallucinogens with antidepressant agents, nitrous oxide (N_2O), and anabolic steroids.

Although these drugs are often categorized as "new drugs of abuse," most of them have been used for many decades, and in the case of N_2O, for two centuries. What makes them appear novel is the fact that their use is generally restricted to small drug subcultures that periodically receive a resurgence of media attention focused on that particular community's drug of choice. For example, GHB and the NMDA antagonists are used by individuals who frequent nightclub settings, while anabolic steroids use is found among serious bodybuilders and athletes. It is difficult to obtain accurate repre-

From: Handbook of Neurotoxicology, Vol. 2
Edited by: E. J. Massaro © Humana Press Inc., Totowa, NJ

Table 1
DAWN "Drug Mentions" in Emergency Department Visits Since 1990[a]

Drug	1990	1991	1992	1993	1994	1995	1996	1997	1998
Ketamine	6	2	16	9	19	150	81	318	209
Dextromethorphan	199	152	228	108	192	176	138	166	213
GHB/GBL	—	—	20	38	55	145	638	762	1282
LSD	3869	3846	3499	3422	5150	5681	4569	5219	—

[a]Note that nitrous oxide and anabolic steroids are not listed in DAWN data as drugs mentioned during ED visits.

sentations of the extent that these drugs are used in the United States because they are often not specifically included in the lists of drugs monitored by the Substance Abuse and Mental Health Services Administration in their annual National Household Survey on Drug Abuse or Monitoring the Future questionnaires. Thus, the degree to which there has been an increase in the use of these drugs is suggested by other measures, such as changes in emergency department (ED) mentions (through the Drug Abuse Warning Network [DAWN]), the MedWatch program at the Food and Drug Administration (FDA), surveillance and drug seizures by the Drug Enforcement Agency (DEA), or police encounters with the drug in question. Table 1 depicts available DAWN data since 1990 for the drugs of abuse discussed in this chapter.

Data from these sources are often difficult to interpret, since the reports are effectively anecdotal in nature. DAWN reports are generated, for example, by a designated ED staff member in a participating ED who culls patient charts for admissions that are determined by that staffer to be the result of drug misuse, regardless of when drug use occurred. Thus, a person admitted for an aspirin overdose, who happened to have mentioned using Drugs Y and Z the day beforehand, could generate emergency-related mentions for Drugs Y and Z that will be counted towards an increase in adverse events associated with those drugs. Within the DAWN system, up to four drug "mentions" can be listed in a report. This reporting system can clearly skew the picture of true negative responses to a particular drug, since DAWN data do not identify if a mentioned drug contributed significantly to the ED visit. The MedWatch program similarly provides limited toxicity information since it is a voluntary reporting system that tracks adverse patient reactions to marketed drug products. Since physicians are not required to participate in this program, there is the possibility that negative effects that are reported will be considered to be far more representative of negative reactions to a certain drug than may be justified.

Adverse events associated with "novel" drugs also often receive press coverage or legal attention that can be out of proportion to the actual frequency of severe reactions related to the biological hazard from use of the drugs. While these sorts of strategies may be effective in mobilizing public opinion or passing new laws, it is questionable whether individuals who are already committed to using a particular drug are influenced by such campaigns in a manner that reduces their drug intake. If the information promoted is seen as inaccurate by the drug using community, based on their direct experience with the drug, the credibility of the source will be reduced.

Yet the ability to disseminate accurate scientific information about these particular drugs has been limited as the result of a research climate that has favored the funding of projects that focus on familiar drugs of abuse. This is a critical fact for a chapter on the neurotoxicity of emerging drugs of abuse. Although some of the drugs discussed in this chapter are associated with morphopathological changes in the central nervous system (CNS) (e.g., ketamine), most are not and their known toxicity is largely limited to acute physiological and behavioral abnormalities that have been primarily documented through ED visits and case reports. Unfortunately, this means it can be suspect to speculate what the actual risk to the brain might be from inappropriate use of these compounds. The information contained in this text reflects what is known to date about the pharmacology of the drugs, including typical adverse effects (whether central or peripheral in origin). From this, it may be possible to identify future areas of research that will demonstrate the degree to which these drugs could pose a neurotoxic risk.

2. "CLUB DRUGS"

In the fall of 1999, the National Institute on Drug Abuse (NIDA) launched a campaign to draw attention to the use and misuse of what they termed "Club Drugs"— drugs that were often used illicitly by "young adults at all-night dance parties such as 'raves' or 'trances,' dance clubs, and bars" (www.clubdrugs.org). Two drugs prominently featured under this classification—ketamine (2-(2-chlorophenyl)-(methylamino)-cyclohexanone) and GHB—will be the focus of this section. A drug with similar properties to ketamine that also has an underground following, dextromethorphan (3-methoxy-17-methylmorphinan), will also be discussed. MDMA (3,4-Methylenedioxymethamphetamine; "Ecstasy"), another drug associated with the rave scene, is discussed in a separate chapter in this volume.

2.1. NMDA Antagonists: Ketamine and Dextromethorphan

2.1.1. Overview

The classic NMDA antagonists, phencyclidine (1-(1-phencyclohexyl)piperidine, PCP) and ketamine, were developed as non-narcotic, nonbarbiturate anesthetic agents. These NMDA antagonists were termed "dissociative anesthetics" because early EEG research in animals indicated they produced a functional dissociation between thalamocortical and limbic systems, resulting in a loss of awareness of the environment *(1)*. Ketamine was approved for general clinical use in 1970. Like PCP, clinical use of ketamine has been limited by long-lasting "emergence reactions" *(2)*. This term describes the hallucinogen-like effects that can occur upon emergence from general anesthesia, which can include euphoria, hallucinations, delusions, blunting of affect, apathy, catatonia, and thought disorder *(3,4)*. Many of these same effects also occur at subanesthetic doses and are considered desirable by illicit users. Table 2 lists possible adverse events resulting from NDMA antagonist overdosage.

NMDA antagonists have effects that mirror not only the positive but also the negative symptoms of schizophrenia *(5,6)*, suggesting an apparently better "model psychosis" than either hallucinogens or psychostimulants. The discovery that PCP acted at the glutamate NMDA receptor *(7)* led to the revival of the hypothesis that endogenous psychosis might be the result of hypoactivity of the glutamate transmitter system *(8)*.

Table 2
Possible Adverse Events Resulting from NDMA-Antagonist Overdosage

Nausea/vomiting
Memory impairment
Ataxia/loss of coordination
Dizziness
Confusion
Excessive salivation
Hyperexcitability
Psychological dissociation
Hallucination
Anesthesia
Psychological dependence
Putative withdrawal syndrome

Since NMDA blockade increases dopamine, this concept functions in a complementary fashion to the dopamine hypothesis of schizophrenia *(9)*.

Aside from their use as an experimental model of reversible psychosis, NMDA antagonists have received considerable attention for their abilities to act as neuroprotectants *(10)* and to prevent the development of physical and psychological tolerance to opioids *(11)*. NMDA antagonists have also been investigated as a treatment for drug and alcohol dependence *(12,13)*. It is not clear whether these drugs will prove clinically useful given their potentially distressing cognitive effects and possible neurotoxicity.

Concern about the use of ketamine under illicit conditions, especially in regard to its reported association with sexual assault, led to its placement into Schedule III of the Controlled Substances Act in 1999 through Congressional legislation. This process was notable because it circumvented the scientific evaluation that normally occurs in the Department of Health and Human Services (at the FDA and NIDA) prior to final scheduling by the Department of Justice through the DEA. (This law also placed GHB into Schedule I.)

In contrast, dextromethorphan is an over-the-counter drug that is available without restriction in cough syrup preparations, either alone or in combination with other medications. Nonetheless, high dose dextromethorphan can produce similar effects to ketamine, because its metabolite dextrorphan also has NMDA-antagonist properties. Interestingly, dextromethorphan is the only compound that is specifically mentioned in the Controlled Substances Act as a drug that is exempted from scheduling because it lacks abuse potential. It has been recently reported that illicitly manufactured Ecstasy pills in the United States frequently contain high-dose dextromethorphan rather than the expected MDMA *(14)*. Since dextromethorphan is not detected by standard urine toxicology panels, it may therefore play an unrecognized role in the adverse events attributed to MDMA use.

2.1.2. Pharmacology of NMDA Antagonists

The NMDA receptor-channel complex is activated competitively by the excitatory amino acids glutamate and aspartate. Once activated, the ion channel opens, allowing the flow of calcium into the neuron. This influx of calcium has been suggested as a trigger for long-term potentiation, the proposed neurophysiological substrate for memory formation and subsequent learning. Thus, it is not surprising that drugs that alter NMDA receptor functioning should impair memory and memory-dependent sensory processing *(15)*, which may contribute to the characteristic sensory distortions and alterations in consciousness. More generally, NMDA receptors are thought to be involved in perceptual, affective, and cognitive processes.

Two other sites mediate activation of the NMDA receptor: an extracellular site that binds glycine or serine as a coagonist, and an intracellular polyamine site, which can allosterically modify how glutamate and aspartate activate the NMDA receptor. Deep within the channel there is another site, that binds such drugs as PCP, ketamine, and dextromethorphan in a noncompetitive manner. Therefore, when this noncompetitive site is occupied, a functional blockade of the NDMA channel occurs. The clinical potency of NMDA antagonists parallels their ability to bind to the noncompetitive site.

At higher doses, NMDA antagonists can block monoamine transporters. This has led to the intriguing demonstration that NMDA antagonists can function as antidepressants *(16)*. Ketamine can also interact with a number of opioid receptors (mu, delta, and kappa) while dextromethorphan binds with high affinity to sigma receptors. The effects at kappa opioid and sigma receptors may contribute to the responses that are sought by illicit users, since activation of these receptors are thought to produce hallucinogenic-like states of consciousness.

Although dextromethorphan is the D-isomer of the semisynthetic opioid levorphanol, it does not itself produce classic opioid-like psychoactive responses *(17)*. The psychoactive effects of high-dose dextromethorphan are primarily from its metabolite, dextrorphan. Dextrorphan has high affinity for the NMDA channel site and a low affinity for sigma receptors *(18)*. The metabolism of dextromethorphan to dextrorphan is catalyzed by the cytochrome P-450 isozyme 2D6 (CYP2D6). The expression of CYP2D6 is genetically controlled and, due to gene deletion or mutation, is absent in 5–10% of the Caucasian population *(19)*. The absence of CYP2D6 leads to deficient metabolism of dextromethorphan to dextrorphan, which may prolong the action of the drug and lead to an increase in adverse effects.

2.1.3. Ketamine

2.1.3.1. Use Patterns of Ketamine

Illicit access to ketamine typically occurs through diversion of the drug from legitimate use as an injectable solution for use in veterinary medicine and long-term pain management. As packaged for medical use, a pharmaceutical vial of ketamine in solution contains approx 1 g of the drug. Although a vial is sold to veterinarians for about $7, mark-up on the street can be as high as $30–45 per vial to drug dealers and $100–200 per vial to individual users. In the past few years, law-enforcement agencies have encountered ketamine powder packaged in small plastic bags, folded paper, aluminum foil, and capsules. These small packets are known as "bumps" and commonly contain 200 mg of ketamine, sold for approx $20. Recently, packaged doses of 70 mg have also been reported.

Ketamine is most frequently administered in powder form intranasally, although intramuscular injection is sometimes practiced. Oral use is less common due to a low

(17%) oral bioavailability *(20)*. Reported intranasal doses range from 50–250 mg, while intramuscular doses do not usually exceed 150 mg. Some users inhale about 20 mg in each nostril, repeated in 5–10-min intervals until the desired state is reached. Thus, a vial of pharmaceutical ketamine containing 1 g of powder can provide 4–20 doses (at $10–25 per dose), depending on route of administration and desired effect. Use of higher doses is reported among chronic users, since tolerance tends to develop with prolonged use *(21,22)*. Psychological dependence and compulsive use may also occur *(22–24)*.

2.1.3.2. EFFECTS OF KETAMINE

2.1.3.2.1. Acute and Chronic Behavioral Responses

An intranasal dose of 70 mg of ketamine may produce sedation and intoxication. As with other sedatives, loss of coordination and memory impairment are common. Other adverse effects include ataxia, nausea, slurring of speech, dizziness, confusion, excessive salivation, and hyperexcitability *(5,25)*. There appears to be no threshold dose for the appearance of dissociative and hallucinogenic-like effects. Instead, distortions in body image, floating sensations, and visual disturbances such as blurring and tunnel vision can be present at lower doses and become more prominent with increasing dose *(26)*. A larger intranasal dose of 200–500 mg can produce full anaesthesia and loss of awareness of surroundings, a state referred to as a "K-hole" by users. Some have compared this state to a "near-death experience" and described perceived contact with spiritual or alien entities *(27,28)*.

Because of the interest in NMDA antagonists as a model of reversible psychosis, extensive research has documented the cognitive and behavioral effects of subanesthetic ketamine in healthy volunteers. Studies using the Brief Psychiatric Rating Scale (BPRS) and similar instruments have documented increased positive symptoms of schizophrenia (such as hallucinatory behavior, conceptual disorganization, suspiciousness, and unusual thought content) as well as negative symptoms (blunted affect, emotional withdrawal, and motor retardation) during ketamine intoxication *(5)*. Proverb interpretation tasks indicate that ketamine decreases capacity for abstract thought and produces a prominent thought disorder *(29)*. In cognitive performance tasks, ketamine causes impairments in verbal and nonverbal declarative memory, impairment on the serial sevens counting task, decreased acquisition of abstract procedural learning, and increased distractibility *(5,30,31)*. These changes are reportedly similar to the symptoms of schizophrenia. Furthermore, studies administering NMDA antagonists to schizophrenics demonstrate that this population has increased sensitivity to the psychotomimetic effects of NMDA receptor blockade *(25,32)*.

In addition to cognitive and behavioral responses, ketamine produces sympathomimetic effects such as increased blood pressure and heart rate and is contraindicated in individuals with cardiovascular disease *(3)*. Bolus intravenous injection of ketamine is sometimes associated with respiratory depression.

Although no controlled studies appear to have been published, chronic ketamine users have reported impairments in speech, memory and attention, as well as visual alterations *(21–23)*. Recurrent hallucinations have also been reported *(33)*. Similar symptoms have been better documented in PCP users *(33,34)*, lending support to these user reports.

Table 3
Neurotoxic Responses to Ketamine

Acute, low-dose ketamine → Reversible cytoplasmic vacuoles in pyramidal neurons of the posterior cingulate and retrosplenial cortex
Repeated, high-dose ketamine → Persistent cytoplasmic vacuoles in pyramidal neurons of the posterior cingulate and retrosplenial cortex; neuronal necrosis in neocortical and limbic regions

2.1.3.2.2. Serious Adverse Events

Clinical toxicity after ketamine use mainly involves behavioral signs such as confused or irrational behavior. Nausea, vomiting, respiratory stimulation or depression, tachycardia or bradycardia, hypertension or hypotension, and cardiac arrythmias are other possible complications. Treatment of ketamine-induced acute behavioral toxicity can be managed by administration of GABA agonists such as benzodiazepines or barbiturates. There may be a pharmacological explanation underlying the ability of this treatment to control adverse events. Under normal conditions in the brain, it is hypothesized that glutamate acts through NMDA receptors on GABA neurons to maintain tonic inhibition over excitatory pathways. When NMDA receptors are blocked with antagonists, there is an inability to prevent excitotoxicity. Thus, GABA agonists may reestablish inhibitory control and reduce behavioral toxicity.

Reports of toxic psychosis following chronic NMDA antagonist abuse have been published, with symptoms persisting up to 90 d after drug use in some cases *(35)*. In addition to the toxic psychosis sometimes noted in NMDA-antagonist users, a lasting functioning psychosis indistinguishable from schizophrenia has been associated with chronic PCP use *(36)*. The extent to which this psychosis depends on preexisting pathology remains unclear *(37)*.

2.1.3.2.3. Neurotoxicity

Acute, low doses of ketamine can induce reversible morphological changes characterized by cytoplasmic vacuoles in pyramidal neurons in the posterior cingulate and retrosplenal cortex of rats. Higher and repeated doses produce a similar but persisting result, with neuronal necrosis extending into neocortical and limbic brain regions, including the cingulate cortex, hippocampus, parahippocampal gyrus, and entorhinal cortex *(38,39)*. Table 3 lists these adverse events from ketamine use. The mechanism of these changes is unknown but has been hypothesized to be the result of disinhibition and consequent overexcitation of cortical pyramidal cells produced by blockade of NMDA receptors on GABAergic inhibitory neurons *(40)*. The anatomical distribution of limbic changes does not correlate with the distribution of NMDA receptors and may be the result of a dual neurodegenerative and neuroprotective effect of NMDA antagonists *(41)*. The relation of these morphopathological changes to the adverse effects of chronic NMDA antagonist use is not yet clear. However, it is suggestive that a relatively brief period of NMDA receptor inactivity can produce lasting structural changes in brain regions that also show alterations in schizophrenia *(42)*.

A number of drugs have been reported to prevent or reduce these changes including GABA agonists (barbiturates, benzodiazepines), muscarinic antagonists, typical and atypical antipsychotics, sigma receptor ligands, and alpha$_2$-adrenergic agonists *(40)*.

Table 4
Adverse Events with Dextromethorphan Products

Adverse drug interactions with dextromethorphan

Dextromethorphan	+	terfenidine	
		quinidine	→ Inhibition of CYP2D6 functioning,
		SSRIs	leading to possible fatality
	+	MAO inhibitors	→ Serotonin syndrome (hyperthermia, hypertonus)

Overdosage of drugs formulated with dextromethorphan

Guaifenesin	→	Vomiting
Decongestants	→	Hypertension
Antihistamines	→	Dizziness, hypertension
Acetaminophen	→	Liver damage

Female rats and mice appear more sensitive than male animals *(43)*, while adult rats are more vulnerable than young ones *(44)*. This age-dependent vulnerability may be the result of NDMA receptors not being fully functional in younger animals.

2.1.4. Dextromethorphan

2.1.4.1. Use Patterns of Dextromethorphan

As the primary over-the-counter cough suppressant in the United States, dextromethorphan is readily availability for would-be abusers. Use of dextromethorphan as an intoxicant has been reported with varying degrees of vigilance and alarm since the early 1960s *(45)*. Dextromethorphan users tend to be young, with a mean age of 16.3 yr reported in one series of intentional dextromethorphan abuse cases at a Western poison control center *(46)*. Dextromethorphan is used almost exclusively by oral administration, although intranasal administration has been recently reported. Dextromethorphan is typically found in cough syrups in a concentration of 3 mg/mL (15 mg per cutlery teaspoon), with 360 mg per 4-oz bottle and 720 mg per 8-oz bottle. Gelcaps are also available, containing 30 mg each.

2.1.4.2. Effects of Dextromethorphan

2.1.4.2.1. Acute Intoxication

According to a frequently asked questions (FAQ) document on the Internet *(47)*, dextromethorphan responses can be characterized into plateaus. According to this report, the first plateau (100–200 mg) is a mild stimulant effect and has been compared to a mild psychedelic. The second plateau (200–500 mg) is more intoxicating and has been compared to being drunk on alcohol and stoned on marijuana at the same time. The third plateau (500–1000 mg) is dissociative, like a lower dose of ketamine. The fourth plateau (above 1000 mg) is fully dissociative like a higher dose of ketamine. Adverse effects of high dose dextromethorphan include hyperexcitability or lethargy, confusion, and tactile or visual hallucinations, ataxia, seizures, nystagmus, diaphoresis, hypertension, and tachycardia.

Treatment of dextromethorphan overdose primarily consists of supportive management of symptoms. Naloxone is reportedly useful for reversing dextromethorphan-induced respiratory depression *(48)*. Tolerance to dextromethorphan has been reported by chronic users but injury or fatalities resulting from occasional dextromethorphan ingestion are rarely reported *(49)*. Controlled clinical studies have employed doses as high as 10 mg/kg/d without significant morbidity or mortality, although side effects have been significant *(50)*.

2.1.4.2.2. Adverse Drug Interactions

Aside from behavioral toxicity related to the psychotomimetic effects of high-dose dextromethorphan, the primary risks associated with dextromethorphan use appear to come from interactions with other drugs. Table 4 depicts these adverse events associated with use of products that contain dextromethorphan as one of their ingredients. For example, fatalities following co-administration of the prescription antihistamine terfenadine with dextromethorphan have been reported. This effect was probably the result of the ability of terfenadine to occupy CYP2D6 (either as a substrate or an inhibitor) and thus prevent metabolism of dextromethorphan. A similar response may occur from coadministration of dextromethorphan with quinidine or with serotonin selective reuptake inhibitors (SSRIs), which are also CYP2D6 inhibitors. Since dextromethorphan itself has the ability to act as a SSRI, coadministration with MAOIs or other SSRIs may produce the "serotonin syndrome," which is characterized by hyperreflexia, confusion, myoclonus, hyperthermia, ataxia, and diaphoresis *(51)*.

Drugs that are formulated with dextromethorphan in cough syrups and other cold medications can also produce adverse effects if taken in large quantities. These other drugs (and their overdose potential) include guaifenesin (which may cause vomiting), decongestants like phenylpropanolamine or pseudoephedrine (which may induce hypertension), antihistamines (which may cause dizziness and hypertension), and acetaminophen (which can produce liver damage). Because dextromethorphan is commonly available in hydrobromide form, bromism may occur in chronic users, characterized by memory impairment, drowsiness, tremors and ataxia, frequent skin eruptions, and organic mental disorder, such as delirium or psychosis *(52)*.

2.2. Gamma-Hydroxybutyrate (GHB)

2.2.1. Overview

Gamma hydroxybutyrate (GHB, also known as sodium oxybate) is a putative inhibitory neurotransmitter that is structurally related to GABA. It was initially synthesized as a GABA analog in 1964 to facilitate research investigations, since GABA itself does not easily cross the blood-brain barrier (BBB). The ability of GHB to induce sleep and reversible coma led to its initial use outside of the United States in the 1960s as a surgical anesthetic. However, the high incidence of vomiting, and an association with petite mal (absence) and grand mal seizures limited this use. GHB has been used experimentally in animals as a model for absence seizures *(53)*, but the induction of genuine absence seizure in humans as the result of GHB ingestion is unclear.

GHB has tissue-protectant properties and can reduce cellular damage during certain kinds of shock, ischemia, and hypoxia *(54)*. The mechanism of action of these protective effects are not fully understood, but has been suggested to be the result of a reduction in adenine nucleotide catabolism, glycolysis, lipolysis, lipid peroxidation *(55)*, or lactic acidosis *(56)*.

Beginning in the 1970s, GHB was used outside of the United States as a treatment for narcolepsy. Trials in the United States began more recently, after the FDA approved clinical investigations of GHB for narcolepsy under an Investigational New Drug application *(57)*. A dose of 2–3 g each night is recommended as a starting dose for individuals being treated for narcolepsy *(58)*. GHB is generally started at 25–50 mg/kg (1.75–3.50 g) twice during the night, with patients deliberately waking after 4 h to take the second dose *(59,60)*. There are no reports of tolerance when GHB is given in clinical trials and there are no reports of hangover-like symptoms the following morning *(61)*. More recently, GHB has been investigated as a neuroprotectant and as an experimental treatment for drug dependence *(62,63)*.

In early 2000, GHB was placed into Schedule I under the Controlled Substances Act. As mentioned above, this was accomplished through political legislation entitled the "Date-Rape Drug Prohibition Act," rather than through scientific evaluation in the Department of Health and Human Services. If an approved product containing GHB is marketed, the legislation allowed for that product to be removed from Schedule I and to be placed into Schedule III. However, diversion of medicinal GHB for illicit purposes will still be prosecuted under Schedule I laws, as will use or possession of illegally produced GHB.

Previous to this legislation, attempts to limit GHB use were undermined by the availability of precursors. GHB is easily produced from gammabutyrolactone (GBL) or from 1,4-butanediol, both of which are metabolized to GHB in vivo. Synthetic-chemical conversion of GBL to GHB also frequently occurred, using "GHB kits." GBL itself was also marketed, although the FDA called for a voluntary withdrawal of these products in 1999. Under the legislation that scheduled GHB, GBL is now classified as a List I chemical (a chemical that is used in the manufacturing of a controlled substance), which severely restricts its sale and availability.

2.2.2. Pharmacology of GHB

GHB is found endogenously in the brain, formed from GABA through a series of enzymatic reactions. Succinate semialdehyde (SSA) is formed as an intermediary, which is either reduced to create GHB or oxidized to produce succinic acid (which then enters the Krebs cycle) *(64,65)*. GHB is also produced endogenously following administration of GBL, through conversion by peripheral lactonase outside of the BBB *(66)*.

A rare genetic disorder, 4-hydroxybutyric aciduria, can also result in abnormal accumulation of endogenous GHB *(67)*. This disease is characterized by mild to moderate retardation, ataxia, convulsions, and speech disorders, symptoms that are reminiscent of those seen in individuals who have consumed extremely high doses of GHB.

Following exogenous administration of GHB, the primary route of excretion is through expired air as carbon dioxide *(68)* although GHB can be detected in plasma and urine. Orally administered GHB has an elimination half-life of 20–27 min before it is metabolized back to SSA and then to GABA, with peak plasma concentrations of GHB occuring after 20–60 min *(69)*.

Endogenous GHB is concentrated in the substantia nigra, thalamus. and hypothalamus *(70)*. GHB does not bind to $GABA_A$ receptors and does not function as an agonist at these sites like benzodiazepines or barbiturates do *(71)*. Distinct binding sites exist for GHB, separate from GABA systems, that appear to be stimulated by lower doses of GHB *(72)*. These are found predominantly in the cortical areas, septum, amygdala, and thalamus. At higher doses of GHB, the compound is converted to a functional pool of GABA that has high affinity for $GABA_B$ receptors. GHB itself has low affinity for $GABA_B$ receptors *(73)* while GABA has an affinity that is 1000 times greater for this site. A high-affinity transporter system for GHB has also been demonstrated that can be inhibited by GABA *(74)*.

GHB produces a biphasic response on dopamine release: low doses inhibit release but higher doses promote release *(75)*. This increase in dopamine release may be secondary to the stimulation of tyrosine hydroxylase activity, which subsequently increases dopamine synthesis. It has been hypothesized that GHB regulates dopaminergic firing and release via a reduction of impulse flow in nigro-striatal and meso-cortico-limbic pathways. Interestingly, naloxone can block the increase in striatal dopamine and catalepsy induced by high doses of GBL *(76)*, but it does not inhibit the changes in dopamine or behavioral induced by GHB *(77)*.

Although GHB does not alter absolute levels of serotonin *(78)*, there is evidence of an increase in serotonin turnover, possibly from an increase in availability of the precursor tryptophan. There is an increase in serotonin release following administration of GBL in freely moving rats *(79)*, possibly from the tryptophan increase. This was not true in anesthetized rats, where there was a biphasic temporal response, such that serotonin first was reduced and then recovered to higher than baseline levels *(79)*.

GHB induces a EEG profile and behavior that resembles slow-wave sleep and paradoxical sleep in animals and humans *(80)*. At higher doses of GHB, this has been interpreted as being more like petit mal (absence) seizures than sleep, especially following evidence that this response can be blocked with drugs used to treat absence seizures (such as valproic acid) *(81)*. As stated earlier, though, absence seizures resulting from GHB administration in humans are controversial, since brain concentrations of GHB must reach a level of greater than 240 μM in order to induce a seizure *(82)*.

It has therefore been suggested that GHB is a precursor for a pool of GABA that is responsible for the absence seizure response, acting through $GABA_B$ receptors *(83)*. Therefore, GABA tone is increased by GHB via $GABA_B$ sites, which generates burst discharges, perhaps in the thalamus *(66)*. Interestingly, $GABA_B$ agonists worsen GHB-induced absence-like seizures in animals while $GABA_B$ antagonists reduce them. $GABA_A$ agonists are not as potent in potentiating these seizures and $GABA_A$ antagonists do not alter the seizure response *(66)*.

2.2.3. Use Patterns of GHB

GHB was frequently used among body builders and health enthusiasts as a "fat burner" based on scientific evidence showing that it could increase growth hormone *(84)*. In this context it was often used in conjunction with anabolic steroids. Unfortunately, there are no data demonstrating that GHB can reduce obesity or increase muscle mass. GHB was also promoted as a sleep aid until the FDA halted over-the-counter sales in 1990 and subsequently issued consumer and physician warnings about life-threatening toxicities.

Despite this history, the ability of GHB to induce a euphoria led to its continuing use as an intoxicant in association with "raves" and the club scene. ED cases suggest that most users are young Caucasians and are predominantly male. GHB is sold under a

Table 5
Possible Adverse Events Resulting from GHB Overdosage

Nausea/vomiting
Weakness
Twitching
Decreased heart rate
Decreased respiration
Delirium
Hallucinations
Nonresponsiveness to pain
Fixed pupils
Unconsciousness (reversible coma)
Psychological dependence
Putative withdrawal syndrome

variety of street names, including "Liquid X," "Georgia Home Boy," and "Grievous Bodily Harm," while GBL has been marketed as "Blue Nitro" and "Renewtrient." GHB is typically available as a clear liquid for oral ingestion, where its soapy, salty taste is easily masked with flavorings and/or dilution. GHB is also available in powder form, but the drug is often placed into solution before consumption since oral ingestion of a gram of powder in capsule form can be daunting to users.

2.2.4. Effects of GHB

The response to GHB is highly dose-dependent. According to user reports on the Internet, low doses (0.5–1.5 g) can induce classic depressant effects, not unlike alcohol, such as relaxation, impaired motor skills, vertigo, and heightened sociability. At doses up to 2.5 g, these depressant effects are increased while additional effects, such as grogginess and increased erotic response, begin to emerge. Above 2.5 g, some individuals experience deep euphoria and vaguely hallucinogenic states of consciousness. This experience can be quite unpleasant to some users because it can involve feelings of disequilibrium, nausea, and vomiting.

The steep dose-response curve for GHB can mean moving quickly from a moderate dose to one that produces unconsciousness. At 40–50 mg/kg (2.8–3.5 g), GHB taken orally induces arousable sleep, while 60–70 mg/kg (4.2–4.9 g) induces reversible coma for 1–3 h *(85,86)*. Animal research has placed the median lethal dose at 5–15 times that required to induce coma *(87)*. Since there are broad variations in the amount of GHB in a "teaspoon"—a level measuring teaspoon of pure GHB reportedly provides 2.5 g, while a rounded cutlery teaspoon of GHB can provided 4.4 g—there is a high risk of overdose when users self-administer GHB in powder form. GHB in solution is even more dangerous since the concentration will rarely be known to the user.

2.2.5. Adverse Effects of GHB

There are currently no studies that have been conducted indicating that GHB produces neurotoxicity. Adverse events following GHB ingestion have been reported and can include weakness or twitching, depressed heart rate and respiration, nausea/vomiting, delirium (confusion, agitation), and hallucinations *(57)*. More problematic signs can include the onset of nonresponsiveness to pain and fixed pupils. Coadministration of depressants or other drugs may increase the incidence of adverse events. In one series of 61 case reports *(88)*, more than one-third of patients had coadministered alcohol and more than one-fourth had coadministered other drugs (most frequently amphetamines or MDMA). Repeated, high dose use of GHB under illicit conditions has been reported to induce tolerance and physical dependence, producing a withdrawal syndrome consisting of muscle cramping, anxious reactions, and insomnia. Table 5 lists possible adverse events resulting from GHB overdosage.

Management of GHB toxicity is largely supportive *(89)* and patients generally recover consciousness spontaneously. Neostigmine or physostigmine appear promising in reversing GHB-induced sedation and have been reported as effective in at least one report *(90)*. In rats, flumazenil, a GABA antagonist, can reverse the antianxiety effects of GHB *(91)* and can block the onset of GHB response when given as a pretreatment. Naloxone has also been tested and found to be ineffective in reversing the effects of GHB coma *(89)*.

3. HALLUCINOGENS

3.1. Overview

Any discussion of hallucinogens is hampered by the difficulty in defining this class of drug. At various times, such structurally and pharmacologically disparate compounds as lysergic acid diethylamine (LSD), marijuana, scopolamine, and ketamine have been classified as hallucinogens. Increased understanding of the pharmacology of hallucinogens has narrowed the definition of classical hallucinogens to those drugs that produce their psychoactive effects by acting primarily at $5HT_2$ receptors *(92,93)*. Classical hallucinogens include simple tryptamines (such as N,N-dimethyltryptamine, DMT; psilocybin, ["shrooms"]), the structurally more complex and rigid ergolines (such as LSD ["acid"]), and phenethylamines (such as mescaline or DOM). All of these hallucinogens are classified as Schedule I compounds.

Acute adverse events after hallucinogen ingestion are rarely life-threatening and generally consist of panic, anxiety, and a profound sense of loss of control *(94)*. These symptoms usually resolve within several hours in a quiet, supportive environment but are sometimes treated with benzodiazepines. Like psychostimulants, some hallucinogens can have significant sympathomimetic effects such as tachycardia and peripheral vasoconstriction, which can lead to acute hypertension. Differences between hallucinogens in their ability to induce sympathomimetic effects may be characteristic of those drugs that act at transporter sites to release neurotransmitter (e.g., methylenedioxyamphetamine [MDA]) in contrast to those drugs that act primarily at receptors (e.g., LSD). Stimulation of $5HT_2$ receptors is also known to produce minor hyperthermia in some settings *(95)*.

A recent review of the scientific literature concluded that there were few, if any, long-term neurocognitive deficits attributable to hallucinogen use *(96)*. Although some individuals have experienced persisting adverse psychiatric or neurological reactions to hallucinogens, an extensive review of scientific papers concluded that LSD only played, at most, a nonspecific precipitatory role in these cases *(94)*. The more recently described posthallucinogen perceptual disorder *(97)* appears to be rare among hallucinogen users, but can be more chronic in those individuals who experience it than the well known transient "flashback."

3.2. Interactions of Hallucinogens with Pharmacological Compounds

Individuals who use hallucinogens often have extensive knowledge of the drugs they use. This high degree of scientific education reflects the demographics of hallucinogen users and stems in part from a 30-yr layperson literature that describes the varieties of the psychedelic experience. Internet newsgroups and websites frequently have posting that discuss how to apply pharmacological principles in order to potentiate the effects of hallucinogens through the coadministration of nonhallucinogenic substances. Given that commonly administered doses of serotonergic hallucinogens very rarely produce serious adverse effects, hallucinogen users have often been somewhat cavalier in combining hallucinogens with other drugs to alter the quality of the intoxication produced. Antidepressant agents such as MAO inhibitors, SSRIs, tricyclic antidepressants (TCAs) and lithium have all been described in their ability to increase or decrease the hallucinogenic response.

In addition, hallucinogens are sometimes taken with other reinforcing drugs. The combination of LSD and MDMA has become sufficiently common to earn a name, "candyflipping." Drug-discrimination studies in rats support user reports that this combination synergistically potentiates the effects of the individual drugs *(98)*. This combination would also be expected to potentiate the neurotoxic effects of MDMA since other $5HT_2$ agonists reportedly potentiate the long-term serotonin depletions produced by MDMA *(99)*.

3.2.1. Interactions of Hallucinogens and Acutely Administered MAO Inhibitors

Acute pretreatment with a monoamine oxidase inhibitor (MAOI) can potentiate the effects of hallucinogens. This practice reflects an awareness of the components in the traditional Brazilian hallucinogen, ayahuasca (also known as yage), which is an admixture of the plants *Banisteriopsis caapi* (containing the MAOI, harmaline) and *Psychotria viridis* (containing the hallucinogen DMT) *(100)*. DMT is not orally active because it is metabolized by peripheral MAO. Co-administration of an MAOI prevents this metabolism, resulting in psychoactive effects *(101)*. Modern application of this principle has led to the term "pharmahuasca" *(102)*, reflecting attempts to increase the effects of both tryptamine and phenethylamine hallucinogens with MAOIs in the form of naturally occurring sources (such as seeds from the grass Syrian rue) or pharmaceutical antidepressants.

Syrian rue, the common name for *Peganum harmala*, contains harmaline and other beta-carboline alkaloids in its seeds at a concentration of 2–6% by weight. At the reported dosage of 1–3 g of ground seeds (half to one full teaspoon) taken orally, this translates to approx 60–180 mg of alkaloids. Aqueous extraction of beta-carboline alkaloids is also sometimes practiced. Syrian rue seeds are available legally through many underground catalogs that offer live or dried plant products with psychoactive properties. Syrian rue also grows wild in the southwest United States. Harmaline is available as a crystaline powder from chemical companies for use in research, but access to purchase the drug is restricted to laboratory workers.

Harmaline was first extracted from Syrian rue seeds in the laboratory in 1841. It has long been known to block the actions of MAO, but is now recognized as a reversible inhibitor of MAO_A (RIMA) *(103)*. Most pharmaceutical MAOIs are mechanistically irreversible, leading to potentially serious interactions with stimulant drugs or certain foodstuffs containing tyramine or phenylalanine that require MAO for metabolism. As a RIMA, harmaline may pose less of a possibility for such interactions.

The use of harmaline in potentiating the effects of hallucinogens other than DMT is intriguing, since most hallucinogens available from illicit sources are orally active by themselves and would not seem to significantly benefit from peripheral MAO inhibition in the gut. This suggests that harmaline might have actions on its own that could pharmacologically contribute to the hallucinogenic response. As a beta-carboline, with some structural similarities to tryptamine hallucinogens, harmaline has been shown to have behavioral properties in animals that resemble those of classic hallucinogens. Animals trained in drug-discrimination procedures to the effects of harmaline identify DOM ((-)-2,5-dimethoxy-4-methylamphetamine; a phenethylamine hallucinogen) as being similar to the effects of harmaline *(104)*. Strangely, rats trained to the effects of tryptamine hallucinogens do not generalize the effects of harmaline to those of LSD *(105)* and only partly generalize the effects of harmaline to those of ibogaine *(106)*, a structurally similar hallucinogen. Investigations have also shown that harmaline has inverse agonist properties at the NDMA channel *(107)*.

In addition to harmaline, pharmaceutical MAOIs have also been used illicitly to potentiate the effects of LSD and other hallucinogens. Examples include irreversible MAOIs like the hydrazides ipronidizid and phenelzine as well as the newer RIMAs like moclobemide. These MAOIs were developed as antidepressant agents because of their ability to block the action of MAO_A in the brain. This mechanism prevents the metabolism of the monoamine neurotransmitters serotonin, norepinephrine, and dopamine, which allows for these chemicals to act for a longer time at their respective receptors. Antidepressants are not scheduled as potentially abusable drugs, but access is restricted through a doctor's prescription, limiting their use with hallucinogens.

3.2.2. Interactions of Hallucinogens and Acutely Administered SSRI

Acute co-administration of SSRIs in combination with hallucinogens has also been reported. We initially published a case report of an individual who ingested fluoxetine prior to ingesting LSD and noted a potentiation of the hallucinogenic responses *(108)* and have had numerous individuals subsequently report that a variety of SSRIs can increase the response to both tryptamine and phenethylamine hallucinogens.

SSRIs block the serotonin transporter from recycling serotonin back into the presynaptic bouton, increasing serotonin in the synapse. Among the SSRIs are fluoxetine, paroxetine, sertraline, and fluvoxamine. The acute potentiating effect between hallucinogens and SSRIs may not be surprising given that there are a handful of case reports in the medical literature indicating that SSRIs have been self-administered acutely by individuals with drug-abuse histories for their reinforcing effects *(109–113)*. In fact, many of the respondents in our study noted that during the early phase of taking an SSRI as treatment for depression, they experienced sensations that they identified as distinctly similar to the first hour or two following hallucinogen administration. Although hallucinogen action is clearly correlated to stimulation of $5HT_2$ receptors, the ability of SSRIs to induce symptoms reminiscent of hallucinogens in experienced users suggests the intriguing prospect that the serotonin transporter may play a role in hallucinogenesis.

Acute SSRIs are also reported to be taken in conjunction with MDMA, shortly after the peak subjective effects of MDMA have subsided. This practice originated after the publication of animal data demonstrating that the neurotoxic effects of extremely high doses of MDMA could be reduced or prevented through the administration of fluoxetine, even several hours after MDMA administration *(114)*. Thus, individuals who follow this routine are seeking neuroprotection, even though it has not been definitively demonstrated that acute MDMA use induces neurotoxicity at commonly administered doses. Clinical studies have shown that SSRI pretreatment reduces the acute effects of MDMA in healthy volunteers *(115)*, consistent with the known pharmacology of MDMA that requires the serotonin transporter for psychoactive effects.

3.2.3. Interactions of Hallucinogens and Chronically Administered Antidepressants

Chronic administration of antidepressants have vastly different effects on the hallucinogenic response than acute administration of antidepressants, suggesting that adaptive neural changes are responsible. Although acute administration of SSRIs or MAOIs can increase the response to hallucinogens, individuals who have taken an SSRI or an MAOI for at least 3 wk have a dramatic reduction or complete abolishment of the hallucinogenic effects from LSD *(108,116)*. Users reported that this lack of response led to confusion and disappointment, since friends who had taken the same dose of LSD but were not taking antidepressants had a full hallucinogenic experience. In contrast, prolonged use of lithium or TCAs produce an exacerbation of the hallucinogenic response, often to a very unpleasant degree. The course of this reaction led to disturbed behaviors such as being unable to communicate with friends, hearing self-critical auditory hallucinations, and travelling to another city while in an apparent fugue state. All of the individuals who participated in our study reported changes in response that were strictly psychological in nature; none of the responses could be characterized as physical distress.

The differential effect of various antidepressant agents on the response to LSD, dependent on duration of treatment, is pharmacologically complex. As stated earlier, the hallucinogenic effect of LSD is thought to primarily result from stimulation at $5HT_{2A}$ receptors, with additional input from $5\text{-}HT_{2C}$ receptors and other sites, including $5\text{-}HT_{1A}$ *(117)*, $5\text{-}HT_{1B}$ *(117)*, $5\text{-}HT_{1D}$ *(117)*, $5\text{-}HT_{1E}$ *(118)*, $5\text{-}HT_5$ *(119)*, $5\text{-}HT_6$ *(120)*, $5\text{-}HT_7$ *(121)*, and dopamine D_1 and D_2 receptors *(122)*. LSD is a partial agonist at serotonergic sites *(123)*, however, suggesting that different effects can occur dependent on local concentrations of serotonin. The four classes of antidepressants differentially affect the response to LSD such that:

- Chronic administration of SSRIs reduce the responsiveness of $5HT_2$ *(124)* and $5\text{-}HT_{1A}$ *(125)* receptors. They also increase serotonin levels in the brain *(126)*, creating a condition where a partial agonist like LSD would act as an antagonist, eliminating its hallucinogenic effect.
- Chronic administration of MAOIs decrease $5HT_2$ receptor number *(127)* as well as increase serotonin levels *(128,129)*, which dually could reduce the hallucinogenic response. Human studies also indicate that MAOIs can reduce hallucinations in schizophrenic patients *(130)*.

Table 6
Effect of Antidepressants on Responses to Hallucinogenic Drugs

Acute administration

MAO inhibitor	+	LSD, other hallucinogens	→	Potentiated response
	+	MDMA	→	Hypertensive crisis, death
SSRI	+	LSD, other hallucinogens	→	Potentiated response
	+	MDMA	→	Reduced response

Chronic administration

MAOI	+	LSD	→	Reduced or abolished response
	+	MDMA	→	Hypertensive crisis, death
SSRI	+	LSD	→	Reduced or abolished response
Lithium	+	LSD	→	Unpleasant potentiated response
TCAs	+	LSD	→	Unpleasant potentiated response

- Chronic administration of TCAs sensitize neurons in the forebrain and limbic system to the effects of LSD *(131,132)*, suggesting a mechanism for the potentiation of hallucinogenic effects in humans. Historical case reports also note that TCAs can exacerbate the symptoms of schizophrenia *(133)*.
- The ability of lithium to potentiate the hallucinogenic response to LSD is difficult to explain, given that studies consistently show no change or a reduction in $5HT_2$ receptors *(134,135)*. Since lithium increases serotonin levels in most studies, LSD as a partial agonist should show a reduced response, which it does not.

Table 6 summarizes these changes in hallucinogenic response resulting from concurrent use with antidepressants.

3.2.4. Serious Adverse Antidepressant-Hallucinogen Interactions

Although the interactions of TCAs or lithium plus hallucinogens can lead to an unpleasant psychological experience, life-threatening physical risks can occur when an MAOI is combined with MDMA (or any other sympathomimetic). There are numerous reports in the medical literature of a dangerous increase in blood pressure known as a hypertensive crisis when these drugs are taken together *(136,137)*. Extreme hypertension requires immediate attention to cardiac, neurological, and renal functioning in order to prevent irreversible damage to vital organs *(138)*. Parenteral use of sodium nitroprusside, labetalol, diazoxide, and hydralazine can reduce blood pressure but do not always maintain cardiac homeostasis. Nitroprusside and nifedipine can also produce additional toxicity *(139)*. Newer choices, such as calcium antagonists, such as nicardipine, may offer more optimal management of a drug-induced hypertensive crisis *(138,140)*. Individuals should be severely cautioned against exposing themselves to the risks associated with consuming MDMA in combination with an MAOI.

4. NITROUS OXIDE

4.1. Overview

Nitrous oxide (N_2O) is a colorless, sweet-smelling gas that was first synthesized by Priestley in 1776 and described by Sir Humphrey Davy in 1800 as an agent that could induce both anesthesia and euphoria. It was first used to produce anesthesia in a medical context by Colton in 1844 during dental surgery. It is still used by itself in dental procedures *(141)* and during the first stages of labor *(142)*, although it is more often used in conjunction with other anesthetic agents. As the sole agent, N_2O can induce analgesia equivalent to that of morphine when patients continuously breath as little as a 20% gas concentration. When 30% N_2O is given in continuous administration, many individuals will lose consciousness and will become fully unconscious at an 80% concentration *(143)*.

As a drug of abuse, N_2O has an illustrious history spanning two centuries. Sir Davy was famous at the beginning of the 19th century for hosting N_2O parties with guests that included the potter Wedgwood, the poet Coleridge and Roget of the Thesaurus. Almost one hundred years later, in 1898, the eminent psychologist William James wrote in the scientific literature of his own experience with N_2O, exclaiming, "...My God! I knew everything! A vast rush of obvious and absolutely satisfying solutions to all possible problems overwhelmed my entire being, which was succeeded by a state of moral ecstasy—I was seized with an immense yearning to take back this truth to the feeble, sorrowing, struggling world *(143a)*."

4.2. Pharmacology of N_2O

There are three primary neurotransmitters that have been identified in the mechanism of action of N_2O: opioids, GABA, and NMDA. Of these, the effects of N_2O on opioid systems are the best characterized. According to Quock and Vaughn *(144)*, N_2O fulfills the criteria for classification as a drug with opioid agonist properties, based on stereospecific antagonism by opioid inhibitors *(145)*, cross-tolerance with morphine *(146)*, potentiation by enkephalinase inhibition *(147)*, provocation of the release of endogenous opioids *(148)*, interfering with specific opioid binding at low concentrations *(149)*, and antagonism by antisera to opioid peptides *(147,150)*. It appears from behavioral testing that the kappa opioid receptor, rather than the mu opioid receptor, may be the site of action, especially in relation to antinociception *(151)*. Drug-discrimination studies also indicate that animals generalize the effects of N_2O to those of kappa agonists but not mu agonists *(152)*. Tolerance to the antinociceptive effects of N_2O has been reported *(153)*.

Many anesthetics are recognized as acting as GABA agonists (such as barbiturates) and N_2O appears to have pharmacological effects on this system as well. As a putative GABA agonist, N_2O produces behavioral effects similar to those of chlordiazepoxide, such as an increase in arm entry in the plus maze *(154)*. The effects of N_2O on these behaviors could be inhibited by the benzodiazepine inverse agonist flumazenil and were similarly reduced in animals that were tolerant to benzodiazepines. N_2O also produces a prolongation of GABA receptor-mediated postsynaptic currents *(155)*. These data showing that N_2O induces behavioral effects similar to anti-anxiety agents provide a rationale for its use to reduce anxiety during dental surgery or childbirth.

However, N_2O may also be acting as an NMDA agonist. Under normal conditions, an increase in NMDA neurotransmission increases the activity of nitric oxide synthase (NOS), which converts L-arginine to nitric oxide (NO). Inhibition of NOS, leading to a decrease in NO, can block both the behavioral effects *(156)* and antinociception *(157)* from N_2O. Administration of L-arginine will reverse these effects or will potentiate the effects of N_2O when NOS inhibitors are not administered *(157)*. These data provide further evidence that the chain of events mediated by NMDA are involved in the effects of N_2O.

4.3. Use Pattern of N_2O

In the last decade, it has become clear that N_2O is still frequently used within certain drug subcultures, especially those that favor hallucinogens. Users typically inhale a large bolus of high-concentration N_2O gas, which is then held in the lungs for as long as possible. Because of the short duration of action, users typically readminister the drug repeatedly in a series of rounds. This has earned N_2O the nickname of "hippie crack." Some measure of tolerance can develop to the effects of N_2O upon repeated use, but there are no known withdrawal symptoms *(158)*.

N_2O is readily available as the propellant for whipping-cream production, either in already prepared aerosol canisters or in 6.5 cm cylinders ("Whippets"™) for use in reusable cylinders at home. Although each of these forms contains the gas at a 87–90% concentration, the aerosol canister will dispense 3 L of N_2O while each cylinder contains 4.3–5.0 L *(159)*. Users recognize that it is therefore more cost-efficient to purchase a box of 10 cylinders at approx $6.00–8.00 instead of a single canister at $1.50–3.00. N_2O is also available illicitly in oversize steel tanks from medical/research or industrial sources. Up to 20% of medical and dental students have admitted using N_2O to get high *(160)*, which is a rate of chemical use greater than the 10–14% of physicians who admit to being drug-dependent *(161)*. N_2O tanks have also found their way to rock concerts and surrounding parking lots, where N_2O is dispensed into 12 inch balloons that sell for approx $5.00 each.

4.4. Effects of N_2O

4.4.1. Acute Intoxication

The psychoactive effects are described by users as being similar to the effects of hallucinogens. Responses may also include sensations of being "spaced out," lightedheaded, stimulated, confused or anxious *(162)*, and "feeling abnormal," dizzy, or drowsy *(163)*. The effects of N_2O begin rapidly after self-administration, peak after 30 s and subside within a minute or so *(162)*. Cognitive testing has shown that 15–30% N_2O can impair consolidation of memory as well as disturb attention and psychomotor performance *(164,165)*. There appears to be no evidence of acute tolerance to N_2O in terms of subjective response or to cognitive/ psychomotor tests when N_2O was administered at concentrations up to 40% for 120 min *(166)*.

4.4.2. Serious Adverse Effects

N_2O is the weakest of the anesthetic agents and therefore the least likely to induce toxic reactions. Even when animals are exposed to N_2O for 4 h a day for 14 wk there is no detectable organ damage or changes in P450 enzymes *(167)*. Although N_2O has some opioid activity, it does not appear to produce respiratory depression *(143)*. However, there is a real risk of hypoxia in those who use N_2O because the high gas concentrations can leave little room for air. Hypoxic reactions are familiar to users because of prominent cyanosis of the lips following inhalation. This effect resolves rapidly upon exhalation as long as breathable air is freely available. Accidental death has occurred when users attempt to to heighten the response to N_2O by placing a plastic bag over the

Table 7
Adverse Events Resulting from N₂O Administration

Acute use of N₂O (relevant to illicit use)

    Reversible hypoxia, leading to cyanosis of the lips and face

Chronic use of N₂O (continuous exposure for hours, may not be relevant to occasional illicit use)

(may be due to chemicals contained in N_2O containers, such as trichloroethylene, tolulene, and phenol)
        Swelling of mitochondria → vacuolar changes in pyramidal neurons in posterior
           cingulate
        Reversible polyneuropathy (amnesia, aphasia, weakness, numbness, incoordination of
           extremities)
        Inactivation of vitamin B_{12} (cobalamin) → inactivation of methionine synthase
           → megaloblastic anemia or reduced fertility in women

head to encourage rebreathing of N_2O, leading to suffocation. N_2O does produce slight depressions in heart rate and cardiac output, but this response is similar the cardiovascular effects from inhaling 100% oxygen. Table 7 depicts adverse events resulting from acute use of nitrous oxide.

4.4.3. Neurotoxicity

At a neural level, the effects of N_2O are still unresolved. One study showing that N_2O has NMDA-antagonist properties suggests that N_2O can prevent the neurodegeneration from NMDA administration, making N_2O neuroprotective *(168)*. However, when given at high concentrations for prolonged periods, it can also be as neurotoxic as the NMDA antagonist MK-801 through its ability to cause vacuolar changes in pyramidal neurons in the posterior cingulate from the swelling of mitochondria *(168)*. These neurotoxic effects were reversible with GABA agonists. Yet, if N_2O is itself a GABA agonist, as detailed earlier, these data are confusing. Concentration and duration of administration are no doubt critical to whether the neurotoxic effects of N_2O emerge. It may well be that conditions of unsustained illicit administration are significantly different than the anesthetic conditions tested in the study demonstrating neurotoxicity.

A polyneuropathy has been described following excessive illicit use of N_2O, involving numbness or paresthesias of the limbs, amnesia, aphasia, weakness, and incoordination *(169,170)*. This syndrome has also been reported in health-care professionals who were occupationally exposed to N_2O *(171)*. Symptoms are often reversible if exposure to N_2O is discontinued *(172)*. This syndrome has been associated with oxidative inactivation of vitamin B_{12} (cobalamin) by N_2O *(173)*, although a possible role for N_2O gas contaminants cannot be excluded *(174,175)*. Since B_{12} is important for proper functioning of methionine synthase *(176)*, inactivation of the vitamin cofactor can lead to a loss of enzyme activity, impairing methylation reactions and nucleic acid synthesis.

As might be expected from a syndrome that resembles B_{12} deficiency, N_2O toxicity can be clinically manifested as megaloblastic anemia, with the additional presence of leukopenia, and thrombocytpoenia *(177)*. In most individuals, N_2O-induced B_{12} inactivation appears to be of no clinical consequence when exposures last less than 8 h *(178)*. However, in individuals with borderline B_{12} stores even short exposures to N_2O may be sufficient to precipitate deficiency *(179)*. B_{12} supplements have been recommended as preventive against the apparently high incidence of reduced fertility or spontaneous abortion in female dental professionals *(180,181)*. Table 7 depicts adverse events resulting from chronic use of nitrous oxide.

5. ANABOLIC STEROIDS

5.1. Overview

Anabolic-androgenic steroids (AASs) are exogenous hormones that are structurally similar to testosterone. Testosterone is the primary hormone produced by the Leydig cells of the testes, although small amounts are also produced by the ovaries (as a precursor to estrogen) and the adrenal glands of both sexes. At physiological concentrations, testosterone is responsible for male secondary sexual characteristics such as an increase in facial/body hair growth, lowered voice from thickened vocal cords, coarser skin, and growth of the penis (androgenic effects) as well as an increase in tissue growth (anabolic effects). Behaviorally, testosterone plays a critical role in sexual interest and activity in both men and women *(182)*.

Under illicit conditions, AASs are taken in supraphysiological doses for their anabolic effects, typically by bodybuilders and athletes *(183)*. Anabolism is a state when more nitrogen is being taken into the body than is being lost from the body. This "positive nitrogen balance" allows for nitrogen to be incorporated into amino acids, leading to an increase in protein synthesis and thus the growth of tissues. AASs have also been used medically since the 1940s in the treatment of diseases that result in catabolism (breakdown of protein) in order to reduce muscle wasting and to improve the healing process in patients *(184)*. Additionally, AASs are used for their androgenizing effects in male hypogonadism *(185)* and to induce and maintain female-to-male transexual conversion *(186)*.

5.2. Pharmacology of Anabolic Steroids

Oral or parenteral administration of a supraphysiological dose of testosterone has limited efficacy because much of the drug is metabolized in the liver before it can circulate in the body. Structural modification of testosterone to reduce hepatic metabolism has resulted into two classes of synthetic AASs: 17-alpha-alkyls (which are orally active) and 17-beta-esters (which must be injected intramuscularly). The ability of a particular AAS to enter the cells of a target tissue determines its anabolic/androgenic potential. Thus, AASs with greater anabolic action more easily enter muscle cells while AASs with more androgenic action more easily enter cells controlling secondary sexual characteristics. AASs with greater anabolic potential include the 17-alpha-alkyls methandrostenolone and oxymetholone and the 17-beta-esters nandrolone decanoate or nandrolone phenpropionate. Conversely, greater androgenic effects result from the 17-alpha-alkyls ethylestrenol and stanozole and the 17-beta-ester methenolone enanthate.

The action of all androgens is the same once they are in circulation *(187)*. At target tissues, the androgen passes into the cell and binds to steroid receptors in the cytoplasm, forming a hormone-receptor complex. The complex is then translocated into the nucleus of the cell, where it attaches to the nuclear chromatin. This induces production of messenger RNA through gene transcription, followed by ribosomal translation leading to the synthesis of structural or enzymatic protein. This genomic process requires a timeframe of minutes to days before effects are fully realized. Androgens are also known to have nongenomic processes affecting opioid systems, where there appears to be reciprocal parallel regulation *(188,189)*. This may account for an AAS withdrawal syndrome in rodents that resembles some of the signs of opioid withdrawal *(190)*.

5.3. Use Pattern of Anabolic Steroids

As early as 1939, it was suggested that AASs might enhance physical performance, but this point remains controversial. Although athletic ability may not improve in direct relation to steroid use, nearly 60 years of scientific research has demonstrated that AASs can dramatically increase muscle mass *(191)*, but only under conditions where there is satisfactory protein consumption and strenuous muscle exertion. Thus, it is not possible for a person to develop the rippling muscles of Mr. Universe through a regimen of AASs, junk food and "couch potato" behavior. Among elite athletes and bodybuilders, 30–75% have admitted using AASs. In the face of unconvincing scientific data concerning performance enhancement from these drugs, the extent of AAS use might be considered surprising. This suggests either a lack of studies using a protocol representative of street use that would demonstrate performance improvements or the development of a unique mythology among AAS abusers independent of real effects (which is, after all, common among the abusers of many classes of drugs). No matter which is true, use of AASs is strictly forbidden by major amateur and professional athletic organizations, with expulsion occurring after testing positive for AASs use. AASs were placed under the Controlled Substances Act as Schedule III drugs by Congress in 1991, in a legislative process similar to that for ketamine and GHB, which avoided scientific oversight by the Department of Health and Human Services.

As designated drugs of abuse, AASs are unusual in that they do not produce an immediate euphoria or a state of intoxication *(192)*. Although recent reports in rodents demonstrate that AASs can induce a conditioned place preference (i.e., an animal will seek to spend more time on the side of the cage where it received the drug than on the side where it received saline) *(193)*, indicating that the drugs have rewarding properties, human users do not report acute psychological effects. Sex steroids are known to improve a sense of well-being in hospitalized patients, but this is not characterized as similar to the reinforcing effects of abused drugs. However, it has been suggested that users of AASs can meet the Diagnostic and Statistical Manual (DSM) criteria for psychoactive substance dependence, based on an uncontrolled pattern of steroid use that continues despite adverse consequences *(194)*.

The fact that animals do not self-administer AASs suggests that human use of these drugs has less to do with physiological reinforcement than it does with the psychological or sociological effects resulting from the effects of AASs on appearance. It is perhaps not surprising, then, that there is a much greater use of AASs among men than women, since "bulking up" in body size has until recently been a desirable condition only for males. This sex difference is stable even among adolescents, where 6.6% of male teens have used AASs but only 1.3% of female teens have done the same *(195)*. Thus, it is possible to hypothesize that young men abuse AASs to attain a muscular, culturally appropriate masculine appearance, while young women seeking a culturally appropriate feminine appearance (e.g., one that is thin) may be more inclined to abuse stimulants instead.

Typically, AASs are used illicitly in "cycles," meaning they are taken for 6–12 wk or longer, accompanied by intense physical exertion, and then discontinued for period of weeks or months before the cycle repeats. The use pattern of weeks to months is directly related to the mechanism of action of androgens, which requires a lengthy administration period before anabolic effects are seen. Another method of use is called "stacking," where several types of AASs are used over the course of a cycle, often in increasing doses, sometimes in conjunction with each other *(196)*. It has been reported by users that tolerance can develop to AASs ("plateauing"), but it is unclear what might constitute tolerance since AASs do not induce immediate behavioral effects. During discontinuation phases, users have reported withdrawal symptoms including a depression and lethargy that are responsive to SSRIs antidepressants *(197)*. There is also the desire to continue using steroids to reduce those symptoms, all of which are indicative of physical dependence. An animal model of AAS withdrawal has been described, which can be prevented and/or alleviated with SSRIs *(190)*. This could be expected, given prior evidence showing an inverse relationship between androgens and serotonin *(198)*.

5.4. Adverse Effects of Anabolic Steroids

5.4.1. Adverse Physiological Effects

All androgens exert negative feedback on the hypothalamus and pituitary, reducing levels of gonadotropin releasing hormone (GRH), lutenizing hormone (LH), and follicle-stimulating hormone (FSH) and causing reduced production of endogenous testosterone. At supraphysiological doses (10–30 times higher than those required for replacement therapy), androgens can cause a myriad of adverse effects. Peripheral responses to AASs include acne exacerbation as well as feminization in men in the form of gynecomastia resulting from the conversion of high levels of androgens to excess estrogen *(199)*. Women taking AASs also report enlargement of the clitoris, cessation of menstrual cycles, and male-pattern baldness *(200)*. More severely, an increased risk of heart disease can occur from a reduction in serum high-density lipoprotein (HDL) ("good") cholesterol and an increase in low-density lipoprotein (LDL) ("bad") cholesterol *(201)*. Liver disorders are especially associated with oral (17-alpha-alkyl) AASs, including jaundice and peliosis hepatis in which liver tissue dies and is replaced by blood-filled cysts *(202)*. Table 8 depicts adverse physiological events resulting from chronic use of anabolic steroids.

5.4.2. Adverse Behavioral Effects

Adverse behavioral responses resulting from AAS abuse are frequently reported within the athletic community. The most prominent anecdotal report is that of increased physical aggressiveness, known colloquially as "roid rage." This is often accompanied by an increase in irritability or impulsivity directed towards other people or inanimate objects, without provocation. Although it is difficult to investigate a tendency towards physical violence under laboratory conditions, supraphysiological doses of an AAS have been shown to induce a higher degree of "aggressive responding" in a mock competitive task using button presses *(203)*. Animal studies similarly show that AASs can

Table 8
Adverse Events Resulting from Chronic Use of Anabolic Steroids

Decreased sperm production/shrinking of testes
Gynecomastia
Acne
Increased clitoral size/decreased breast size
Reduced menstrual cycles
Male pattern baldness
Increased high-density lipoprotein (HDL) ("bad cholesterol")
Decreased low-density lipoprotein (LDL) ("good cholesterol")
Jaundice
Peliosis hepatis (blood filled cysts in the liver)
Increased aggression ("roid rage")
Psychological dependence
Putative withdrawal syndrome (depression)

induce aggression and dominance when given at very high doses, behaviors that could be reduced through administration of the 5-HT$_{1A}$ agonist anxiolytic, buspirone *(204)*.

Other inventories of AAS users have reported higher scores for narcissism but lower scores for empathy *(205)* and symptoms of mania, hypomania, or major depression in 23% of participants *(206)*. However, controlled scientific studies have not been able to demonstrate a relationship between administration of supraphysiological doses of androgens and psychiatric symptoms. At doses of five times that needed for physiological replacement, AASs have not been shown to alter mood, behavior, or psychosexual functioning in healthy men after 14 wk except minimally *(207)*. Even at six times the physiological dose, where some AAS abusers had symptoms of mania or aggressiveness, 84% of repondants had only minimal psychiatric effects *(208)* and there was no increase in angry behavior *(209)*. The discrepancy between the clinical studies and street use reports may speak to the fact that abusers typically self-administer doses 10–100 times the medically necessary dose *(210)*.

6. SUMMARY

6.1. General

Although all drugs of abuse can induce short-lived behavioral toxicities, those drugs that are primarily used within smaller subcultural groups are often less well characterized in terms of their neurotoxic potential than drugs of abuse with a more ubiquitous use profile. This necessarily limits the ability of science to inform public debate and decision-making about the possible biological hazards of these compounds under the conditions that they are used on the street.

6.2. Club Drugs: Ketamine, Dextromethorphan, and GHB

Ketamine can induce a reversible vacuolization in pyramidal neurons of the posterior cingulate and retrosplenial cortex of rats follow acute administration of low doses of the drug, while chronic, high-dose use of ketamine can induce persistent vacuoles and neuronal necrosis in neocortical and limbic regions.

The main risk associated with illicit dextromethorphan use comes from interactions with other drugs. Drugs that inhibit the P450 CYP2D6 enzyme can prevent metabolism of dextromethorphan, while MAOIs can induce the "serotonin syndrome." Overdosage of drugs formulated with dextromethorphan in cough syrups is also possible when large quantities of dextromethorphan are consumed.

While there are no studies that suggest that GHB can produce neurotoxicity, the threat of overdose among illicit users can be high since GHB is often sold as a liquid with unknown drug concentrations.

6.3. Hallucinogens Combined with Antidepressants

No toxicity research has been conducted on the interaction between hallucinogens and antidepressants, but the combination of an MAOI plus the substituted amphetamine, MDMA, can produce a predictable and life-threatening hypertensive crisis.

6.4. Nitrous Oxide (N_2O)

Prolonged exposure to high doses of N_2O can induce vacuolar changes in the pyramidal neurons of the posterior cingulate, an inactivation of vitamin B_{12} (leading to a loss of activity of methionine synthase), and a polyneuropathy syndrome. Since illicit users of N_2O seldom expose themselves to more than acute doses, neurotoxicity is unlikely.

6.5. Anabolic Steroids

Supraphysiological doses of anabolic steroids taken chronically can induce a variety of physical and psychological disorders, including reports of aggressiveness and withdrawal depression, but it has yet to be shown that these are neurotoxic responses to drug use.

ACKNOWLEDGMENT

The authors wish to acknowledge the research contributions from Joshua Buckholtz and Dr. A. Potrezebie.

REFERENCES

1. Corssen, G., Miyasaka, M., and Domino, E. F. (1968) Changing concepts in pain control during surgery: dissociative anesthesia with CI–581. A progress report. *Anesth, Analg.* **47**, 746–759.
2. Johnstone, M., Evans, V., and Baigel, S. (1958) Sernyl (CI–395) in clinical anesthesia. *Br. J. Anaeth.* **31**, 433–439.
3. White, P. F., Ham, J., Way, W. L., and Trevor, A. J. (1980) Pharmacology of ketamine isomers in surgical patients. *Anesthesiology* **52**, 231–239.
4. Fine, J. and Finestone, S. C. (1973) Sensory disturbances following ketamine anesthesia: recurrent hallucinations. *Anesth. Analg.* **52**, 428–430.
5. Krystal, J. H., Karper, L. P., Seibyl, J. P., Freeman, G. K., Delaney, R., Bremner, J. D., et al. (1994) Subanesthetic effects of the noncompetitive NMDA antagonist, ketamine, in humans. Psychotomimetic, perceptual, cognitive, and neuroendocrine responses. *Arch. Gen. Psychiatry* **51**, 199–214.
6. Luby, E. D., Cohen, B. D., Rosenbaum, G., Gottlieb, J. S., and Kelley, R. (1959) Study of a new schizophrenomimetic drug: sernyl. *Arch. Neurol. Psychiatry* **81**, 363–369.

7. Lodge, D. and Anis, N. A. (1982) Effects of phencyclidine on excitatory amino acid activation of spinal interneurones in the cat. *Eur. J. Pharmacol.* **77**, 203–204.

8. Kim, J. S., Kornhuber, H. H., Schmid-Burgk, W, and Holzmuller, B. (1980) Low cerebrospinal fluid glutamate in schizophrenic patients and a new hypothesis on schizophrenia. *Neurosci. Lett.* **20**, 379–382.

9. Carlsson, A. (1988) The current status of the dopamine hypothesis of schizophrenia. *Neuropsychopharmacology* **1**, 179–186.

10. Choi, D. W., Koh, J. Y., and Peters, S. (1988) Pharmacology of glutamate neurotoxicity in cortical cell culture: attenuation by NMDA antagonists. *J. Neurosci.* **8**, 185–196.

11. Marek, P., Ben-Eliyahu, S., Gold, M., and Liebeskind, J. C. (1991) Excitatory amino acid antagonists (kynurenic acid and MK-801) attenuate the development of morphine tolerance in the rat. *Brain Res.* **547**, 77–81.

12. Bisaga, A. and Popik, P. (2000) In search of a new pharmacological treatment for drug and alcohol addiction: N-methyl-D-aspartate (NMDA) antagonists. *Drug Alcohol Depend.* **59**, 1–15.

13. Krupitsky, E. M. and Grinenko, A. Y. (1997) Ketamine psychedelic therapy (KPT): a review of the results of ten years of research. *J. Psychoactive Drugs* **29**, 165–183.

14. Baggott, M., Sferios, E., Zhender, J., Heifets, B., Jones, R. T., and Mendelson, J. (2000) Chemical analysis of ecstasy pills. *JAMA* **284**, 2190.

15. Morris, R. G., Anderson, E., Lynch, G. S., and Baudry, M. (1986) Selective impairment of learning and blockade of long-term potentiation by an N-methyl-D-aspartate receptor antagonist, AP5. *Nature* **319**, 774–776.

16. Berman, R. M., Cappiello, A., Anand, A., Oren, D. A., Heninger, G. R., Charney, D. S., and Krystal, J. H. (2000) Antidepressant effects of ketamine in depressed patients. *Biol. Psychiatry* **47**, 351–354

17. Isbell, H. and Fraser, H. F. (1953) Actions and addiction liabilities of Dromoran derivatives in man. *J. Pharmacol. Exp. Ther.* **107**, 524–530.

18. Franklin P. H., Murray T. F. (1992) High affinity [3H]dextrorphan binding in rat brain is localized to a noncompetitive antagonist site of the activated N-methyl-D-aspartate receptor-cation channel. *Mol. Pharmacol.* **41**, 134–146.

19. Gough, A. C., Miles, J. S., Spurr, N. K., Moss, J. E., Gaedigk, A., Eichelbaum, M., and Wolf, C. R. (1990) Identification of the primary gene defect at the cytochrome P450 CYP2D6 locus. *Nature* **347**, 773–776.

20. Clements, J. A., Nimmo, W. S., and Grant, I. S. (1982) Bioavailability, pharmacokinetics, and analgesic activity of ketamine in humans. *J. Pharm. Sci.* **71**, 539–542.

21. Siegel, R. K. (1978) Phencyclidine and ketamine intoxication: a study of four populations of recreational users. *NIDA Res. Monogr.* **21**, 119–147.

22. Kamaya, H., Krishna, P. R. (1987) Ketamine addiction. *Anesthesiology* 67, 861–862.

23. Jansen, K. L. (1990a) Ketamine: can chronic use impair memory? *Int. J. Addict.* **25**, 133–139.

24. Ahmed, S. N. and Petchkovsky, L. (1980) Abuse of ketamine. *Br. J. Psychiatry* **137**, 303.

25. Malhotra, A. K., Pinals, D. A., Weingartner, H., Sirocco, K., Missar, C. D., Pickar, D., and Breier, A. (1996) NMDA receptor function and human cognition: the effects of ketamine in healthy volunteers. *Neuropsychopharmacology* **14**, 301–307.

26. Bowdle, T. A., Radant, A. D., Cowley, D. S., Kharasch, E. D., Strassman, R. J., and Roy-Byrne, P. P. (1998) Psychedelic effects of ketamine in healthy volunteers: relationship to steady-state plasma concentrations. *Anesthesiology* **88**, 82–88.

27. Jansen, K. L. (1990b) Neuroscience and the near-death experience: roles for the NMSA-PCP receptor, the sigma receptor and the endopsychosins. *Med. Hypotheses* **31**, 25–29.

28. Lilly, J. C. (1972) *Center of the Cyclone*. Julian Press, New York.

29. Adler, C. M., Malhotra, A. K., Elman, I., Goldberg, T., Egan, M., Pickar, D., and Breier, A. (1999) Comparison of ketamine-induced thought disorder in healthy volunteers and thought disorder in schizophrenia. *Am. J. Psychiatry* **156**, 1646–1649.

30. Krystal, J. H., Bennett, A., Abi-Saab, D., Belger, A., Karper, L. P., D'Souza, D. C., et al. (2000) Dissociation of ketamine effects on rule acquisition and rule implementation: possible relevance to NMDA receptor contributions to executive cognitive functions. *Biol. Psychiatry* **47,** 137–143

31. Newcomer, J. W., Farber, N. B., Jevtovic-Todorovic, V., Selke, G., Melson, A. K., Hershey, T., et al. (1999) Ketamine-induced NMDA receptor hypofunction as a model of memory impairment and psychosis. *Neuropsychopharmacology* **20,** 106–118.

32. Lahti, A. C., Koffel, B., LaPorte, D., and Tamminga, C. A. (1995) Subanesthetic doses of ketamine stimulate psychosis in schizophrenia. *Neuropsychopharmacology* **13,** 9–19.

33. Perel, A. and Davidson, J. T. (1976) Recurrent hallucinations following ketamine. *Anaesthesia* **31,** 1081–1083.

34. Cosgrove, J. and Newell, T. G. (1991) Recovery of neuropsychological functions during reduction in use of phencyclidine. *J. Clin. Psychol.* **47,** 159–169.

35. Allen, R. M. and Young, S. J. (1978) Phencyclidine-induced psychosis. *Am. J. Psychiatry* **135,** 1081–1084.

36. Luisada, P. V.(1978) The phencyclidine psychosis: phenomenology and treatment. *NIDA Res. Monogr.* **21,** 241–253.

37. Erard, R., Luisada, P. V., and Peele. R. (1980) The PCP psychosis: prolonged intoxication or drug-precipitated functional illness? *J. Psychedelic Drugs* **12,** 235–251.

38. Allen, H. L. and Iversen, L. L. (1990) Phencyclidine, dizocilpine, and cerebrocortical neurons. *Science* **247,** 221.

39. Fix, A. S., Horn, J. W., Wightman, K. A., Johnson, C. A., Long, G. G., Storts, R. W., et al. (1993) Neuronal vacuolization and necrosis induced by the noncompetitive N-methyl-D-aspartate (NMDA) antagonist MK(+)801 (dizocilpine maleate): a light and electron microscopic evaluation of the rat retrosplenial cortex. *Exp. Neurol.* **123,** 204–215.

40. Olney, J. W., Labruyere, J., Wang, G., Wozniak, D. F., Price, M. T., and Sesma, M. A. (1991) NMDA antagonist neurotoxicity: mechanism and prevention. *Science* **254,** 1515–1518.

41. Ellison, G. (1995) The N-methyl-D-aspartate antagonists phencyclidine, ketamine and dizocilpine as both behavioral and anatomical models of the dementias. *Brain Res. Brain Res. Rev.* **20,** 250–267

42. Bogerts, B. (1993) Recent advances in the neuropathology of schizophrenia. *Schizophr. Bull.* **19,** 431–445.

43. Honack, D. and Loscher, W. (1993) Sex differences in NMDA receptor mediated responses in rats. *Brain Res.* **620,** 167–170.

44. Farber, N. B., Wozniak, D. F., Price, M. T., Labruyere, J., Huss, J., St. Peter, H., and Olney, J. W. (1995) Age-specific neurotoxicity in the rat associated with NMDA receptor blockade: potential relevance to schizophrenia? *Biol. Psychiatry* **38,** 788–796.

45. Bem, J. L. and Peck, R. (1992) Dextromethorphan. An overview of safety issues. *Drug Saf.* **7,** 190–199.

46. McElwee, N. E. and Veltri, J. C. (1990) Intentional abuse of dextromethorphan (DM) products: 1985 to 1988 statewide data. *Vet. Hum. Toxicol.* **32,** 355.

47. White, W. E. (1997) Answers to frequently ssked wuestions about fextromethorphan (DXM), *http://www.erowid.org/chemicals/dxm/faq/dxm_faq.shtml*

48. Schneider, S. M., Michelson, E. A., Boucek, C. D., and Ilkhanipour, K. (1991) Dextromethorphan poisoning reversed by naloxone. *Am. J. Emerg. Med.* **9,** 237–238.

49. Office of Applied Studies (1999) Year-End 1998 Emergency Department Data from the Drug Abuse Warning Network. SAMHSA, Office of Applied Studies, Rockville, MD.

50. Hollander, D., Pradas, J., Kaplan, R., McLeod, H. L., Evans, W. E., and Munsat, T. L. (1994) High-dose dextromethorphan in amyotrophic lateral sclerosis: phase I safety and pharmacokinetic studies. *Ann. Neurol.* **36,** 920–924.

51. Sternbach, H. (1991) The serotonin syndrome. *Am. J. Psychiatry* **148,** 705–713.

52. Ng, Y. Y., Lin, W. L., Chen, T. W., Lin, B. C., Tsai, S. H., Chang, C. C., and Huang, T. P. (1992) Spurious hyperchloremia and decreased anion gap in a patient with dextromethorphan bromide. *Am. J. Nephrol.* **12**, 268–270

53. Hu, R. Q., Banerjee, P. K., and Snead, O. C. 3rd. (2000) Regulation of gamma-aminobutyric acid (GABA) release in cerebral cortex in the gamma-hydroxybutyric acid (GHB) model of absence seizures in rat. *Neuropharmacology* **39**, 427–439.

54. Artru, A. A., Steen, P. A., and Michenfelder, J. D. (1980) Gamma-Hydroxybutyrate: cerebral metabolic, vascular, and protective effects. *J. Neurochem.* **35**, 1114–1119.

55. Petrin, I. N., Dolgikh, V. T., and Krolevets, I. P. (1993) The use of sodium gamma-oxybutyrate and gutimine for decreasing metabolic disorders in the heart, caused by exotoxic shock in acetic acid poisoning. *Vopr. Med. Khim.* **39**, 36–39.

56. Lopatin, A. F., Riabtseva, E. G., and Riabova, W. (1984) Effect of sodium oxybate on metabolic indices in ishchemic hypoxia of muscle tissue. *Farmakol. Toksikol.* **47**, 53–55.

57. Dyer, J. E. (1991) Gamma-Hydroxybutyrate: a health-food product producing coma and seizurelike activity. *Am. J. Emerg. Med.* **9**, 321–324.

58. Broughton, R. and Mamelak, M.. (1979) The treatment of narcolepsy-cataplexy with nocturnal gamma-hydroxybutyrate. *Can. J. Neurol. Sci.* **6**, 1–6.

59. Mamelak, M., Scharf, M. B., and Woods, M. (1986) Treatment of narcolepsy with gamma-hydroxybutyrate. A review of clinical and sleep laboratory findings. *Sleep* **9**, 285–289.

60. Scrima, L., Hartman, P. G., Johnson, F. H., Jr., and Hiller, F. C. (1989) Efficacy of gamma-hydroxybutyrate versus placebo in treating narcolepsy-cataplexy: double-blind subjective measures. *Biol. Psychiatry* **26**, 331–343

61. Scharf, M. B., Brown, D., Woods, M., Brown, L., and Hirschowitz, J. (1985) The effects and effectiveness of gamma-hydroxybutyrate in patients with narcolepsy. *J. Clin. Psychiatry* **46**, 222–225

62. Poldrugo, F. and Addolorato, G. (1999) The role of gamma-hydroxybutyric acid in the treatment of alcoholism: from animal to clinical studies. *Alcohol Alcohol* **34**, 15–24.

63. Gallimberti, L., Schifano, F., Forza, G., Miconi, L., and Ferrara, S. D. (1994) Clinical efficacy of gamma-hydroxybutyric acid in treatment of opiate withdrawal. *Eur. Arch. Psychiatry Clin. Neurosci* **244**, 113–114.

64. Mamelak, M. (1989) Gammahydroxybutyrate: an endogenous regulator of energy metabolism. *Neurosci. Biobehav Rev.* **13**, 187–198

65. Roth, R. H. and Giarman, N. J. (1969) Conversion in vivo of gamma-aminobutyric to gamma-hydroxybutyric acid in the rat. *Biochem. Pharmacol.* **18**, 247–250.

66. Maitre, M. (1997) The gamma-hydroxybutyrate signalling system in brain: organization and functional implications. *Prog. Neurobiol.* **51**, 337–361.

67. Rahbeeni, Z., Ozand, P. T., Rashed, M., Gascon, G. G., al Nasser M, al Odaib A, et al. (1994) 4-Hydroxybutyric aciduria. *Brain Dev.* **16(Suppl.),** 64–71.

68. Laborit, H. Sodium 4 hydroxybutyrate. (1964) *Intl. J. Neuropharmacol.* **43**, 433–452.

69. Vickers, M. (1969) Gamma hydroxybutyric acid. *Intl. Anesthesia Clin.* **7**, 75–89.

70. Vayer, P. and Maitre, M. (1988) Regional differences in depolarization-induced release of gamma-hydroxybutyrate from rat brain slices. *Neurosci. Lett.* **87**, 99–103.

71. Serra, M., Sanna, E., Foddi, C., Concas, A., and Biggio, G. (1991) Failure of gamma-hydroxybutyrate to alter the function of the GABAA receptor complex in the rat cerebral cortex. *Psychopharmacology* **104**, 351–355.

72. Hechler, V., Gobaille, S., and Maitre, M. (1992) Selective distribution pattern of gamma-hydroxybutyrate receptors in the rat forebrain and midbrain as revealed by quantitative autoradiography. *Brain Res.* **572**, 345–348.

73. Hill, D. R. and Bowery, N. G. (1981) ^{3}H-baclofen and 3H-GABA bind to bicuculline-insensitive GABA B sites in rat brain. *Nature* **290**, 149–152

74. Benavides, J., Rumigny, J. F., Bourguignon, J. J., Wermuth, C. G., Mandel, P., and Maitre, M. (1982) A high-affinity, Na^+-dependent uptake system for gamma-hydroxybutyrate in membrane vesicles prepared from rat brain. *J. Neurochem.* **38**, 1570–1575.

75. Cheramy, A., Nieoullon, A., and Glowinski, J. (1977) Stimulating effects of gamma-hydroxybutyrate on dopamine release from the caudate nucleus and the substantia nigra of the cat. *J. Pharmacol. Exp. Ther.* **203,** 283–293.

76. Snead, O. C., 3d and Bearden, L. J. (1980) Naloxone overcomes the dopaminergic, EEG, and behavioral effects of gamma-hydroxybutyrate. *Neurology* **30,** 832–828.

77. Devoto, P., Colombo, G., Cappai, F., and Gessa GL. (1994) Naloxone antagonizes ethanol—but not gamma-hydroxybutyrate-induced sleep in mice. *Eur. J. Pharmacol.* **252,** 321–324.

78. Miguez, I., Aldegunde, M., Duran, R., and Veira, J. A. (1988) Effect of low doses of gamma-hydroxybutyric acid on serotonin, noradrenaline, and dopamine concentrations in rat brain areas. *Neurochem. Res.* **13,** 531–533.

79. Broderick, P. A. and Phelix, C. F. (1997) I. Serotonin (5-HT) within dopamine reward circuits signals open-field behavior. II. Basis for 5-HT—DA interaction in cocaine dysfunctional behavior. *Neurosci. Biobehav. Rev.* **21,** 227–260.

80. Lapierre, O., Montplaisir, J., Lamarre, M., and Bedard, M. A. (1990) The effect of gamma-hydroxybutyrate on nocturnal and diurnal sleep of normal subjects: further considerations on REM sleep-triggering mechanisms. *Sleep* **13,** 24–30.

81. Godschalk, M., Dzoljic, M. R., and Bonta, I. L. (1976) Antagonism of gamma hydroxybutyrate induced hypersynchronisation in the EEG of the rat by anti-petit mal drugs. *Neurosci. Lett.* **3,** 145–150.

82. Snead, O. C., 3d (1991) The gamma-hydroxybutyrate model of absence seizures: correlation of regional brain levels of gamma-hydroxybutyric acid and gamma-butyrolactone with spike wave discharges. *Neuropharmacology* **30,** 161–167.

83. Misgeld, U., Bijak, M., and Jarolimek, W. (1995) A physiological role for GABAB receptors and the effects of baclofen in the mammalian central nervous system. *Prog. Neurobiol.* **46,** 423–462.

84. Bluet-Pajot, M. T., Schaub, C., and Nassiet, J. (1978) Growth hormone response to hypoglycemia under gamma-hydroxybutyrate narco-analgesia in the rat. *Neuroendocrinology* **26,** 141–149.

85. Galloway, G. P., Frederick, S. L., Staggers, F. E. Jr., Gonzales, M., Stalcup, S. A., and Smith, D. E. (1997) Gamma-hydroxybutyrate: an emerging drug of abuse that causes physical dependence. *Addiction* **92,** 89–96.

86. Hunter, A. S., Long, W. J., and Ryrie, C. G. (1971) An evaluation of gamma-hydroxybutyric acid in paediatric practice. *Br. J. Anaesth.* **43,** 620–628.

87. Series, F., Series, I., and Cormier, Y. (1992) Effects of enhancing slow-wave sleep by gamma hydroxybutyrate on obstructive sleep apnea. *Am. Rev. Respir. Dis.* **145,** 1378–1383.

88. Chin, R. L., Sporer, K. A., Cullison, B., Dyer, J. E., and Wu, T. D. (1998) Clinical course of gamma-hydroxybutyrate overdose. *Ann. Emerg. Med.* **31,** 716–722.

89. Li, J., Stokes, S. A., and Woeckener, A. (1998) A tale of novel intoxication: a review of the effects of gamma hydroxybutyric acid with recommendations for management. *Ann. Emerg. Med.* **31,** 729–736.

90. Yates, S. W. and Viera, A. J. (2000) Physostigmine in the treatment of gamma-hydroxybutyric acid overdose. *Mayo Clin. Proc.* **75,** 401–402.

91. Schmidt-Mutter, C., Pain, L., Sandner, G., Gobaille, S., and Maitre, M. (1998) The anxiolytic effect of gamma-hydroxybutyrate in the elevated plus maze is reversed by the benzodiazepine receptor antagonist, flumazenil. *Eur. J. Pharmacol.* **342,** 21–27.

92. Teitler, M., Leonhardt, S., Appel, N. M., De Souza, E. B., and Glennon, R. A. (1990) Receptor pharmacology of MDMA and related hallucinogens. *Ann. NY Acad. Sci.* **600,** 626–638.

93. Vollenweider, F. X., Vollenweider-Scherpenhuyzen, M. F., Babler, A., Vogel, H., and Hell, D. (1998) Psilocybin induces schizophrenia-like psychosis in humans via a serotonin-2 agonist action. *NeuroReport* **9,** 3897–3902.

94. Strassman, R. J. (1984) Adverse reactions to psychedelic drugs. A review of the literature. *J. Nerv. Ment. Dis.* **172**, 577–595.

95. Aulakh, C. S., Mazzola-Pomietto, P., Wozniak, K. M., Hill, J. L., and Murphy, D. L. (1994) Evidence that 1-(2,5-dimethoxy-4-methylphenyl)-2-aminopropane-induced hypophagia and hyperthermia in rats is mediated by serotonin–2A receptors. *J. Pharmacol. Exp. Ther.* **270**, 127–132

96. Halpern, J. H. and Pope, H. G., Jr. (1999) Do hallucinogens cause residual neuropsychological toxicity? *Drug Alcohol Depend.* **53**, 247–256.

97. Abraham, H. D. and Aldridge, A. M. (1993) Adverse consequences of lysergic acid diethylamide. *Addiction* **8**, 1327–1334.

98. Schechter, M. D. (1998) 'Candyflipping': synergistic discriminative effect of LSD and MDMA. *Eur. J. Pharmacol.* **341**, 131–134.

99. Gudelsky, G. A., Yamamoto, B. K., and Nash, J. F. (1994) Potentiation of 3,4-methylenedioxymethamphetamine-induced dopamine release and serotonin neurotoxicity by 5-HT2 receptor agonists. *Eur. J. Pharmacol.* **264**, 325–330.

100. Naranjo, C. (1967) Ayahuasca, caapi, yage. Psychotropic properties of the harmala alkaloids. *Psychopharmacol Bull.* **4**, 16–17.

101. McKenna, D. J., Towers, G. H., and Abbott, F. (1984) Monoamine oxidase inhibitors in South American hallucinogenic plants: tryptamine and beta-carboline constituents of ayahuasca. *J. Ethnopharmacol.* **10**, 195–223.

102. Ott, J. (1999) Pharmahuasca: human pharmacology of oral DMT plus harmine. *J. Psychoactive Drugs* **31**, 171–177.

103. Ask, A. L., Fagervall, I., and Ross, S. B. (1983) Selective inhibition of monoamine oxidase in monoaminergic neurons in the rat brain. *Naunyn Schmiedebergs Arch. Pharmacol.* **324**, 79–87.

104. Grella, B., Dukat, M., Young, R., Teitler, M., Herrick-Davis, K., Gauthier, C. B., and Glennon, R. A. (1998) Investigation of hallucinogenic and related beta-carbolines. *Drug Alcohol Depend.* **50**, 99–107.

105. Helsley, S., Fiorella, D., Rabin, R. A., and Winter, J. C. (1998a) A comparison of N,N-dimethyltryptamine, harmaline, and selected congeners in rats trained with LSD as a discriminative stimulus. *Prog. Neuropsychopharmacol. Biol. Psychiatry* **22**, 649–663.

106. Helsley, S., Fiorella, D., Rabin, R. A., and Winter, J. C. (1998b) Behavioral and biochemical evidence for a nonessential 5-HT2A component of the ibogaine-induced discriminative stimulus. *Pharmacol. Biochem. Behav.* **59**, 419–425.

107. Du, W., Aloyo, V. J., and Harvey, J. A. (1997) Harmaline competitively inhibits [3H]MK-801 binding to the NMDA receptor in rabbit brain. *Brain Res.* **770**, 26–29.

108. Bonson, K. R., Buckholtz, J. W., and Murphy, D. L. (1996) Chronic administration of serotonergic antidepressants attenuate the subjective effects of LSD in humans. *Neuropsychopharmacology* **14**, 425–436.

109. Wilcox, J. A. (1987) Abuse of fluoxetine by a patient with anorexia nervosa. *Am. J. Psychiatry* **144**, 1100.

110. Goldman, M. J., Grinspoon, L., and Hunter-Jones, S. (1990) Ritualistic use of fluoxetine by a former substance abuser. *Am. J. Psychiatry* **147**, 1377.

111. Pagliaro, L. A. and Pagliaro, A. M. (1993) Fluoxetine abuse by an intravenous drug user. *Am. J. Psychiatry* **150**, 1898.

112. Gross, R. (1994) Abuse of fluoxetine. *Mayo Clin. Proc.* **69**, 914.

113. Tinsley, J. A., Olsen, M. W., Laroche, R. R., and Palmen, M. A. (1994) Fluoxetine abuse. *Mayo Clin. Proc.* **69**, 166–168.

114. Schmidt, C. J. (1987) Neurotoxicity of the psychedelic amphetamine, methylenedioxymethamphetamine. *J. Pharmacol. Exp. Ther.* **240**, 1–7.

115. Liechti, M. E., Baumann, C., Gamma, A., Vollenweider, F. X. (2000) Acute psychological effects of 3,4-methylenedioxymethamphetamine (MDMA, "Ecstasy") are attenuated by the serotonin uptake inhibitor citalopram. *Neuropsychopharmacology* **22**, 513–552.

116. Bonson, KR and Murphy, DL. (1996) Alterations in responses to LSD in humans associated with chronic administration of tricyclic antidepressants, monoamine oxidase inhibitors or lithium. *Behav. Brain Res.* **73**, 229–233.

117. Hoyer D (1989) 5-Hydroxytryptamine receptors and effector coupling mechanisms in peripheral tissues, in *The Peripheral Actions of 5-Hydroxytryptamine* (Fozard, J. R., ed.), Oxford University Press, Oxford, pp. 72–99.

118. Lovenberg, T. W., Erlander, M. G., Baron, B. M., Racke, M., Slone, A. L., Siegel, B. W., et al. (1993a) Molecular cloning and functional expression of 5-HT1E-like rat and human 5-hydroxytryptamine receptor genes. *Proc. Natl. Acad. Sci. USA* **90**, 2184–2188.

119. Erlander, M. G., Lovenberg, T. W., Baron, B. M., de Lecea, L., Danielson, P. E., Racke, M., et al. (1993) Two members of a distinct subfamily of 5-hydroxytryptamine receptors differentially expressed in rat brain. *Proc. Natl. Acad. Sci. USA* **90**, 3452–3456.

120. Monsma, F. J., Jr., Shen, Y., Ward, R. P., Hamblin, M. W., and Sibley, D. R. (1993) Cloning and expression of a novel serotonin receptor with high affinity for tricyclic psychotropic drugs. *Mol. Pharmacol.* **43**, 320–327.

121. Lovenberg, T. W., Baron, B. M., de Lecea, L., Miller, J. D., Prosser, R. A., Rea, M. A., et al. (1993b) A novel adenylyl cyclase-activating serotonin receptor (5-HT7) implicated in the regulation of mammalian circadian rhythms. *Neuron* **11**, 449–458.

122. Watts, V. J., Lawler, C. P., Fox, D. R., Neve, K. A., Nichols, D. E., and Mailman, R. B. (1995) LSD and structural analogs: pharmacological evaluation at D1 dopamine receptors. *Psychopharmacology (Berl.)* **118**, 401–409.

123. Glennon, R. A. (1990) Do classical hallucinogens act as 5-HT2 agonists or antagonists? *Neuropsychopharmacology* **3**, 509–517.

124. Goodwin, G. M., Green, A. R., and Johnson, P. (1984) 5-HT2 receptor characteristics in frontal cortex and 5-HT2 receptor-mediated head-twitch behaviour following antidepressant treatment to mice. *Br. J. Pharmacol.* **83**, 235–242.

125. Maj, J. and Moryl, E. (1992) Effects of sertraline and citalopram given repeatedly on the responsiveness of 5-HT receptor subpopulations. *J. Neural Transm. Gen. Sect.* **88**, 143–156.

126. Fuller, R. W. (1994) Uptake inhibitors increase extracellular serotonin concentration measured by brain microdialysis. *Life Sci.* **55**, 163–167.

127. Murphy, D. L., Aulakh, C. S., Garrick, N. A., and Sunderland, T. (1987) Monoamine oxidase inhibitors as antidepressants, in *Psychopharmacology* (Meltzer, H. Y., ed.), Raven Press, New York, pp. 545–552.

128. Mousseau, D. D. and Greenshaw, A. J. (1989) Chronic effects of clomipramine and clorgyline on regional levels of brain amines and acid metabolites in rats. *J. Neural Transm.* **75**, 73–79.

129. Hrdina, P. D. (1987) Regulation of high- and low-affinity [3H]imipramine recognition sites in rat brain by chronic treatment with antidepressants. *Eur. J. Pharmacol.* **138**, 159–168.

130. Brenner, R. and Shopsin, B. (1980) The use of monoamine oxidase inhibitors in schizophrenia. *Biol. Psychiatry* **15**, 633–647.

131. de Montigny, C. and Aghajanian, G. K. (1978) Tricyclic antidepressants: long-term treatment increases responsivity of rat forebrain neurons to serotonin. *Science* **202**, 1303–1306.

132. Wang, R. Y. and Aghajanian, G. K. (1989) Enhanced sensitivity of amygdaloid neurons to serotonin and norepinephrine after chronic antidepressant administration. *Commun. Psychopharmacol.* **4**, 83–90.

133. Gershon, S., Holmberg, G., Mattsson, E., Mattsson, N., and Marshall, A. (1962) Imipramine hydrochloride. *Arch. Gen. Psychiatry* **6,** 96–101.

134. Hotta, I., Yamawaki, S., and Segawa, T. (1986) Long-term lithium treatment causes serotonin receptor down-regulation via serotonergic presynapses in rat brain. *Neuropsychobiology* **16,** 19–26.

135. Odagaki, Y., Koyama, T., Matsubara, S., Matsubara, R., and Yamashita, I. (1990) Effects of chronic lithium treatment on serotonin binding sites in rat brain. *J. Psychiatr. Res.* **24,** 271–277.

136. Bonson, K. R., Buckholtz, J. W., and Murphy, D. L. (1999) Antidepressant treatments differentially alter human subjective responses to MDMA, psilocybin and other psychedelics. Society for Neuroscience Abstract.

137. Smilkstein, M. J., Smolinske, S. C., and Rumack, B. H. (1987) A case of MAO inhibitor/MDMA interaction: agony after ecstasy. *J. Toxicol. Clin. Toxicol.* **25,** 149–159.

138. Ram, C. V. (1991) Management of hypertensive emergencies: changing therapeutic options. *Am. Heart J.* **122,** 356–363.

139. Varon, J. and Marik, P. E. (2000) The diagnosis and management of hypertensive crises. *Chest* **118,** 214–227.

140. Bolognesi, R., Tsialtas, D., Straneo, U., Conti, M., and Manca, C. (1990) Effects of i.v. nicardipine in the treatment of hypertensive crisis. *Minerva Cardioangiol.* **38,** 299–303.

141. Berge, T. I. (1999) Acceptance and side effects of nitrous oxide oxygen sedation for oral surgical procedures. *Acta Odontol. Scand.* **57,** 201–206.

142. Carstoniu, J., Levytam, S., Norman, P., Daley, D., Katz, J., and Sandler, A. N. (1994) Nitrous oxide in early labor. Safety and analgesic efficacy assessed by a double-blind, placebo-controlled study. *Anesthesiology* **80,** 30–35.

143. Marshall, B. E. and Longnecker, D. E. (1996) General anesthetics, in *The Pharmacological Basis of Therapeutics* (Hardman, J. G. and Limbird, L. E., eds), McGraw-Hill, New York, p. 319.

143a. James, W. (1998) Consciousness under nitrous oxide. *Psychol. Rev.* **5,** 194–196.

144. Quock, R. M. and Vaughn, L. K. (1995) Nitrous oxide: mechanism of its antinociceptive action. *Analgesia* **1,** 151–159.

145. Quock, R. M., Curtis, B. A., Reynolds, B J., and Quock, R. M. (1993) Dose-dependent antagonism and potentiation of nitrous oxide antinociception by naloxone in mice. *J. Pharmacol. Exp. Ther.* **267,** 117–122.

146. Berkowitz, B. A., Finck, A. D., Hynes, M. D., and Ngai, S. H. (1979) Tolerance to nitrous oxide analgesia in rats and mice. *Anesthesiology* **51,** 309–312.

147. Branda, E. M., Ramza, J. T., Cahill, F. J., Tseng, L. F., and Quock, R. M. (2000) Role of brain dynorphin in nitrous oxide antinociception in mice. *Pharmacol. Biochem. Behav.* **65,** 217–221.

148. Quock, R. M., Kouchich, F. J., and Tseng, L. F. (1985) Does nitrous oxide induce release of brain opioid peptides? *Pharmacology* **30,** 95–99.

149. Daras, C., Cantrill, R. C., and Gillman, M. A. (1983) [3H]Naloxone displacement: evidence for nitrous oxide as opioid receptor agonist. *Eur. J. Pharmacol.* **89,** 177–178.

150. Hara, S., Gagnon, M. J., Quock, R. M., and Shibuya, T. (1994) Effect of opioid peptide antisera on nitrous oxide antinociception in rats. *Pharmacol. Biochem. Behav.* **48,** 699–702.

151. Quock, R. M. and Mueller, J. (1991) Protection by U–50,488H against beta-chlornaltrexamine antagonism of nitrous oxide antinociception in mice. *Brain Res.* **549,** 162–164.

152. Hynes, M. D. and Hymson, D. L. (1984) Nitrous oxide generalizes to a discriminative stimulus produced by ethylketocyclazocine but not morphine. *Eur. J. Pharmacol.* **105,** 155–159.

153. Rupreht, J., Dworacek, B., Bonke, B., Dzoljic, M. R., van Eijndhoven, J. H., and de

Vlieger, M. (1985) Tolerance to nitrous oxide in volunteers. *Acta Anaesthesiol. Scand.* **29**, 635–638.

154. Emmanouil, D. E., Johnson, C. H. and Quock, R. M. (1994) Nitrous oxide anxiolytic effect in mice in the elevated plus maze: mediation by benzodiazepine receptors. *Psychopharmacology* **115**, 167–172.

155. Mennerick, S., Jevtovic-Todorovic, V., Todorovic, S. M., Shen, W., Olney, J. W., and Zorumski, C. F. (1998) Effect of nitrous oxide on excitatory and inhibitory synaptic transmission in hippocampal cultures. *J. Neurosci.* **18**, 9716–9726.

156. Caton, P. W., Tousman, S. A., and Quock, R. M. (1994) Involvement of nitric oxide in nitrous oxide anxiolysis in the elevated plus-maze. *Pharmacol. Biochem. Behav.* **48**, 689–692.

157. McDonald, C. E., Gagnon, M. J., Ellenberger, E. A., Hodges, B. L., Ream, J. K., Tousman, S. A., and Quock, R. M. (1994) Inhibitors of nitric oxide synthesis antagonize nitrous oxide antinociception in mice and rats. *J. Pharmacol. Exp. Ther.* **269**, 601–608.

158. Dzoljic, M., Rupreht, J., Erdmann, W., Stijnen, T. H., van Briemen, L. J., and Dzoljic, M. R. (1994) Behavioral and electrophysiological aspects of nitrous oxide dependence. *Brain Res. Bull.* **33**, 25–31.

159. Murray, M. J. and Murray, W. J. (1980) Nitrous oxide availability. *J. Clin. Pharmacol.* **20**, 202–205.

160. Rosenberg, H., Orkin, F. K., and Springstead, J. (1979) Abuse of nitrous oxide. *Anesth. Analg.* **58**, 104–106.

161. Spiegelman, W. G., Saunders, L., and Mazze, R. I. (1984) Addiction and anesthesiology. *Anesthesiology* **60**, 335–341.

162. Zacny, J. P., Coalson, D. W., Lichtor, J. L., Yajnik, S., and Thapar, P. (1994) Effects of naloxone on the subjective and psychomotor effects of nitrous oxide in humans. *Pharmacol. Biochem. Behav.* **49**, 573–578.

163. Tiplady, B., Sinclair, W. A., and Morrison, L. M. (1992) Effects of nitrous oxide on psychological performance. *Psychopharmacol. Bull.* **28**, 207–211.

164. Armstrong, P. J., Morton, C., Sinclair, W., and Tiplady, B. (1995) Effects of nitrous oxide on psychological performance. A dose-response study using inhalation of concentrations up to 15%. *Psychopharmacology* **117**, 486–490.

165. Mewaldt, S. P., Ghoneim, M. M., Choi, W. W., Korttila, K., and Peterson, R. C. (1988) Nitrous oxide and human state-dependent memory. *Pharmacol. Biochem. Behav.* **30**, 83–87.

166. Yajnik, S., Zacny, J. P., Young, C. J., Lichtor, J. L., Rupani, G., Klafta, J. M., Coalson, D. W., and Apfelbaum, J. L. (1996) Lack of acute tolerance development to the subjective, cognitive, and psychomotor effects of nitrous oxide in healthy volunteers. *Pharmacol. Biochem. Behav.* **54**, 501–508.

167. Rice, S. A., Mazze, R. I., and Baden, J. M. (1985) Effects of subchronic intermittent exposure to nitrous oxide in Swiss Webster mice. *J. Environ. Pathol. Toxicol. Oncol.* **6**, 271–281.

168. Jevtovic-Todorovic, V., Todorovic, S. M., Mennerick, S., Powell, S., Dikranian, K., Benshoff, N., et al. (1998) Nitrous oxide (laughing gas) is an NMDA antagonist, neuroprotectant and neurotoxin. *Nat. Med.* **4**, 460–463.

169. Paulson, G. W. (1979) "Recreational" misuse of nitrous oxide. *J. Am. Dent. Assoc.* **98**, 410–411.

170. Layzer, R. B., Fishman, R. A., and Schafer, J. A. (1978) Neuropathy following abuse of nitrous oxide. *Neurology* **28**, 504–506.

171. Brodsky JB, Cohen EN, Brown BW Jr, Wu ML, Whitcher CE. (1981) Exposure to nitrous oxide and neurologic disease among dental professionals. *Anesth Analg* **60**, 297–301

172. Gutmann, L., Farrell, B., Crosby, T. W., and Johnsen, D. (1979) Nitrous oxide-induced

myelopathy-neuropathy: potential for chronic misuse by dentists. *J. Am. Dent. Assoc.* **98,** 58–59.

173. Sweeney, B., Bingham, R. M., Amos, R. J., Petty, A. C., and Cole, P. V.(1985) Toxicity of bone marrow in dentists exposed to nitrous oxide. *Br. Med. J. (Clin. Res. Ed.)* **291,** 567–569.

174. Sahenk, Z., Mendell, J. R., Couri, D., and Nachtman, J. (1978) Polyneuropathy from inhalation of N_2O cartridges through a whipped-cream dispenser. *Neurology* **28,** 485–487.

175. Jastak, J. T. and Greenfield, W. Trace contamination of anesthetic gases: a brief review. *J. Am. Dent. Assoc.* **95,** 758–762.

176. Marsh, E. N. (1999) Coenzyme B12 (cobalamin)-dependent enzymes. *Essays Biochem.* **34,** 139–154.

177. Frasca, V., Riazzi, B. S., and Matthews, R. G. (1986) In vitro inactivation of methionine synthase by nitrous oxide. *J. Biol. Chem.* **261,** 15,823–15,826.

178. Rupreht, J., Erdmann, W., Dzoljic, M., and van Stolk, M. A. (1989) Nitrous oxide in anesthesia—present status of the use of nitrous oxide, risks for patients and personnel and treatment of side effects. *Anaesthesiol. Reanim.* **14,** 251–259.

179. Marie, R. M., Le Biez, E., Busson, P., Schaeffer, S., Boiteau, L., Dupuy, B., and Viader, F. (2000) Nitrous oxide anesthesia-associated myelopathy. *Arch. Neurol.* **57,** 380–382.

180. Ostreicher, D. S. (1994) Vitamin B12 supplements as protection against nitrous oxide inhalation. *NY State Dent. J.* **60,** 47–49.

181. Rowland, A. S., Baird, D. D., Shore, D. L., Weinberg, C. R., Savitz, D. A., and Wilcox, A. J. (1995) Nitrous oxide and spontaneous abortion in female dental assistants. *Am. J. Epidemiol.* **141,** 531–538.

182. Anderson, R. A., Bancroft, J., and Wu, F. C. (1992) The effects of exogenous testosterone on sexuality and mood of normal men. *J. Clin. Endocrinol. Metab.* **75,** 1503–1507.

183. Strauss, R. H. and Yesalis, C. E. (1991) Anaboic steroids in the athlete. *Ann. Rev. Med* **42,** 449–457.

184. Demling, R. H. and DeSanti, L. (1999) Involuntary weight loss and the nonhealing wound: the role of anabolic agents. *Adv. Wound Care* **12**(1 Suppl.), 1–14.

185. Zitzmann, M. and Nieschlag, E. (2000) Hormone substitution in male hypogonadism. *Mol. Cell Endocrinol.* **161,** 73–88.

186. Schlatterer, K., von Werder, K., and Stalla, G. K. (1996) Multistep treatment concept of transsexual patients. *Exp. Clin. Endocrinol. Diabetes* **104,** 413–419.

187. Beato, M. (1989) Gene regulation by steroid hormones. *Cell* **56,** 335–344.

188. Cicero, T. J., Schainker, B. A., and Meyer, E. R. (1979) Endogenous opioids participate in the regulation of the hypothalamus-pituitary-luteinizing hormone axis and testosterone's negative feedback control of luteinizing hormone. *Endocrinology* **104,** 1286–1291.

189. Takayama, H., Ogawa, N., Asanuma, M., and Ota, Z. (1990) Regional responses of rat brain opioid receptors upon castration and testosterone replacement. *Res. Commun. Chem. Pathol. Pharmacol.* **70,** 355–358.

190. Bonson, K. R. and Murphy, D. L. (1994) Evidence for a withdrawal syndrome resulting from chronic administration of anabolic steroids to Wistar and Fawn-Hooded rats. Society for Neuroscience Abstract, 503.23, **20,**1235.

191. Hickson, R. C. and Kurowski, T. G. Anabolic steroids and training. *Clin. Sports Med.* **5,** 461–469.

192. Fingerhood, M. I., Sullivan, J. T., Testa, M., and Jasinski, D. R. (1997) Abuse liability of testosterone. *J. Psychopharmacol.* **11,** 59–63.

193. de Beun, R., Jansen, E., Slangen, J. L., Van de Poll, N. E. (1992) Testosterone as appetitive and discriminative stimulus in rats: sex- and dose-dependent effects. *Physiol. Behav.* **52,** 629–634.

194. Kashkin, K. B. and Kleber, H. D. (1989) Hooked on hormones? An anabolic steroid addiction hypothesis. *JAMA* **262,** 3166–3170.

195. Johnston, R. (1990) *Monitoring the Future: a continuing study of the lifestyles and values of youth.* University of Michigan Institute for Social Research, Ann Arbor.

196. Tatro, D. S. (1985) Use of steroids by athletes. *Drug Newslett.* **4**, 33–34.

197. Malone, D. A., Jr. and Dimeff, R. J. (1992) The use of fluoxetine in depression associated with anabolic steroid withdrawal: a case series. *J. Clin. Psychiatry* **53**, 130–132.

198. Bonson, K. R. and Winter, J. C. (1992) Reversal of testosterone-induced dominance by the serotonergic agonist quipazine. *Pharmacol. Biochem. Behav.* **42**, 809–813.

199. Evans, N. A. (1997) Gym and tonic: a profile of 100 male steroid users. *Br. J. Sports Med.* **31**, 54–58.

200. Strauss, R. H., Liggett, M. T., and Lanese, R. R. (1985) Anabolic steroid use and perceived effects in ten weight-trained women athletes. *JAMA* **253**, 2871–2873.

201. Webb, O. L., Laskarzewski, P. M., and Glueck, C. J. (1984) Severe depression of high-density lipoprotein cholesterol levels in weight lifters and body builders by self-administered exogenous testosterone and anabolic-androgenic steroids. *Metabolism* **33**, 971–975.

202. Bagheri, S. A. and Boyer, J. L. (1974) Peliosis hepatis associated with androgenic-anabolic steroid therapy. A severe form of hepatic injury. *Ann. Intern. Med.* **81**, 610–618.

203. Kouri, E. M., Lukas, S. E., Pope, H. G., Jr,, and Oliva, P. S. (1995) Increased aggressive responding in male volunteers following the administration of gradually increasing doses of testosterone cypionate. *Drug Alcohol Depend.* **40**, 73–79.

204. Bonson, K. R., Johnson, R. G., Fiorella, D., Rabin, R. A., and Winter, J. C. (1994) Serotonergic control of androgen-induced dominance. *Pharmacol. Biochem. Behav.* **49**, 313–322.

205. Porcerelli, J. H. and Sandler, B. A. (1995) Narcissism and empathy in steroid users. *Am. J. Psychiatry* **152**, 1672–1674.

206. Pope, H. G., Jr., Katz, D. L. (1994) Psychiatric and medical effects of anabolic-androgenic steroid use. A controlled study of 160 athletes. *Arch. Gen. Psychiatry* **51**, 375–382.

207. Yates, W. R., Perry, P. J., MacIndoe, J., Holman, T., and Ellingrod, V. (1999) Psychosexual effects of three doses of testosterone cycling in normal men. *Biol. Psychiatry* **45**, 254–260.

208. Pope, H. G., Jr., Kouri, E. M., and Hudson, J. I. (2000) Effects of supraphysiologic doses of testosterone on mood and aggression in normal men: a randomized controlled trial. *Arch. Gen. Psychiatry* **57**, 133–140.

209. Tricker, R., Casaburi, R., Storer, T. W., Clevenger, B., Berman, N., Shirazi, A., and Bhasin, S. (1996) The effects of supraphysiological doses of testosterone on angry behavior in healthy eugonadal men—a clinical research center study. *J. Clin. Endocrinol. Metab.* **81**, 3754–3758.

210. Pope, H. G., Jr. and Katz, D. L. (1988) Affective and psychotic symptoms associated with anabolic steroid use. *Am. J. Psychiatry* **145**, 487–490.

10

Mechanisms of Methamphetamine-Induced Neurotoxicity

Jean Lud Cadet and Christie Brannock

1. BRIEF OVERVIEW OF METHAMPHETAMINE USE

Methamphetamine (METH) was first synthesized in Japan in 1919 and then used medically in Germany in the 1930s (1). After its introduction into the medical community, METH has been used as an appetite suppressant and as an energy booster, as well as in the treatment of narcolepsy (2).

During World War II, METH was used by soldiers and factory workers in the warring countries because of its stimulant properties. After the war ended, a surplus of METH was legally released into the world market. An epidemic emerged, peaking in Japan in 1954 and peaking in the United States in 1965 (3,4).

METH is a long-lasting stimulant that affects the central nervous system (CNS). METH has become increasingly more popular because of its low production costs and its longer-lasting euphoric effects when compared with cocaine, often lasting between 8 and 24 h. METH has many names (Chalk, Crank, Crystal, Ice, Speed, Splash, Methedrine) and can be taken via many routes (i.e., smoke, snort, ingest, intravenous [IV]) (5,6).

While the administration of METH in humans is accompanied by acute experiences of euphoria, increased energy, and increased confidence, the long-term use of the drug is associated with psychotic symptoms as well as withdrawal-induced depression to the point of suicide. In animals, the acute administration of METH is associated with increased release of dopamine (DA) in the striatum and nucleus accumbens. The repeated use of and the use of large dosages of the drug can cause marked depletion of DA, serotonin (5-HT), and their metabolites (7–10).

2. MOLECULAR AND CELLULAR PATHWAYS OF METH-INDUCED TOXICITY

2.1. Toxic Effects of Methamphetamine

As noted earlier, METH can cause neurotoxic damage to monoaminergic systems of rats, mice, and nonhuman primates. Several markers of DA and 5-HT terminals are severely affected by these drugs. These include neostriatal DA levels, striatal tyrosine hydroxylase activity, and DA uptake sites *(8–14)*. A number of studies have indicated that the toxicity of the amphetamine analogs might be dependent on DA levels *(8–11)*, on intact DA and 5-HT uptake sites *(15)*, and on the activation of DA receptors *(16)*, as well as on the stimulation of glutamate receptors *(17)*. Moreover, a number of investigators have hinted to a role for oxygen-based free radicals in the actions of this drug. Specifically, administration of antioxidants, such as ascorbic acid or vitamin E, can attenuate, whereas inhibition of superoxide dismutase (SOD) by diethyldithiocarbamate can increase METH-induced toxicity *(18)*.

2.2. The Role of Reactive Species in METH-Induced Toxicity

In order to test the involvement of superoxide radicals in the neurotoxic effects of METH, we used transgenic (Tg) mice that express the human CuZnSOD gene *(7,19)*. These mice have much higher CuZnSOD activity than wild-type animals from similar backgrounds with homozygous SOD-Tg mice, having a mean increase of about 5.7-fold and heterozygous SOD-Tg mice having a mean increase of about 2.5-fold in comparison to wild-type mice. Hirata et al. *(7)* showed that a low dose of METH (2.5 mg/kg) which caused a 48% decrease of DA uptake sites in the striata of male nontransgenic (NonTg) mice, caused only 7% and 2% decreases in heterozygous and homozygous SOD-Tg mice, respectively. Higher doses of METH caused greater magnitude of losses in striatal DA uptake site; these decreases were significantly attenuated in SOD-Tg mice *(7)*. Similar observations were obtained for the serotonin system *(20)*.

These results suggest that superoxide radicals are, indeed, involved in the causation of METH-induced DA-terminal damage. This increase in the production of superoxide radicals could occur subsequent to the oxidation of the massive amount of DA released in the brain after METH *(21,22)*. Further redox-cycling of dopaquinone formed during DA catabolism would also enhance the concentration of oxygen-based radicals within DA terminals. These series of events could then cause the demise of DA terminals through membrane destabilization or through changes in calcium homeostasis.

In order to further test the role of oxidative stress in the toxic effects of METH, we made use of the pineal hormone, melatonin, which has been shown to have neuroprotective effects against toxic quinones and monoamine-induced oxidative stress *(23)*. Four dosages (5, 20, 40, 80 mg/kg) of melatonin were administered to mice intraperitoneally 30 min prior to the injections of METH (4 × 5 mg/kg) given at 2-h intervals. Mice were sacrificed 2 wk later and the status of DA and 5-HT terminals were investigated by using receptor autoradiographic techniques. The lowest doses of melatonin (5 mg/kg) had no significant effects against METH-induced toxicity. However, higher doses (40 or 80 mg/kg) of melatonin significantly attenuated METH-induced toxic effects on both dopamine and serotonin systems. These data provide further evidence for a possible role of oxidative stress in METH-induced toxicity. Itzhak et al. *(24)* have also reported that melatonin can attenuate the toxic effects of METH on striatal dopaminergic systems.

If METH were causing its toxic effects through the production of free radicals, it would be highly likely that the administration of toxic doses of the agent could alter the brain antioxidant defense systems. In addition, because METH-induced toxicity is known to be attenuated in copper/zinc-SOD transgenic (Cu/Zn-SOD-Tg) mice, we sought to determine if METH had differential effects on antioxidant enzymes on these mice in comparison to non-Tg mice *(25)*. Our results substantiated these predictions. Specifically, the administration of METH caused a significant decrease in Cu/Zn-SOD activity in the cortical region without altering enzyme activity in the striata of non-Tg mice. CuZn SOD activity was not affected in the brains of heterozygous SOD-Tg mice, whereas there was a small increase in the striata of homozygous SOD-Tg mice. In addition, METH caused decreases in catalase (CAT) activity in the striatum of non-Tg mice and significant increase in the cortex of homozygous SOD-Tg mice. METH also induced decreases in glutathione peroxidase (GSH-Px) in both cortical and striatal regions of non-Tg mice and in the striatum of heterozygous SOD-Tg mice, whereas this enzyme was not affected in the homozygous SOD-Tg mice. More interestingly, lipid peroxidation was markedly increased in both cortices and striata of non-Tg and heterozygous SOD-Tg mice, but not in the homozygous SOD-Tg. Glutathione levels were also reported to be decreased by repeated administration of this drug *(26)*.

When taken together, the accumulated data suggest that the toxic effects of METH involve not only superoxide radicals but also a cascade that also includes hydrogen peroxide and hydroxyl radicals. In vitro studies in this laboratory have now documented the production of both superoxide radicals and hydrogen peroxide during exposure of cells to METH. Observations from other laboratories have recently provided ample evidence that superoxide radicals and hydroxyl radicals are also involved in METH-induced toxicity *(25,27)*.

In addition for the role of reactive oxygen species (ROS), a number of investigators had documented a role for the glutamatergic system in METH-induced neurotoxicity *(17)*. Recent lines of evidence have also suggested that excitotoxic damage might occur through the production of nitric oxide (NO) via the action of nitric oxide synthase (NOS) *(28)*. Some investigators have provided supporting evidence for an interaction of the oxygen-based pathways and the NO-based pathways in the causation of degenerative changes in the brain *(29,30)*. If this were true in the case of METH, this might explain the demonstration that CuZnSOD transgenic mice *(7,19)* as well as animals treated with glutamate antagonists *(17,31,32)* are protected against the toxic effects of the drug. We thus decided to test the idea that NO production might be linked to METH-induced neurotoxic effects by using an in vitro model of fetal mesencephalic cultures.

In this culture system, METH was found to cause dose-dependent increases in toxicity over a 24-h period. Specifically, 1.5 mM of METH caused about 50% cell loss, whereas 3.5 mM of METH caused an almost complete disappearance of neurons in the cultures. Both nitro-arginine and monomethyl-L-arginine, which block the synthesis of NO, were able to attenuate METH-induced death of mesencephalic neurons *(33)*. These ideas have also been tested in vivo by other investigators. Specifically, Ali et al. *(34)* had reported that 7-nitroindazole, which is a blocker of NO synthetase, can protect against the toxic effects of METH while Itzhak et al. *(24)* had used NOS knockout mice to show similar findings.

These results indicate that blocking of NO formation can result in attenuation of the toxic effects of this illicit agent. The present data are also consistent with those of others that have shown that NO is toxic to a number of cell types in vitro. In any case, when taken together with the data obtained using the CuZnSOD-Tg mice *(7,19)*, these in vitro data provide possible evidence for interactions of NO and O_2^- for the causation of METH-induced damage in mammalian brains.

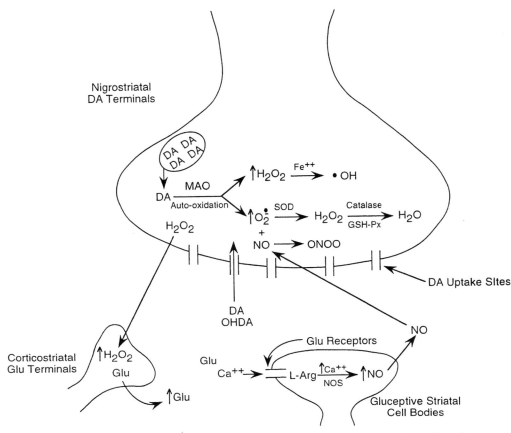

Fig. 1. Interactions of catecholamines and glutamate in nigrotriatal dopaminergic system degeneration.

2.3. METH-Induced Toxicity Involves Activation of Poly (ADP-Ribose) Polymerase (PARP)

The production of ROS is known to be associated with DNA damage. Consequent to this damage, there is activation of the enzyme poly (ADP-ribose) polymerase (PARP) that activates a series of events that cause depletion of cellular energy stores and subsequent cell death. NO is thought to cause its damage in a similar way. Recent observations from our lab suggest that the deleterious effects of METH also involve activation of PARS because benzamide, nicotinamide, 3-aminobenzamide, and theophylline, which all block the activity of the enzyme, also block METH-induced cell death. It is interesting to note that benzamide also prevents METH-induced gliosis in vitro. Recent in vivo data have also shown that pre-treatment of rodents with the PARP inhibitor, benzamide, can also protect the animals against the toxic effects of METH *(35)*.

Another aspect of METH-induced neurotoxicity is that it is associated with extensive gliosis in the rodent brain *(8)*. Using the in vitro model of cultures of fetal mesencephalic cells, we also showed that exposure to METH causes a hyperplastic response in glial fibrillary acidic protein (GFAP)-positive cells *(36)*. The GFAP cells became enlarged and put out large processes, thus suggesting that METH can cause reactive

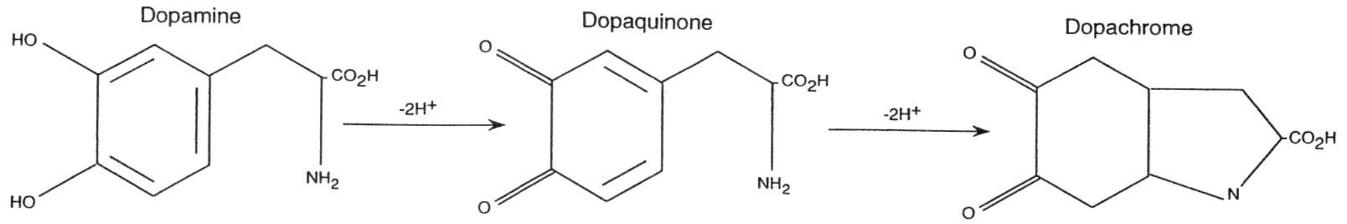

Fig. 2. Formation of quinone from dopamine. Dopamine can also undergo redox-cycling with generation of free radicals.

gliosis in vitro. However, in the same cultures, TH-immunopositive cells were exquisitely sensitive to the toxic effects of the drug. Both the toxic effects on TH+ cells and the hyperplastic response of the GFAP+ cells were blocked by the PARP inhibitor, benzamide *(36)*.

In summary, these studies show that superoxide radicals, hydrogen peroxide hydroxyl radicals, and NO play an integral part in METH-induced toxicity. This toxic cascade also appears to involve PARP activation. Figures 1 and 2 provide a working model for METH-induced toxicity for the studies summarized earlier.

2.4. Involvement of Cell Death-Related Genes in the Toxic Effects of Methamphetamine

As reported earlier, the accumulated evidence implicates free radicals in METH-associated neurodegeneration. These include superoxides, hydroxyl radicals, and NO. Degenerative processes in the CNS are thought to occur through either necrosis or apoptosis. Necrosis often follows severe insults and results in early membrane damage, cellular swelling, spilling of intracellular contents, and inflammatory responses in the penumbra of the damage. Apoptosis, on the other hand, is usually caused by mild to moderate toxic injuries, participates in the normal process of tissue regulation, and results in cell shrinkage, vacuolar formation, but no inflammatory changes in surrounding cells. Both apoptosis and necrosis can be caused by the same agents depending on the doses used to cause the damage. Several manipulations have been shown to abrogate the apoptotic process. Among the most interesting of these manipulations is the use of bcl$_2$. Bcl$_2$ is a proto-oncogene that was first identified at the chromosomal breakpoint t(14;18) in B-cell lymphomas. Subsequent studies have revealed that bcl$_2$ could promote cell survival, block apoptosis, and prevent cellular damage caused by oxidative stress. It was thus of interest to determine if bcl$_2$ could protect against toxic damage caused by METH in view of our previous suggestions that superoxide radicals are involved in the toxic manifestations of the drug.

Our studies also show that METH caused dose-dependent loss of cellular viability in immortalized neural cells while bcl$_2$-expressing neural cells were protected against these deleterious effects *(37)*. Using flow cytometry, immunofluorescent staining, and DNA electrophoresis, we also showed that METH exposure can cause DNA strand breaks, chromatin condensation, nuclear fragmentation, and DNA laddering. All these changes were prevented by bcl$_2$ expression. These data implicate apoptosis as one of the molecular mechanisms involved in the deleterious effects of amphetamine analogs. It is to be pointed out that the majority of the studies conducted in the effects of METH have concentrated on its effects on DA and 5-HT terminals. This is most likely due to the ease with which the effects of the drug can be determined by the measurements of monoamine levels or of DA transporter binding *(19,24,34)*. Our in vitro studies with the immortalized cells raise the possibility that METH might have other effects that need to be more thoroughly investigated. This idea is supported by the recent report that METH can cause significant cortical cell-body damage *(38)*. Our recent findings that METH can cause decreases in striatal DA D_1 binding sites also suggest that the drug might have toxic effects on striatal cell bodies that express these receptors *(39)*.

Cell death can occur by the activation of a number of cell death-related genes. One such gene is the tumor suppressor p53. Mutations in the p53 gene have been identified in both inherited and sporadic forms of cancer. This discovery has galvanized research on the mode of action of the p53 protein. For example, the wild-type p53 protein is involved in both apoptosis and cell-cycle arrest after toxic insults. Exposure of cells to gamma irradiation or etoposide causes DNA damage that is associated with accumulation of p53. This accumulation stimulates increases in Waf1/Cip1 (p21), an inhibitor of Cdk, which can induce cell-cycle arrest. Depending on the extent of DNA damage, p53 activation can cause apoptosis instead of cell cycle arrest. Although the involvement of p53 in cell death has been assessed mostly through in vitro experiments, we reasoned that this process might also be involved in the causation of METH-induced neurotoxicity and apoptosis. We postulated that if p53 protein is an important determinant of METH-induced neurotoxicity, animals lacking the gene for p53 protein should show protection against the toxic effects of the drug. Our results support this prediction and demonstrate that the p53 knockout phenotype does, in fact, attenuate the neurotoxic effects of METH on striatal dopaminergic terminals *(39)*.

P53-knockout mice provide a useful model to test the role of p53 in the neurotoxic effects of drugs in vivo. To test the involvement of p53 in METH-induced toxicity, wild-type mice, as well as heterozygous and homozygous p53-knockout male mice, were administered four injections of three different doses (2.5, 5.0, and 10.0 mg/kg) of the drug given at 2-h intervals within the space of 1 d. METH caused a marked dose-dependent loss of dopamine transporters in both the striatum and the nucleus accumbens of wild-type mice killed 2 wk after drug administration. However, this METH-induced decrease in dopamine transporters was attenuated in both homozygous and heterozygous p53-knockout mice with homozygous animals showing significantly greater protection. Moreover, METH treatment caused significant decreases in dopamine transporter mRNA and the number of tyrosine hydroxylase-positive cells in the substantia nigra pars compacta and the ventral tegmental area of wild-type mice, but not of homozygous p53-knockout mice killed 2 wk after cessation of METH administration. Further evidence for the involvement of p53 was provided by immunohistochemical experiments demonstrating an increase in p53-like immunoreactivity in the brains of METH-treated wild-type mice. We have also recently shown that p53 mRNA is increased by METH-treatment (unpublished results). These results provide concordant evidence for a role of the tumor suppressor, p53, in the long-term deleterious effects of drugs acting on the brain dopamine system.

3. CONCLUDING REMARKS

Finally, the data summarized previously have provided substantial evidence for a role of reactive species (O_2^-, H_2O_2, $^\cdot OH$, and NO) in the neurotoxicity caused by METH.

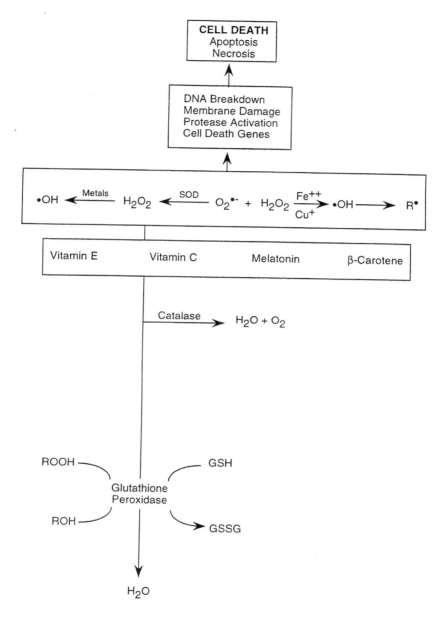

Fig. 3. Mammalian antioxidant defenses in the brain.

In addition, these studies have also implicated the involvement of cell-death related genes in the process of neurodegeneration that occur through apoptosis, since bcl_2 overexpression and a lack of p53 can protect against these toxic manifestations of METH usage. These studies, thus, suggest that p53-mediated downstream events as well as those associated with the process of apoptosis might be activated during METH abuse (*see* Fig. 3 for a working model). Our future plans are thus to continue to dissect these pathways further.

REFERENCES

1. Ogata, A. (1919) Preparation by reducing the condensation product of benzyl methyl ketone and methylamine. *J. Pharm. Soc. Japn.* **451,** 751.
2. Lynch, J. and House, M. (1992) Cardiovascular effects of methamphetamine. *J. Cardiovasc. Nurs.* **6(2),** 12–18.
3. Greberman, S. B. and Wada, K. (1994) Social and legal factors related to drug abuse in the United States and Japan. *Pub. Health Rep.* **109(6),** 731–737.
4. Cox, C. and Smart, R. (1972) Social and psychological aspects of speed use. A study of types of speed users in Toronto. *J. Addict.* **7(2),** 201–217.
5. Derlet, R. W. and Heischober, B. (1990) Methamphetamine. Stimulant of the 1990s? *West J. Med.* **153,** 625–628.
6. Beebe, D. and Walley, E. (1995) Smokable methamphetamine ('ice'): an old drug in a different form. *Am. Family Phys.* **51(2),** 449–453.
7. Hirata, H. H., Ladenheim, B., Carlson, E., Epstein, C., and Cadet, J. L. (1996) Autoradiographic evidence for methamphetamine-induced striatal dopaminergic loss in mouse brain: attenuation in CuZn-superoxide dismutase transgenic mice. *Brain Res.* **714,** 95–103.
8. O'Callaghan, J. P. and Miller, D. E. (1994) Neurotoxicity profiles of substituted amphetamines in the C57BL/6J mouse. *J. Pharmacol. Exp. Ther.* **270,** 741–751.
9. Ricaurte, G. A., Schuster, C. R., and Seiden, L. S. (1980) Long-term effects of repeated methylamphetamine administration on dopamine and serotonin neurons in the rat brain: a regional study. *Brain Res.* **193,** 153–163.
10. Wagner, G. C., Ricaurte, G. A., Seiden, L. S., Schuster, C. R., Miller, R. J., and Westley, J. (1980) Long-lasting depletions of striatal dopamine and loss of dopamine uptake sites following repeated administration of methamphetamine. *Brain Res.* **181,** 151–160.
11. Cadet, J. L., Sheng, P., Ali, S., Rothman, R., Carlson, E., and Epstein, C. (1994) *J. Neurochem.* **62,** 380–383.
12. Hotchkiss, A. J. and Gibb, J. W. (1980) Long-term effects of multiple doses of methamphetamine on tryptophan hydroxylase and tyrosine hydroxylase activity in rat brain. *J. Pharmacol. Exp. Ther.* **214,** 257–262.
13. Nakayama M., Loyama T. and Yamashita I. (1992) Long-lasting decrease in dopamine uptake sites following repeated administration of methamphetamine in the rat striatum. *Brain Res.* **601,** 209–212.
14. Steranka, L. R. and Sanders-Bush, E. (1980) Long-term effects of continuous exposure to amphetamine on brain dopamine concentration and synaptosomal uptake in mice. *Eur. J. Pharmacol.* **65,** 439–443.
15. Fumagalli, F., Gainetdinov, R. R., Valenzano, K. J., and Caron, M. G. (1998) Role of dopamine transporter in methamphetamine-induced neurotoxicity: evidence from mice lacking the transporter. *J. Neurosci.* **18(13),** 4861–4869.
16. Sonsalla, P. K., Gibb, J. W., and Hanson, G. R. (1986) Roles of D1 and D2 dopamine receptor subtypes in mediating the methamphetamine-induced changes in monoamine systems. *J. Pharmacol. Exp. Ther.* **238(3),** 932–937.
17. Weihmuller, F. B., O'Dell, S. J., and Marshall, J. F. (1992) MK–801 protection against methamphetamine-induced striatal dopamine terminal injury is associated with attenuated dopamine overflow. *Synapse* **11,** 155–163.
18. DeVito, M. J. and Wagner, G. C. (1989) Methamphetamine-induced neuronal damage: a possible role for free radicals. *Neuropharmacology* **28,** 1145–1150.
19. Cadet, J. L., Ali, S., and Epstein, C. (1994) Involvement of oxygen-based radicals in methamphetamine-induced neurotoxicity: evidence from the use of CuZnSOD transgenic mice. *Ann. NY Acad. Sci.* **17(738),** 388–391.

20. Hirata, H., Ladenheim, B., Rothman, R. B., Epstein, C., and Cadet, J. L. (1995) Metham-phetamine-induced serotonin neurotoxicity is mediated by superoxide radicals. *Brain Res.* **677(2)**, 345–347.

21. Baldwin, H. A., Colado, M. I., Murry, T. K, De Souza, R. J., and Green, A. R. (1993) Striatal dopamine release in vivo following neurotoxic doses of methamphetamine and effect of the neuroprotective drugs, chlormethiazole and dizocilpine. *Br. J. Pharmacol.* **108**, 590–596.

22. Marshall, J. F., O'Dell, S. J., and Weihmuller, F. B. (1993) Dopamine-glutamate interac-tions in methamphetamine-induced neurotoxicity. *J. Neural. Transm.* **91**, 241–254.

23. Hirata, H., Asanuma, M., and Cadet, J. L. (1998) Melatonin attenuates methamphetamine-induced toxic effects on dopamine and serotonin terminals in mouse brain. *Synapse* **30(2)**, 150–155.

24. ltzhak, Y., Gandia, C., Huang, P. L., and Ali, S. F. (1998) Resistance of neuronal nitric oxide synthase-deficient mice to methamphetamine-induced dopaminergic neurotoxicity. *J. Pharmacol. Exp. Ther.* **284(3)**, 1040–1047.

25. Jayanthi, S., Ladenheim, B., and Cadet, J. L. (1998) Methamphetamine-induced changes in antioxidant enzymes and lipid peroxidation in copper/zinc-superoxide dismutase transgenic mice *Ann. NY Acad. Sci.* **844**, 92–102.

26. Moszczynska, A., Turenne, S., and Kish, S. J. (1998) Rat striatal levels of the antioxidant glutathione are decreased following binge administration of methamphetamine. *Neurosci. Lett.* **255(1)**, 49–52.

27. Yokoyama, H., Tsuchihashi, N., Kasai, N., Matsue, T., Uchida, I., Mori, N., et al. (1997) Hydrogen peroxide augmentation in a rat striatum after methamphetamine injection as monitored in vivo by a Pt-disk microelectrode. *Biosens. Bioelectron.* **12(9–10)**, 1037–1041.

28. Dawson, V. L., Dawson, T. M., Bartley, D. A., Uhl, G. R., and Snyder, S. M. (1993) Mechanisms of nitric oxide-mediated neurotoxicity in primary brain cultures. *Neuroscience* **13**, 2651–2661.

29. Beckman, J. S. (1991) The double-edged role of nitric oxide in brain function and superox-ide-mediated injury. *J. Dev. Physiol.* **15**, 53–59.

30. Radi, R., Beckman, J. S., Bush, K. M., and Freeman, B. A. (1991) Peroxynitrite oxidation of sulfhydryls. The cytotoxic potential of superoxide and nitric oxide. *J. Biol. Chem.* **266**, 4244–4250.

31. Sonsalla, P. K., Nicklas, W. J., and Heikkila, R. E. (1989) Role for excitatory amino acids in methamphetamine-induced nigrostriatal dopaminergic toxicity. *Science* **243**, 398–400.

32. Sonsalla, P. K., Riordan, D. E., and Heikkila, R. E. (1991) Competitive and noncompeti-tive antagonists at N-methyl-D-aspartate receptors protect against methamphetamine-in-duced dopaminergic damage in mice. *J. Pharmacol. Exp. Ther.* **256**, 506–512.

33. Sheng, P., Cerruti, C., Ali, S., and Cadet, J. L. (1996) Nitric oxide is a mediator of metham-phetamine (METH)-induced neurotoxicity. In vitro evidence from primary cultures of mesencephalic cells. *Ann. NY Acad. Sci.* **801**, 174–186.

34. Ali, S. F. and Itzhak, Y. (1998) Effects of 7-nitroindazole, an NOS inhibitor on metham-phetamine-induced dopaminergic and serotonergic neurotoxicity in mice. *Ann. NY Acad. Sci.* **844**, 122–130.

35. Cosi, C., Chopin, P., and Marien, M. (1996) Benzamide, an inhibitor of poly(ADP-ribose) polymerase, attenuates methamphetamine-induced dopamine neurotoxicity in the C57B1/6N mouse. *Brain Res.* **735(2)**, 343–348.

36. Cerruti, C., Sheng, P., Ladenheim, B., Epstein, C. J., and Cadet, J. L. (1995) Involvement of oxidative and L-arginine-NO pathways in the neurotoxicity of drugs of abuse in vitro. *Clin. Exp. Pharmacol. Physiol.* **22(5)**, 381–382.

37. Cadet, J. L., Ordonez, S. V., and Ordonez, J. V. (1997) Methamphetamine induces apoptosis in immortalized neural cells: protection by the proto-oncogene, bcl–2. *Synapse* **25(2)**, 176–184.

38. Eisch, A. J. and Marshall, J. F. (1998) Methamphetamine neurotoxicity: dissociation of striatal dopamine terminal damage from parietal cortical cell body injury. *Synapse* **30(4),** 433–445.

39. Cadet, J. L., Ladenheim, B., and Hirata, H. (1998) Effects of toxic doses of methamphetamine (METH) on dopamine D1 receptors in the mouse brain. *Brain Res.* **786(1–2),** 240–242.

40. Hirata, H. and Cadet, J. L. (1997) Methamphetamine-induced serotonin neurotoxicity is attenuated in p53-knockout mice. *Brain Res.* **768(1–2),** 345–348.

11

Neurotoxic Effects of Substituted Amphetamines in Rats and Mice

Challenges to the Current Dogma

James P. O'Callaghan and Diane B. Miller

1. INTRODUCTION

Whether you read about it in the popular press or in the scientific literature, there is no lack of coverage of the issue of amphetamine-induced neurotoxicity. Included among these articles are reports on the adverse effects in both animals and humans of methamphetamine *(1–3)* and methylenedioxymethamphetamine (MDMA; "Ecstasy") *(4–7)*. Until it was withdrawn from the market for the potential to affect heart valvular function, the anorectic agent dexfenfluramine drew attention in the experimental and clinical literature for reported neurotoxic effects, even at the prescribed anorectic dosage *(8)*. Lastly and most recently, attention has been focused on the fact that a large percentage of school-age children are maintained on stimulants, including amphetamines, for the treatment of attention deficit/hyperactivity disorder (ADHD) *(9)*. The potential for neurotoxic effects associated with such long-term human exposures is just now being raised *(10)*. Clearly, the term "neurotoxicity" has been very broadly applied to describe the effects of these drugs in both humans and experimental animals. Unfortunately, emphasis has been placed on documenting effects of these agents without distinguishing how and why these effects should be considered "neurotoxic." Thus, there are many descriptions of drug-induced neurotoxicity but there are very few attempts to link these purported neurotoxic effects to pathological actions on the nervous system or to functional changes meaningful to the human condition. Here, we will briefly review the current status of our understanding of the neurotoxic effects of substituted amphetamines. Emphasis will be placed on defining the neurotoxic condition beyond effects attributable to the neuropharmacological actions of a specific compound. In so doing, we will challenge current dogma with regard to describing neurotoxic effects of this class of drugs. A detailed and comprehensive review of methamphetamine and amphetamine neurotoxicity recently has appeared *(2)* and it should be considered the authoritative source on this topic, especially with reference to effects in rats and the modulating role of body temperature. We will cover some of the

From: Handbook of Neurotoxicology, Vol. 2
Edited by: E. J. Massaro © Humana Press Inc., Totowa, NJ

issues raised by Bowyer and Holson *(2)*, and agree with all of their points, but we will discuss effects of amphetamines in the context of the toxic actions of many known and potential chemical neurotoxicants *(11)*.

2. CURRENT DOGMA

2.1. Amphetamines Cause Dopamine and Serotonin Neurotoxicity

Amphetamines, taken here to include amphetamine (AMP), methamphetamine (METH), methylenedioxyamphetamine (MDA), methylenedioxymethamphetamine (MDMA) and fenfluramine/dexfenfluramine (FEN), are known to result in protracted decrements in the levels of the neurotransmitters dopamine and/or serotonin *(1,2,12– 14)*. The degree to which one transmitter is affected more than the other is species dependent *(see* below). In general, AMP and METH are regarded as preferentially affecting dopamine whereas the other amphetamines affect serotonin. High-dose exposure regimens with any of these compounds also decreases the activity and/or levels of the respective biosynthetic enzymes, tryptophan hydroxylase (TPH) *(15,16)* and tyrosine hydroxylase (TH) *(15,17)* as well as the dopamine *(18)* and serotonin transporters *(17,19)*. Continued presence of the drug is not required to maintain a protracted decrease in these markers of serotonergic and dopaminergic nerve terminals. Loss of these markers occurs in the nerve-terminal fields/plexus with sparing of the same markers in the neuronal perikarya. Retrograde transport and classic Nissl or H & E stains also reveal preservation of neuronal cell bodies *(1,20,21)*. Together, these data, whether from biochemical or morphological assessments, have been taken as evidence for dopaminergic or serotonergic neurotoxicity of the respective substituted amphetamines. As a result, the terms "dopamine neurotoxicity" and "serotonin neurotoxicity" have crept into the literature on substituted amphetamines and are used to describe the purported axonal pathology induced by the compound in question (e.g., *see* ref. *8)*. Until recently, little consideration has been given to the possibility that decrements in serotonin and dopamine nerve-terminal markers may reflect a downregulation of components of the specific transmitter system in question rather than loss of the nerve terminals or axons *(1,2,14,22)*. In other words, the possibility exists that decreases in these "axonal markers" may not be indicative of nerve terminal or axonal loss.

2.2. Neurotoxicity Profiles for Amphetamines Are Shared Across Species

Historically, the rat has been the model of choice for demonstrating the effects of amphetamines on dopaminergic or serotonergic neurons. In large measure, the effects of various dosing regimens in rats have been shown to be extended to a number of nonhuman primate models; moreover, data from postmortem tissue of chronic users of METH *(3)* and MDMA *(6)* confirms effects in rats and monkeys *(23)*. Thus, by extension, it is not surprising that most of the effects observed in rat and monkey have been presumed to occur in humans *(8)*. With the advent of transgenic models, mice have come into play in studies of substituted amphetamine neurotoxicity. Their historical absence from this area of research likely is a reflection of the lack of a behavioral database for effects of amphetamines, such as exists for the rat. While the effects of most substituted amphetamines in the mouse appear "rat-like," some compounds appear to have transmitter-related effects distinct from those seen in the rat (e.g., *1*; also *see* below). Rat vs mouse differences (not counting differences attributable to different strains) are not uncommon in monoaminergic neurotoxicity studies. One needs only to consider the fact that the meperidine analog, 1-methy-4-phenyl-1,2,3,6-tetra-hydropyridine (MPTP), was found to be toxic to dopaminergic neurons of humans and several strains of mice but was devoid of such effects in the rat *(24–27)*.

2.3. Temperature Plays Some Role in Amphetamine Neurotoxicity

As early as the 1940s, body temperature has been known to be a factor in AMP and METH-induced lethality in humans as well as experimental animals *(2,14,28–30)*. Only recently however, has the role of this "nuisance" variable been appreciated as a major determinant of the effects of amphetamines on the nervous system *(2,14,31–36)*. It is now generally accepted that hyperthermia is required for the transmitter depleting and neurodegenerative effects of METH in the rat. Conversely, any means used to lower core temperature (during the period of amphetamine dosing) is protective against the transmitter-depleting actions of amphetamines *(2,14,31,33,36–38)*. Bowyer and colleagues *(2)* are responsible for the seminal findings surrounding this "new" awareness of the role of temperature in amphetamine "neurotoxicity." Most of the key findings that link temperature to the effects of amphetamines in the rat are documented in Bowyer and Holson *(2)*. The role of temperature in the effects of amphetamines in the mouse is similar to what has been reported for the rat (and humans), but differs in a few important respects that are documented below. Among the many key experimental findings of Bowyer and colleagues *(2)*, two stand out: First, altered pharmacokinetics is not the explanation for the role of temperature in the actions of amphetamines; rats administered dosages that would be lethal at room temperature are without effect at lowered ambient temperature but result in higher brain levels of drug than seen at room temperature *(2,22)*. Thus, increased brain levels of amphetamines have no effect when dosages are administered at lower than ambient temperature. A second key observation of Bowyer and co-workers is that a wide variety of neuropharmacological agents result in lowered core temperatures when co-administered with METH *(2)*. Thus, the apparent "neuroprotective" effects of these agents against the "neurotoxic" effects of amphetamines likely can be attributed to lowered body temperature rather than any specific mechanism ascribed to the drug in question (e.g., "excitotoxicity, *see* refs. *14,39*). Supporting this notion are data showing that these compounds do not protect against the effects of amphetamines when ambient temperature is raised and hyperthermia occurs *(14,40)*. Although painful to consider, what these data suggest is that the results of all "mechanistic" studies of amphetamine neuropharmacology or neurotoxicity are compromised unless temperature can be ruled out as a contributing factor. Unfortunately, only recently has there been widespread acceptance of the dominant role of temperature in the effects of amphetamines on serotonergic and dopaminergic systems. Only those studies where temperature has first been taken into consideration (and measured) can other "mechanisms" of amphetamine toxicity be considered to play a role.

3. CRITERIA FOR ASSESSING NEUROTOXICITY

3.1. Brain Damage vs "Neurotoxicity"

Certainly it is not uncommon to see all substituted amphetamines labeled as potentially or outright "neurotoxic" compounds *(4,5,8,12,17,41,42)*. What is implied by the term "neurotoxicity," if not expressly stated, is that the agent causing this (neurotoxic) effect is causing brain damage (e.g., *see* refs. *8,43*). We agree that damage to, or destruction of, neural elements of the nervous system, regardless of the cause, constitutes neurotoxicity *(11)*. It is our contention, however, that the term neurotoxicity has been too broadly applied to the action of amphetamines, so much so that "neurotoxic" effects attributed to these agents are not necessarily associated with brain damage *(11,43,44)*. We place an emphasis on "damage" as a criteria for labeling an effect neurotoxic, because it allows for a more scientifically unambiguous definition of neurotoxicity, one that encompasses a destructive nature of the effect that eventually will have an adverse functional consequence to the organism *(11,43–46)*.

When one refers to brain damage, in general terms, what does this mean? Brain damage is a condition normally thought to be synonymous with neuropathology. Thus, there is little argument that neuropathological changes that accompany traumatic brain injury (TBI), stroke or neurological disease (e.g., Alzheimer's disease [AD], Parkinson's disease [PD], Creutzfeldt-Jakob's disease, multiple sclerosis [MS] or Huntington's disease [HD]) constitute brain damage *(47,48)*. In all of these cases, neuroanatomical hallmarks serve as the cellular (structural) basis for the functional deficits associated with a given condition or disease. When patients come to autopsy, their brains have well-defined signs of cell loss and damage with the appearance of distinct neuropathological features that allow for the appropriate diagnosis, using criteria that have been established for decades. Of course, under these circumstances one is dealing with an end-stage condition where brain damage is the most obvious. Does that mean that underlying neuropathology (i.e., brain damage) is not present years earlier or even in the absence of neurological symptoms? Unfortunately, that is hardly the case. Owing to the functional reserve of the central nervous system (CNS), damage or even near complete destruction of a given brain area is not necessarily associated with loss of brain function. The classic example of this situation is PD, where upwards of 70% loss of the target dopaminergic neurons is required for the characteristic symptoms of the disease to emerge *(49–51)*. Likewise, in the MPTP model of PD, marked damage to dopaminergic nerve terminals resulting from exposure to this agent can occur in the absence of behavioral deficits *(52)*. Thus, it is likely that subtle, nearly lifelong neuronal damage can occur without evidence of functional impairment. Complicating this diagnosis of underlying brain damage is the fact that injury to certain elements of the brain may not have obvious functional consequences because we lack a complete understanding of the neurobiology of the system. For example, even severe damage to the serotonergic nervous system, a putative target of amphetamines, may only result in subtle pathology that is manifested in minor changes in mood, appetite, and sexual behavior *(53–55)*.

Is there general acceptance of the potential for chemicals/drugs to damage the brain? Certainly, for decades the neuroscience/neuropharmacology research community has employed specific chemicals as denervation tools (for examples *see* ref. *56*), including chemicals used to selectively damage the dopaminergic and serotonergic pathways such as MPTP and 5,7-dihydroxytryptamine (5,7-DHT), respectively. Thus, it is not in doubt that chemicals have the potential to damage the nervous system, including the monoamine-containing neurons that serve as putative targets of amphetamine neurotoxicity. Chemically induced brain damage goes far beyond the experimental arena, however, and is not confined to concerns related to self-administration of drugs of abuse. The now classic text by Spencer and Schaumburg *(57)* documented the broad array of toxicants that damage the nervous system. In one compendium, this text shows the variety of neurotoxic episodes that have occurred in humans, including exposures as diverse as ingestion of tainted food (e.g., cresyl phosphates in cooking oil), dermal application of tainted acne medication, water-borne exposure to harmful bacteria, and the exposure to industrial solvents and metals. Whether these compounds were truly neurotoxic was not in question as the exposures were associated with deaths and (brain tissue could be examined for neuropathological changes) were accompanied by neuropathological changes. The revised edition *(58)* updates the list of agents that damage the nervous system to both a greater number and to even more diverse types of chemicals and mixtures. Again, the point is not whether chemicals can damage the nervous system, but rather what changes or markers of cell damage are adequate to indicate that damage has occurred.

One of the principles of toxicology is that the dose makes the poison *(59)*. Clearly, pharmaceuticals that act on the nervous system can be neurotoxic at high dosages *(11)*. One cannot assume, however, that toxic effects of a drug on the nervous system are simply dose-related extensions of its pharmacology. For example, therapeutic dosages of dizocilpine (MK-801) antagonize the toxic actions of excessive levels of the neurotransmitter glutamate by blocking its receptors throughout the brain *(60)*. At higher dosages, however, MK-801 has been shown to destroy neurons in a small area of cerebral cortex, a brain region unrelated to the sites of its neuroprotective (therapeutic) actions *(61–63)*. Likewise, drugs known to inhibit acetylcholinesterase are used therapeutically for the treatment of myasthenia gravis or AD. High dosages of organophosphate pesticides, compounds designed to inhibit aceytlcholinesterase, cause toxicity secondary to neuromuscular paralysis and neurotoxicity secondary to seizures *(64)* but nerve damage is not necessarily associated with regions of cholinergic innervation in the CNS *(64–66)*. By analogy, even though substituted amphetamines may act on biogenic amine neurotransmitter systems, there is no *a priori* reason to assume that these same neuronal pathways would be preferentially damaged by high dosages of these compounds.

In summary, a large variety of chemicals are neurotoxic (i.e., can cause damage) to the nervous system *(11,44–46,65,67)*. The inherent complexity of the nervous system makes it likely that desired pharmacological effects of a given drug may not be mediated through the same neurobiological substrates as potential neurotoxic effects of the same compound. The discrete nature of chemical/drug interactions with neurobiological systems, combined with the functional reserve of the nervous system, suggests that damage can occur in experimental animals and in humans in the absence of overt symptoms.

3.2. *Argyrophilia, Degeneration Flurochromes, and Glial Activation*

In the previous section, we reaffirmed the fact that chemicals can damage the brain and that damage constitutes the most scientifically sound and widely accepted conceptual basis for defining neurotoxicity. From this view follows the notion that techniques used to assess brain damage should be applied for detecting neurotoxicity. As with the evaluation of stroke, neurotrauma, or diseased brains, neuroanatomical methods have remained the dominant means for detection and characterization of neurotoxicity *(11)*.

Where large numbers of brain cells are killed outright by the offending agent, it is possible to visualize the damaged areas with tissue stains that have been in common usage for more than a century. Of course, under these circumstances, the functional deficits associated with the loss of cells already may have provided the clues to point to a neurotoxic exposure. Indeed, most neurotoxins known to humans have first been discovered by human poisonings (57). Sites of brain pathology resulting from such exposures, therefore, have been identified based on hindsight knowledge that brain damage likely had occurred. This situation is hardly the desirable approach for protecting humans from exposure to neurotoxic agents. Even more alarming is the possibility that chronic low level exposure to neurotoxicants (i.e., real-world exposure scenarios) may cause subtle neural damage that is not likely to be manifested by clinical symptoms. Thus, the greatest concern should be directed toward detecting and preventing the cumulative damage that occurs following protracted exposures to chemicals or drugs whose damage is not detectable using traditional neuroanatomical stains. Examples would be drugs or chemicals that kill only a few cells, where the surviving cells would be in far greater numbers than those that were destroyed (i.e., like looking for the "needle in the haystack"). Perhaps an even more likely situation would be chemical destruction of parts of neurons or glia with sparing of the cell itself. Under both of these scenarios, the selective and discrete nature of neurotoxic effects dictates the need for special techniques/indicators to identify cells damaged (but not necessarily killed) by a given neurotoxic agent (68). This is not an easy task because, as mentioned earlier, while the targets of neurotoxic insults may be limited to a very small area of the nervous system, any area of the nervous system may be affected. For the small drop of damaged brain to be detected within the sea of unaffected tissue, requires an indicator of neurotoxicity (i.e., damage) to fulfill several criteria, as follows: (1) it must reveal diverse types of damage to any cell type in any area of the nervous system, (2) it must be sensitive to low levels of damage, (3) it must be specific to the damage (neurotoxic) condition so that therapeutic effects of drugs are not scored positive. Succinctly stated, the ideal neurotoxicity endpoint would be an indicator of damage at any level anywhere in the nervous system that would not pick up therapeutic actions of drugs (11).

As indicated earlier, traditional neuroanatomical stains such as Hemotoxylin and Eosin or stains of Nissl elements are not sufficient to identify damaged neural cells unless a massive die-off has occurred. This is not so much a lack of sensitivity problem as it is a problem of signal to noise (for an excellent discussion, see ref. 65). Thus, where targets of brain damage are unknown, as is generally the case, techniques are needed that give a positive signal against a negative background, (i.e., a high signal to noise ratio). Two classes of endpoints fulfill such a requirement: selective degeneration stains and markers of glial activation.

3.2.1. Degeneration Stains

For many years, silver-based stains were used to trace neuronal fiber paths in the intact nervous system (see ref. 65). More recently, background suppression of normal staining has been employed to identify argyrophilic neurons undergoing degeneration. Where these selective silver degeneration stains have been used in neurotoxicology they have shown excellent sensitivity. Very discrete regions and small numbers of damaged neurons can be revealed with these stains following neurotoxic exposures (for

Table 1
Examples of Target-Appropriate Effects of Prototypical Neurotoxicants as Assessed by Selective Degeneration Stains and the Induction of GFAP

| Compound | Regional target | Species | Degeneration stains[a] | | Induction of GFAP[a] | | |
			Silver	F-J[b]	IR[b]	Assay	Ref.
Cadmium	Striatum	Rat				+	*(71)*
IDPN	Olfactory bulb, cortex	Rat	+			+	*(72)*
TMT	Hippocampus, cortex, many non-limbic areas	Rat	+		+	+	*(73,74)*
MPTP	Neostriatum	Mouse	+	+	+	+	*(67,68,75)*
Kainic acid	Hippocampus amygdala	Rat		+		+	*(67,76)*
Domoic acid	Hippocampus	Rat	+		+	+	*(77,78)*
3-NPA	Striatum hippocampus	Rat	+	+			*(67,79)*
Bilirubin	Cerebellum	Rat				+	*(80)*
6-OHDA	Substantia nigra, striatum	Rat	+			Fig. 1	*(81)*
5,7-DHT	Cortex, striatum, hippocampus	Rat	Fig. 3		+	+	*(44,82,83)*
3-Acetyl- pyridine	Inferior olive	Rat	+				*(84)*
TOCP	Spinal cord, brain stem, cerebellum	Chicken	+				*(66)*
MK-801	Retrosplenial cortex	Rat			+	+	*(61,63)*
Ampheta- mines	Striatum, cortex	Mouse	+			+	*(1)*
Ibogaine	Cerebellum	Rat				+	*(85)*
Ethanol	Cortex	Rat			+	+	*(86)*
Methylazo- oxymethanol	Cortex	Rat				+	*(87)*
TET	Hippocampus, forebrain, cerebellum	Rat				+	*(88)*

[a]The lack of a positive (+) score for a given indice does not necessarily imply a negative outcome; it indicates that this technique may not have been applied to the toxicant in question or was not shown as an example.
[b]F-J, Flouro-Jade; IR, immunoreactivity.

reviews, *see* refs. *65,68–70*). Moreover, silver staining reveals not only damaged neuronal perikarya but also degenerating axons and terminals. Furthermore, these effects are seen in the absence of overt cytopathology, as assessed by traditional neuroanatomical methods; i.e., these stains are sensitive. Neuropharmacological agents administered at therapeutic dosages, in the limited cases examined, do not screen positive with these methods, i.e., these stains are selective for neurotoxicity. Some of the neurotoxic compounds and their targets revealed by silver stains are listed in Table 1.

Recently, two anionic fluorescein derivatives, denoted Fluoro-Jade and Fluoro-Jade B, have been shown to reveal sites of neuronal degeneration *(67,89)*. The main advantage of these stains over silver-staining techniques resides in their ease of application and their reproducibility. A number of prototypical neurotoxicants have been used to validate these stains as sensitive indicators of neural damage (*see* Table 1). Perhaps the only drawback of these stains is that they do not appear to reveal damage to nerve terminals. An even more recent histochemical stain, termed black gold, has been developed to stain normal and toxicant-damage myelin *(90)*. While the mechanism through which these degeneration stains reveal damage to neurons and myelin remains unknown, all of these stains satisfy the criteria for an ideal indicator of neurotoxicity listed earlier. That these stains have been validated with a fairly extensive number and type of neurotoxic agents suggests that their combined application may lend a high degree of confidence for determining the potential for a given chemical to cause neurotoxicity.

3.2.2. Glial Activation

The propensity of the damaged brain to activate two resident glial cell types, astroglia and microglia *(91–93)*, can be exploited for detection and quantification of neurotoxicity. Astrogliosis, often termed reactive gliosis, is characterized by hypertrophy of astrocytes and represents the generic reaction of this neural cell to all types of brain injury *(11,44,46,94–97)*. The hallmark of this response is the accumulation of a protein within astrocytes known as glial fibrillary acidic protein (GFAP) *(98)*. Increases in GFAP, therefore, serve as an indicator of astrogliosis and, by extension, of neurotoxicity *(11,44,46,97)*. Enhanced expression of GFAP can readily be assessed by immunohistochemistry using widely available monoclonal and polyclonal antibodies (MAbs/PAbs). This approach has been applied for over two decades to establish astrogliosis as a dominant response to brain damage associated with neurological disease states, such as AD and MS, and more recently, to show similar associations with damage resulting from toxic insult *(11,44,46,97)*. This approach often is sufficient to detect even discrete sites of damage to the brain *(63)*. However, low-level astrocytic hypertrophy that accompanies subtle damage to the brain, including low-level damage due to chemical exposures, can escape detection by immunohistochemistry of GFAP, because of background expression of this protein by resident astrocytes *(99)*. An alternate approach that can be combined with GFAP immunohistochemistry *(99,100)* is measurement of GFAP by sensitive immunoassays *(101)*. We have used this approach to characterize, quantitatively, the astroglial response engendered by a wide variety of prototype chemical neurotoxicants *(11,44–46,97)*. These include agents that damage many regions of the brain and many different cell types within a brain region, as would be expected to occur under "real-world" conditions. Moreover, increases in GFAP reveal subtle damage to neurons, such as loss of nerve endings, under conditions where traditional neuropathological stains fail to reveal the damage *(1,11,44,46,68)*. Importantly, GFAP levels do not change with pharmacological agents administered at therapeutic dosages *(11,46)*. Thus, GFAP assessments fulfill the desired requirements for an indicator of neurotoxicity. It should be emphasized, however, that astrogliosis (assessed by GFAP immunohistochemistry or GFAP immunoassay) is linked to the onset and duration of neural damage *(11,44)*. Because neural damage is the stimulus for astrogliosis, once toxicant exposure is terminated the stimulus for astrogliosis subsides *(11,44)*. In practical terms this means that toxicant-induced gliosis (including gliosis induced by amphetamines) is transient in nature *(11,46)*. Therefore, a time-course analysis should be included in evaluations of amphetamine-induced gliosis to avoid false negative results. Some prototypical toxicants used to validate GFAP as an indirect indicator of neural damage are listed in Table 1.

While not as well-documented as reactive astrogliosis, the response of microglia to disease, injury, and toxic exposures of the brain also represents a sensitive index of brain damage *(91–93)*. Activation of this glial-cell type, thought to be the resident macrophage of the brain, often occurs before astroglial activation *(91–93,102)*, making it one of the earliest "sensors" of brain damage regardless of the source. Moreover, unlike astrocyte expression of GFAP, little background staining is observed for microglia in the intact brain as revealed by lectin staining or antibodies directed toward microglial complement receptors *(91,92)*. Thus, when microglia are activated by injury, high signal to noise ratios often make these cell types very sensitive indicators of neurotoxicity. Beyond image analysis, however, no approach exists to quantify microglial activation, because few molecular entities have been identified that can be assayed when this cell type reacts to brain damage. The rapid and sensitive nature of the microglial reaction to brain damage suggests that future neurotoxicological studies, including those on substituted amphetamines, should include examinations of microglia as a part of any comprehensive characterization of the neurotoxic condition. Again, as with astrogliosis, microglial activation is transient in nature, which dictates the need for a time-course analysis to detect this cellular response to neural damage *(102)*.

In the first two sections of this chapter, we have briefly reviewed the current dogma with respect to amphetamine neurotoxicity and we have hinted that confusion exists with respect to understanding what is meant by amphetamine "neurotoxicity." We have argued that a damage perspective provides the most scientifically defensible view toward defining whether neurotoxicity has indeed occurred, because criteria exist for defining and quantifying damage, regardless of the source of neurotoxic insult. Finally, we have briefly discussed some of the indices of damage and how they serve as valuable indicators of chemically induced neurotoxicity. We belabored these points because they serve to establish a context within which various effects of amphetamines can be categorized. This compartmentalization of effects, while not clearly "black and white," does allow one to distinguish between effects associated with neural damage ("bad") vs effects (even protracted effects) that only represent a change from baseline. In so doing, we hope to shift the research paradigm from a focus on defining virtually any effect of a substituted amphetamine as "neurotoxic" to an emphasis on understanding mechanisms of substituted amphetamine-induced neural damage that are likely to differ from mechanisms underlying protracted long-term effects (e.g., downregulation of transporters, etc.) of these agents, because they can occur in the absence of damage. Distinguishing biochemical events related to amphetamine-induced neural damage from mechanisms that are regulatory in nature offers the potential for implementing intervention strategies that are neuroprotective, not just neuro-active. Below we will briefly review some of the purported features of amphetamine neurotoxicity in the rat and mouse, distinguishing where possible, those effects implicated in neuronal damage from those that are not.

4. RAT DATA

By far, the largest amount of data on substituted amphetamine neurotoxicity, including effects of AMP, METH, MDA, MDMA, and FEN, has been obtained using a rat model. For decades, most work on these compounds has centered on the effects of a high single dose or to up to 6 injections in a single day on various parameters thought to reflect the integrity of the dopamine or serotonin containing neurons *(2)*. Bowyer and Holson *(2)* cover all the relevant features surrounding METH neurotoxicity as a model for the effects of most substituted amphetamines. They review in detail the fact that METH effects are probably a mixture of regulatory actions on monoamine synthesis and dopaminergic (possibly serotonergic) axonal damage and point out the critical role of body temperature in these actions. While progress has been made in our understanding of the toxic actions of METH and other amphetamines (e.g., *see* below), no studies have provided definitive data on mechanisms of neurotoxicity not already discussed in detail by Bowyer and Holson *(2)*. Their review, therefore, should be considered the authoritative source for information on amphetamine neurotoxicity in the rat. Below, we briefly outline the types of data that have been reported to link exposure to amphetamines with neurodegenerative changes.

4.1. Dopamine and Serotonin "Neurotoxicity"

Amphetamine neurotoxicity has been the object of intense research for over two decades. In large measure, this effort has been driven by the bulk of data, obtained from the rat, showing persistent reductions in markers thought to reflect the structural integrity of the dopamine and serotonin-containing neurons (*see* citations above in Subheading 2.1. and ref. *2*. These endpoints include the transmitters themselves (dopamine and serotonin), their respective biosynthetic enzymes (TH and TPH), their reuptake transporters, and the vesicular monoamine transporters. Both immunohistochemical and biochemical assessments of these indices have shown them to be persistently decreased days to months postdrug administration. In aggregate, these data have been used to support the notion that amphetamines result in dopamine and serotonin "neurotoxicity." What is not clear is how these "neurotoxic" effects relate to the potential of these compounds to cause damage to dopaminergic or serotonergic neurons. There is fairly general agreement that dopamine and serotonin neuronal perykarya are spared by dosing regimens of amphetamines that produce long-lasting decrements in transmitter markers in the nerve terminal fields. What remain at issue are the circumstances under which decreases in monoamine markers reflect damage to the nerve terminals (i.e., true serotonin and dopamine axonal pathology). Clearly, months-long decreases in these endpoints, even with an eventual return to baseline, are suggestive of a derangement of the biosynthetic capacity of these neurons. Such effects may reflect inhibition of protein synthesis *(103)*, in general, or intraneuronal modification of proteins that result in loss of biosynthetic capacity of monoaminergic neurons *(104–106)* and/or reprogramming of intracellular biosynthetic capacity *(107,108)*. On the basis of these types of effects, the actions of amphetamines could be considered neurotoxic. These changes, however, cannot be equated with neuronal damage and are not necessarily reflective of the expected functional deficits associated with loss of a specific transmitter. For example, human brains obtained from METH users show marked reduction in dopamine, tyrosine hydroxylase, and the dopamine transporter *(3)*. Decrease in these

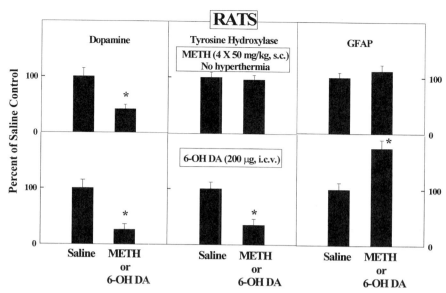

Fig. 1. Multiple, high-dose exposure of rats to methamphetamine (METH), in the absence of hyperthermia, results in depletion of striatal dopamine without affecting levels of tyrosine hydroxylase, a marker of dopaminergic nerve terminals in the striatum, or GFAP, a marker of reactive gliosis (upper panels). A single intracerebroventricular injection of the known dopaminergic neurotoxicant, 6-hydroxydopamine, depletes dopamine and results in the loss of TH and the induction of gliosis as evidence by an increase in GFAP (lower panels). METH was administered four times in a single day and rats were sacrificed at 48 h after the last dose. Rats were single-housed in wire-bottom cages at an ambient temperature of approx 21°C. to prevent METH-induced hyperthermia. At 7 d postdosing with METH, dopamine levels returned to control and TH and GFAP remained unchanged, findings indicative of the regulatory, not toxicological, nature of even this high-dosage regimen of METH in the absence of hyperthermia. Dopamine, TH, and GFAP data were obtained from the same rats. A lack of an effect of METH on TH and GFAP could not be attributed to a lack of responsiveness of this indicators to dopaminergic nerve-terminal damage as 6-hydroxydopamine (given in 1% ascorbate and after pretreatment with desmethylimipramine to protect noradrenergic fibers) caused the expected loss of TH and the induction of GFAP. These latter data were obtained at 3 d postdosing but persisted for at least 2 wk (data not shown). Dopamine, TH, and GFAP data from these experiments also were obtained from the same rats. Dopamine, TH, and GFAP were determined as described in O'Callaghan and Miller *(1)* *Significantly different from saline controls, $p < 0.05$. METH data are modified from O'Callaghan and Miller *(44)*.

markers were at levels so low that they resemble those associated with PD but these individuals were not parkinsonian. Moreover, the vesicular transporter and dopa decarboxylase, markers reduced in PD, were at normal levels, suggesting that the dopaminergic pathway, despite severe reductions in other markers, remained intact. We have obtained similar data in the rat for both METH and MDMA, i.e., changes in neurotransmitter levels without corresponding changes in markers of damage (Figs. 1 and 2; discussed below). Data such as these indicate that marked decreases in markers of dopaminergic and serotonergic neurons can occur in the absence of neuronal degeneration. Indeed, the potential for amphetamines to downregulate transmitter biomarkers rather than destroy nerve terminals was raised by Bowyer and colleagues as early as

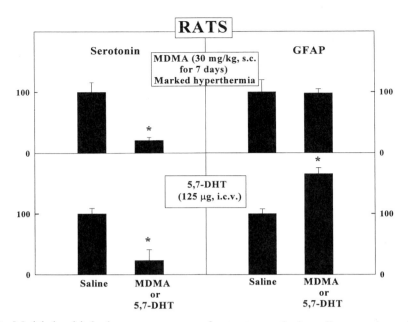

Fig. 2. Multiple, high-dose exposures of rats to methylenedioxymethamphetamine (MDMA), in the presence of extreme hyperthermia, results in marked depletion of cortical serotonin without affecting levels of GFAP, a marker of reactive gliosis (upper panels). A single intracerebroventricular injection of the known serotonergic neurotoxicant, 5,7-dihydroxytryptamine (5,7-DHT), depletes serotonin and results in the induction of gliosis, as evidenced by an increase in GFAP (lower panels). MDMA was administered once daily for 7 d and rats were sacrificed at 48 h after the last dose. Rats were group-housed (5 per cage) in bedding at an ambient temperature of approx 21°C. Core temperature was monitored prior to and throughout the dosing period and was found to be elevated but rats were noticeably warm to the touch and spot checks over the initial 2–3 d of dosing revealed core temperatures in the 39.5–40.5°C range. Mortality in the 10–20% range was common. Serotonin and GFAP data were obtained from the same rats. A lack of an effect of MDMA on GFAP could not be attributed to a lack of responsiveness of this indicator neural damage because 5,7-DHT (given in 1% ascorbate) caused the expected induction of GFAP. These latter data were obtained at 7 d postdosing but gliosis (increased GFAP) was observed as early as 2 d post 5,7-DHT (data not shown). Serotonin and GFAP data in these experiments also were obtained from the same rats. Serotonin and GFAP were determined as described in O'Callaghan and Miller *(1)*. *Significantly different from saline controls, $p < 0.05$. Data are modified from O'Callaghan and Miller *(44)*.

1992 *(109)*. A regulatory rather than a toxic action of these compounds should not be unexpected, given that recent data indicate that dopamine and serotonin transporters, as well as their respective biosynthetic enzymes, are subject to pharmacological regulation *(110–113)*.

4.2. Neural Damage Markers

4.2.1. Transmitter-Related Immunohistochemistry and Autoradiography

For over a decade, immunohistochemistry has been used to visualize the dopamine and serotonin neurons affected by "neurotoxic" regimens of various substituted amphetamines. Tyrosine hydroxylase frequently is the antigen of choice for identifying dopaminergic processes *(114)*, whereas the low relative abundance of serotonin innervation has restricted analysis of this system to antibodies directed against the transmitter itself *(115)*, often in animals pretreated with drugs to "boost" the serotonin signal *(116)*. With respect to amphetamines that primarily affect serotonin-containing neurons (e.g., DEX and MDMA), it is not an understatement to conclude that serotonin immunohistochemistry constitutes the bulk of evidence for the "neurotoxic" effects of these compounds. Despite numerous claims to the contrary, serotonin immunohistochemistry in amphetamine-treated rats does not provide evidence for axonal pathology or loss. It only provides a morphological verification for what can be quantified by high-performance liquid chromatography (HPLC), i.e., reductions in the levels of the transmitter not reductions in the number of serotonin positive nerve fibers. Thus, presentation of control micrographs of serotonin immunostaining patterns along side micrographs that appear to show near complete MDMA- or FEN-induced destruction of the serotonergic plexus, is highly misleading but, nevertheless, is a very common practice *(8,23,116,117)*. Further claims that serotonin immunohistochemisty can reveal aberrant (i.e., pathological) neuronal profiles due to amphetamine exposure (e.g., *see* ref. *116*) also appear to be without merit because drugs that target the brain serotonin system but do not deplete serotonin result in the same "aberrant" profiles *(20)*. Ligands for the serotonin transporter (as well as the dopamine and norepinephrine transporters) also have been used to provide a "quantitative" index of terminal loss as assessed by autoradiography *(19,118)*. The subsequent widespread demonstration that these transporters are subject to pharmacological and even dietary regulation (*see* refs. *110–113*) indicates that transporter analysis cannot be used to assess damage to monoaminergic nerve terminals. What data such as these illustrate is that protein constituents of monoaminergic neurons are dynamic and subject to a variety of regulatory controls. They cannot simply be viewed as structural elements, the loss of which would be indicative of cell loss or damage. Instead, changes in the levels (or activity) of, for example, tyrosine hydroxylase, must be viewed in concert with other changes reflective of damage (for a detailed discussion, *see* refs. *1,3,44*), in order to obtain the most comprehensive and accurate picture as to whether monoaminergic neuronal damage occurs with a given amphetamine exposure regimen.

4.2.2. Oxidative Stress Markers

A variety of reactive chemical species have been implicated in the etiology of neurodegenerative diseases states (HD, PD, amyotrophic lateral sclerosis [ALS], etc.) *(48)*. Because of the linkage between certain reactive chemical events and brain damage, markers of oxidative stress have been pursued as indices of amphetamine-induced neurotoxicity. Hydroxyl radicals, peroxynitrite, superoxide radicals, sulfhydral oxidants, and reactive quinones all have been proposed to play a role in the dopamine and serotonin neurotoxicity of amphetamines *(104–106,119–123)*. Methods exist to either directly or indirectly measure these reactive species. The results of these studies show that oxidizing conditions inactivate tyrosine hydroxylase and tryptophan hydroxylase. Conversely, antioxidants, reducing conditions and radical scavengers protect against oxidative damage to these key biosynthetic enzymes (e.g., *see* refs. *120,121,124,125*). The effects of these reactive processes, especially those involving covalent modification of enzymes at active sites, can result in their inactivation with subsequent functional consequences that may lead to nerve terminal damage. While ample evidence exits to document such processes, in vitro, few attempts have been made to correlate oxidative stress with the evolution of neural damage in the rat, even though methods now exist to explore such possibilities. Thus, it is not clear whether the effects of oxidative "damage," if they occur, in vivo, actually result in damage and loss of serotonergic or dopaminergic nerve terminals. The possibility exists that these effects may instead be responsible for protracted decrements in biogenic amine markers that eventually recover to control levels in an otherwise intact neuron (see earlier discussion). It is hoped that data emerging from the use of transgenic mice (see below) will shed some light on specific processes involved in amphetamine-induced oxidative stress related to the potential to cause neuronal damage and degeneration.

4.2.3. Silver Stains

Silver degeneration stains have been shown to reveal amphetamine-induced damage to neurons. As early as 1982, Ricaurte and colleagues (13) used the Fink-Heimer silver stain to demonstrate that nerve-terminal degeneration accompanied the prolonged decreases in striatal dopamine following administration of METH to rats. Other reports of cortical damage due to AMP, including loss of pyramidal neurons, were demonstrated with this technique (126). Because of the association of degeneration staining with protracted loss (weeks to months) of dopamine, it was easy to assume (and more practical to determine) that amphetamine-induced decreases in dopamine were a reflection of nerve-terminal damage. Using a modified de Olmos silver stain, Bowyer also showed a METH-induced degeneration of striatal nerve terminals to be accompanied by long-term decreases in dopamine (22). More importantly, Bowyer demonstrated that decreases in the transmitter could occur in the absence of evidence for damage and indicated the requirement for hyperthermia (22) (see below). The implication of these findings was that dopamine depletion per se was not sufficient evidence for nerve terminal damage, findings consistent with our data (44) (see also Subheading 4.2.5. and Fig. 1).

As with METH, MDMA has been shown to cause a silver-degeneration reaction (42,127). Also consistent with data for METH and its target transmitter (dopamine), persistent decreases in the target transmitter of MDMA (serotonin), can occur in the absence of silver staining (44,127). Moreover, silver staining, when it occurred, was not associated with serotonergic axons, as only cortical neurons (perikarya) were shown to undergo degeneration (42,127). Finally, hyperthermia was not a concomitant for silver impregnation to occur (see below).

The implication of the findings with MDMA are: (1) long-term decreases in serotonin can occur in the absence of evidence for neuronal damage or degeneration (silver staining); (2) when damage is demonstrated after MDMA based on silver-degeneration staining, it is not a high-dose extension of its pharmacological effects, because serotonin neurons do not stain; and (3) hyperthermia is not required to observe degeneration (see discussion below on the role of hyperthermia in amphetamine-induced neurotoxicity in rats; Subheading 4.3.). A lack of sensitivity of the silver method is not at issue because administration of the known serotonergic neurotoxicant, 5,7-DHT, results in serotonin depletions equal to those seen with MDMA (Fig. 2) along with an accompanying silver-degeneration stain in the target regions (cortex) (Fig. 3).

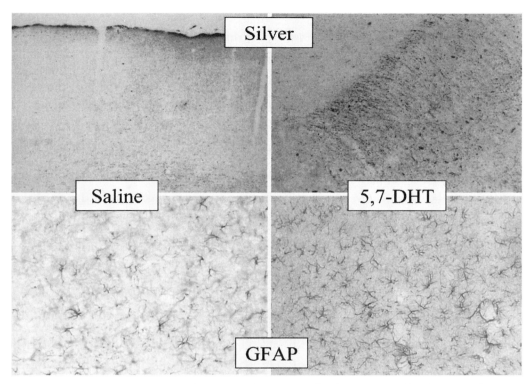

Fig. 3. The known serotonergic neurotoxicant, 5,7-dihydroxytryptamine (5,7-DHT) causes a silver degeneration-staining pattern in cortex characterized by the presence of argyrophilic debris (upper right panel) and the induction of hypertrophied astrocytes characteristic of gliosis (lower right panel). Controls, dosing regimen, and survival times were the same as those described in the legend to Fig. 2. Evidence of argyrophilia after 5,7-DHT was most prevalent in cortex (upper right panel) with saline controls showing only sparse background staining in all areas of cortex (upper left panel, lower magnification). Evidence of gliosis, characterized by an apparent greater number of astrocytes but, more typically, by astrocytes with swollen and elongated processes, was most prevalent in cortex (lower right panel vs lower left panel). The Cupric silver degeneration-staining procedure and GFAP immunohistochemistry were performed as described in Jensen et al. *(127)* and O'Callaghan and Jensen *(68)*, respectively. (*See* color plate 2 appearing in the insert following p. 368.)

4.2.4. Fluoro-Jade

Staining with Fluoro-Jade, which reveals degenerating neurons, has been used to examine damage due to METH and FEN *(67,89,128,129)*. While Fluoro-Jade does not stain degenerating nerve terminals and, therefore, does not delineate METH-induced damage to dopaminergic neurons, its sensitivity has proven useful for detecting novel sites of METH-induced neurodegeneration in areas of cortex and thalamus *(67,128,129)*. Fluoro-Jade also is useful for demonstrating the conditions under which FEN can cause neuronal damage. Even high dosages of FEN do not cause Fluoro-Jade staining in the brains of rats housed at ambient temperature despite the fact that such exposures are associated with prolonged decreases in serotonin *(129)*. Only small numbers of Fluoro-Jade positive neurons are seen with FEN in animals housed at 37°C and that exhibit greatly elevated core temperature *(129)*. Even under these circumstances, serotonin neurons in the raphe nucleus are spared suggesting that the serotonin decreases observed in these animals are not the result of degeneration of the serotonin-containing neurons. Overall, the data indicate that Fluoro-Jade is a very sensitive indicator for identifying subtle neuronal damage following exposure to amphetamines. When combined with silver staining for axonal and synaptic damage, it should be useful for identifying even the most discrete areas of neuronal damage, regardless of the amphetamine regimen or presence of susceptibility factors (e.g. temperature/stress) that contribute to or protect from neurotoxic outcomes (e.g., *see* ref. *14*).

4.2.5. GFAP

Astrocytic hypertrophy in the rat, as evidenced by increases in the levels or immunostaining of GFAP go hand in hand with silver degeneration staining and Fluoro-Jade staining (e.g., *see* refs. *11,65,67*). Thus, METH-associated silver staining in the neostriatum is accompanied by astrocytic activation *(22)*. Likewise, regimens of MDMA that result in silver staining in cortex and striatum also result in increases in GFAP in the same region *(44,127)*. In the absence of evidence for astrogliosis, METH-induced decrements in dopamine and MDMA-induced decreases in serotonin can still occur (Figs. 1 and 2), data that are consistent with corresponding negative results for silver staining for the two compounds *(22,44,127)*. Again, sensitivity does not appear to be at issue because known dopamine and serotonin neurotoxins, 6-OH DA (Fig. 1) and 5,7-DHT (Figs. 2 and 3), respectively, cause target appropriate increases in GFAP (Figs. 1 and 2) or GFAP immunoreactivity (Fig. 3) and/or silver degeneration staining (Fig. 3) *(see also* refs. *82,83,130)*.

It is now more widely known that METH-induced striatal damage in the rat requires sustained METH-induced hyperthermia (*see* Subheading 4.3.). Knowledge of this requirement has made it easier to demonstrate METH-induced astrogliosis in the rat (e.g., *see* refs. *131,132*). GFAP immunohistochemistry often is the method of choice for assessing this effect *(133)*, although the GFAP enzyme-linked immunosorbent assay (ELISA) also has been employed to obtain a quantitative assessment of this marker of neural damage *(131)*. As noted earlier, induction of GFAP as a measure of gliosis frequently has been shown to be accompanied by other accepted indices of neural damage, such as selective degeneration stains (Table 1). Thus, generally speaking, enhanced expression of GFAP can be taken as a stand-alone measure for neural damage. GFAP, however, is subject to physiological regulation (e.g., *see* ref. *134*), and it is possible, under as yet certain unforeseen circumstances, that its expression (increased or decreased) may not be a reflection of neural damage. The unexpected role of temperature in METH neurotoxicity provides but one example of an unforeseen factor playing a major role in neurotoxic outcomes. Therefore, as we stress throughout this chapter, it is important to obtain as many multiple independent measures of damage as possible to distinguish amphetamine-induced damage from effects that are unrelated to the damage condition.

4.2.6. Microglia

Injury-induced microglial activation (microgliosis) (for a review, *see* ref. *91*) almost always accompanies (and often precedes) the activation of astroglia, therefore, amphetamine regimens that increase GFAP should have an accompanying microgliosis. Such activation can occur with damage to dopaminergic neurons in the rat (6-OH-DA)

(135), but relatively little attention has been given to the potential for microglial activation following exposures to amphetamines. METH regimens that are accompanied by hyperthermia can produce microglial activation as evidenced by enhanced staining with B4 isolectin or OX-42 (J. F. Bowyer and T. G. Hastings, personal communication). Serotonin-depleting regimens of parachloroamphetamine have been reported to cause a small microglial activation in the rat *(136)*. Core temperature was not recorded in this study and other indices of neural damage (e.g., GFAP increases, silver-degeneration stains) were not documented. It is notable that few reports of microglial activation have been observed following serotonin-depleting regimens of substituted amphetamines. Destruction of the serotonin plexus by 5,7-DHT has been shown to elicit an astroglial activation *(44,82,83)* and also is accompanied by silver-degeneration staining in the affected area (Figs. 2 and 3). Therefore, damage to the serotonergic pathway engenders the expected damage response. The lack of similar effects of amphetamines, even in the face of long-term reductions in serotonin levels and serotonin immunostaining, suggests that serotonergic neurons are resistant to damage by amphetamines. The neurotoxicological significance of serotonin depletion in the absence of evidence of damage remains an attractive area for future research.

4.3. Effects of Temperature

A persistent (hours) elevation in core temperature (to 39.5–41°C) appears to be an absolute requirement for METH-induced damage to dopaminergic nerve terminals in the rat *(2)*. This level of hypothermia is severe enough to require hypothermic intervention to prevent lethality. Hyperthermia alone is not sufficient to cause neural damage or dopamine depletion. Although a significant body of evidence suggests that the degree of striatal dopamine depletion because of METH is related to the amount of elevation of temperature above baseline, a similar relationship has not been established for the degree METH-induced dopaminergic nerve terminal damage and temperature. Thus, while METH exposures that result in elevated core temperature requiring hypothermic rescue clearly result in gliosis and silver degeneration staining *(2,22)*, little evidence exists to show that less severe increases in core temperature are associated with evidence of neural damage, even though dopamine levels are persistently decreased. (*see* Fig. 1). These data suggest that, at least with respect to effects on dopaminergic neurons, amphetamines can exert a persistent regulatory effect on dopamine levels in the absence of evidence of damage to dopaminergic nerve terminals in the neostriatum (for an extended discussion, *see* ref. *2*). Amphetamine-induced damage to forebrain neurons, as assessed by Fluro-Jade staining of neurons and iso-lectin staining of activated microglia, appears to have a requirement for severe hyperthermia, but seizure severity and age appear to be the more relevant covariates for damage *(137)*.

As with substituted-amphetamines that affect dopamine in the rat, amphetamines that act on the serotonergic system (e.g., MDMA, parachlroamphetamine) also result in hyperthermia. A greater degree of hyperthermia also results in a greater degree of depletion of serotonin for these compounds *(37)*. In contrast, persistent FEN-induced reductions in serotonin are not associated with hyperthermia, indeed, hypothermia often is the result (D. B. Miller and J. P. O'Callaghan, unpublished observation). Data such as these indicate that the relationship between body temperature and the propensity of certain amphetamines to decrease serotonin is complex. It should not be surprising, therefore, to find that the relationship between body temperature and the propensity of these same compounds to cause neural damage also is complex. For example, we used a 7 d/b.i.d. exposure regimen of MDMA that caused a large (sometimes lethal) elevation in core temperature and a large and persistent reduction in serotonin (44). This same regimen failed to increase GFAP (Fig. 2) or result in silver-degeneration staining in the serotonin-containing brain regions. In contrast, when rats were given a very high b.i.d. regimen of MDMA for 2 d but did not become hyperthermic, because they were housed singly in wire-bottom cages, reductions in serotonin were not as great as observed for the 7-d regimen (44). In this case, however, large increases in GFAP were observed and silver-degeneration staining was found in the same areas exhibiting enhanced expression of GFAP (44). These data indicated that neural degeneration was independent of hyperthermia and the degree of depletion of serotonin. Indeed, it was unlikely that serotonergic neurons were damaged because the patterns of silver staining were suggestive of damage to intrinsic neurons of the cortex not the projection fields of serotonin-containing neurons (127). Large (50%) and persistent (>6 mo) decreases in serotonin due to FEN were not associated with evidence of neural degeneration in the serotonin terminal fields (D. B. Miller and J. P. O'Callaghan, unpublished observation). As noted earlier, only by employing elevated ambient temperatures to raise core temperature can FEN be shown to cause neural damage based on F-J staining. Moreover, even under these circumstances, damage is slight and sparsely scattered and does not appear to involve serotonin containing neurons, nor is there glial activation in the serotonin-projection field (138).

It is difficult to summarize the relationship between core temperature and the propensity of amphetamines to cause neural damage in the rat. A marked elevation in core temperature appears to be required for damage to dopaminergic neurons and any means to prevent exposure-related hypothermia will be partially to fully protective. The involvement of temperature in the effects of amphetamines on serotonin-containing neurons is far less clear. Indeed, little evidence exists to link even high-level exposures to amphetamines and damage to serotonergic neurons. These data, or the lack thereof, are suggestive of a complex role for temperature in the transmitter depleting actions of amphetamines. Hyperthermia clearly plays some role in the damage response of dopaminergic neurons to amphetamines, therefore, a more rigorous and systematic evaluation of temperature responses in relationship to damage responses would be of value in future investigation of amphetamine-mediated dopaminergic neurotoxicity. Amphetamine-mediated damage to serotonergic neurons has been difficult to demonstrate and core temperature appears to have compound-specific effects on serotonin depletion. Thus, it is even more difficult to assign a role to temperature for neural damage associated with administration of serotonin depleting amphetamines to the rat.

5. MOUSE DATA

Compared to the large database for effects of amphetamines on the brain and behavior of rats, relatively little data has been accumulated for the effects of these compounds in the mouse. By far the greatest number of studies using the mouse as a model have focused on the effects of METH but, until recently, little attention has been directed toward an understanding of the potential for METH-induced neurotoxicity in this species (see, however, refs. 39,139). Most work on METH neurotoxicity in the mouse, as in the rat, has utilized a protocol of four injections in a single day with subsequent examination of various endpoints thought to reflect the integrity of the nigral-striatal dopaminergic pathway; the serotonergic system has received less attention because it does not appear to be as affected in the mouse (e.g., *see* refs. *1,14*). The lack of effects of amphetamines on the serotonin system, in general, and the shift of certain amphetamine (e.g., MDMA) from an action on serotonin systems in the rat to dopamine system in the mouse *(1,11,14,36)* point to strong species-dependent effects that have heretofore not been widely acknowledged (or investigated). Moreover, despite the concerns raised by Bowyer and colleagues *(2)* that neurotransmitter changes due to amphetamines may reflect a combination of both regulatory and damage-induced changes, little attention has been devoted to this issue in studies of amphetamine neurotoxicity in the mouse. As in the rat, body temperature has been found to play a role in most of the effects of these compounds that are suspected to reflect "neurotoxicity" *(14,31)*. It is clear, however, that an elevation in body temperature to near lethal levels in not a critical requirement for amphetamine-mediated damage to dopaminergic nerve terminals *(14)*.

5.1. Dopamine and Serotonin "Neurotoxicity"

Research on substituted amphetamine neurotoxicity has been ongoing for more than two decades, yet only recently has there been an effort to evaluate neurotoxicity patterns in the mouse. The bulk of the data obtained using the mouse model concerns the effects of METH on monoaminergic systems. As in the rat, it is now well-established that repeated exposure to high dosages results in persistent reductions in endpoints thought to reflect the integrity of dopamine neurons. METH causes persistent decrements in striatal and cortical dopamine and its metabolites, as well as the activity, immunostaining, and levels of TH *(1,14,31,35,36,39,139–142)*. In these respects, the effects in mice are similar to those reported for the hyperthermic rat. In large measure, however, there are as many differences as there are similarities, even without taking into consideration the enormous potential for strain differences among mice *(34,35,142)*. For example, METH does not produce persistent depletions of serotonin in the mouse as it does in the rat *(1)*. Further, agents such as MDMA and MDA, known mainly for their effects on serotonergic markers in the rat, fail to have their main effects on the serotonergic system in the mouse *(1)*. Instead, nearly all amphetamines examined to date, with the exception of fenfluramine, cause protracted decreases exclusive to the dopaminergic system in striatum and cortex *(1)*. Limited evaluation of neural damage markers (*see* discussion below) suggest that all of these compounds cause dopaminergic-nerve terminal degeneration with the exception of FEN, which appears to deplete serotonin without damaging serotonergic neurons *(1,14)*, just as it does in the rat *(138)*. Of potential significance is the fact that the shift of MDMA from a serotonergic-acting compound in the rat to a dopaminergic neurotoxicant in the mouse does not simply reflect a high-dose extension of its neuropharmacological actions in the latter species. Single, low to high dosages of MDMA in the mouse do not affect dopamine levels or turnover (J. P. O'Callaghan and D. B. Miller, unpublished observation). Thus, the damaging effects of high multiple dosages that are accompanied by dopamine depletions in the mouse may reflect toxicity mechanisms unrelated to dopamine release, in contrast to neurotoxicity mechanisms proposed for the effects of METH in the rat *(143)*.

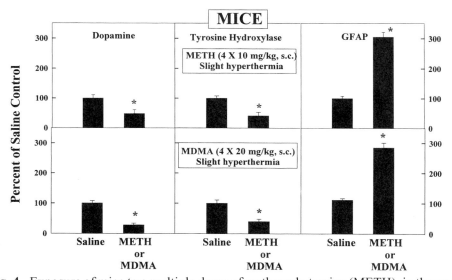

Fig. 4. Exposure of mice to a multiple doses of methamphetamine (METH), in the presence of slight hyperthermia, results in depletion of striatal dopamine, loss of tyrosine hydroxylase (TH), a marker of dopaminergic nerve terminals in the striatum and the induction of GFAP, a marker of reactive gliosis (upper panels). Exposure of mice to multiple doses of methylenedioxymethamphetamine (MDMA), in the presence of slight hyperthermia, also results in results in depletion of striatal dopamine, loss of TH, and the induction of GFAP (lower panels). METH and MDMA were administered four times in a single day at the dosages specified and the mice were sacrificed at 72 h after the last dose. Mice were housed in groups of 6 in bedded cages at an ambient temperature of approx 21°C. At 21 d postdosing with METH or MDMA, dopamine and TH levels remained reduced. At this time GFAP levels had returned to near-control values, data consistent with the transient nature of toxicant-induced reactive gliosis *(46)*. Silver-degeneration staining in the striatum accompanied the induction of GFAP and loss of dopamine and TH for both compounds (data not shown). The data are consistent with METH—and MDMA-induced damage to striatal dopaminergic nerve terminals in the mouse striatum. Dopamine, TH, and GFAP data from these experiments were obtained from the same mice. Dopamine, TH, and GFAP were determined as described in O'Callaghan and Miller *(1)*. *Significantly different from saline controls, $p < 0.05$. Data are modified from O'Callaghan and Miller *(1)*.

5.2. Neural Damage Markers

5.2.1. Transmitter-Related Immunohistochemistry and Autoradiography

Immunohistochemistry has not frequently been used to assess damage to dopamine and serotonin neurons in the mouse following neurotoxic regimens of substituted amphetamines (*see*, however, refs. *139,140*). As dopamine nerve terminals appear to be the primary target of the effects of substituted amphetamines in the mouse, tyrosine hydroxylase has been the most common antigen examined. Decreases in TH immunoreactivity, consistent with loss of dopamine and TH activity, often are taken as evidence of loss of the dopaminergic nerve terminals *(139,140)*. In the absence of other evidence for neural damage, just as in rats and humans, the possibility exists that the observed changes are regulatory in nature. Thus, as emphasized above for the rat, a constellation of neural damage markers should be used to obtain a true picture of the damage profiles of substituted amphetamines in the mouse *(1,14,139,140)*. Autoradiography data for the mouse has centered on ligands for the dopamine transporter *(140,144)*. The same caveats that applied to the use of autoradiography in the rat also apply to studies of amphetamine neurotoxicity in the mouse. Despite the potential for drawing erroneous conclusions from immunhistochemical and autoradiographic approaches, it is notable in the mouse that changes in monoamine markers often go hand in hand with changes in other markers linked to the damage condition *(see* Fig. 4 and discussion below) *(1,11,36,44,139–141,144)*. The general absence of such data in the rat model suggests that amphetamine-induced neural damage is more readily obtained in the mouse.

5.2.2. Oxidative Stress Markers

Evidence suggests the amphetamines may effect their degenerative properties through the production of reactive compounds generated by the presence of nonsequestered dopamine (e.g., *see* ref. *145)*. This suggests that amphetamine-induced changes in these reactive species (e.g., hydroxyl or superoxide free radicals, quinones, etc.) would be accompanied by changes in endpoints indicative of degeneration (e.g., argryophilia, astrogliosis, etc.). However, no studies utilizing the mouse have directly examined dopamine oxidation or lipid peroxidation products nor has there been direct evidence for amphetamine-related production of free radicals. What has been reported, however, is a linkage between oxidative stress and amphetamine neurotoxicity using indirect measures (e.g., measurement of 3-nitrotyrosine as a marker of peroxynitrite generation), transgenic mice with modifications of oxidative pathways (e.g., overexpression of superoxide dismutase [SOD]), or the use of antioxidants or free radical spin-trapping agents (e.g., melatonin, selenium, etc.) *(124,145–153)*. Thus, methamphetamine exposure increases striatal levels of 3-nitrotyrosine *(148)* and increases n-NOS *(146)*. Amphetamines decrease the level of scavenging enzymes like SOD, catalase, or glutathione peroxidase *(152)*. Methamphetamine-induced decrements in dopamine can be blocked or decreased by antioxidants *(147,149)*. The depleting actions are blocked as well in mice overexpressing SOD *(145,151)*, the enzyme responsible for the scavenging of superoxide radicals. What has been rare in these oxidative stress studies is to examine the indirect measures of oxidative stress in tandem with endpoints linked to neural degeneration, such as glial activation and silver-degeneration staining. While these studies link indirect measures of oxidative stress to the dopamine depleting actions of the amphetamines, and provide support for the idea that reactive oxygen species (ROS) play a role in these effects, they do not confirm a link between ROS action and the degenerative actions of the amphetamines. Little consideration has been given to the possibility that the transmitter-depleting actions of amphetamines may relate to oxidative processes distinct from neurodegenerative actions of these compounds.

5.2.3. Silver

Silver-degeneration staining has seen limited use in the assessment of amphetamine-induced neural damage. We employed the de Olmos cupric silver method to demonstrate argyrophilic debris in the striatum of C57Bl6/J mice treated with four doses of METH, MDMA, and MDA over a 6-h period *(1)*. The onset of argyrophilia was consistent with the onset of glial activation *(see* below) as well as a decrease in dopamine and

TH levels. All changes were limited to the projection field of the nigral striatal pathway; neuronal perikarya were spared in the nigra based on Nissl staining and the lack of glial activation. Together these data paint a fairly clear picture of METH-, MDMA-, and MDA-induced dopaminergic neurotoxicity. Despite small but persistent decreases in cortical levels of 5-HT following a four-dose regimen of FEN, this compound did not result in silver staining in any brain region, findings suggestive of a regulatory action on 5-HT-containing neurons in the absence of neural damage *(1)*. Using a newer version of the de Olmos stain *(154)*, Schmued and Bowyer *(155)* confirmed the aforementioned findings for METH and extended them to include evidence of degeneration in the indusium griseum and fasciola cinerea with minor evidence apparent in tinea tectum. Blockade of these latter effects by phenobarbital was suggestive of a role of seizures in the observed damage.

5.2.4. Fluoro-Jade

Fluoro-Jade staining after METH revealed cell death in the hippocampal remnants: indusium griseum, fasciola cinerea, and tinea tectum *(155)*. The damage areas were consistent with those seen after staining with cupric-silver *(155)*. Fluoro-Jade should be utilized to analyze patterns of neural damage in the mouse that are induced by other substituted amphetamines.

5.2.5. GFAP

A decade ago, Hess and colleagues *(139)* showed a striking astroglial response to METH in the mouse as evidence by GFAP immunohistochemistry. Recent studies have confirmed these subjective data *(140)*. We have utilized the GFAP ELISA *(101)* to quantify the astroglial response to METH, MDMA, and MDA *(1)*. The region-specific pattern and the time-course of the GFAP response are consistent with decrements in TH *(1)*, TH activity *(39)*, dopamine *(1,39)* (*see* Fig. 4) and the patterns of silver *(1)* and Fluoro-Jade staining *(155)*. Consistent with the silver staining data, FEN did not result in an increase in GFAP *(1)*. All of these data portray METH, MDMA, and MDA, but not FEN, as dopaminergic neurotoxicants. GFAP levels also can be used to demonstrate not only the dosage-dependent nature of the apparent nerve-terminal damage *(1)* but the neuroprotective role of reduced body temperature (*see* below). The effects of METH, MDMA, and MDA are in marked contrast to the effects of these compounds in the rat where 5-HT pathways are partially (METH or MDA) or nearly exclusively (MDMA) targeted.

5.2.6. Microglia

Neurotoxic regimens of METH in the mouse have not been reported to engender a microglial activation. Although short-lived, the microglial response should occur just prior to the induction of astrogliosis, based on data obtained from existing toxicant-exposure models (e.g., *see* refs. *91,102*). Using a neurotoxic regimen of METH, we have obtained preliminary evidence for activation of microglial signaling elements, in vivo, prior to the induction of GFAP *(156)*. A greater understanding of the signaling mechanisms underlying gliosis may lead to earlier detection of neural damage and offer greater potential for therapeutic intervention *(156)*.

5.3. Effects of Temperature

As Bowyer has so elegantly documented *(2)*, an elevation in body temperature to or above 41°C is necessary for METH to produce striatal dopamine-terminal degeneration in the rat. Core temperatures of this degree are at or near that producing lethal hyperthermia and METH can cause temperatures to spike above this level. Therefore, rats must be carefully monitored and their temperatures rapidly reduced by immersion in ice water or other reduced temperature environments to ensure their survival. Although amphetamines can cause striatal dopaminergic nerve-terminal degeneration in the mouse, the role of core-temperature elevation in this damage response to drug exposure is uncertain. We do know that damage can occur in the mouse at core temperatures well below those required to produce degeneration in the rat *(see* Fig. 4) *(1,14,34,35)*. We also know that any manipulation capable of reducing body temperature during the period of treatment is capable of reducing or completely blocking the terminal degeneration associated with exposure to the amphetamines *(1,14,31,33,34)*. This includes pharmacological treatments such as MK-801, pentobarbital, ethanol, and even fenfluramine *(14)*; a reduction in ambient temperature from 22 to 15°C *(14,31)*; removal of the adrenal *(35)*; and whole-body restraint *(14)*. Although this data reinforces the idea that there is a link between body temperature and amphetamine neurotoxicity, the exact nature of the link is far from clear. Thus, some compounds can lower body temperature quite significantly during the period of dosing but provide only partial neuroprotection *(see* Fig. 6 in ref. *14)*. Reserpine, for example, administered to mice 18 h. prior to METH exposure results in a dramatically lowered basal temperature and an even lower temperature when given in combination with METH *(33)*. It provides, however, no protection against the METH-induced striatal dopamine depletion *(33)*. The difficulty in determining the exact role of body temperature in the neurotoxic effects of amphetamines is because of the lack of knowledge concerning the exact mechanism by which the amphetamines can cause terminal degeneration. Furthermore, complicating this issue is the lack of information as to the role of core temperature relative to brain temperature in the neurotoxicity of the amphetamines. However, continued study of the role of temperature, especially in situations where neurotoxicity occurs and body temperature is not elevated, may provide important clues as to the mechanism by which amphetamines exact their neurotoxic effects.

6. SUMMARY AND CONCLUSIONS

We have briefly reviewed the current dogma ascribed to the "neurotoxic" effects of substituted amphetamines. We also have provided an overview of criteria that need to be satisfied to demonstrate that a compound has damaged the brain. In so doing we have challenged the contention that many substituted amphetamines are serotonin and dopamine neurotoxins because not all amphetamine-induced decreases in serotonin and dopamine markers are associated with evidence of neural damage. Based on the points we have made, we conclude:

1. Amphetamine-induced alterations in dopaminergic and serotonergic markers can occur in the absence of evidence of neural damage. This conclusion is based on the observation that amphetamines can exert long-term effects on dopamine and serotonin systems that are regulatory in nature or, at the least, that occur without destruction of the serotonin or dopamine nerve-terminal fields.

2. Damage profiles of different amphetamines differ between rats and mice. Compounds that deplete, for example serotonin, in the rat (e.g., MDMA) appear to selectively destroy dopamine terminals in the mouse. In general, damage is easier to induce in mice and expression of damage markers almost exclusively is associated with the dopaminergic system.

3. Core temperature (hyperthermia and hypothermia) plays an important role in amphetamine-induced brain damage. Sustained elevations in core temperature in the rat (i.e., lethal elevations in the absence of a cold "rescue") are required for damage to dopaminergic nerve terminals. Sustained elevations in core temperature in the rat enhance amphetamine-induced decreases in serotonin but do not lead to damage to serotonergic nerve terminals. Amphetamine-induced damage to the dopaminergic neurons in the mouse is associated with only minor elevations in core temperature. Most agents or conditions that lower core temperature in the presence of an amphetamine afford at least a partial neuroprotective action. These observations underscore the importance of species-dependent aspects of neurodegenerative responses to amphetamines and the complex and poorly understood role of body temperature.

A great deal of data has been accumulated over the past decades concerning aspects of amphetamine action that have been viewed as evidence for "neurotoxicity." Some amphetamine-related changes may in fact be reflective of neuronal damage, whereas other changes may reflect downregulation of monoamine markers. Future research would benefit from an emphasis on defining the damage as opposed to the "changed" condition associated with exposures to substituted amphetamines. To understand the potential for these compounds to adversely affect the nervous system, we must understand the significance of long-term changes in relation to changes reflective of neural damage.

ACKNOWLEDGMENTS

The authors acknowledge Dr. George R. Breese for teaching us the i.c.v. injection procedure and Dr. Karl F. Jensen for performing the cupric silver staining and GFAP immunohistochemistry on the 5,7-DHT-treated rats. Drs. E. Anne Johnson and Stanley A. Benkovic are thanked for a critical review of the manuscript. We thank Dr. John F. Bowyer for his sound advice and Ms. Beth Ann Walker and Dr. Stanley A. Benkovic for excellent assistance in preparing the figures and table. This work was supported in part by NIDA IAG RA-ND-89-4.

REFERENCES

1. O'Callaghan, J. P. and D. B. Miller. (1994) Neurotoxicity profiles of substituted amphetamines in the C57BL/6J mouse. *J. Pharmacol. Exp. Ther.* **270,** 741–751.

2. Bowyer, J. F. and Holson, R. R. (1995) Methamphetamine and amphetamine neurotoxicity, in *Handbook of Neurotoxicology* (Chang, L. W. and Dyer, R. S., eds.), Marcel Dekker, New York, pp. 845–870.

3. Wilson, J. M., Kalasinsky, K. S., Levey, A. I., Bergeron, C., Reiber, G., Anthony, R. M., et al. (1996) Striatal dopamine nerve terminal markers in human, chronic methamphetamine users. *Nat. Med.* **2,** 699–703.

4. Steele, T. D., McCann, U. D., and Ricaurte, G. A. (1994) 3,4-Methylenedioxymethamphetamine (MDMA, "Ecstasy"): pharmacology and toxicology in animals and humans. *Addiction* **89,** 539–551.

5. Schmidt, C. J. and Kehne, J. H. (1990) Neurotoxicity of MDMA: neurochemical effects. *Ann. NY Acad. Sci.* **600,** 665–680.

6. Kish, S. J., Furukawa, Y., Ang, L., Vorce, S. P., and Kalasinsky, K. S. (2000) Striatal serotonin is depleted in brain of a human MDMA (Ecstasy) user. *Neurology* **55,** 294–296.

7. Gouzoulis-Mayfrank, E., Daumann, J., Tuchtenhagen, F., Pelz, S., Becker, S., Kunert, H. J., et al. (2000) Impaired cognitive performance in drug free users of recreational ecstasy (MDMA). *J. Neurol. Neurosurg. Psychiatry* **68,** 719–725.

8. McCann, U. D., Seiden, L. S., Rubin, L. J., and Ricaurte, G. A. (1997) Brain serotonin neurotoxicity and primary pulmonary hypertension from fenfluramine and dexfenfluramine. A systematic review of the evidence. *JAMA* **278,** 666–672.

9. Angold, A., Erkanli, A., Egger, H. L., and Costello, E. J. (2000) Stimulant treatment for children: a community perspective. *J. Am. Acad. Child Adolesc. Psychiatry* **39,** 975–984.

10. Rowland, A. S., Umbach, D. M., O'Callaghan, J. P., Miller, D. B., and Dunnick, J. K. (2001) Public health and toxicological issues concerning stimulant treatment of ADHD, in *Diagnosis and Treatment of Attention-Deficit/Hyperactivity Disorder: An Evidence-Based Approach* (Jensen, P., ed.), AMA Press, Chicago, in press.

11. O'Callaghan, J. P., Jensen, K. F., and Miller, D. B. (1995) Quantitative aspects of drug and toxicant-induced astrogliosis. *Neurochem. Int.* **26,** 115–124.

12. Ricaurte, G. A., Schuster, C. R., and Seiden, L. S. (1980) Long-term effects of repeated methylamphetamine administration on dopamine and serotonin neurons in the rat brain: a regional study. *Brain Res.* **193,** 153–163.

13. Ricaurte, G. A., Guillery, R. W., Seiden, L. S., Schuster, C. R., and Moore, R. Y. (1982) Dopamine nerve terminal degeneration produced by high doses of methylamphetamine in the rat brain. *Brain Res.* **235,** 93–103.

14. Miller, D. B. and O'Callaghan, J. P. (1994) Environment-, drug- and stress- induced alterations in body temperature affect the neurotoxicity of substituted amphetamines in the C57BL/6J mouse. *J. Pharmacol. Exp. Ther.* **270,** 752–760.

15. Hotchkiss, A. J. and Gibb, J. W. (1980) Long-term effects of multiple doses of methamphetamine on tryptophan hydroxylase and tyrosine hydroxylase activity in rat brain. *J. Pharmacol. Exp. Ther.* **214,** 257–262.

16. Schmidt, C. J. and Taylor, V. L. (1987) Depression of rat brain tryptophan hydroxylase activity following the acute administration of methylenedioxymethamphetamine. *Biochem. Pharmacol.* **36,** 4095–4102.

17. Fleckenstein, A. E., Haughey, H. M., Metzger, R. R., Kokoshka, J. M., Riddle, E. L., Hanson, J. E., et al. (1999) Differential effects of psychostimulants and related agents on dopaminergic and serotonergic transporter function. *Eur. J. Pharmacol.* **382,** 45–49.

18. Kim, S., Westphalen, R., Callahan, B., Hatzidimitriou, G., Yuan, J., and Ricaurte, G. A. (2000) Toward development of an in vitro model of methamphetamine-induced dopamine nerve terminal toxicity. *J. Pharmacol. Exp. Ther.* **293,** 625–633.

19. Battaglia, G., Yeh, S. Y., O'Hearn, E., Molliver, M. E., Kuhar, M. J., and De Souza, E. B. (1987) 3,4-Methylenedioxymethamphetamine and 3,4-methylenedioxyamphetamine destroy serotonin terminals in rat brain: quantification of neurodegeneration by measurement of [3H]paroxetine-labeled serotonin uptake sites. *J. Pharmacol. Exp. Ther.* **242,** 911–916.

20. Kalia, M., O'Callaghan, J. P., Miller, D. B., and Kramer, M. (2000) Comparative study of fluoxetine, sibutramine, sertraline and dexfenfluramine on the morphology of serotonergic nerve terminals using serotonin immunohistochemistry. *Brain Res.* **858,** 92–105.

21. Kalia, M. (1991) Reversible, short-lasting, and dose-dependent effect of (+)–fenfluramine on neocortical serotonergic axons. *Brain Res.* **548,** 111–125.

22. Bowyer, J. F., Davies, D. L., Schmued, L., Broening, H. W., Newport, G. D., Slikker, Jr., W., and Holson, R. R. (1994) Further studies of the role of hyperthermia in methamphetamine neurotoxicity. *J. Pharmacol. Exp. Ther.* **268,** 1571–1580.

23. Ricaurte, G. A., Forno, L. S., Wilson, M. A., Delanney, L. E., Irwin, I., Molliver, M. E., and Langston, J. W. (1988) (+/-)3,4-Methylenedioxymethamphetamine selectively damages central serotonergic neurons in nonhuman primates. *JAMA* **260,** 51–55.

24. Johannessen, J. N., Chiueh, C. C., Burns, R. S., and Markey, S. P. (1985) Differences in the metabolism of MPTP in the rodent and primate parallel differences in sensitivity to its neurotoxic effects. *Life Sci.* **36,** 219–224.

25. Chiueh, C. C., Markey, S. P., Burns, R. S., Johannessen, J. N., Jacobowitz, D. M., and Kopin, I. J. (1984) Neurochemical and behavioral effects of 1-methyl-4-phenyl-1,2,3,6-tetrahydropyridine (MPTP) in rat, guinea pig, and monkey. *Psychopharmacol. Bull.* **20,** 548–553.

26. Giovanni, A., Sonsalla, P. K., and Heikkila, R. E. (1994) Studies on species sensitivity to the dopaminergic neurotoxin 1-methyl-4-phenyl-1,2,3,6-tetrahydropyridine. Part 2: Central administration of 1-methyl-4-phenylpyridinium. *J. Pharmacol. Exp. Ther.* **270,** 1008–1014.

27. Giovanni, A., Sieber, B. A., Heikkila, R. E., and Sonsalla, P. K. (1994) Studies on species sensitivity to the dopaminergic neurotoxin 1-methyl-4-phenyl-1,2,3,6-tetrahydropyridine. Part 1: Systemic administration. *J. Pharmacol. Exp. Ther.* **270,** 1000–1007.

28. Chance, M. R. A. (1946) Aggregation as a factor influencing the toxicity of sympathomimetic amines in mice. *J. Pharmacol. Exp. Ther.* **87,** 214–219.

29. Askew, B. M. (1962) Hyperpyrexia as a contributory factor in the toxicity of amphetamine to aggregated mice. *Eur. J. Pharmacol.* **19,** 245–257.

30. Gordon, C. J., Watkinson, W. P., O'Callaghan, J. P., and Miller, D. B. (1991) Effects of 3,4-methylenedioxymethamphetamine on autonomic thermoregulatory responses of the rat. *Pharmacol. Biochem. Behav.* **38,** 339–344.

31. Ali, S. F., Newport, G. D., Holson, R. R., Slikker, Jr., W., and Bowyer, J. F. (1994) Low environmental temperatures or pharmacologic agents that produce hypothermia decrease methamphetamine neurotoxicity in mice. *Brain Res.* **658,** 33–38.

32. Ali, S. F., Newport, R. R., Holson, W., Slikker, Jr., W., and Bowyer, J. F. (1995) Low environmental temperatures or pharmacologic agents that produce hyperthermia decrease methamphetamine neurotoxicity in mice. *Ann. NY Acad. Sci.* **765,** 338.

33. Albers, D. S. and Sonsalla, P. K. (1995) Methamphetamine-induced hyperthermia and dopaminergic neurotoxicity in mice: pharmacological profile of protective and nonprotective agents. *J. Pharmacol. Exp. Ther.* **275,** 1104–1114.

34. Miller, D. B. and O'Callaghan, J. P. (1995) The role of temperature, stress, and other factors in the neurotoxicity of the substituted amphetamines 3,4-methylenedioxymethamphetamine and fenfluramine. *Mol. Neurobiol.* **11,** 177–192.

35. Miller, D. B. and O'Callaghan, J. P. (1996) Neurotoxicity of d-amphetamine in the C57BL/6J and CD-1 mouse. Interactions with stress and the adrenal system. *Ann. NY Acad. Sci.* **801,** 148–167.

36. Johnson, E. A., Sharp, D. S., and Miller, D. B. (2000) Restraint as a stressor in mice against the dopaminergic neurotoxicity of D-MDMA, low body weight mitigates restraint-induced hypothermia and consequent neuroprotection. *Brain Res.* **895,** 107–118.

37. Malberg, J. E. and Seiden, L. S. (1998) Small changes in ambient temperature cause large changes in 3,4-methylenedioxymethamphetamine (MDMA)-induced serotonin neurotoxicity and core body temperature in the rat. *J. Neurosci.* **18,** 5086–5094.

38. Malberg, J. E., Sabol, K. E., and Seiden, L. S. (1996) Co-administration of MDMA with drugs that protect against MDMA neurotoxicity produces different effects on body temperature in the rat. *J. Pharmacol. Exp. Ther.* **278,** 258–267.

39. Sonsalla, P. K., Nicklas, W. J., and Heikkila R. E. (1989) Role for excitatory amino acids in methamphetamine-induced nigrostriatal dopaminergic toxicity. *Science* **243,** 398–400.

40. Miller, D. B. and O'Callaghan, J. P. (1993) The interactions of MK-801 with the amphetamine analogues D-methamphetamine (D-METH), 3,4-methylenedioxymethamphetamine

(D-MDMA) or D-fenfluramine (D-FEN): neural damage and neural protection. *Ann. NY Acad. Sci.* **679,** 321–324.

41. Wagner, G. C., Ricaurte, G. A., Seiden, L. S., Schuster, C. R., Miller, R. J., and Westley, J. (1980) Long-lasting depletions of striatal dopamine and loss of dopamine uptake sites following repeated administration of methamphetamine. *Brain Res.* **181,** 151–160.

42. Commins, D. L., Vosmer, G., Virus, R. M., Woolverton, W. L., Schuster, C. R., and Seiden, L. S. (1987) Biochemical and histological evidence that methylenedioxymethylamphetamine (MDMA) is toxic to neurons in the rat brain. *J. Pharmacol. Exp. Ther.* **241,** 338–345.

43. O'Callaghan, J. P. and Miller, D. B. (1997) Brain serotonin neurotoxicity and fenfluramine and dexfenfluramine. *JAMA* **278,** 2141–2142.

44. O'Callaghan, J. P. and Miller, D. B. (1993) Quantification of reactive gliosis as an approach to neurotoxicity assessment. *NIDA Res. Monogr.* **136,** 188–212.

45. O'Callaghan, J. P. (1994) Biochemical analysis of glial fibrillary acidic protein as a quantitative approach to neurotoxicity assessment: advantages, disadvantages and application to the assessment of NMDA receptor antagonist-induced neurotoxicity. *Psychopharmacol. Bull.* **30,** 549–554.

46. O'Callaghan, J. P. (1993) Quantitative features of reactive gliosis following toxicant-induced damage of the CNS. *Ann. NY Acad. Sci.* **679,** 195–210.

47. Adams, J. H. and Duchen, L. W. (eds.) (1992) *Greenfield's Neuropathology,* 5th ed. Oxford University Press, Oxford, UK.

48. Clark, C. M. and Trojanowski, J. Q. (eds.) (2000) *Neurodegenerative Dementias.* McGraw-Hill, New York.

49. Jellinger, K. (1987) The pathology of parkinsonism, in *Movement Disorders* (Marsden, C. D. and Fahn, S., eds.), Butterworth Press, London, pp. 124–165.

50. Dunnett, S. B. and Bjorklund, A. (1999) Prospects for new restorative and neuroprotective treatments in Parkinson's disease. *Nature* **399,** A32–A39.

51. Simuni, T. and Hurtig, H. I. (2000) Parkinson's disease: the clinical picture, in *Neurodegenerative Dementias* (Clark, C. M. and Trojanowski, J. Q., eds.), McGraw-Hill, New York, pp. 219–228.

52. Miller, D. B., Reinhard, Jr., J. F., Daniels, A. J., and O'Callaghan, J. P. (1991) Diethyldithiocarbamate potentiates the neurotoxicity of in vivo 1-methyl-4-phenyl–1,2,3,6-tetrahydropyridine and of in vitro 1-methyl-4-phenylpyridinium. *J. Neurochem.* **57,** 541–549.

53. Curzon, G. (1990) Serotonin and appetite. *Ann. NY Acad. Sci.* **600,** 521–530.

54. Gorzalka, B. B., Mendelson, S. D., and Watson, N. V. (1990) Serotonin receptor subtypes and sexual behavior. *Ann. NY Acad. Sci.* **600,** 435–444.

55. Meltzer, H. Y. (1990) Role of serotonin in depression. *Ann. NY Acad. Sci.* **600,** 486–499.

56. Cooper, J. R., Bloom, F. E., and Roth, R. H. (eds.) (1996) *The Biochemical Basis of Neuropharmacology,* 7th ed. Oxford University Press, New York.

57. Spencer, P. S. and Schaumburg, H. H. (eds.) (1980) *Experimental and Clinical Neurotoxicology,* 1st ed. Williams and Wilkins, Baltimore.

58. Spencer, P. S. and Schaumburg, H. H. (eds.) (2000) *Experimental and Clinical Neurotoxicology,* 2nd ed. Oxford University Press, New York.

59. Klaassen, C. D. (ed.) (1996) *Cassarett & Doull's Toxicology,* 5th ed. McGraw-Hill, New York.

60. Monaghan, D. T., Bridges, R. J., and Cotman, C. W. (1989) The excitatory amino acid receptors: their classes, pharmacology, and distinct properties in the function of the central nervous system. *Annu. Rev. Pharmacol. Toxicol.* **29,** 365–402.

61. Fix, A. S., Stitzel, S. R., Ridder, G. M., and Switzer, R. C. (2000) MK-801 neurotoxicity in cupric silver-stained sections: lesion reconstruction by 3-dimensional computer image analysis. *Toxicol. Pathol.* **28,** 84–90.

62. Wozniak, D. F., Dikranian, K., Ishimaru, M. J., Nardi, A., Corso, T. D., Tenkova, T., et al. (1998) Disseminated corticolimbic neuronal degeneration induced in rat brain by MK-801: potential relevance to Alzheimer's disease. *Neurobiol. Dis.* **5**, 305–322.

63. Fix, A. S., Wightman, K. A., and O'Callaghan, J. P. (1995) Reactive gliosis induced by MK–801 in the rat posterior cingulate/retrosplenial cortex: GFAP evaluation by sandwich ELISA and immunocytochemistry. *Neurotoxicology* **16**, 229–237.

64. Switzer, R. C., Murphy, M. R., Campbell, S. K., Kerenyi, S. A., and Miller, S. A. (1988) Soman in multiple low doses: famage to selected populations of neurons in rat brain. *Soc.Neurosci. Abstr.* **14**, 774–774.

65. Switzer, R. C., III. (2000) Application of silver degeneration stains for neurotoxicity testing. *Toxicol. Pathol.* **28**, 70–83.

66. Tanaka, D., Jr. and Bursian, S. J. (1989) Degeneration patterns in the chicken central nervous system induced by ingestion of the organophosphorus delayed neurotoxin tri-ortho-tolyl phosphate. A silver impregnation study. *Brain Res.* **484**, 240–256.

67. Schmued, L. C. and Hopkins, K. J. (2000) Fluoro-Jade: novel fluorochromes for detecting toxicant-induced neuronal degeneration. *Toxicol. Pathol.* **28**, 91–99.

68. O'Callaghan, J. P. and Jensen, K. F. (1992) Enhanced expression of glial fibrillary acidic protein and the cupric silver degeneration reaction can be used as sensitive and early indicators of neurotoxicity. *Neurotoxicology* **13**, 113–122.

69. Switzer, R. C., III (1993) Silver staining methods: their role in detecting neurotoxicity. *Ann. NY Acad. Sci.* **679**, 341–348.

70. Switzer, R. C., III (1991) Strategies for assessing neurotoxicity. *Neurosci. Biobehav. Rev.* **15**, 89–93.

71. O'Callaghan, J. P. and Miller, D. B. (1986) Diethyldithiocarbamate increases distribution of cadmium to brain but prevents cadmium-induced neurotoxicity. *Brain Res.* **370**, 354–358.

72. Llorens, J., Crofton, K. M., and O'Callaghan, J. P. (1993) Administration of 3,3'-iminodipropionitrile to the rat results in region-dependent damage to the central nervous system at levels above the brain stem. *J. Pharmacol. Exp. Ther.* **265**, 1492–1498.

73. Balaban, C. D., O'Callaghan, J. P., and Billingsley, M. L. (1988) Trimethyltin-induced neuronal damage in the rat brain: comparative studies using silver degeneration stains, immunocytochemistry and immunoassay for neuronotypic and gliotypic proteins. *Neuroscience* **26**, 337–361.

74. Brock, T. O. and O'Callaghan, J. P. (1987) Quantitative changes in the synaptic vesicle proteins synapsin I and p38 and the astrocyte-specific protein glial fibrillary acidic protein are associated with chemical-induced injury to the rat central nervous system. *J. Neurosci.* **7**, 931–942.

75. O'Callaghan, J. P., Miller, D. B., and Reinhard, Jr. J. F. (1990) 1-Methyl-4-phenyl-1,2,3,6-tetrahydropyridine (MPTP)-induced damage of striatal dopaminergic fibers attenuates subsequent astrocyte response to MPTP. *Neurosci. Lett.* **117**, 228–233.

76. Gramsbergen, J. B. and Van Den Berg, K. J. (1994) Regional and temporal profiles of calcium accumulation and glial fibrillary acidic protein levels in rat brain after systemic injection of kainic acid. *Brain Res.* **667**, 216–228.

77. Appel, N. M., Rapoport, S. I., O'Callaghan, J. P., Bell, J. M., and Freed, L. M. (1997) Sequelae of parenteral domoic acid administration in rats: comparison of effects on different metabolic markers in brain. *Brain Res.* **754**, 55–64.

78. Appel, N. M., Rapoport, S. I., and O'Callaghan, J. P. (1997) Sequelae of parenteral domoic acid administration in rats: comparison of effects on different anatomical markers in brain. *Synapse* **25**, 350–358.

79. Miller, P. J. and Zaborszky, L. (1997) 3-Nitropropionic acid neurotoxicity: visualization by silver staining and implications for use as an animal model of Huntington's disease. *Exp. Neurol.* **146**, 212–229.

80. O'Callaghan, J. P. and Miller, D. B. (1985) Cerebellar hypoplasia in the Gunn rat is associated with quantitative changes in neurotypic and gliotypic proteins. *J. Pharmacol. Exp. Ther.* **234,** 522–533.

81. Hedreen, J. C. and Chalmers, J. P. (1972) Neuronal degeneration in rat brain induced by 6-hydroxydopamine; a histological and biochemical study. *Brain Res.* **47,** 1–36.

82. Frankfurt, M., O'Callaghan, J., and Beaudet, A. (1991) 5,7-Dihydroxytryptamine injections increase glial fibrillary acidic protein in the hypothalamus of adult rats. *Brain Res.* **549,** 138–140.

83. Dugar, A., Patanow, C., O'Callaghan, J. P., and Lakoski, J. M. (1998) Immunohistochemical localization and quantification of glial fibrillary acidic protein and synaptosomal-associated protein (mol. wt 25000) in the ageing hippocampus following administration of 5,7-dihydroxytryptamine. *Neuroscience* **85,** 123–133.

84. Desclin, J. C. and Escubi, J. (1974) Effects of 3-acetylpyridine on the central nervous system of the rat, as demonstrated by silver methods. *Brain Res.* **77,** 349–364.

85. O'Callaghan, J. P., Rogers, T. S., Rodman, L. E., and Page, J. G. (1996) Acute and chronic administration of ibogaine to the rat results in astrogliosis that is not confined to the cerebellar vermis. *Ann. NY Acad. Sci.* **801,** 205–216.

86. Goodlett, C. R., Leo, J. T., O'Callaghan, J. P., Mahoney, J. C., and West, J. R. (1993) Transient cortical astrogliosis induced by alcohol exposure during the neonatal brain growth spurt in rats. *Brain Res. Dev. Brain Res.* **72,** 85–97.

87. Goldey, E. S., O'Callaghan, J. P., Stanton, M. E., Barone, Jr., S., and Crofton, K. M. (1994) Developmental neurotoxicity: evaluation of testing procedures with methylazoxymethanol and methylmercury. *Fundam. Appl. Toxicol.* **23,** 447–464.

88. O'Callaghan, J. P. and Miller, D. B. (1988) Acute exposure of the neonatal rat to triethyltin results in persistent changes in neurotypic and gliotypic proteins. *J. Pharmacol. Exp. Ther.* **244,** 368–378.

89. Schmued, L. and Hopkins K.J. (2000) Fluoro-Jade B: A high affinity fluorescent marker for the localization of neuronal degeneration. *Brain Res.* **874,** 123–130.

90. Schmued, L. and Slikker, Jr., W. (1999) Black-gold: a simple, high-resolution histochemical label for normal and pathological myelin in brain tissue sections. *Brain Res.* **837,** 289–297.

91. Streit, W. J., Walter, S. A., and Pennell, N. A. (1999) Reactive microgliosis. *Prog. Neurobiol.* **57,** 563–581.

92. Streit, W. J. (1996) The role of microglia in brain injury. *Neurotoxicology* **17,** 671–678.

93. Kreutzberg, G. W. (1996) Microglia: a sensor for pathological events in the CNS. *Trends Neurosci.* **19,** 312–318.

94. Eng, L. F. (1988) Regulation of glial intermediate filaments in astrogliosis, in *Biochemical Pathology of Astrocytes* (Norenberg, M. D., Hertz, L., and Schousboe, A., eds.), Alan R. Liss, New York, pp. 79–90.

95. Norton, W. T., Aquino, D. A., Hozumi, I., Chiu, F. C., and Brosnan, C. F. (1992) Quantitative aspects of reactive gliosis: a review. *Neurochem. Res.* **17,** 877–885.

96. Bignami, A. and Dahl, D. (1995) Gliosis, in *Neuroglia* (Kettenmann, H. and Ransom B. R., eds.), Oxford University Press, New York, pp. 843–858.

97. Little, A. R. and O'Callaghan, J. P. (2001) The astrocyte response to neural injury: a review and reconsideration of key features, in *Site-Selective Neurotoxicity* (Lester, D., Slikker, Jr., W., Johannessen, J. N., and Lazarovici, P., eds.), Harwood Academic Publishers, Amsterdam, Netherlands.

98. Eng, L. F. (1985) Glial fibrillary acidic protein (GFAP): the major protein of glial intermediate filaments in differentiated astrocytes. *J. Neuroimmunol.* **8,** 203–214.

99. Martin, P. M. and O'Callaghan, J. P. (1995) A direct comparison of GFAP immunocytochemistry and GFAP concentration in various regions of ethanol-fixed rat and mouse brain. *J. Neurosci. Methods* **58,** 181–192.

100. Martin, P. M. and O'Callaghan, J. P. (1995) Biochemical immunohistology, in *Central Nervous System Trauma-Research Techniques* (Ohnishi, S. T. and Ohnishi, T., eds.), CRC Press, Boca Raton, FL, 509–516.

101. O'Callaghan, J. P. (1991) Quantification of glial fibrillary acidic protein: comparison of slot-immunobinding assays with a novel sandwich ELISA. *Neurotoxicol. Teratol.* **13**, 275–281.

102. McCann, M. J., O'Callaghan, J. P., Martin, P. M., Bertram, T., and Streit, W. J. (1996) Differential activation of microglia and astrocytes following trimethyl tin-induced neurodegeneration. *Neuroscience* **72**, 273–281.

103. Moskowitz, M. A., Rubin, D., Nowak, Jr., T. S., Baliga, B. S., and Munro, H. N. (1978) Site of action of neurotoxins on protein synthesis. *Ann. NY Acad. Sci.* **305**, 96–106.

104. Stone, D. M., Johnson, M., Hanson, G. R., and Gibb, J. W. (1989) Acute inactivation of tryptophan hydroxylase by amphetamine analogs involves the oxidation of sulfhydryl sites. *Eur. J. Pharmacol.* **172**, 93–97.

105. Kuhn, D. M. and Arthur, Jr., R. (1998) Dopamine inactivates tryptophan hydroxylase and forms a redox-cycling quinoprotein: possible endogenous toxin to serotonin neurons. *J. Neurosci.* **18**, 7111–7117.

106. Lavoie, M. J. and Hastings, T. G. (1999) Dopamine quinone formation and protein modification associated with the striatal neurotoxicity of methamphetamine: evidence against a role for extracellular dopamine. *J. Neurosci.* **19**, 1484–1491.

107. Pennypacker, K. R., Hong, J. S., and McMillian, M. K. (1995) Implications of prolonged expression of Fos-related antigens. *Trends Pharmacol. Sci.* **16**, 317–321.

108. Pennypacker, K. R. (1995) AP-1 transcription factor complexes in CNS disorders and development. *J. Fla. Med. Assoc.* **82**, 551–554.

109. Bowyer, J. F., Tank, A. W., Newport, G. D., Slikker, W., Jr., Ali, S. F., and Holson, R. R. (1992) The influence of environmental temperature on the transient effects of methamphetamine on dopamine levels and dopamine release in rat striatum. *J. Pharmacol. Exp. Ther.* **260**, 817–824.

110. Kekuda, R., Torres-Zamorano, V., Leibach, F. H., and Ganapathy, V. (1997) Human serotonin transporter: regulation by the neuroprotective agent aurintricarboxylic acid and by epidermal growth factor. *J. Neurochem.* **68**, 1443–1450.

111. Lesch, K. P., Aulakh, C. S., Wolozin, B. L., Tolliver, T. J., Hill, J. L., and Murphy, D. L. (1993) Regional brain expression of serotonin transporter mRNA and its regulation by reuptake inhibiting antidepressants. *Brain Res. Mol. Brain Res.* **17**, 31–35.

112. Wilson, J. M. and Kish, S. J. (1996) The vesicular monoamine transporter, in contrast to the dopamine transporter, is not altered by chronic cocaine self-administration in the rat. *J. Neurosci.* **16**, 3507–3510.

113. Zhou, D., Huether, G., Wiltfang, J., Hajak, G., and Ruther, E. (1996) Serotonin transporters in the rat frontal cortex: lack of circadian rhythmicity but down-regulation by food restriction. *J. Neurochem.* **67**, 656–661.

114. Ryan, L. J., Martone, M. E., Linder, J. C., and Groves, P. M. (1988) Continuous amphetamine administration induces tyrosine hydroxylase immunoreactive patches in the adult rat neostriatum. *Brain Res. Bull.* **21**, 133–137.

115. Molliver, M. E., Berger, U. V., Mamounas, L. A., Molliver, D. C., O'Hearn, E., and Wilson, M. A. (1990) Neurotoxicity of MDMA and related compounds: anatomic studies. *Ann. NY Acad. Sci.* **600**, 649–661.

116. O'Hearn, E., Battaglia, G., De Souza, E. B., Kuhar, M. J., and Molliver, M. E. (1988) Methylenedioxyamphetamine (MDA) and methylenedioxymethamphetamine (MDMA) cause selective ablation of serotonergic axon terminals in forebrain: immunocytochemical evidence for neurotoxicity. *J. Neurosci.* **8**, 2788–2803.

117. Fischer, C., Hatzidimitriou, G., Wlos, J., Katz, J., and Ricaurte, G. (1995) Reorganization of ascending 5-HT axon projections in animals previously exposed to the recreational

drug (+/-)3,4-methylenedioxymethamphetamine (MDMA, "ecstasy"). *J. Neurosci.* **15**, 5476–5485.

118. Appel, N. M., Contrera, J. F., and De Souza, E. B. (1989) Fenfluramine selectively and differentially decreases the density of serotonergic nerve terminals in rat brain: evidence from immunocytochemical studies. *J. Pharmacol. Exp. Ther.* **249**, 928–943.

119. Cubells, J. F., Rayport, S., Rajendran, G., and Sulzer, D. (1994) Methamphetamine neurotoxicity involves vacuolation of endocytic organelles and dopamine-dependent intracellular oxidative stress. *J. Neurosci.* **14**, 2260–2271.

120. Kuhn, D. M., Aretha, C. W., and Geddes, T. J. (1999) Peroxynitrite inactivation of tyrosine hydroxylase: mediation by sulfhydryl oxidation, not tyrosine nitration. *J. Neurosci.* **19**, 10,289–10,294.

121. Kuhn, D. M. and Geddes, T. J. (1999) Peroxynitrite inactivates tryptophan hydroxylase via sulfhydryl oxidation. Coincident nitration of enzyme tyrosyl residues has minimal impact on catalytic activity. *J. Biol. Chem.* **274**, 29,726–29,732.

122. Tsao, L. I., Ladenheim, B., Andrews, A. M., Chiueh, C. C., Cadet, J. L., and Su, T. P. (1998) Delta opioid peptide [D-Ala2,D-leu5]enkephalin blocks the long-term loss of dopamine transporters induced by multiple administrations of methamphetamine: involvement of opioid receptors and reactive oxygen species. *J. Pharmacol. Exp. Ther.* **287**, 322–331.

123. Kita, T., Takahashi M., Kubo K., Wagner G. C., and Nakashima T. (1999) Hydroxyl radical formation following methamphetamine administration to rats. *Pharmacol. Toxicol.* **85**, 133–137.

124. Ali, S. F., Martin, J. L., Black, M. D., and Itzhak, Y. (1999) Neuroprotective role of melatonin in methampheta. *Ann. NY Acad. Sci.* **890**, 119.

125. Stone, D. M., Hanson, G. R., and Gibb, J. W. (1989) In vitro reactivation of rat cortical tryptophan hydroxylase following in vivo inactivation by methylenedioxymethamphetamine. *J. Neurochem.* **53**, 572–581.

126. Ryan, L. J., Linder, J. C., Martone, M. E., and Groves, P. M. (1990) Histological and ultrastructural evidence that D-amphetamine causes degeneration in neostriatum and frontal cortex of rats. *Brain Res.* **518**, 67–77.

127. Jensen, K. F., Olin, J., Haykal-Coates, N., O'Callaghan, J., Miller, D. B., and De Olmos, J. S. (1993) Mapping toxicant-induced nervous system damage with a cupric silver stain: a quantitative analysis of neural degeneration induced by 3,4-methylenedioxymethamphetamine. *NIDA Res. Monogr.* **136**, 133–149.

128. Eisch, A. J., Schmued, L. C., and Marshall, J. F. (1998) Characterizing cortical neuron injury with Fluoro-Jade labeling after a neurotoxic regimen of methamphetamine. *Synapse* **30**, 329–333.

129. Schmued, L., Slikker, W., Clausing, P., and Bowyer, J. (1999) d-Fenfluramine produces neuronal degeneration in localized regions of the cortex, thalamus, and cerebellum of the rat. *Toxicol. Sci.* **48**, 100–106.

130. Gordon, M. N., Schreier, W. A., Ou, X., Holcomb, L. A., and Morgan, D. G. (1997) Exaggerated astrocyte reactivity after nigrostriatal deafferentation in the aged rat. *J. Comp Neurol.* **388**, 106–119.

131. Cappon, G. D., Pu, C., and Vorhees, C. V. (2000) Time-course of methamphetamine-induced neurotoxicity in rat caudate-putamen after single-dose treatment. *Brain Res.* **863**, 106–111.

132. Fukumura, M., Cappon, G. D., Pu, C., Broening, H. W., and Vorhees, C. V. (1998) A single dose model of methamphetamine-induced neurotoxicity in rats: effects on neostriatal monoamines and glial fibrillary acidic protein. *Brain Res.* **806**, 1–7.

133. Pu, C. and Vorhees, C. V. (1993) Developmental dissociation of methamphetamine-induced depletion of dopaminergic terminals and astrocyte reaction in rat striatum. *Brain Res. Dev. Brain Res.* **72**, 325–328.

134. O'Callaghan, J. P., Brinton, R. E., and McEwen, B. S. (1991) Glucocorticoids regulate the synthesis of glial fibrillary acidic protein in intact and adrenalectomized rats but do not affect its expression following brain injury. *J. Neurochem.* **57,** 860–869.

135. Akiyama, H. and McGeer, P. L. (1989) Microglial response to 6-hydroxydopamine-induced substantia nigra lesions. *Brain Res.* **489,** 247–253.

136. Wilson, M. A. and Molliver, M. E. (1994) Microglial response to degeneration of serotonergic axon terminals. *Glia* **11,** 18–34.

137. Bowyer, J. F., Peterson, S. L., Rountree, R. L., Tor-Agbidye, J., and Wang, G. J. (1998) Neuronal degeneration in rat forebrain resulting from D-amphetamine-induced convulsions is dependent on seizure severity and age. *Brain Res.* **809,** 77–90.

138. Stewart, C. W. and Slikker, Jr., W. (1999) Hyperthermia-enhanced serotonin (5-HT) depletion resulting from D-fenfluramine (D-Fen) exposure does not evoke a glial-cell response in the central nervous system of rats. *Brain Res.* **839,** 279–282.

139. Hess, A., Desiderio, C., and McAuliffe, W. G. (1990) Acute neuropathological changes in the caudate nucleus caused by MPTP and methamphetamine: immunohistochemical studies. *J. Neurocytol.* **19,** 338–342.

140. Deng, X., Ladenheim, B., Tsao, L. I., and Cadet, J. L. (1999) Null mutation of c-fos causes exacerbation of methamphetamine-induced neurotoxicity. *J. Neurosci.* **19,** 10,107–10,115.

141. Fumagalli, F., Gainetdinov, R. R., Valenzano, K. J., and Caron, M. G. (1998) Role of dopamine transporter in methamphetamine-induced neurotoxicity: evidence from mice lacking the transporter. *J. Neurosci.* **18,** 4861–4869.

142. Kita, T., Paku S., Takahashi M., Kubo K., Wagner G. C., and Nakashima T. (1998) Methamphetamine-induced neurotoxicity in BALB/c, DBA/2N and C57BL/6N mice. *Neuropharmacology* **37,** 1177–1184.

143. O'Dell, S. J., Weihmuller, F. B., and Marshall, J. F. (1991) Multiple methamphetamine injections induce marked increases in extracellular striatal dopamine which correlate with subsequent neurotoxicity. *Brain Res.* **564,** 256–260.

144. Miller, G. W., Gainetdinov, R. R., Levey, A. I., and Caron, M. G. (1999) Dopamine transporters and neuronal injury. *Trends Pharmacol. Sci.* **20,** 424–429.

145. Cadet, J. L., Ali, S. F., Rothman, R. B., and Epstein, C. J. (1995) Neurotoxicity, drugs and abuse, and the CuZn-superoxide dismutase transgenic mice. *Mol. Neurobiol.* **11,** 155–163.

146. Deng, X. and Cadet, J. L. (1999) Methamphetamine administration causes overexpression of nNOS in the mouse striatum. *Brain Res.* **851,** 254–257.

147. Imam, S. Z. and Ali, S. F. (2000) Selenium, an antioxidant, attenuates methamphetamine-induced dopaminergic toxicity and peroxynitrite generation. *Brain Res.* **855,** 186–191.

148. Imam, S. Z., Crow, J. P., Newport, G. D., Islam, F., Slikker, Jr., W., and Ali, S. F. (1999) Methamphetamine generates peroxynitrite and produces dopaminergic neurotoxicity in mice: protective effects of peroxynitrite decomposition catalyst. *Brain Res.* **837,** 15–21.

149. Imam, S. Z., Newport, G. D., Islam, F., Slikker, Jr., W., and Ali, S. F. (1999) Selenium, an antioxidant, protects against methamphetamine-induced dopaminergic neurotoxicity. *Brain Res.* **818,** 575–578.

150. Itzhak, Y., Gandia, C., Huang, P. L., and Ali, S. F. (1998) Resistance of neuronal nitric oxide synthase-deficient mice to methamphetamine-induced dopaminergic neurotoxicity. *J. Pharmacol. Exp. Ther.* **284,** 1040–1047.

151. Jayanthi, S., Ladenheim, B., Andrews, A. M., and Cadet, J. L. (1999) Overexpression of human copper/zinc superoxide dismutase in transgenic mice attenuates oxidative stress caused by methylenedioxymethamphetamine (Ecstasy). *Neuroscience* **91,** 1379–1387.

152. Jayanthi, S., Ladenheim, B., and Cadet, J. L. (1998) Methamphetamine-induced changes in antioxidant enzymes and lipid peroxidation in copper/zinc-superoxide dismutase transgenic mice. *Ann. NY Acad. Sci.* **844,** 92–102.

153. Kim, H., Jhoo, W., Shin, E., and Bing, G. (2000) Selenium deficiency potentiates meth-amphetamine-induced nigral neuronal loss; comparison with MPTP model. *Brain Res.* **862,** 247–252.

154. De Olmos, J. S., Beltramino, C. A., and De Olmos, D. L. (1994) Use of an amino-cupric-silver technique for the detection of early and semiacute neuronal degeneration caused by neurotoxicants, hypoxia, and physical trauma. *Neurotoxicol. Teratol.* **16,** 545–561.

155. Schmued, L. C. and Bowyer, J. F. (1997) Methamphetamine exposure can produce neuronal degeneration in mouse hippocampal remnants. *Brain Res.* **759,** 135–140.

156. Hebert, M. A. and O'Callaghan, J. P. (2000) Protein phosphorylation cascades associated with methamphetamine-induced glial activation. *Ann. NY Acad. Sci.* **914,** 238–262.

12

Studies of Neural Degeneration Indicate that Fasciculus Retroflexus Is a Weak Link in Brain for Many Drugs of Abuse

Gaylord Ellison

1. GOALS OF THIS CHAPTER

The research to be described in this chapter has followed a distinctively different historical path than most neurotoxic research, and this is because of the underlying goals that have guided it. A fundamental question is why one would study the neurotoxic effects of drugs of abuse. One obvious answer is because this is an issue of great relevance to society. Another is because most of the closest models of mental disorders such as schizophrenia, or compulsive disorders, or depression, are based on drug models from addicts. This leads to the hope that understanding the effects of addiction will shed light on many other psychopathologies as well.

However, these goals are frequently forgotten in the race for scientific "progress." Because any compound will have neurotoxic effects on brain if given in sufficient quantities, many workers in this field subscribe to the "more is better" strategy: Give as much drug as one possibly can without killing the animal, or at least too many of the animals, and study the huge effects on brain. This strategy has led to enormous wastes of scientific resources, such as with the methamphetamine neurotoxicity research (reviewed elsewhere in this book and also briefly in this chapter). The experiments to be described in this chapter are based on what I think is a better scientific strategy:

1. To study the literature on addicts, then administer the drugs to animals in the same way addicts take them;
2. While giving the lowest effective dose possible, study the behaviors in the animals, attempting to determine when "breaks" in behavioral reactions occur that seem to mimic those of the addicts, and then;
3. Search for alterations in brain produced by the drugs, scanning the entire brain rather than focusing on only one's favorite structures; and
4. Find, it is hoped, "weak links" in brain for drugs of abuse (i.e., structures that degenerate after a variety of different compounds). Further research can then attempt to determine if these same structures are altered in the comparable endogeneous psychopathologies.

From: Handbook of Neurotoxicology, Vol. 2
Edited by: E. J. Massaro © Humana Press Inc., Totowa, NJ

Table 1
Two Drug Models of Psychosis

1. Stimulant psychoses
   Produced by chronic amphetamine or cocaine abuse
   Well-documented in addicts who develop "speed runs" and in controlled hospital studies
      involving continuously administered amphetamines
   Chief symptoms are stereotypies, paranoid delusions, parasitosis and other sensory
      hallucinations, and loosening of associations
   Evidence of persisting alterations in nervous system ("reactivation")
2. Phencyclidine and ketamine psychosis
   Produced by NMDA antagonists (phencyclidine, ketamine)
   "Bingeing" intake pattern develops in addicts
   Chief symptoms are flat affect, depersonalization, body-image distortion, amnesia,
      catatonia, thought disturbances
   Evidence of persisting memory deficits

2. STIMULANT PSYCHOSES AND "SPEED RUNS"

Many of the experiments to be described here have grown out of attempts to develop animal models of psychosis, and especially of schizophrenia. Because the studies to be described in this chapter have been guided by an attempt to mimic human psychotic states in animals in an effort to develop animal models of schizophrenia, the toxicological implications of this research were not planned—the research dictated this direction. As such, these studies represent an interesting intersection of psychopathology, neuropharmacology, and neurotoxicology. They lead to the suggestion that certain neural pathways in brain may be the "weak links" in psychopathological disorders. Because they are based in part on observations from human drug addicts, the "weak-link pathways" they discover will be only a subset of those pathways in brain that are especially susceptible to neurotoxic effects, i.e., those with a reward component. But compared to the alternative strategies, this approach can have strong implications for the psychiatric clinic, and for the neural foundations of psychopathology.

In humans, there are certain drug-induced states that can be indistinguishable, to the untrained observer, from an endogenous psychosis, such as occurs in acute schizophrenic episodes. In order to develop animal models of these states, one attempts to mimic them by inducing similar drug-induced states in animals and, in controlled studies, thereby clarifying the altered neural mechanisms that underlie these abnormal states. It is generally recognized that there are two principle drug models of psychosis in humans: the stimulant-induced psychoses and phencyclidine-induced psychosis (Table 1). The stimulant psychoses are observed following chronic amphetamine or cocaine abuse. We have previously reviewed *(1–3)* the extensive literature indicating the emergence of a paranoid-like psychosis in chronic amphetamine and cocaine addicts, the chief symptoms of which are motor stereotypies, paranoid delusions, sensory hallucinations, and a loosening of associations. This literature on amphetamine abuse has also been reviewed by Connell *(4)*, Bell *(5)*, and Ellinwood *(6)*, and for cocaine abuse by Siegal *(7)*, Lesko et al. *(8)*, Gawin *(9)*, and Manschreck et al. *(10)*. A particularly interesting feature of this psychosis is the pronounced parasitosis, or the delusion of bugs or snakes on the skin *(11–13)*.

In order to induce a model stimulant psychosis in animals, it is of paramount importance not only to give the proper drugs but also to do so in the proper drug regimen. The development of "speed runs" appear to be a key factor for the induction of stimulant psychoses. It was recognized long ago *(4)* that a true amphetamine psychosis only appears in chronic addicts; that most amphetamine addicts eventually come to self-administer amphetamine every few hours (in binges lasting 5 d or even more); and that towards the end of these binges, they reliably develop paranoid delusions and hallucinations *(14)*. In fact, every controlled study eliciting an overt amphetamine psychosis in humans has involved continuous, low-dose administration of the drug every hour for days (e.g., *see* ref. 15). As the number of binges increases, the paranoia appears earlier and earlier during the binge and can eventually appear upon initial drug exposure (*16*; discussed in ref. *3*). This fact suggests persisting alterations in brain have occurred. Virtually all of these conclusions can be extended to cocaine as well. There is a similarly extensive literature from cocaine addict populations of "runs" that eventually lead to paranoia. Satel et al. *(17)* found that every one of their subjects who had experienced cocaine-induced paranoia did so while on a "binge" of from 6 h to 5 d in duration.

Many years ago, in an effort to mimic amphetamine "speed runs" in animals, we developed a slow-release silicone pellet containing amphetamine base (releasing 20 mg over a 5-d period), and found that rats and nonhuman primates implanted with this pellet showed stages of behavioral alterations that were similar in sequence to those that had been reported in the controlled studies in humans, although the precise behaviors elicited were much more complex in the higher organisms. In rats, continuous amphetamine administration initially resulted in a period during which a sensitization to motor stereotypies elicited by amphetamine developed *(18)* followed by a "late stage" (3–5 d after pellet implantation) in which the motor stereotypies decreased and certain distinctive "late-stage" behaviors emerged, including limb-flicks, wet-dog shakes, spontaneous startle responses, and abnormal social behaviors *(19)*. A similar progression, but with even more distinctive and varied late-stage behaviors occur in monkeys *(1,20)*. Many of these behaviors have been called "hallucinogen-like" because they are normally induced by hallucinogens, whereas they are suppressed by acute injections of amphetamine. Another distinctive late-stage behavior is excited parasitotic grooming episodes. In monkeys this is expressed as rapid, slapping hand movements directed at the skin surface moving from limb to limb *(20)*; in rats this is expressed as a change from the normal body washing and grooming sequence to a body-biting sequence similar to that of a dog inflicted with fleas *(21)*. There are close similarities between the amphetamine and cocaine-induced parasitotic effects in humans and in these animal studies *(22)*.

3. NEUROTOXIC EFFECTS OF CONTINUOUS *D*-AMPHETAMINE IN CAUDATE

These late-stage behaviors induced by continuous amphetamine have a number of distinct neurochemical correlates in brain. Amphetamine continuously administered for 5 d induces alterations including a downregulation of D_2 dopamine receptors in striatum *(23)* and a progressive shift of heightened glucose metabolism away from striatal and towards mesolimbic structures *(1)*. But one of the most striking effects of continuously administered amphetamine is its well-documented neurotoxic effects on dopamine terminals in caudate. Studies of catecholamine fluorescence in animals administered continuous amphetamine *(24–26)* reveal the appearance of swollen, distinct axons with multiple enlarged varicosities and stump-like endings; similar observations were made using silver stains for degenerating axons *(27)*. Furthermore, rats given this pellet showed extremely persisting alterations in tyrosine hydroxylase activity in caudate. The continuous amphetamine was inducing degeneration in dopamine terminals in caudate (but, surprisingly, not in dopamine terminals in accumbens and frontal cortex, nor in norepinephrine terminals anywhere in brain).

4. ESPECIALLY POTENT NEUROTOXIC EFFECTS OF INCESSANT DRUGS

One of the most interesting aspects of this neurotoxic effect is that only continuous amphetamine induces it. If the same amount of amphetamine (20 mg over 5 d, or about 12 mg/kg/d) is given as five daily injections, once each day, there is no neurotoxicity observed. This was initially a rather surprising finding, for the peak brain levels, and behavioral reactions, achieved after such large single injections are enormously greater than those when the drug is administered around-the-clock. However, it now appears that, for a number of pharmacological agents, prolonged plasma levels are more crucial for producing neurotoxicity than are much larger but more transient plasma levels. Apparently neuronal systems have developed more effective ways to cope with sudden and brief insults than with progressive, more prolonged ones. If neurons are given huge amounts of drug, but a period to recover, they do not die. But if not allowed a recovery period, toxicological effects are immense. In retrospect, this is not surprising when considered from the drug model of psychopathology viewpoint. Psychopathologies are typically incessant, around-the-clock disorders, not once a day, extreme disruptions.

5. EXTREME DOSE METHAMPHETAMINE MODEL

The unique capability of continuous amphetamine administration to induce degeneration of dopamine terminals in the caudate nucleus has been validated using a variety of techniques, as reviewed elsewhere in this book. The amphetamine can be delivered by slow-release silicone pellets, minipumps, very frequent injections, or as substantial and frequent doses of methamphetamine, which has a slower rate of clearance and is considerably more potent at releasing dopamine *(28–30)*. Furthermore, Fuller and Hemrick-Luecke *(31)* found that an amphetamine injection administered in combination with drugs that slow its metabolism becomes neurotoxic to caudate dopamine terminals. The amphetamine or methamphetamine-induced damage to dopamine endings can be prevented by pretreatments or concurrent administration of drugs such as a tyrosine hydroxylase inhibitor *(32)*, dopamine uptake inhibitors *(33,34)*, and noncompetitive antagonists of NMDA *(35,36)*.

But most investigators of this effect have employed an "easy" way of getting the neurotoxic effects: giving extremely high doses of methamphetamine every 2 h for a total of five injections. Studies of this high dose methamphetamine-induced neurotoxicity (reviewed in ref. *37*), employ extreme doses. These induce death in 25–30% of the rats, and the rats are in terrible shape behaviorally. In spite of the large number of studies that have employed this drug regimen, it remains problematical to what extent this extreme high-dose strategy has shed light on the mechanisms underlying amphetamine-induced neurotoxicity. Hyperthermia contributes extensively to this degeneration, and this extremely vigorous methamphetamine regimen is probably a poor way to investigate selective neurotoxicity and discover "weak links." Rats given the much lower plasma levels induced by the slow-release silicone pellet containing *d*-amphetamine show zero lethality, and are no more hyperthermic than a normal rat during the active periods of the day. For example, what real conclusions about aftereffects of specific caudate dopamine neurotoxicity can be drawn if persisting motor deficits are found in animals given this extreme high-dose methamphetamine regimen, for these doses also induce damage to serotonin cells, and induce widespread neuronal degeneration in a variety of other structures? Ellison and Switzer *(38)* found degeneration following this extreme high-dose methamphetamine regimen in virtually every white-matter tract in brain, including cerebellum, corpus callosum, and the optic tract.

6. A WEAK LINK: NEUROTOXIC EFFECTS OF ALL CONTINUOUS "DOPAMINERGIC" STIMULANTS IN FASCICULUS RETROFLEXUS

We recently attempted to determine if these findings with amphetamine could be generalized to cocaine psychosis. Cocaine, like amphetamine, also potentiates dopamine at the receptor, is a sympathomimetic, and leads to "speed runs" in chronic addicts who, in some cases, develop a paranoid psychosis similar in many aspects to that induced by amphetamine. The question for the dopamine model of psychosis that grew out of the amphetamine literature was whether continuous cocaine would also have a neurotoxic effect on dopamine terminals in caudate, i.e., if this was an anatomical correlate of the paranoia. Since continuous cocaine cannot be reliably administered via osmotic minipumps due to local vasoconstrictive and necrosis-inducing properties, an alternative drug-delivery system was needed. Consequently, we developed *(39)* a cocaine silicone pellet with a release rate of 103 mg cocaine base over 5 d and found it to induce behavioral stages similar to those caused by continuous amphetamine (initial hyperactivity, the evolution of stereotypies, a crash stage, and finally late-stage behaviors including limb flicks, wet-dog shakes, and parasitotic grooming episodes; *see* ref. *39).* We then looked for persisting alterations in dopamine receptors produced by continuous cocaine, as would be expected following dopamine (DA) terminal damage in striatum. We found no such changes at 14 d following continuous cocaine administration, although a parallel group that had received continuous amphetamine showed large changes in striatal dopamine D_1 and D_2 receptors *(40).* However, the rats which had received continuous cocaine did show persisting alterations in acetylcholine (ACh) and GABA receptors in caudate, perhaps indicating that continuous cocaine had produced a somewhat different kind of neurotoxicity in caudate, perhaps one postsynaptic to dopamine receptors. And so, in collaborative studies with Robert Switzer of Neuroscience Associates, this issue was investigated using silver-stain studies to assess neural degeneration *(41,42).* By using minimally toxic doses and then searching for selective degeneration in brain, one can search for the weak links in neuronal circuitry induced by continuous stimulants with the assumption that these "weak" or "especially vulnerable" pathways, when overdriven by incessant stimulant-induced activity, eventually degenerate, leaving the brain in a persistently altered state.

Rats were given continuous amphetamine, continuous cocaine, or no drugs for 5 d, and then their brains were removed and examined for degeneration at various times

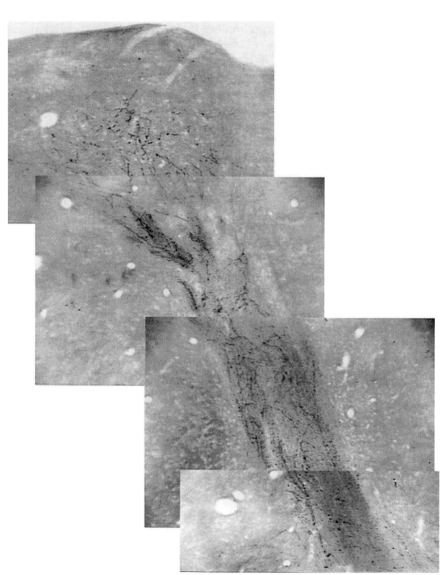

Fig. 1. Photomontage showing degeneration in habenula and fasciculus retroflexus following 5 d of continuous cocaine. At the top of the figure is lateral habenula; the more ventral three sections follow fasciculus retroflexus. Because fasciculus retroflexus moves slightly laterally as it projects more ventrally, the bottom two sections are from a section slightly more lateral than the top two. Multiple, long, darkly stained axons and swollen varicosities can be traced throughout fasciculus retroflexus.

following cessation of drug administration *(43)*. The entire brain from the olfactory nucleus to the mesencephalon was screened. The continuous amphetamine animals were found to evidence quite substantial degeneration in caudate. However, there was essentially no degeneration observed in caudate in the cocaine animals. But a very distinctive pattern of extensive degeneration was observed after either continuous amphetamine or cocaine in a totally unexpected brain region: the lateral habenula (LHb) and fasciculus retroflexus (FR). Many of these long degenerating axons, when observed after several days had elapsed following pellet removal, showed classical anatomical signs of disintegration, such as axons beginning to fragment and the appearance of corkscrew or stump-like endings. These degenerating axons were almost exclusively in the mantle, or sheath of FR (as opposed to the core). Figure 1 shows this dramatic degeneration of FR after 5 d of continuous cocaine in a saggital section.

These results, coupled with the existing literature, have implications for models of stimulant-produced psychosis and paranoia. It is clear that amphetamine and cocaine are similar in that they are both strong stimulants with potent actions in potentiating dopamine, and both lead to a pattern of drug intake in addicts in which the drug is taken repeatedly over prolonged periods. For both drugs, these "runs" or binges produce a progressive dysphoria and paranoia followed by a rebound depression upon drug discontinuation. Furthermore, when given continuously to animals, both drugs eventually induce comparable late-stage behaviors. However these two drugs are markedly different in their persisting effects in caudate. Continuous amphetamine has neurotoxic effects on dopamine terminals and dopamine receptors in caudate; continuous cocaine does not. Continuous cocaine produces persisting alterations in GABA and ACh receptors, whereas continuous amphetamine does not. However, the two drugs are quite similar in their ability to induce degeneration of axons in LHb extending ventrally into FR. A logical conclusion would be that it is the neurotoxic alterations in LHb and FR that play a critical role in mediating the paranoid psychosis that follows the continuous use of these stimulants and the persistently altered paranoid reactions to the drug which develop in chronic addicts. We have now found this degeneration in FR following every stimulant we have tested which predominantly acts by potentiating dopamine, including amphetamine, methylenedioxymethamphetamine (MDMA), cathinone, and methamphetamine, each given at a 5-d, relatively low continuous dose.

7. HABENULA, FR, AND ANATOMY OF PARANOIA

These recent findings suggest a need to reevaluate the role of the LHb and FR in the mediation of dopamine-related circuitry. Figure 2 illustrates the principle connections of the habenula as described in the classical anatomical studies by Herkenham and Nauta *(44,45)* and others. The inputs consist predominantly of pathways traveling in stria medullaris terminating in either the medial habenular (Mhb) or LHb nuclei, with two subdivisions: a medial "septal-limbic" and a lateral "pallidal-limbic" one. The principal input for medial habenula is cholinergic fibers arising from the septal area (nearly every septal cell projects to the medial habenula), but there are also projections from nucleus accumbens and the diagonal band of Broca. The major input to LHb are GABA fibers from the medial (or internal) globus pallidus (in primates) or its homologue in rat, the entopeduncular nucleus, but there are also inputs from limbic forebrain, including the lateral hypothalamus, diagonal band of Broca, substantia innominata, lateral

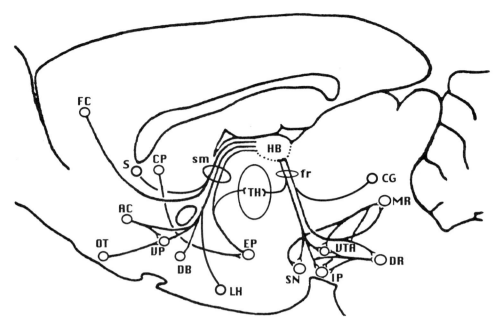

Fig. 2. Schematic representation of some of the chief inputs and outputs of the habenular complex. Abbreviations: FC, frontal cortex; OT, olfactory tubercle; AC, nucleus accumbens; CP, caudate-putamen; DB, nucleus of the diagonal band; VP, ventral pallidum; sm, stria medullaris thalami; EP, entopeduncular nucleus; FR, fasciculus retroflexus; TH, thalamic nuclei, including dorsalmedial, ventral anterior, and ventral lateral; HB, habenula; SN, substantia nigra; VTA, ventral tegmental area; IP, interpeduncular nucleus; MR, medial raphe nucleus; DR, dorsal raphe nucleus. Major descending pathways as shown entering sm, passing through or synapsing in habenula, and descending in FR to a variety of mesencephalic structures. Collaterals from EP and HB to thalamus are also shown.

preoptic area, nucleus accumbens, frontal cortex, and the suprachiasmatic nucleus. Both nuclei also receive less extensive ascending afferents from the central gray and medial raphe, and the LHb receives dopaminergic inputs from the substantia nigra and ventral tegmental area.

The principal efferent fibers from the medial habenula, including cholinergic, glutaminergic, and substance P fibers, travel in the core of FR principally to the interpeduncular nucleus, but also somewhat to the ventral tegmental area, raphe nuclei, and substantia nigra. The LHb has more varied outputs, with axons travelling principally in the periphery or mantle region of the FR sending projections to several thalamic (mediodorsal and ventromedial) and hypothalamic (lateral, septal, and preoptic) nuclei. But the principal efferents from LHb are to midbrain nuclei such as the dorsal and medial raphe nuclei (constituting one of the major inputs to raphe), to ventral tegmental area and substantia nigra pars compacta, and also to central gray.

Sutherland *(46)* described some of the functional roles of what he termed this "dorsal diencephalic conduction system." It has anatomical and functional connections to modulate important functions such as sensory gating through the thalamus, pain gating through the central gray and raphe, and mediation of motor stereotypies and reward mechanisms through the substantia nigra and the ventral tegmental area. Lesions of habenula produce a wide variety of behavioral alterations, including alterations in self-stimulation, pain inhibition, avoidance learning, and sexual and maternal behaviors *(3)*.

Studies of glucose utilization have consistently shown the habenula to be highly sensitive to dopamine agonists and antagonists, and in fact is the most sensitive region in brain to agonists such as cocaine *(47)*. The dorsal diencephalic system has major and predominantly inhibitory connections onto dopamine-containing cells. The descending control of monoamine and other mesencephalic cells carried in FR appears to consist largely of inhibitory influences. Sasaki et al. *(48)* found that they could markedly attenuate methamphetamine-induced inhibition of substantia nigra cells by making lesions of the habenula, of the entopeduncular nucleus, or transections of the stria medullaris. These studies support an important role of the dorsal diencephalic conduction system in inhibiting dopamine cell bodies and in mediating part of the negative feedback from limbic and striatal dopamine receptors onto dopamine cell bodies. These are ideal connections for the mediation of psychosis on both anatomical and functional grounds. The descending influences from dopamine-rich and limbic structures are quite unique in brain in that striatal and limbic inputs directly converge. In addition, this circuitry apparently mediates a major part of the descending control over serotonin cells of the raphe complex (in fact, FR carries the chief inputs from all of brain to raphe). An implication of this is that due to the amphetamine or cocaine-induced degeneration of the FR fibers, the higher brain areas might no longer be able to regulate dopaminergic and serotoninergic cell firing, and especially to inhibit these midbrain cells.

8. DO THE FIBERS IN FR THAT DEGENERATE AFTER COCAINE BINGES CARRY NEGATIVE FEEDBACK FROM DA-RICH REGIONS ONTO DA CELL BODIES?

There is additional evidence that the LHb and FR mediate part of the negative feedback from dopamine-rich regions onto dopamine-cell bodies. Lesions of either stria medullaris, LHb, or FR increase dopamine turnover in prefrontal cortex, nucleus accumbens, and striatum *(49,50)*, and electrical stimulation of the habenula inhibits dopamine-containing cells in substantia nigra (SN) and ventral tegmented area (VTA) *(51)*. Several recent observations from this laboratory clarify some of the long-lasting effects of continuous cocaine administration and also provide indirect evidence consistent with the hypothesis that the degenerating axons carry part of the DA-mediated negative feedback. We have found that there are long-lasting sequelae of 5 d of continuous treatment with the cocaine pellet that suggest correlates of the neurotoxicity observed in brain. Cocaine pellet-pretreated rats, when tested several weeks following pellet explant, act frightened in open-field tests. At the beginning of the test they initially "freeze," remaining immobile for prolonged periods *(40)*, and when tested over prolonged periods in novel environments they remain hyperactive far longer than the controls. This suggests a lack of habituation to novel sensory stimulation in these animals. Both of these observations are highly consistent with increased DA turnover after lesions of LHb. We recently attempted to test the hypothesis that the axons that degenerate in FR and LHb following continuous cocaine mediate part of the negative feedback from DA receptors onto DA cell bodies using microdialysis techniques *(52)*.

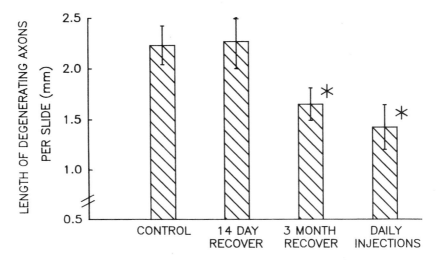

Fig. 3. Total amount of degeneration (sum of all axon lengths) in from one slide unilaterally. A blind observer sketched degenerating fibers using camera lucida and the resulting ink traces were quantified using NIMH Image. * Means significantly less than Control, $p < .05$.

Rats were pretreated with either cocaine or control pellets for 5 d, and then 14 d later, microdialysis probes were lowered into the caudate nucleus. Baseline dopamine and GABA levels were not significantly different in the two groups. However, when the animals were perfused locally with the D_1 agonist SKF38393, the controls showed a large decrease in striatal dopamine overflow and dopaminergic metabolites compared to the cocaine animals. Because D_1 receptors are largely postsynaptic in caudate, where dopamine release is governed largely by presynaptic mechanisms, this result suggests a deficiency in the negative feedback pathways extending from caudate onto SN and VTA cell bodies, or locally within striatum.

It has also been reported that FR lesions in rats lead to decreased spontaneous alternation *(53)*. Similarly, we found that cocaine pellet-pretreated rats evidence long-lasting deficits in spontaneous alteration. Thus, animals treated with the cocaine pellet and then given a recovery period show a number of behavioral and biochemical alterations similar to those of animals following lesions of LHb or FR.

9. REPEATED COCAINE BOUTS: PROGRESSIVE EFFECTS ON BEHAVIOR AND TOXICITY

We have reported *(54)* that prior drug exposure alters this degeneration in FR. The total extent of degeneration in FR was quantified by tracing, via camera lucida, all degenerating axons following various drug insults. The 5-d cocaine pellet induced substantial degeneration in FR. Rats given the 5-d pellet, a 3-mo recovery period, and then a second 5-d pellet showed new degeneration, but it was less than with the first pellet.

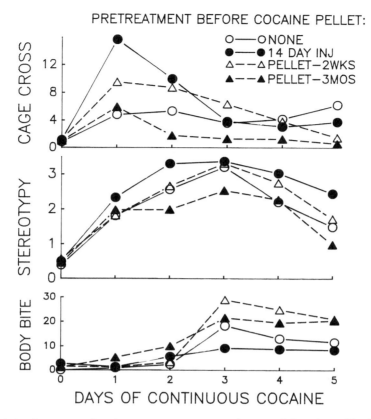

Fig. 4. Activity (cage crossings), motor stereotypy ratings, and duration of body biting, etc. in the four groups. When rats are pretreated with daily injections of cocaine and then implanted with a cocaine pellet, they show more initial hyperactivity and then motor stereotypies than any other group, but less "late-stage" behaviors.

Apparently some tolerance can occur, or the axons had already been lesioned. But surprisingly, when rats were given this 5-d pellet, then a 14-d recovery period, then a second 5-d pellet, there was again about the same amount of degeneration induced as by the first pellet, and this was fresh (new) degeneration (Fig. 3). Two clear conclusions emerge: one bout of the 5-d cocaine pellet is not causing degeneration in all of the susceptible axons, but even more interestingly, frequently repeated binges are especially neurotoxic.

One other group in this experiment was given 14 daily injections of cocaine (in the "sensitization" or "inverse tolerance" paradigm, and then, 2 wk later, a 5-d cocaine pellet. These animals showed an enormous behavioral potentiation of stereotypies during the pellet, but fewer "late-stage" behaviors (Fig. 4). However, they showed appreciably less degeneration than rats receiving their first pellet. Prior drug exposure can exaggerate the initial behavioral reactions, but attenuate the neurotoxicity. This is an interesting example of the clear difference between continuously induced, neurotoxic, "late-stage" hallucinatory behaviors, and intermittent-regimen, sensitized, motor stereotypies.

It thus appears that repeated bouts of cocaine exposure in rats may produce progressively summating alterations in brain and behavior and that we have never really observed the fully developed "late-stage" hallucinatory syndrome of behavior, nor investigated the full ramifications of how extensive the correlated alterations in brain can be. Yet a highly recurrent theme in studies of both amphetamine and cocaine addicts (e.g., *147*) is how paranoia and parasitosis progressively evolve in the confirmed addict, eventually reaching the point where the initial drug intake can induce them. The cocaine addicts studied by Satel et al., who showed the full syndrome of binge-limited paranoia, had been addicts for over 2 yr and had consumed an enormous estimated quantity of cocaine each (1.34 ± 1.7 kg). The repeated pellet preparation may develop into an extraordinarily interesting paradigm not only for the study of chronic cocaine abuse but also for more general models of sensory hallucinations such as parasitosis and of paranoia. These findings may have therapeutic implications as well as general scientific ones, for the progressive development of parasitosis and paranoia is often cited by addicts as critical for their seeking treatment. This "repeated binge" preparation should prove perfect for the study of metabolic and other regional brain changes correlated with "late-stage" behaviors.

10. WHERE ARE THE CELL BODIES THAT GIVE RISE TO FR DEGENERATION?

There are two distinct possibilities for where the cell bodies that give rise to the degenerating axons following continuous amphetamine or cocaine are located. They could be in LHb, projecting ventrally through FR, but they could also be in midbrain cell groups. The dopaminergic cells of the SN or VTA give rise to ascending dopamine axons terminating in habenula, and the raphe nuclei also project to habenula, as does the central gray.

Three lines of evidence point to the cell bodies in LHb as the source. The first is related to the fact that the degenerating axons are quite highly concentrated in the mantle of FR. When the anterograde tracer PHAL is injected into LHb *(55)* the pattern of staining observed mirrors almost exactly that seen in the degenerating fibers: a high concentration of descending fibers in the mantle of FR, with some fibers then entering thalamic nuclei but the majority terminating in regions such as VTA. The ascending fibers such as from SN and VTA projecting to LHb are not so rigidly confined to FR. Some of the degenerating axons in FR following cocaine show a morphological pattern identical to those described by Araki et al. *(55)* in normal animals labeled with injections into LHb.

A second line of evidence comes from studies in our laboratory. Rats were injected with PHAL in LHb using the Araki et al. *(55)* protocol, then given 7 d for anterograde transport to occur, and then implanted with either amphetamine or cocaine pellets for 5 d. When the animals were sacrificed 2 d after pellet removal, PHAL-stained fibers were observed in FR that had the distinctive characteristics of degenerating fibers (fragmented axons, cork-screw shaped axons, and "end-stumps"). This finding means that at least some of the degenerating axons have cell bodies in LHb.

The third line of evidence comes from the study described previously of animals given repeated cocaine bouts. When these animals were stained for degeneration, only a few stained cell bodies were observed (principally in the repeated pellet groups), but of these most were concentrated in the most lateral part of the LHb, with a few in the more medial portion of LHb. When considered altogether, these data support the hypothesis that most, if not all, of the degenerating axons are from cells in LHb.

11. WHAT ARE THE MECHANISMS OF THIS NEUROTOXICITY?

In most cases of neurotoxicity induced by drugs of abuse, the neurotoxic effects are observed in brain regions where glucose metabolism is markedly heightened by the drug. Examples are the neurotoxicity produced in caudate by continuous amphetamine *(3)* and the toxicity in several limbic regions produced by N-methyl-D-aspartate (NMDA) antagonists such as phencyclidine *(56)*.

The neurotoxic effects of continuous cocaine and amphetamine in LHb and FR are unusual in that they are so strongly correlated with a decrease in glucose metabolism in the affected structures. An immense number of studies of glucose utilization have consistently shown that while virtually all dopamine agonists increase glucose metabolism in dopamine-rich regions such as caudate nucleus, nucleus accumbens, SN, and VTA, they markedly decrease glucose metabolism in the habenula (this literature is reviewed in ref. *3*). Indeed, in some studies glucose metabolism in the habenula is the most sensitive region in all of brain to low doses of dopamine agonists such as cocaine. Another characteristic of the toxicity in LHb is that the conditions of drug administration sufficient to induce this effect must be continuous and extremely prolonged, on the order of many days. This was dramatically validated when it was found that very high doses of methamphetamine given for 8–10 h, while producing extraordinary degeneration in caudate-putamen and many other brain regions, were relatively ineffective in producing degeneration in LHb and FR *(38)*.

Recent data suggest a reason for this, as well as a proposed mechanism for the toxicity. Glucose metabolism, as reflected by 2DG uptake, typically reflects the summed activity in terminals, whereas CFOS induction represents the heightened activity in cell bodies *(57)*. Consequently, it is possible that striatal GABAergic efferents to the entopeduncular nucleus are stimulated by the DA agonist administration and, thus, produce a strong inhibition of the entopeduncular efferents to the LHb, which are also largely GABAergic. The reduced activity in the terminals of these GABA projections to LHb would result in both the reduction of 2DG uptake and the disinhibition of habenular cells.

This hypothesis, reviewed by Wirtshafter et al. *(58)*, is supported by their finding that dopamine agonists induce Fos-like immunoreactivity in cells in the most lateral LHb. In fact, the pattern of induction produced by amphetamine in their study was almost identical to the pattern of cells staining for degeneration. Wirshafter et al. *(58)* further found that this Fos-like induction could be abolished by 6-OHDA lesions of the nigrostriatal bundle. These findings suggest that the neurotoxicity induced by continuous amphetamine or cocaine in the LHb and FR may be due to the prolonged hyperactivity in the LHb cells produced by the removal of GABAergic inhibitory influences, which then lead to a prolonged overstimulation of these cells and eventual excitotoxic neurotoxicity.

This is an unusual kind of neurotoxicity, however. Almost if not all of the silver-stained degeneration in LHb and FR is of axons. In other cases of neurotoxicity, the

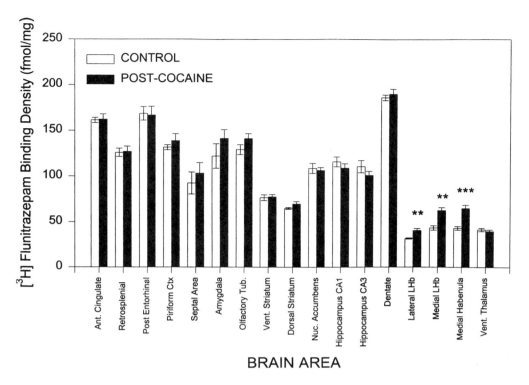

Fig. 5. Flunitrazepam binding at 14 d after final pellet removal. The largest changes in all of brain, for 6 different ligands, are of increased flunitrazepam binding in all three subdivisions of the habenula.

specific microanatomy of the degeneration provides clues as to what the mechanisms underlying the neurotoxicity might be. For example, with prolonged amphetamine, the degeneration is predominantly dopamine terminals in caudate, and this correlates with other evidence that this neurotoxicity is mediated by the conversion of dopamine to a neurotoxic substance, or the production of some other neurotoxin, which is then taken up by the dopamine terminals. Similarly, with prolonged phencyclidine and other NMDA antagonists, the predominant silver-staining is of entire cells, with all of their processes stained. This correlates with evidence that this neurotoxicity is mediated by increases in the production of glutamate following the blockade of NMDA receptors, which then induce excitotoxic damage via the nonblocked AMPA receptors. What mechanisms would lead to degeneration of axons only? This question represents a major intellectual challenge to be solved.

In a recent study *(59)*, this selective neurotoxicity in habenula was validated using an entirely different methodology. Rats were given two bouts of cocaine spaced by 10 d apart, a 14-d recovery period, and then sacrificed for autoradiographic studies using a variety of ligands for GABA, muscarinic, AMPA, serotonergic, and other receptors, as well as for the dopamine transporter. The largest change in receptor density for any ligand and any brain region was GABA (flunitrazepam) receptors in habenula (Fig. 5). This is a striking confirmation of the neurotoxicity in habenula using an en-

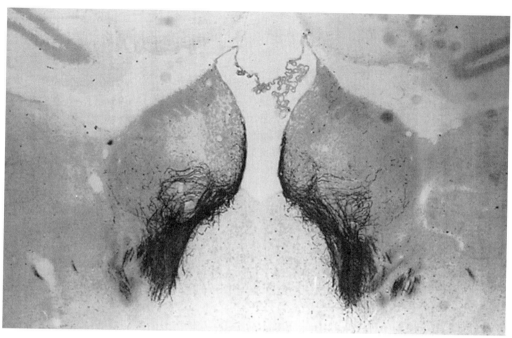

Fig. 6. Degeneration in FR induced by nicotine. (*See* color plate 3 appearing in the insert following p. 368.)

tirely independent measure, and one which is much more amenable to quantification than silver staining. Electron microscopic studies *(60)* confirmed the finding that continuous cocaine selectively induces changes in GABA cells in LhB.

12. STUDIES OF DEGENERATION FOLLOWING NICOTINE VALIDATE THE "WEAK LINK" HYPOTHESIS

In further studies, we have studied degeneration in brain following a variety of drugs of abuse given continuously. One drug also tested was the effects of continuous nicotine on degeneration in brain. In one group, nicotine base was administered via minipump to 6 rats for 5 d continuously at a dose (3.9 mg/d of nicotine base, i.e., 13 mg/kg/d) that had been found previously to induce long-lasting alterations in behavior, including as an enhancement of performance in the 8-arm maze *(61,62)*, or a persisting elevation of sucrose intake *(63)* or alcohol intake *(64)*. In four further groups, nicotine was administered as the salt (nicotine bitartrate) via minipump at varying doses in order to study the dose-dependancy of any effects. In these rats, the nicotine was administered for 5 d at various doses to groups of four rats each: a "very high" dose like that in the nicotine base animals (11 mg/d of the tartrate, equivalent to 3.9 mg/d of nicotine base).

We were astounded to find extremely selective degeneration in brain following nicotine. Virtually only one tract was affected by nicotine: FR. But in this case it was the other half of the tract: the cholinergic part. Degenerating axons could be traced from medial habenula, entering the core of FR, and the degeneration could be traced all the way into the interpeduncular nucleus (Fig. 6).

But the most remarkable aspects of these findings is that two broad classes of addictive compounds both have their major neurodegenerative effects in brain on the same anatomical complex, although different parts of this pathway are involved following dopaminergic and nicotinic stimulants. Some of these results are highly consistent with other neurochemical evidence, such as the observation that the LHb is one of the most sensitive structures in brain to alterations in 2-deoxyglucose uptake induced by dopaminergic compounds, or that the medial habenula-FR-interpeduncular system contains one of the highest concentrations of nicotinic receptors in brain *(65,66)*. But these results with FR, taken as a whole, constitute strong evidence that alterations in this descending pathway from forebrain, one that exerts important control over lower midbrain structures, may constitute a "weak link" in brain for chronic drug effects, including addiction and relapse. Lesions of habenula or of FR induce alterations in a wide variety of behaviors, including general activity levels, feeding behavior, avoidance and maze learning, social and maternal behaviors, sleep patterns, and seizure thresholds. Much of these data, as well as the neuroanatomical connections of FR, have been previously reviewed *(3)*, but there are more recent reports of effects on food intake *(67)*, avoidance behavior *(68)*, maternal behavior *(69)*, rapid eye movement (REM) sleep *(70)*, and schizophrenia *(69)*. More attention needs to be paid to this system in studies of drug addiction.

REFERENCES

1. Ellison, G. D. and Eison, M. S. (1983) Continuous amphetamine intoxication: an animal model of the acute psychotic episode. *Psychol. Med.* **13**, 751–761.
2. Ellison, G. (1991) Animal models of hallucinations: continuous stimulants, in *Neuromethods, vol 18: Animal Models in Psychiatry* (Boulton, A., Baker, G., and Martin-Iverson, M., eds.), pp. 151–196.
3. Ellison, G. (1994) Stimulant-induced psychosis, the dopamine theory, and the habenula. *Brain Res. Rev.* **19**, 223–239.
4. Connell, P. (1958) *Amphetamine Psychosis*. Maudsley Monographs No. 5. Oxford University Press, London.
5. Bell, D. (1965) Comparison of amphetamine psychosis and schizophrenia. *Am. J. Psychiatry* **111**, 701–707.
6. Ellinwood, E. H. Jr., (1967) Amphetamine psychosis: I. Description of the individuals and the process. *J. Nerv. Mental Dis.* **144**, 273–283.
7. Siegal, R. K. (1977) Cocaine: recreational use and intoxication, in *NIDA Research Monograph 13* (Petersen, R. C. and Stillman, R. C., eds.), US Government Printing Office, Washington, DC.
8. Lesko, L. M., Fischman, M., Javaid, J., and Davis, J. (1982) Iatrogenous cocaine psychosis. *N. Engl. J. Med.* **307**, 1153–1156.
9. Gawin, F. H. (1986) Neuroleptic reduction of cocaine-induced paranoia but not euphoria? *Psychopharmacology* **90**, 142–143.
10. Manschreck, T. C., Laughery, J. A., Weisstein, C. C., Allen, D., Humblestone, B., Neville, M., et al. (1988) Characteristics of freebase cocaine psychosis. *Yale J. Biol. Med.* **61**, 115–122.
11. Brady, K., Lydiard, R., Malcolm, R., and Ballenger, J. (1991) Cocaine-induced psychosis. *J. Clin. Psychiatry* **52**, 509–512.
12. Elpern, D. (1988) Cocaine abuse and delusions of parasitosis. *Cutis* **42**, 273–274.
13. Mitchell, J. and Vierkant, A. (1991) Delusions and hallucinations of cocaine abusers and paranoid schizophrenics: a comparative study. *J. Psychiatry* **125**, 301–310.

14. Kramer, J. C., Gischman, V., and Littlefield, D. (1967) Amphetamine abuse: pattern and effects of high doses taken intravenously. *J. Am. Med. Assoc.* **201,** 89–93.
15. Griffith, J., Cavanaugh, J., Held, N., and Oates, J. (1972) D-amphetamine: evaluation of psychotomimetic properties in man. *Arch. Gen. Psychiatry* **26,** 97–100.
16. Bell, D. (1973) The experimental reproduction of amphetamine psychosis. *Arch. Gen. Psychiatry* **29,** 35–40.
17. Satel, S., Southwick, S., and Gawin, F., (1992) Clinical features of cocaine-induced paranoia. *Am. J. Psychiatry* **148,** 495–498.
18. Ellison, G. and Morris, W. (1981) Opposed stages of continuous amphetamine administration: parallel alterations in motor sterotypies and in vivo spiroperidol accumulation. *Eur. J. Pharmacol.* **74,** 207–214.
19. Ellison, G. D., Eison, M. S., and Huberman, H. (1978b) Stages of constant amphetamine intoxication: delayed appearance of abnormal social behaviors in rat colonies. *Psychopharmacology* **56,** 293–299.
20. Ellison, G. D., Nielsen, E. B., and Lyon, M. (1981) Animal models of psychosis: hallucinatory behaviors in monkeys during the late stage of continuous amphetamine intoxication. *J. Psychiatry Res.* **16,** 13–22.
21. Nielsen, E., Lee, T., and Ellison, G. (1980b) Following several days of continuous administration d-amphetamine acquires hallucinogen-like properties. *Psychopharmacology* **68,** 197–200.
22. de Leon, J., Antelo, R., and Simpson, G. (1992) Delusion of parasitosis or chronic hallucinosis: hypothesis about their brain physiopathology. *Compr. Psychiatry* **33,** 25–33.
23. Nielsen, E. B., Neilsen, M., Ellison, G., and Braestrup, E. (1980a) Decreased spiroperidol and LSD binding in rat brain after continuous amphetamine. *Eur. J. Pharmacol.* **66,** 149–154.
24. Ellison, G. D., Eison, M., Huberman, H., and Daniel, F. (1978a) Long term changes in dopaminergic innervation of caudate nucleus after continuous amphetamine administration. *Science* **201,** 276–278.
25. Nwanze, E. and Jonsson, G. (1981) Amphetamine neurotoxicity on dopamine nerve terminals in the caudate nucleus of mice. *Neurosci. Lett.* **26,** 163–168
26. Ryan, L., Martone, M., Linder, J., and Groves, P. (1990) Histological and ultrastructural evidence that d-amphetamine causes degeneration in neostriatum and frontal cortex of rats. *Brain Res.* **518,** 67–77.
27. Ryan, L. J., Martone, M., Linder, J., and Groves, P. M. (1988) Cocaine, in contrast to d-amphetamine, does not cause axonal terminal degeneration in neostriatum and agranular frontal cortex of long-evans rats. *Life Sci.* **43,** 1403–1409.
28. Hotchkiss, A. and Gibb, J. (1980) Long-term effects of multiple doses of methamphetamine on tryptophan hydroxylase and tyrosine hydroxylase activity in rat brain. *J. Pharmacol. Exp. Ther.* **214,** 257–262.
29. Ricaurte, G. A., Schuster, C. R., and Seiden, L. S. (1980) Long-term effects of repeated methylamphetamine administration on dopamine and serotonin neurons in the rat brain: a regional study. *Brain Res.* **193,** 153–163.
30. Steranka, L. and Sanders-Bush, E. (1980) Long-term effects of continuous exposure to amphetamine on brain dopamine concentration and synaptosomal uptake in mice. *Eur. J. Pharmacol.* **65,** 439–443.
31. Fuller, R. and Hemrick-Luecke, S. (1980) Long-lasting depletion of striatal dopamine by a single injection of amphetamine in iprindole-treated rats. *Science* **209,** 305–306.
32. Wagner, G., Lucot, J., Chuster, C., and Seiden, L. (1983) Alpha-methyltyrosine attenuates and reserpine increases methamphetamine-induced neuronal changes. *Brain Res.* **270,** 285–288.
33. Fuller, R. and Hemrick-Luecke, S. (1982) Further studies on the long-term depletion of

striatal dopamine in iprindole-treated rats by amphetamine. *Neuropharmacology* **21,** 433–438.

34. Hanson, G. R., Matsuda, L., and Gibb, J. W. (1987) Effects of cocaine on methamphetamine-induced neurochemical changes: characterization of cocaine as a monoamine uptake blocker. *J. Pharmacol. Exp. Ther.* **242,** 507–513.

35. Sonsalla, P., Nicklas, W., and Heikkila, R. (1989) Role for excitatory amino acits in methamphetamine-induced nigrostriatal dopaminergic toxicity. *Science* **243,** 398–400.

36. Fuller, R., Hemrick-Luecke, S., and Ornstein, P. (1992) Protection against amphetamine-induced neurotoxicity toward striatal dopamine neurons in rodents by LY274614, an excitatory amino acid antagonist. *Neuropharmacology* **31,** 1027–1032 .

37. Seiden, L. and Ricaurte, G. (1987) Neurotoxicity of methamphetamine and related drugs, in *Psychopharmacology: The Third Generation of Progress* (Meltzer, H., ed.), Raven Press, New York, pp. 359–366.

38. Ellison, G. and Switzer, R. III (199e) Dissimilar patterns of degeneration in brain following four different addictive stimulants. *NeuroReport* **5,** 17–20.

39. Lipton, J., Zeigler, S., Wilkins, J., and Ellison, G. (1991) Silicone pellet for continuous cocaine administration: heightened late-stage behaviors compared to continuous amphetamine. *Pharmacol. Biochem. Behav.* **38,** 927–930.

40. Zeigler, S., Lipton, J., Toga, A., and Ellison, G. (1991) Continuous cocaine produces persistent changes in brain neurochemistry and behavior different from amphetamine. *Brain Res.* **552,** 27–35.

41. Switzer, R. C. (1991) Strategies for assessing neurotoxicity. *Neurosci. Biobehav. Rev.* **15,** 89–93.

42. de Olmos, J., Ebbesson, S., and Heimer, L. (1981) Silver methods for the impregnation of degenerating axoplasm, in *Neuroanatomical Tract-tracing Methods* (Heimer, L. and Robards, N., eds.), Plenum Press, New York, pp. 117–168.

43. Ellison, G. (1992) Continuous amphetamine and cocaine have similar neurotoxic effects in lateral habenular nucleus and fasciculus retroflexus. *Brain Res.* **598,** 353–356.

44. Herkenham, M. and Nauta, W. J. H. (1977) Afferent connections of the habenular nuclei in the rat. *J. Comp. Neurol.* **173,** 123–146.

45. Herkenham, M. and Nauta, W. J. H. (1979) Efferent connections of the habenular nuclei in the rat. *J. Comp. Neurol.* **187,** 19–48.

46. Sutherland, R. J. (1982) The dorsal diencephalic conduction system: a review of the anatomy and functions of the habenular complex. *Neurosci. Biobehav. Rev.* **6,** 1–13.

47. London, E., Wilkerson, G., Goldberg, S., and Risner, M. (1986) Effects of L-cocaine on local cerebral glucose utilization in the rat. *Neurosc. Lett.* **68,** 73–78.

48. Sasaki, K., Suda, H., Watanabe, H., and Yagi, H. (1990) Involvement of the entopeduncular nucleus and the habenula in methamphetamine-induced inhibition of dopamine neurons in the substantia nigra of rats. *Brain Res. Bull.* **25,** 121–127.

49. Lisoprawski, A., Herve, D., Blanc, G., Glowinski, J., and Tassin, J. (1980) Selective activation of the mesocortico-frontal dopaminergic neurons induced by lesions of the habenula in the rat. *Brain Res.* **183,** 229–234.

50. Nishikawa, T., Fage, D., and Scatton, B. (1986) Evidence for, and nature, of the tonic inhibitory influence of habenulointerpeduncular pathways upon cerebral dopaminergic transmission in the rat. *Brain Res.* **373,** 324–336.

51. Christoph, C., Leonzio, R., and Wilcox, K. (1986) Stimulation of the lateral habenula inhibits dopamine-containing neurons in the substantia nigra and ventral tegmental area of the rat. *J. Neurosci.* **6,** 613–619.

52. Keys, A. and Ellison, G. (1994) Continuous cocaine induces persisting alterations in dopamine overflow in caudate following perfusion with a D1 agonist. *J. Neur. Trans. Gen. Sect.* **97,** 225–233.

53. Corodimas, K., Rosenblatt, J., and Morrell, J. (1992) The habenular complex mediates hormonal stimulation of maternal behavior in rats. *Behav. Neurosci.* **106,** 853–865

54. Ellison, G. D., Irwin, S., Keys, A., Noguchi, K., and Sulur, G. (1996) The neurotoxic effects of continuous cocaine and amphetamine in habenula: implications for the substrates of psychosis, in *Neurotoxicity and Neuropathology Associated with Cocaine Abuse* (Majewska, M., ed.), NIDA Research Monograph, National Institute on Drug Abuse, Rockville MD, p. 163.

55. Araki, M., McGeer, P., and Kimura, H. (1988) The efferent projections of the rat lateral habenular nucleus revealed by the PHA-L anterograde tracing method. *Brain Res.* **441,** 319–330.

56. Ellison, G. (1995) The NMDA antagonists phencyclidine, ketamine, and dizocilpine as both behavioral and anatomical models of the dementias. *Brain Res. Rev.* **20,** 250–267.

57. Sharp, F., Sagar, S., and Swanson, R. (1993) Metabolic mapping with cellular resolution: c-fos vs. 2-deoxyglucose. *Crit. Rev. Neurobiol.* **679,** 205–228.

58. Wirtshafter, D., Asin, K., and Pitzer, M. (1994) Dopamine agonists and stress produce different patterns of Fos-like immunoreactivity in the lateral habenula. *Brain Res.* **633,** 21–26.

59. Keys, A. and Ellison, G. (1999) Long-term alterations in benzodiazepine, muscarinic and alpha-amino–3-hydroxy–5-methylisoxazole–4-propionic acid (AMPA) receptor density following continuous cocaine administration. *Pharmacol. Toxicol.* **85,** 144–150.

60. Meshul, C. K., Noguchi, K., Emire, N., and Ellison, G. (1998) Cocaine-induced changes in glutamate and GABA immunolabeling within rat habenula and nucleus accumbens. *Synapse* **30,** 211–220.

61. Levin, E., Kim, P., Meray, R., Levin, E. D., Kim, P., and Meray, R. (1996) Chronic nicotine working and reference memory effects in the 16-arm radial maze: interactions with D_1 agonist and antagonist drugs. *Psychopharmacology* **127,** 25–30.

62. Levin, E., Lee, C., Rose, J. E., Reyes, A., Ellison, G., Jarvik, M., and Gritz, E. (1990) Chronic nicotine and withdrawal effects on radial-arm maze performance in rats. *Behav. Neural Biol.* **53,** 269–276.

63. Jias, L. M. and Ellison, G. (1990) Chronic nicotine induces a specific appetite for sucrose in rats. *Pharmacol. Biochem. Behav.* **35,** 489–491.

64. Potthoff, A. D., Ellison, G., and Nelson, L. (1983) Ethanol intake increases during continuous administration of amphetamine and nicotine, but not several other drugs. *Pharmacol. Biochem. Behav.* **18,** 489–493.

65. London, E. D., Waller, S. B., and Wamsley, J. K. (1985) Autoradiographic Localization of [3H]Nicotine Binding Sites in the Rat Brain. *Neurosci. Lett.* **53,** 179–184.

66. Perry, D. C. and Kellar, K. J. (1995) [^{3}H]Epibatidine labels nicotinic receptors in rat brain: an autoradiographic study. *J. Pharmacol. Exp. Ther.* **275,** 1030–1034.

67. Wolinsky, T. D., Carr, K. D., Hiller, J. M., and Simon, E. J. (1994) Effects of chronic food restriction on mu and kappa opioid binding in rat forebrain: a quantitative autoradiographic study. *Brain Res.* **656,** 274–280.

68. Thornton, E. W., Murray, M., Connors-Eckenrode, T., and Haun, F. (1994) Dissociation of behavioral changes in rats resulting from lesions of the habenula versus fasciculus retroflexus and their possible anatomical substrates. *Behav. Neurosci.* **108,** 1150–1162.

69. Felton, T. M., Linton, L., Rosenblatt, J. S., and Morrell, J. I. (1998) Intact neurons of the lateral habenular nucleus are necessary for the nonhormonal, pup-mediated display of maternal behavior in sensitized virgin female rats. *Behav. Neurosci.* **112,** 1458–1465.

70. Valjakka, A., Vartiainen, J., Tuomisto, L., Tuomisto, J. T., Olkkonen, H., and Airaksinen, M. M. (1998) The fasciculus retroflexus controls the integrity of rem sleep by supporting the generation of hippocampal theta rhythm and rapid eye movements in rats. *Brain Res. Bull.* **47,** 171–184.

13

Microsensors Detect Neuroadaptation by Cocaine

Serotonin Released in Motor Basal Ganglia
Is Not Rhythmic with Movement

Patricia A. Broderick

1. GOALS

At the beginning of this twenty-first century, this millennium year, we are seeing the fruits of our labors from previous animal models developed to elucidate the neurochemistry underlying brain reward in drug addiction. Behavioral animal models such as stimulant self-administration has lent some explanation. Nonetheless, there are major, yet, subtle neurochemical changes that occur during these processes that are not amenable to detection by current methods.

In fact, critically subtle neurochemical changes are not detected by current methods. Such is the case with the microdialysis method because of its limited temporal resolution (time sensitivity) as well as its spatial resolution (space sensitivity) *(1)*. One problem, which has confronted the microdialysis method, is that it does not actually perform the detection *per se*. Instead, the method uses high-performance liquid chromatography (HPLC) to detect neurochemicals in the perfusate, collected by a microdialysis membrane. Another problem that microdialysis has been faced with is that the method does not operate in real time since real time is defined as "viewing events as they happen."

The goal of this chapter is to present a unique, real time, in vivo biotechnology that overcomes limitations inherent in previous methods. With the development of novel miniature sensors, BRODERICK PROBE® Microelectrodes, neurotransmitters, precursors, metabolites, and peptides are detected, selectively, on-line, and within seconds, at precisely the same time as behavior is monitored in the freely moving animal. This biotechnology is unique because: (1) natural/normal (often called basal or endogenous) release of neurotransmitters within specific neuroanatomic substrates in brain can be detected in the freely moving animal while the animal is behaving, while behavior is monitored, and (2) the release of neurotransmitters can be detected within the same specific brain neuroanatomic substrate of the same animal while cocaine is altering neurotransmission, while cocaine is altering animal behavior at the same time.

From: Handbook of Neurotoxicology, Vol. 2
Edited by: E. J. Massaro © Humana Press Inc., Totowa, NJ

This chapter first presents empirical animal data showing the detection of serotonin (5-HT), released during open-field movement behaviors (normal locomotion/exploratory and stereotypy) without cocaine, while the same animal is monitored for behavior via infrared photobeams. Serotonin is studied as it is released within the basal ganglia (nuclei), (A_9) striatum (DStr) and (A_{10}) nucleus accumbens (NAcc), and within the brain-stem nucleus (A_{10}), somatodendrites, ventral tegmental area (VTA). Then, empirical data is presented that is in direct comparison to neurochemistry and behavior studied in the normal state, e.g., 5-HT released in the same basal nuclei and in A_{10} somatodendrites is detected while the animal is experiencing the psychomotor stimulant effects of cocaine. The technology presented here, is a technology wherein the miniature sensors, BRODERICK PROBES® actually perform the in vivo electrochemical detection.

Subtle changes in neurochemical function can be detected directly with these miniature electrochemical probes or sensors, in vivo so that new insight can be gained into neuroadaptation or neural injury, possibly leading to neurotoxicity, even before neuronal degeneration can be seen. Neurotoxicity from drug abuse can come from neuroadaptive changes and this is an area of research that is deserving of study *(2)*, especially since cocaine-induced neuronal degeneration in dopamine (DA) basal ganglia or DA cell bodies has not been revealed with previous neurochemical and histological techniques. Reflecting on knowledge garnered over the years about the basal ganglia disease Parkinson's disease (PD), the necessity of early intervention is clear because it is known that a significant amount of DA neurons in nigrostriatum have degenerated before this devastating movement disorder can be observed.

Oftentimes, movement circuits are conceptualized to be physically separate from their neuromodulatory systems. But, unique data is presented here, wherein the neurotransmitter, 5-HT within basal nuclei (A_9 and A_{10}) and within somatodendrites for basal nuclei in A_{10}, appears to rhythmically modulate the synaptic properties of the same circuit that is responsible for motor performance. Within the same circuit, cocaine is shown to disrupt the 5-HT-modulated control of rhythmic movement. The data show that time-dependent changes occur in neuroadaptative processses within motor circuits via 5-HT after the administration of the psychomotor stimulant, cocaine.

2. INTRODUCTION

2.1. Background and History: Brain Reward, Monoamines, and Cocaine

The very early studies of brain reward neuronal circuitry focused on electrically stimulating the hypothalamic-medial forebrain bundle (MFB) neuronal pathway in the brain of animals, wherein MFB stimulation resulted in a pleasurable experience, so much so that the animal wanted to repeat the experience, an experience called brain reward *(3,4)*. *Psychology Today* popularized this concept of a brain reward mechanism in the 1970s and the notion of a neuronal pathway in mammalian brain that could carry and transmit feelings of "joie de vivre" appealed to the general public. This was an exciting time for the lay person because scientific research had presented a substantive area of discussion and some tangible answers to the often pondered question, "Why do we behave the way we do?"

A possible role for the monoamine, DA, as "neurotransmitter" came about when there were reports that DA was an important constituent of mammalian brain. Scientists began to think that not only did DA constitute a neurotransmitter but DA was a separate neurotransmitter from its sister catecholamine, norepinephrine (NE), because DA and NE were found in mammalian brain in different concentrations *(5–7)*. Now, the excitement was felt in the DA/behavioral sect because the psychomotor stimulant behavior, repetitive and stereotypic, was reported to be restored when DA was injected into the basal nucleus, A_9 striatum, of DA-brain depleted rats *(8–10)* and also when compulsive gnawing behavior was evoked by injection of DA agonists into basal nuclei, striatum, or globus pallidus *(11)*. The compulsive gnawing behavior observed was similar to the stereotyped response described by Randrup et al. *(12)*, which was dependent on DA in basal nuclei. Moreover, neuroleptics, DA antagonists, used in the treatment of human psychosis, were able to block psychomotor-stimulant stereotyped behavior *(13–15)*. It was also during this period that a good amount of research was focusing on cocaine and its ability to reinforce cocaine-induced reward through the neurotransmitter DA in basal nuclei, hence, the psychomotor-stimulant theory of addiction was born *(16)*.

The involvement of the monoamine neurotransmitter, 5-HT in brain reward processes was even more intriguing because 5-HT was believed *a priori,* to be the "punishment" neurotransmitter. Gray ascribed the ascending forebrain septohippocampal 5-HT-ergic pathways, which originate within cell bodies, dorsal raphe (DR) and median raphe (MR), to the transmission of punishment signals predominantly and to signals of reward only secondarily *(17)*. However, the original concept that 5-HT was the punishment neurotransmitter may have been also derived from work by Stein's group, who found that 5, 6, dihydroxytryptamine (5,6 DHT), a 5-HT neurotoxin, was able to allow an animal to better handle behavior that was being punished *(18–20)*. Confirmed by other laboratories *(21–24)*, the general interpretation was that a deficiency in 5-HT function could be directly associated with the ability to better handle punishment or displeasure. But, the secondary corollary to the latter hypothesis, was that an enhanced central 5-HT-ergic function was not directly related to brain reward mechanisms. Instead, enhanced 5-HT function was associated with a diminished ability to withstand punishment or displeasure. Interestingly, it was during this period of time, during the early 1970s, that the older generation anti-anxiety agents, the benzodiazepines (BZDS) were shown to decrease 5-HT function *(25)*. Current evidence also shows that the BZDS and direct acting 5-HT_{1A} agonists decrease 5-HT concentrations in septohippocampal regions of brain *(26–32)*, although recently, low 5-HT levels in the basal nucleus, ventral striatum, were associated with anxiety state *per se (33)*.

Thus, decreased 5-HT function and allowance of punishment, was an idea set in motion from the early behavioral conflict studies. The problem was though, that there might have been an ensuing extrapolation of this concept to cocaine's mechanism of action via 5-HT. Serotonin function in brain after cocaine, via self-administration studies, was thought to act in opposition to the catecholamine, DA. Since DA was the reward neurotransmitter in cocaine mechanisms, one was led to interpret 5-HT as, again, the punishment neurotransmitter in cocaine mechanisms. At least one was led to believe that 5-HT was not involved in the rewarding mechanisms of cocaine *(34–36)*.

The current consensus by neuroscientists on cocaine's action on 5-HT in basal nuclei and their neuronal pathways is that cocaine increases 5-HT efflux in these regions. That cocaine increased 5-HT in basal-nuclei substrates, was reported first less than 10 yr ago, by Broderick's laboratory *(37–40)*. In these studies, DA release was also detected within the same neuroanatomic substrate as was 5-HT in real time, and within seconds, by separate signals for each monoamine and at the same time, locomotor activity and stereotypic behaviors were monitored and found to increase. These studies have been confirmed by others, although in the following studies, neurochemistry was not studied in real time and behaviors were not addressed *(41–43; see* ref. *44* for extensive review of DA cocaine and 5-HT cocaine literature). Further agreement has come from a study published in 1998, wherein the neurochemistry was assayed by high-performance liquid chromatography (HPLC) with electrochemical detection and locomotor activity and stereotypy were monitored, but in separate studies *(45)*.

In the very early literature, from the Wise laboratory, there was a report that cocaine reinforcement was not blocked by antagonists of the catecholamine norepinephrine (NE) *(46)*, leading neuroscientists away from the idea of NE having any importance at all in cocaine's mechanism of action on neuronal circuits in general. This kind of thinking made sense in that the basal ganglia contained significantly lesser amounts of NE than DA. The Wise conceptualization has been maintained in the literature, even recently *(47)*, but now unexpectedly cocaine has been shown to increase NE efflux in the basal nucleus NAcc in freely moving animals *(48)*.

As expected, there is evidence that cocaine acts on various neurotransmitters either alone or in combination with DA and 5-HT and in other neuronal subpathways such as the striatopallidal pathway and the extended amygdala systems *(49)*. Multiple neurotransmitters are involved, e.g., acetylcholine, the excitatory amino acid neurotransmitter glutamate, the inhibitory amino acid neurotransmitter gamma-aminobutyric acid (GABA), and various peptides such as corticotropin-releasing factor (CRF), the details of which are beyond the scope of this chapter *(50,51)*. Glutamate is said to play an important role in cocaine recidivism *(52)*.

3. COCAINE: THE PSYCHOMOTOR STIMULANT

3.1. Cocaine, like Amphetamine, Can Produce Psychosis

3.1.1. Cocaine Can Produce Psychosis in Humans

Albeit complex and multifaceted in its differential diagnosis, schizophrenia may be termed the prototypical psychotic disorder *(53)*. Although amphetamine-induced psychosis was reported clinically as early as 1938 *(54)*, clinical reports of paranoid psychosis induced by cocaine have more recently emerged. Clinical studies using cocaine users as subjects are becoming more common. In 1988, for example, a study wherein a 4-h intravenous infusion of cocaine after a loading dose of cocaine was administered to experienced cocaine users, suspiciousness and paranoia were reported, whereas intravenous infusion of saline after a loading dose of cocaine was unremarkable in producing such effects *(55)*. An equal-opportunity disorder, cocaine-induced psychosis has been seen even in the elderly *(56)*. Emergency Room (or Emergency Department [ED], as this is now called) cases of patients diagnosed with cocaine-induced psychosis, are being considered by some to be alarming *(57–59)*.

Single-photon emission computerized tomography (SPECT) studies have shown that cocaine caused changes in cerebral blood flow that are similar to those seen in patients diagnosed with schizophrenia-induced psychosis *(60)*. Some reports show that the phenomenology of schizophrenic psychosis in the absence of cocaine abuse is similar to cocaine psychosis in the absence of schizophrenia. There are some differences, however, such as: thought broadcasting and thought withdrawal were displayed more prominently in schizophrenia, whereas paranoia and fear of being harmed were displayed more prominently in the cocaine psychotic group *(61)*.

A controlled study comprised of 100 cocaine subjects and 100 schizophrenic subjects in an East Texas State Psychiatric Hospital produced interesting results. Both groups were found to be delusional, but the delusions of the schizophrenic group were more bizarre, e.g., the schizophrenic group exhibited "Capgrass Syndrome," which consists of experiences that are delusional and in which the schizophrenic patient believes that his/her family relations are imposters *(62)*. In the same study, hallucinations were found in both groups, but cocaine abusers had more visual hallucinations distinguished by flashing lights (snow lights); also, the cocaine group experienced "parasitosis" with greater frequency. Parasitosis is a physiological phenomenon where the subject experiences the sensation that bugs are crawling on the skin (also sometimes called "formication" from the Latin, "formica," which means ants). Finally, command hallucinations occurred in both groups but the schizophrenic group commands were, again, more bizarre, e.g., the schizophrenic group experienced a command to commit murder.

Cocaine-induced paranoia has been likened to schizophrenic paranoia *(63)*. Patients who experience paranoia from cocaine abuse are said to be at a higher risk for development of psychosis than their counterparts *(64)*, and prolonged cocaine abusers may have an underlying major psychiatric disorder or one may be implicit *(65)*. There is a report of schizophrenic symptomotology aggravated by cocaine *(66)*, but schizophrenic patients seem to want to use cocaine and the results show that patients who use cocaine and are schizophrenic as well, exhibit fewer negative effects *(67–69)*. Perhaps this is the rationale.

Some have said that the two symptomatologies of cocaine-induced psychosis and schizophrenic-induced psychosis are easily distinguishable; that is, it is easy to see the differences in the symptomatologies *(70,71)*. However, even different types of schizophrenia are said not to be easily distinguishable. Comorbidity makes these issues even more problematic. Dual diagnoses showing that patients have both overlapping symptomatologies of cocaine psychosis and schizophrenia are reported in the literature *(72–74)*.

From both preclinical and clinical points of view, the similarities between the two symptomatologies are relevant. Basal nuclei DA is hypothesized to be a mechanism for producing both schizophrenic symptoms and cocaine's reinforcing and psychomotor stimulant effects *(75; see ref. 76* for review). Lieberman et al. discusses DA issues and further points out the similarities between cocaine and amphetamine-induced psychoses and the ensuing difficulties when psychiatric illness presents concomitantly with stimulant abuse psychosis *(77)*. The importance of the issue of 5-HT/DA interactions in human and animal psychoses is also emerging *(78–79,82,83; see refs. 44,80,81* for reviews).

3.1.2. Cocaine Can Produce "Psychosis" in Animals

How can animals exhibit psychosis? How can animals be psychotic? In humans, the diagnostic criteria for schizophrenia (DSM IV) are: (1) delusions, (2) hallucinations,

(3) disorganized speech, (4) grossly disorganized or catatonic behavior, and (5) negative symptoms (affective flattening of mood, alogia [poverty of speech], avolition [loss of energy]) *(53)*. More simply put, some component(s) of psychosis are as follows: motor stereotypies, paranoid delusions, sensory hallucinations, and loosening of associations.

It seems that the critical feature of psychosis that crosses species and can be adequately studied in animals is motor stereotypies. That the phenomenon of psychosis can cross species from human to animal is not such a grossly anthropomorphic thought. After all, although significant advances have been made in the neurobiology and neurochemistry of schizophrenia, there are still no laboratory assays and no blood or urine tests that diagnose psychosis. We cannot look at the laboratory results and say to the patient, "The results of your blood tests are complete and unfortunately, you have schizophrenia." It is true that we have progressed to the point where metabolites of neurotransmitters can be assayed in body fluids of mentally ill patients and comparisons between groups can be made, post factum. But, for the present at least, we routinely continue to rely on representative clinical signs and we continue to look for the patient's view of reality in specific thought and behavioral processes.

In the animal, the psychomotor stimulants cocaine and amphetamine, reliably produce the behaviors—increased locomotion and stereotypy—that we think are analogous to psychosis. The early studies of locomotion and stereotypy focused primarily on amphetamine. Cocaine studies have been reviewed *(44)*. It is noteworthy and respectfully amusing, however, that a similarity between "animal psychosis" and "human hebephrenic psychosis" (now called "disorganized psychosis") is most unlikely because in this type of psychosis, uncontrollable laughter is exhibited.

Stereotyped behavior, a term that previously described a single drug expression *(84)* has markedly evolved into a term that describes a continuum of discrete and distinct components that can be differentiated both pharmacologically *(85)* and by electrolytic lesion studies *(86)*. Stereotypy is comprised of several different states of repetitive behavior (*see* ref. *87* for an excellent description of these behaviors). The brain monoamine DA has been associated with these behaviors (*see* ref. *88* for review) and the role of 5-HT in stereotypy has been discussed in ref *88*; "The Serotonin Syndrome" has also been described elsewhere *(89)*.

Specifically, 5-HT's mediation in open-field behaviors has been studied by pharmacologic lesioning interventions within 5-HT somatadendrites, the raphe nuclei. When midbrain raphe neurons were no longer viable, open-field locomotor activity was suppressed *(90–94)*. Consistent with these studies, local application of 5-HT and the 5-HT$_{1A}$ agonist, 8-hydroxy-2-(di-n-propylamino)tetralin (8-OH-DPAT) into median raphe neurons also produced hyperactivity *(95)*. The study of stereotypic or fine movement behaviors (grooming and licking) were studied by injecting 5-HT into the basal nucleus, ventrolateral striatum, and vlNAcc, and 5-HT was found to increase with increasing oral stereotypies *(96)*.

3.1.3. Cocaine and Amphetamine Effects Are Similar in Neurochemistry and Behavior

Cocaine and amphetamine are similar in their ability, acutely, to elicit sympathomimetic DA-ergic effects, increased motor activity and increased motor stereotypy *(37,97–99)*.

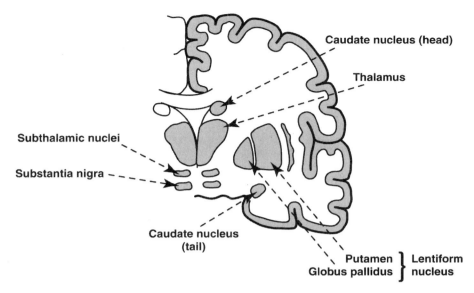

Fig. 1. Schematic diagram representing a coronal section of cerebral hemisphere, showing paired subcortical masses, the deep basal nuclei of gray matter, the extrapyramidal system (EPS). Adapted with permission from ref. *(102)*.

3.1.4. Cocaine and Amphetamine Effects Are Different in Neuronal Degeneration Processes

Cocaine, in contrast to amphetamine, did not produce neuronal degeneration in basal ganglia (nuclei) *(100)*. Cocaine still maintains its reputation of not causing neurotoxic effects on DA and 5-HT in basal nuclei *(101)*.

3.2. The Goal Is Reiterated

A microvoltammetric technology using novel miniature sensors, BRODERICK PROBE® Microelectrodes is presented. The data show empirical evidence that suggests a possible predisposed form of cocaine-induced neurotoxicity in basal nuclei. This is shown by a time-dependent neuroadaptation in 5-HT release within basal nuclei, which occurs at the same time as movement behaviors occur. First, a review of the basal ganglia motor circuits is presented.

4. BASAL GANGLIA (NUCLEI)

4.1. Extrapyramidal System

The extrapyramidal system consists of paired subcortical masses or nuclei of gray matter called basal ganglia, which are also called basal nuclei. The terms basal ganglia or basal nuclei (used interchangeably) are applied to a group of forebrain structures that include the caudate putamen and the globus pallidum. The caudate and putamen are structurally distinct in the human, but they are joined in lower mammals and are generally considered to function as a unit. Closely associated with the basal nuclei are two small brain-stem nuclei, the substantia nigra and the subthalamus *(102)* (Fig. 1).

The control of voluntary movement is executed by the interaction of the pyramidal, cerebellar, and extrapyramidal systems, which interconnect with each other as well as projecting to the anterior horn region or cranial nerve motor nuclei. The connections are highly complex, but what can be observed at first glance about the deep basal nuclei,

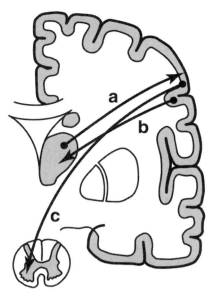

Fig. 2. Schematic diagram showing the interconnections of the deep basal nuclei. **(A)** Thalamus projects information from basal nuclei and cerebellum to motor cortex via thalamocortical circuits and influences corticospinal circuits as well. **(B)** Cortical neurons project to thalamus and serve as a feedback loop between thalamus and cortex, and **(C)** outflow is via corticobulbar and corticospinal (pyramidal) circuits. Adapted with permission from ref. *(102)*.

the basal ganglia, is that: (1) the thalamus plays a vital role in projecting information from the basal nuclei and cerebellum to the motor cortex via the thalamocortical pathways, and also exerts influence on the corticospinal pathway at its origin; (2) the cortical neurons project to the thalamus via feedback; and (3) output from basal ganglia occurs via the corticobulbar and corticospinal (cortical, pyramidal) pathways *(102)* (Fig. 2).

These small gray-matter basal nuclei, although they lie deep within the forebrain and hindbrain and away from the cortex, have complex and multifaceted neuronal connections with the cortex. Electrophysiology studies in primates and locomotor and cognitive-deficit studies in movement-disorder patients have provided suggestions for the functions of the basal nuclei. They include: (1) the determination of force and velocity of movement, (2) preparing for movement, (3) the development of automaticity of movement, (4) promoting sequential movement, (5) inhibiting unwanted movement, (6) adapting to novel or rewarding movement, and (7) motor learning and planning (*see* ref. *103*) for review.

Neuronal circuits, which include a motor loop linking the supplementary motor area (SMA) to primary motor cortex, putamen, globus pallidus and ventrolateral thalamus, and a dorsolateral prefrontal cortical pathway involving the dorsal striatum, the (A_9) caudate, and ventrolateral thalamus, are used by the basal nuclei to execute movement. Two other loops, the anterior cingulate and the orbitofrontal pathways, work to execute motor function via the ventral striatum (A_{10} nucleus accumbens). Supplementary motor area and dorsolateral prefrontal cortical circuits are thought to play a role in voluntary movement *(104,105)*. The loops involving the ventral striatum, also called the nucleus

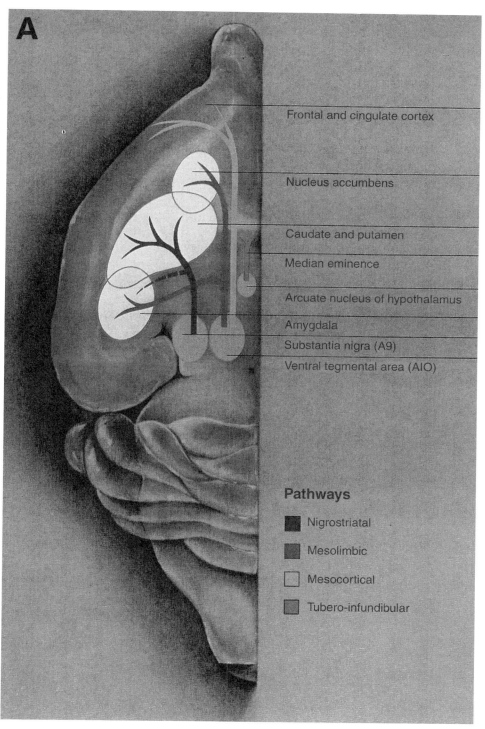

A

Frontal and cingulate cortex

Nucleus accumbens

Caudate and putamen

Median eminence

Arcuate nucleus of hypothalamus

Amygdala

Substantia nigra (A9)

Ventral tegmental area (AIO)

Pathways

Nigrostriatal

Mesolimbic

Mesocortical

Tubero-infundibular

Fig. 3A. (*See* color plate 4 appearing in the insert following p. 368)

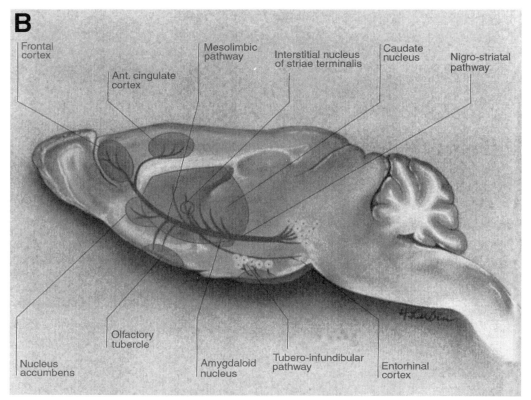

Fig. 3. (A) Schematic diagram of anatomic dopamine (DA) tracts in the rat brain, represented longitudinally. **(B)** Schematic diagram of anatomic dopamine (DA) tracts in the rat brain, represented sagittally. Adapted with permission from ref. *(108)*. (*See* color plate 5 appearing in the insert following p. 368.)

accumbens (NAcc) (A_{10}), are believed to subserve attention and motor responses to novel or rewarding situations, respectively *(106,107)*. Closely related, even physically to the nigrostriatal DA A_9 pathway is the A_{10} pathway, which is a mesencephalic DA projection from the somatodendritic ventral tegmentum (VTA) to the ventral striatum, A_{10} terminals (also called NAcc).

DA-ergic neurons emanate from A_8 and A_9 cell bodies in the pars compacta of the substantia nigra; A_8 and A_9 cell bodies merge imperceptibly with the A_{10} cell bodies in the medial region above the interpeduncular nucleus. The axons of A_8 and A_9 cells form the nigrostriatal pathway, which runs in the crus cerebri and internal capsule to innervate the basal nuclei, the caudate nucleus, putamen and globus pallidus, and possibly the amygdala. This is the pathway that degenerates in idiopathic PD and other diseases that occur after exposure to toxic substances, such as carbon monoxide. This is also the pathway that is involved with the adverse side effects, the motor effects, (extrapyramidal side effects) associated with the use of neuroleptic drugs used in the treatment of schizophrenia. Motor abnormalities (stereotypies), such as those induced by cocaine and amphetamine, originate in this pathway.

The A_{10} cell bodies form the mesolimbic projection system, which runs more medially to terminate in NAcc just anterior to the caudate, olfactory tubercle, septum, and related areas. This tract is believed to act in the regulation of emotional behavior, especially the motor components of emotional behavior, such as the locomotor component of the psychomotor-stimulant behaviors associated with cocaine and amphetamine. Axons from A_{10} neurons and from the medial part of the A_9 group also project to the frontal-cingulate and entorhinal cortices and this extended pathway forms the mesocorticolimbic tract.

In addition, there are several short DA-ergic pathways close to the midline, which run from the central grey area to various nuclei in the thalamus and hypothalamus. One of these is the tuberoinfundibular; its cell bodies are located in the arcuate nucleus and its axons project into the median eminence and pars intermedia of the pituitary (*see* ref. *108*) (Fig. 3A,B).

4.2. Dopamine in Basal Nuclei

Significant amounts of DA were found in basal nuclei terminals, A_9 nerve terminals, and striatum by Bertler and Rosengren in Carlsson's laboratory *(109,110)* and by another group of researchers, Sano and colleagues *(111)*, about the same time. The somatodendrites, the cell bodies for the A_9 region, substantia nigra, were found to contain DA approx 2 yr later *(112)*. The visualization of the monoamines including DA soon followed and DA was visualized in cell bodies and nerve terminals of the A_9 region *(113–115)* by the Falck et al. *(116)* method, with the largest DA-containing pathway originating in the substantia nigra pars compacta. Dopamine in the ventral tegmental pathway, the adjacent pathway to the nigrostriatal pathway, was reported by Anden et al. *(117)*.

The A_9 and A_{10} DA circuits were further distinguished from each other in terms of psychomotor-stimulant behavior. In pioneering studies, the neurotoxin, 6-hydroxy-dopamine (6-OHDA) was used to lesion the basal nucleus A_9 striatum, and the result was to eliminate the classical stereotyped responses of grooming and licking *(118)*. In other pioneering studies, the psychomotor stimulant, amphetamine, was injected into basal nuclei, A_{10} NAcc, and olfactory tubercle; the result was the production of locomotor hyperactivity *(119)*.

There is now an extensive body of empirical evidence pointing to cocaine's potent ability to affect motor function and actually cause movement disorders by affecting DA in basal nuclei and in DA somatodendrites. These are habit-forming responses, which are also DA-dependent *(16)*. Craving for cocaine can re-emerge, even months or years after the last episode of cocaine use, and cocaine craving can occur in association with affective (mood) states (either positive or negative), geographic locations, specific persons or events, intoxication with other substances, or in the presence of various objects directly or indirectly connected with cocaine use *(120)*. Cocaine craving appears to be related to DA, to a reduction in DA neurotransmission *(121)*, to a reduction in 5-HT *(122)*, and to a reduction in both DA and 5-HT simultaneously *(123)*.

4.3. Serotonin in Basal Nuclei

Serotonin was reported to co-exist in DA neurons in basal nuclei about 25 yr ago. An analytical study of 5-HT neuronal organization in brain demonstrated a prominent transtegmental 5-HT fiber pathway in the A_{10} region that begins in median raphe (MR) and dorsal raphe (DR), which then curves ventrally across DA somatodendrites in VTA

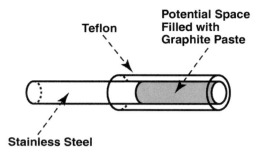

Fig. 4. Schematic diagram of the BRODERICK PROBE® Microelectrodes for the selective electrochemical detection, in vitro, in vivo, and *in situ*, of neurotransmitters, neuromodulators, metabolites, precursors, and peptides in humans and animals, centrally and peripherally. These inventions relate to a variety of unique, patented, and trademarked miniature carbon sensors comprised of a series of selective organic and inorganic compounds. Schematic diagram of microelectrode is greatly oversized; actual sizes range from numbers of microns in single digits to a few hundred microns. For detailed description of microsensors and biotechnology, *see* chapter text and cited references *(37–40,44,133–143)*.

to communicate in MFB *(124,125)*. Both autoradiographic *(124)* and immunohistochemical *(126)* studies and our studies *(44)* show that VTA *per se* contains a dense network of 5-HT axonal varicosities. Ultrastructural evidence from light and electron microscopy show that, after an intraventricular infusion of [^{3}H]-5-HT, 5-HT neurons innervate DA neurons via actual synaptic communication *(127)*. More recent evidence reports the existence of prominent asymmetric junctions, which are formed by 5-HT-labeled terminals in A_{10} DA projections to NAcc, suggesting a cellular basis for 5-HT excitation of A_{10} DA neurons *(128)*. Furthermore, 5-HT axons from DR and MR converge in hypothalamus at the neuroanatomic substrate, MFB; anterograde and retrograde studies have shown that A_9 DStr and A_{10} NAcc as well as hippocampus are major targets of these 5-HT-ergic projections *(129–132)*.

5. NOVEL MICROSENSORS AND BIOTECHNOLOGY

5.1. BRODERICK PROBE® Microelectrodes

These inventions relate to a variety of unique, patented, and trademarked miniature carbon sensors, which are selectively comprised of a series of compounds that includes, among others, classes of molecules in the biochemical categories of lipid, glycolipid, lipoprotein, and saturated and unsaturated fatty acid. These inventions are able to detect electrochemical signals for a vast number of neurotransmitters, neuromodulators, and metabolites, including neuropeptides, hormones, and vitamins *(133–137)*. In this laboratory, we routinely and selectively detect in discrete neuroanatomic substrates of living human and animal brain, the monoamines, DA, NE, and 5-HT, in addition to the precursor to 5-HT, l-tryptophan (l-TP), ascorbic acid (AA), and uric acid (UA) *(138–143)*. This laboratory has also differentiated the catecholamines, DA and NE, electrochemically *(138,143)*. The electrochemical detection of somatostatin and dynorphin A are among our latest discoveries *(141,142)*.

A schematic diagram of the BRODERICK PROBE® Microelectrodes is shown in Fig. 4. Within the field of electrochemistry, this sensor is termed the "indicator" microelectrode and is also called the "working" microelectrode. The readers' attention is directed to the surface of the microelectrode. The surface consisting of carbon, is the electrochemical device.

Capacitance is one of the most important concepts in electrochemistry. Capacitance is important at the surface of the indicator microelectrode. When one changes the surface of the sensor, one changes the capacitance of the surface of the sensor. The surface of the indicator microelectrode is a capacitance diffuse double layer (C_{dt}) that allows potential to accumulate on its surface. Capacitance is a critical aspect of charging (background) current. Charging current is a current pulse that flows through the C_{dt} to allow faradaic electron transfer to begin. Allowing potential to accumulate on the surface of the indicator microelectrode is a necessary requirement to get to the point where faradaic electron transfer can begin. Charging current is proportional to electrode surface area, therefore, these miniature sensors (200 microns and less in diameter) minimize charging current effects.

BRODERICK PROBES® detect basal (normal, natural, endogenous, or steady-state) concentrations of neurotransmitters and other neurochemicals in vivo, in situ, and in vitro, as well as any alterations in these neurotransmitters or neurochemicals in brain or body before and after pharmacological manipulation with drugs and other compounds. Neurochemicals during actual, induced, or even mimicked brain diseases can be detected as well. Neurochemicals in the brain and body of animals and human can be detected. The studies presented in this chapter focus on 5-HT alterations in NAcc in the freely moving animal during normal open-field behaviors of locomotor (exploratory) and stereotypy compared with, in the same animal, cocaine psychomotor-stimulant effects on 5-HT and behavior. However, other disorders can be studied, e.g., (a) in the area of other athetoid, dystonic diseases, such as Lesch Nyhan Syndrome. This is a disease somewhat recently recognized wherein there is severe athetoid and dystonic movements and self-mutilation, and repetitive oral stereotypies. This is a debilitating disease; patients' teeth may have to be removed to avoid oral stereotypies that cause the patient to devour lips, tongues, or fingers. The stereotypies involve DA and 5-HT *(144)*, and high levels of UA levels are involved *(145)*; (b) in the area of other athetoid and dystonic diseases: autism, schizophrenia, epilepsy, and PD are amenable for study with these miniature sensors, even intraoperatively, insofar as epilepsy and PD are concerned; and (c) cancers, both peripheral and central, are amenable for study with these miniature sensors *(133–143)*.

5.2. General Description of the Microvoltammetric Technique

Microvoltammetric indicator microelectrodes do not sense membrane potentials. Instead, indicator microelectrodes pass small but finite currents as neurotransmitters and metabolites close to the microelectrode surface undergo oxidation and/or reduction *(146)*. When an electrode is placed in contact with a solution, any solution, a phase boundary is created that separates out identical solutes into two different types. They are: (1) molecules that are at a distance from the microelectrode, and (2) those molecules that are close enough to participate in mutual interactions between the surface of the microelectrode and the sample-solution interface. Kissinger calls these interactions, whether with macro or microelectrodes, fascinating, and this author agrees *(147)*. Collectively, these interactions are called electrochemistry.

$$i_t = nFAC_0D_0^{1/2}/3.14^{1/2}t^{1/2}$$

where i = current at time t
       n = number of electrons, eq/mol
       F = Faraday's constant, 96,486C/eq
       A = electrode area, cm²
       C = concentration of O, mol/cm³
       D = Diffusion coefficient of O, cm²/s

Fig. 5. The Cottrell Equation: The proportionality between charge and mass of an electrochemical reaction describes the relationship between charge of each neurochemical in the process of oxidation/reduction and concentration of each neurochemical.

Detection of electrochemical signals from solutions and also from anatomic brain sites is termed "faradaic," because the amount of the oxidative and/or reductive species detected at the surface of the microelectrode, is calculated by a derivation of Faraday's Law, the "Cottrell Equation" (Fig. 5). The proportionality between charge and mass of an electrochemical reaction describes the relationship between the charge of each neurochemical in the process of oxidation and/or reduction and the concentration of each neurochemical. The Cottrell Equation relates to quiet solution experiments wherein the potential is instantaneously switched from an initial value E_i to a final potential, then held constant for a fixed time, then switched back to E_i. If material diffuses to a planar electrode surface in only one direction (linear diffusion) then the exact description of the current-time curve is the Cottrell Equation.

Current-time relationships with a circular electrode are defined in electrochemistry by the Cottrell Equation. For a long time, other electrode sizes and experiments using different electrolysis times were considered deviations from the Cottrell Equations that could be considered negligible but Wightman's laboratory pointed out that linear diffusion is not enough to describe the action that takes place at spherical microelectrodes *(148)*. Therefore, it is important to remember that the quiet solution behavior of very small electrodes is different and this is described well in *(146)* where a steady state equation involving the radius of the electrode is taken into account, so that for even a 300 micron diameter electrode, one can calculate that the edge effect or spherical steady-state contribution adds approx 30% "extra" current to the linear diffusion component for an electrolysis time of only one second.

5.3. Microvoltammetric Circuit: The Detector

BRODERICK PROBES® can be used in conjunction with classical electrical circuits used in electrochemistry such as chronoamperometry, differential-pulse voltammetry, and double differential-pulse voltammetry. Another electrical circuit for providing an output signal having a mathematical relationship in operation to an input signal can be semiderivative or semidifferential. These two terms are used interchangeably here, although these two circuits have some technical differences. Semiderivative electroanalysis diminishes nonfaradaic current by the addition of analysis time. In the present studies, a CV 37 detector (BAS, West Lafayette, IN) was equipped with a semiderivative circuit. This circuit uses a linear scanning methodology as its basis. Semiderivative treatment of voltammetric data means that the signals are recorded mathematically as the first half derivative of the linear analog signal. A semiderivative circuit combines an additional series of resistors and capacitors, called a "ladder network" *(149)*, with the traditional linear scanning technology, which then allows more clearly defined waveforms and peak amplitudes of electrochemical signals than was previously possible with linear scanning methodology.

5.4. In Vivo Microvoltammetric (Electrochemical) Method

The main strength of in vivo microvoltammetry (electrochemistry) is that it is considered among neuroscientists to be clearly superior to others, in the sense that it allows the study of the neurochemical time-course of action of normal neurochemistry, as well as the neurochemistry after an administered drug regimen. Temporal resolution is fast, in seconds and milliseconds. Moreover, the attendant microspatial resolution is superior (availability of discrete areas of brain without disruption). Highly sensitive temporal and spatial resolution make these studies ultimately most efficient for mechanism of action studies Another strength lies in the fact that these in vivo microvoltammetric studies are done in the freely moving and behaving animal model, using the same animal as its own control (studies in the living human brain are underway as well). Thus, we can directly determine whether or not we are dealing with an abnormal neurochemical effect because the normal neurochemical effect is seen *a priori*.

The basic in vivo electrochemistry experiment involves the implantation of an indicator electrode in a discrete and specified region of brain, the application of a potential to that electrode, the oxidation or reduction of the selected neurochemical, and the recording of the resultant current. In essence, the potential is applied between the indicator and the reference electrode; the reference electrode provides a relative zero potential. This is an electrochemical technique with which information about an analyte, a neurotransmitter, or its metabolite, including its concentration, is derived from an electrochemical current as a function of a potential difference, a potential difference that is applied to the surface of an electrochemical electrode.

It is necessary to make an important distinction between the detection of signals in microvoltammetry as compared with the detection of signals in microdialysis, i.e., in the microvoltammetric technology, the indicator microelectrodes is the detecting device, whereas in microdialysis methods, the dialysis membrane is a membrane and not the detecting device. The microdialysis membrane is simply a membrane through which perfusate is collected. The perfusate is then brought to the HPLC device, equipped with an electrochemical column that is the actual detecting device. These electrochemical columns range in millimeters in diameter, whereas microvoltammetry-indicator microelectrodes range from single-digit microns to a few hundred microns in diameter.

Currently, there is a grave misconception in the neuroscience community that the microdialysis membrane is the detecting device and, therefore, that this microdialysis membrane can be compared directly with the microvoltammetry indicator-detecting devices. Whether or not microdialysis membranes are the same size as voltammetry microelectrodes is irrelevant because the microdialysis membrane is not the detection

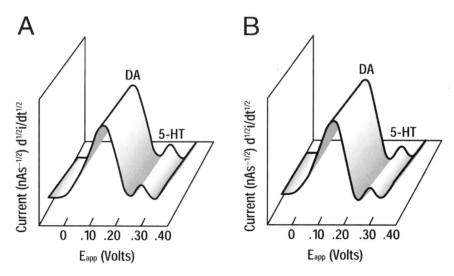

Fig. 6. Microvoltammograms, recorded in vivo and in real time, from NAcc of freely moving and behaving, male, fawn-hooded laboratory rats (*x* axis is oxidation potential in millivolts; *y* axis is current derived from each neurochemical; Current Scale = 25 pAs$^{-1/2}$ 12.5 mm$^{-1/2}$). **(A)** was recorded 2 wk after surgical implantation of BRODERICK PROBES® under sodium pentobarbital anesthesia and **(B)** was recorded 7 mo later. Both voltammograms represent endogenous release of DA and serotonin (5-HT) in the basal nucleus, NAcc, while the animal is exhibiting normal motor activity in the open-field behavioral paradigm. Animal was not treated with drugs at either recording time, nor was the animal treated with drugs during the 7-mo period; recordings taken during the 7-mo period were stable as well.

technology. Microdialysis membranes simply collect perfusate from brain and this perfusate is then analyzed by HPLC.

5.5. Identification of Microvoltammetric Signals

In microvoltammetry, each neurotransmitter, metabolite, precursor to neurotransmitter, etc. is identified by the peak oxidation potential, or half-wave potential at which the neurochemical generates its maximum current. What does this mean? In this chapter, the focus is on the biogenic amines DA and 5-HT. Figure 6A,B show microvoltammetric recordings obtained in vivo from NAcc of a male, fawn-hooded, freely moving and behaving laboratory rat. On the *x* axis, the oxidation potential in millivolts is delineated; current generated is depicted on the *y* axis. It is clear that the oxidation potential at which DA generates its maximum current, in vivo, at physiological pH, and 37.5°C, in NAcc is, +0.140 V (SE derived from over 1000 studies is ±0.015 V). Serotonin, shown as the second electrochemical signal detected, generates its maximum current at a peak oxidation potential of +0.290 V (SE derived from over 1000 studies is ±0.015 V).

What matters in microvoltammetry is that each of these biogenic amines have amine groups that are protonated at neutral pH and therefore, exist as cations, whereas metabolites of the monoamines are deprotonated at neutral pH and exist as anions *(150)*. Thus, the monoamine metabolites such as the metabolites of DA, 3,4 dihydroxyphenylacetic acid (DOPAC), 3,4-dihydroxyphenylglycol (DHPG-DOPEG), and homovanillic acid (HVA) cannot interfere with the detection of DA at the same peak oxidation potential or half-wave potential that is characteristic of DA.

The same principles are applicable to detection of the biogenic amine, 5-HT. Serotonin is detected without interference at the same oxidation potential or half-wave potential from either its metabolite, 5-hydroxyindoleacetic acid (5-HIAA), or UA, which is a constituent of brain with similar electroactive properties to those of 5-HT. Factors such as the significantly lower sensitivity of the indicator microelectrode to anions, the charge and diffusion characteristics of each catecholamine or indoleamine vis-à-vis its metabolites, preclude such interference. Descriptions of each neurochemical detected in this laboratory with BRODERICK PROBES® are published in detail *(37–40,44,133–143)*.

The detection of compounds such as glutamate is a work in progress in this laboratory. Although the detection of glutamate is routinely reported by scientists who utilize the microdialysis method in conjunction with HPLC with electrochemical (EC) detection, these reports are essentially inaccurate. It is the detection of a derivative of glutamate that actually occurs with microdialysis. Acetylcholine, too, often reported to be detected by the microdialysis membrane method, is not really detected at all. It is hydrogen peroxide (H_2O_2) that is detected, instead of the neurotransmitter acetylcholine with microdialysis *(151)*. Moreover, correlation between either the derivative of glutamate or H_2O_2 detected and the Cottrell Equation has never been addressed with microdialysis. Therefore, detection of straight chain carbon compounds by the microdialysis membrane method may be questionable.

5.6. Characteristics of the BRODERICK PROBE® Microelectrodes

5.6.1. Provide Long-Lived and Stable Electrochemical Signals

Figure 6A,B depicts microvoltammograms recorded in *real time* and in vivo from NAcc freely moving and behaving fawn-hooded laboratory rats, at (A) 2 wk postsurgical implantation and (B) 7 mo later, published by this laboratory *(123,152)*. A BRODERICK PROBE® indicator microelectrode was implanted in NAcc and reference and auxiliary microelectrodes were placed in contact with cortex under sodium pentobarbital anesthesia. Separate signals for DA and 5-HT were recorded in the freely moving rat, 2 wk after recovery from surgery (Fig. 6A). Figure 6B shows the detection of DA and 5-HT in NAcc from the same animal, 7 mo later. Both voltammograms represent normal/natural release of the biogenic amines DA and 5-HT in NAcc. The animal was not treated with drugs at either recording time, nor was the animal treated with drugs for any time during the 7 mo-period. Recordings taken during the 7 mo were stable as well. Histology (intracardial 10% formalin-perfusion method) was performed to assess that the indicator microelectrode had not changed position due to increase in animal weight. A 15-yr data base from this laboratory shows that these miniature sensors maintain their integrity and provide reliable reproducible detection of signals long term in chronic implants.

5.6.2. Do Not Promote Bacterial Growth

Studies from Dr. Phil Tierno's laboratory at NYU Medical School show that BRODERICK PROBES® do not promote bacterial growth either before or after sterilization with gamma irradiation. Gamma irradiation treatment was performed by Sterigenics International, Inc. (Haw River, NC).

5.6.3. Can Be Used Effectively for Different Applications in Human and Animal Surgery

Preliminary studies with BRODERICK PROBE® Lauric Acid microelectrodes showed a particularly faster stabilization rate to reach neurotransmitter steady-state levels. This may be important for intraoperative recordings *(133–137,153)*.

5.6.4. Can Be Quantitated

Generally, quantitation of neurochemistry is described as a percentage of a few data points, over hours, used as "control" in microdialysis studies. However, BRODERICK PROBES® are easily calibrated and concentrations are interpolated from calibration curves *(143)*.

5.7. Study Protocol

5.7.1. Implantation of BRODERICK PROBE® Microelectrodes

Stereotaxic surgery was performed under pentobarbital sodium anesthesia, on male, virus-free, Sprague-Dawley laboratory rats for implantation of BRODERICK PROBE® Microelectrodes; the atlas used was Pellegrino et al. *(154)*. Ag/AgCl reference micro-electrodes and stainless steel auxiliary microelectrodes were placed in contact with the cortex, approx 7 mm contralaterally to the placement of the indicator microelectrode *(37,44,133–143)*. The basal nuclei, A_9 dorsal striatum (DStr) and A_{10} ventral striatum (NAcc), were studied, in addition to the brain-stem nucleus, the somatodendritic A_{10} VTA. Stereotaxic coordinates were: DStr, +2.5 mm anterior to Bregma, +2.6 mm lateral to midline and –5.0 mm below skull surface; NAcc, +2.5 mm anterior to Bregma, +2.6 mm lateral to midline and –7.3 mm below skull surface and VTA, +2.8 mm anterior to Bregma, 0.9 mm lateral to midline and –8.6 mm below skull surface.

The three microelectrode assembly, indicator, reference, and auxiliary, enclosed within the animal's prosthetic acrylic cap, was connected to a CV 37 detector by means of a mercury commutator (Brain Res. Instruments, Princeton, NJ), a flexible cable, and a mating connector (BJM Electronics, Staten Island, NY).

Cocaine HCL (Sigma/Aldrich, St. Louis, MO), (10 mg/kg) was dissolved in distilled water, and injected intraperitoneally, following the completion of first, the exploration, and second, the habituation period of behavior.

5.7.2. A Note on the Subdivisions of the NAcc, Core, and Shell

The subterritories of NAcc, core and shell, have been recently delineated based on brain regional distribution of neurochemicals including DA, neuropeptides, and calcium-binding protein. These consist of a central core region, which surrounds the anterior commissure, and a shell region, which is more ventromedial than the core; the shell region partially encases the core *(155–159)*. Core projects to typical motor-related structures of basal nuclei and shell projects primarily to limbic structures of basal nuclei *(160)*. Core region projects to the dorsolateral part of the ventral pallidum, which in turn projects to the subthalamic nucleus and A_9 somatodendrites, substantia nigra (SN), whereas shell projects to the ventromedial ventral pallidum, which in turn projects to the A_{10} somatodendrites VTA *(160–162)*.

The subterritories of the basal nucleus, NAcc, and the amygdala may be key neural sites for the neuroadaptative processes used by cocaine *(163)*. The amygdala exhibits

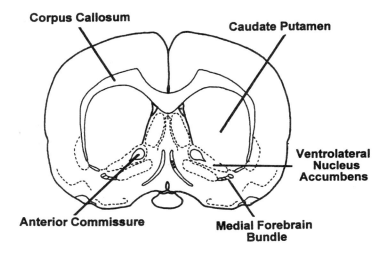

Fig. 7. Schematic diagram of microelectrode placement in vlNAcc. The tip of the arrow denotes the tip of the indicator microelectrode. It is important to note that this particular BRODERICK PROBE® Microelectrode was 200 μm diameter by 500 μm length. These miniature sensors cause virtually no damage to brain tissue because they are the same dimensions throughout their length. It is noteworthy that the carbon-fiber microelectrode *(148)* (although 10 μm in diameter at the tip) actually has a much larger diameter throughout its entire length. It is also noteworthy that the microdialysis membrane, although it is not equivalent to voltammetry electrodes because it is not the detecting device, still has wider dimensions than those reported for the voltammetry electrodes. Adapted from Pellegrino, L.J., Pellegrino, A.S., Cushman, A.J. (1979) *A Stereotaxic Atlas of the Rat Brain,* Plenum Press, NY *(154).*

projections to both core and shell of NAcc *(164–166)*, with patterns of afferent inner-vation of the core exhibiting patch and matrix characteristics similar to that of striatum (DStr) and that of shell exhibiting cell-cluster patches *(165)*. Importantly, 5-HT has been demonstrated in both core and shell subterritories of A_{10} basal nucleus, NAcc, and in VTA *(167–172)*.

5.7.3. A Note on the vlNAcc

The vlNAcc was noted early on by Swanson and Cohen *(173)*. Depicted schemati-cally in Fig. 7, as indicated by Pellegrino et al. *(150)*, we considered the vlNAcc to be a critical substructure to study in both normal and cocaine-induced motor behavior because both anterograde- and retrograde-tract tracing studies have demonstrated a reciprocal connectivity between the vlNAcc and VTA *(173–175)*.

5.7.4. Basal Nuclei, DStr, NAcc Core, and Motor Behavior

Previous studies on DA-ergic neurotransmission have divided striatal behaviors, thought to include fine movements, such as grooming and sniffing, from accumbens behaviors, such as locomotion *(118–119)*. However, new hypotheses have emerged; for example, the hypothesis of Whishaw et al. *(176)* is interesting, although technique and results were limited, wherein DA in frontal cortex and striatum may compete for behavioral expression of locomotor and stereotypic behavior. Moreover, Oades has discussed an hypothesis for DA having the inherent ability to switch between target outputs circuits in CNS to control different motor behaviors *(177)*. Functionally, this "switching" hypothesis could be extrapolated to DA-ergic mechanism in NAcc to switch to cue-directed behaviors also *(178)*.

However, ideas are forming to elucidate a role for the anatomic differences between NAcc core and shell, in relationship to DA and 5-HT in basal nuclei, which may be responsible for switching target output circuits for locomotion and stereotypy from one target nucleus to another. This could mean switching from classically core-directed behaviors to classically shell-dependent behaviors in a time-dependent manner. An extensive treatise that provides evidence for the suggestion that 5-HT may act through DA to inhibit shell neurons, switching to core output and in addition, exciting core neurons to switch from locomotion to stereotypy, is presented in ref. *(44)*. Other functional implications come from the work of Van Bockstaele and Pickel *(179)*, wherein, based on differing sizes of 5-HT terminals in the core vs the shell, they proposed that a phasic rapidly fatigued 5-HT release pattern in the core is consistent with highly repetitive yet, shorter behavioral events, which would typify classical behavioral stereotypy. On the other hand, these authors proposed that a tonic 5-HT release in the shell, would be more consistent with more macro-type movements, e.g., persistent and unchanged, more simple unidirectional movements.

6. BEHAVIORAL METHODOLOGY

Behaviors were studied by infrared photocell beam detection. The faradaic copper-enclosed Plexiglass behavioral chamber [L = 23"; W = 18"; H = 23.5"], was equipped with side-by-side double doors [W = 15.5"; H = 23.5"] to enable a facile injection procedure. This system permits simultaneous monitoring of several different responses both as they occur in space and in time with a resolution of 0.1 s in time and 1.5 inches, spatially *(180)*. A computerized 16×16 array of infrared photobeams was used to define the *xy* position of the animal within a 1.5 inch resolution. Every 100 ms, the computer sampled the status of all the photocell beams in the behavioral chamber. Multiple concurrent measures of the animals' activity were simultaneously assayed. Data were then reduced to individual behavioral components: (1) locomotor activity (Ambulations) and (2) stereotypy, repetitive movements of grooming and sniffing (Fine Movements). Activity patterns were simultaneously assayed while neurochemical detection of each biogenic amine was detected. Behavioral data are presented as frequency (number of behavioral events). The test system was custom built by San Diego Instruments (San Diego, CA).

7. SEROTONIN WITHIN MOTOR CIRCUITS MODULATES RHYTHMIC, EPISODIC MOVEMENT DURING NORMAL BEHAVIOR

7.1. Serotonin within DA Basal Nuclei: DStr. (A_9) and NAcc (A_{10})

In Fig. 8, release of 5-HT within DStr, an A_9 DA basal nucleus and nerve-terminal field, is plotted with Ambulations (top) and Fine Movements (bottom). These studies were performed in real time during open-field locomotor (exploratory) and stereotypic behaviors from time 0 min to time 60 min as movement occurred. Serotonin release in this motor nucleus is rhythmic with movement even as movement waxed and waned. This was an intriguing and exciting result since locomotion is known to be not only

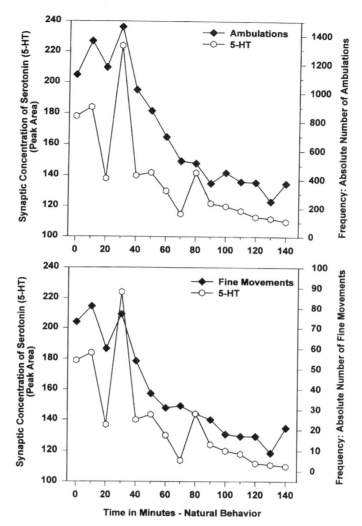

Fig. 8. Normal neurochemistry and behavior: Line graph depicting endogenous 5-HT release (open circles) at basal nucleus, A_9 terminals, DStr, detected in real time, while the freely moving, male, Sprague-Dawley laboratory rat is actually behaving, during normal/natural movement (first hour) and subsequent habituation behavior (second hour). Serotonin, detected within seconds of release, is plotted with a line graph derived from infrared photobeam monitoring of behavior (closed circles): (top) Locomotion (Ambulations); (bottom) Stereotypy (Fine Movements). Open-field behaviors were studied in units of frequency of events recorded every 100 ms during normal/natural behavior. Data show that normal episodic, rhythmic nature of locomotor movement may be neuromodulated by 5-HT within the basal nucleus, A_9 terminals.

rhythmic but, very importantly, it is known to be episodic, unlike most other rhythmic and repetitive behaviors.

In Fig. 9, release of 5-HT within NAcc, an A_{10} DA basal nucleus and nerve-terminal field, is plotted with Ambulations (top) and Fine Movements (bottom). These studies, also performed in real time, show that 5-HT was released in a motor nucleus, again, rhythmically and episodically during the open-field paradigm study, of locomotor

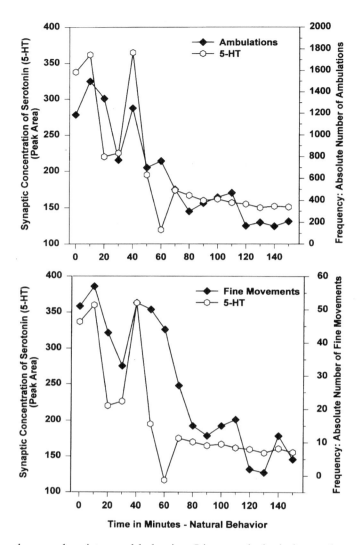

Fig. 9. Normal neurochemistry and behavior: Line graph depicting endogenous 5-HT release (open circles) at basal nucleus A_{10} terminals, vlNAcc, in real time, while the freely moving, male, Sprague-Dawley laboratory rat is actually behaving, during normal/natural movement (first hour) and subsequent habituation behavior (second hour). Serotonin, detected within seconds of release, is plotted with a line graph derived from simultaneous infrared photobeam monitoring of behavior (closed circles): (top) Locomotions (Ambulations); (bottom) Stereotypy (Fine Movements). Open-field behaviors were studied in units of frequency of events, which were recorded every 100 ms during normal/natural locomotor behavior. Data show that normal episodic, rhythmic nature of locomotor movement may be neuromodulated by 5-HT within the basal nucleus, A_{10} terminals.

(exploratoy) and stereotypic behaviors as movement occurred, and again, even as movement's episodic nature was clear. Notice, in both figures, that as the habituation period was initiated and continued from time 60 min to time 120 min, 5-HT release was rhythmic with both movement and cessation of movement. Also very interesting is that, although the frequency of Ambulations and Fine Movements was not significantly different between studies shown in Figs. 8 and 9, the extent of 5-HT released in A_9 was less than that released in A_{10} basal nucleus.

The data show a co-relationship between the 5-HT released within basal nuclei and the motor performance of the animal in the open-field paradigm. Moreover, the rhythm between 5-HT released within A_9 basal nucleus and motor behavior is remarkably similar to that rhythm seen between 5-HT released within A_{10} basal nucleus and motor behavior.

Thus, 5-HT within terminal basal nuclei affects rhythmic movement during the normal/natural operation of repetitive motor behaviors. Serotonin, released within the A_9 terminal field, DStr, and the A_{10} terminal field, vlNAcc, increased as each open field behavior increased. But, the fact that 5-HT increased as movement increased, is not the "cutting edge" story. The cutting edge story is that 5-HT is released within basal nuclei in a time-course fashion, with the time-course changes in motor behavior controlled by the same nuclei that are responsible for the movement. This demonstrates that 5-HT released within terminal basal nuclei may direct open-field episodic, locomotor (exploratory), and stereotypic movement behaviors.

Lucki, in a review as recent as 1998, states that, "diminished 5-HT causes increased exploratory or locomotor activity" *(181)*. However, there is considerable data that show that 5-HT increases as exploratory or locomotor movement increases (e.g., *90–96*). The technology presented here enables scientists to move away from gross behavioral studies that simply average events over long periods of time and space.

7.2. Serotonin Within DA (A_{10}) Cell Bodies, the Somatodendrites VTA

In Fig. 10, 5-HT, released within A_{10} somatodendrites, is plotted with Ambulations (top) and Fine Movements (bottom). These studies were also performed in real time, and show that 5-HT was released in a motor brain-stem nucleus, again, rhythmically and episodically during the usual, normal/natural operation of movement behaviors as movement occurred, without cocaine, and again, even as movement's episodic nature was clear. Habituation brought about a decrease in 5-HT release as well as a decrease in locomotor and stereotypic behaviors. Serotonin release in VTA was less than that seen in the basal nuclei.

Within DA somatodendrites, release of 5-HT dramatically increased in a synchronous and rhythmic manner with Ambulations and Fine Movement behaviors of grooming and sniffing. Yet, the temporal relationship between 5-HT released within A_{10} somatodendrites, VTA, with movement, is different from that 5-HT released in A_{10} terminals and in A_9 terminals, with movement. Still highly rhythmic, 5-HT released within A_{10} somatodendrites, affects movement in a juxtaposed pattern that was not seen in basal nuclei DA nerve terminals, A_9 DStr, or within A_{10} NAc. This was also an intriguing and exciting result since A_{10} somatodendrites are not basal nuclei; A_{10} cell

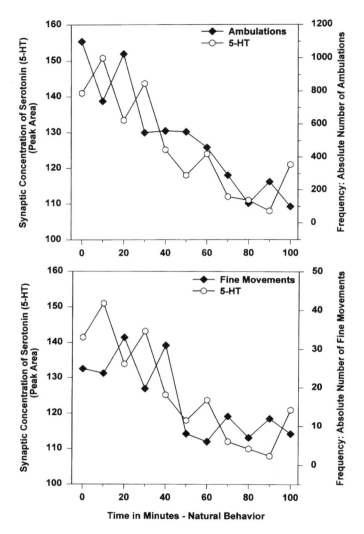

Fig. 10. Normal neurochemistry and behavior: Line graph depicting endogenous 5-HT release (open circles) at basal stem nucleus, DA A_{10} terminals, somatodendrites, VTA, in real time, while the freely moving, male, Sprague-Dawley laboratory rat is actually behaving, during normal/natural movement (first hour) and subsequent habituation behavior (second hour). Serotonin, detected within seconds of release, is plotted with a line graph derived from simultaneous infrared photobeam monitoring of behavior (closed circles): (top) Locomotion (Ambulations); (bottom) Stereotypy (Fine Movements). Open-field behaviors were studied in units of frequency of events, which were recorded every 100 ms during normal/natural locomotor behavior. Data show that normal episodic, rhythmic nature of locomotor movement is exhibited and can be detected with this biotechnology. However, still very rhythmic 5-HT neuromodulation of movement in VTA exhibits a different pattern of rhythm with movement than that pattern seen in basal nuclei.

bodies is a brain stem nucleus, comprised of DA somatodendritic neurons projecting to A_{10} basal nuclei.

What may be an important mechanism, managing the communication between 5-HT released within DA somatodendrites during concurrent open-field Ambulatory and Fine Movement behavior, is the increase in somatodendritic 5-HT cell firing within 5-HT somatodendrites that occurs before movement behavior occurs *(182)*, which influences DA interactions within terminal basal nuclei *(44)*. Also realized, among other possible mechanisms that could be operating here, is that an important component of DA neuronal responsiveness is dendritic release properties of DA somatodendritic autoreceptors on DA cells *(183)* with calcium-conductance properties, typical of cells exhibiting dendritic release of neurotransmitter *(184)*. Influenced by DR stimulation, *(185)* the time-lag could be due to suppressed DA somatodendritic excitability.

From Figs. 8–10, a synopsis of important messages about normal/natural 5-HT release within two basal nuclei, a brain stem nucleus and movement behaviors, follows:

- 5-HT released within A_9 and A_{10} basal nuclei and A_{10} somatodendrites increased with locomotor behavior and with the fine movement stereotypic behaviors of grooming and sniffing; 5-HT decreased during habituation when movement had essentially ceased.
- 5-HT released within A_9 and A_{10} basal nuclei, exhibits rhythmicity, in synchrony with locomotion and stereotypic behavior; dramatically similar rhythmic patterns occurred within both basal nuclei.
- 5-HT released within A_{10} somatodendrites, DA cell bodies, and VTA also showed remarkable rhythmicity with movement and stereotypic behavior, but the rhythmic control by 5-HT in A_{10} somatodendrites assumes a different pattern that that pattern observed when basal nuclei were studied. VTA is brain stem nucleus and not a basal nucleus.
- Data demonstrate normal/natural rhythmic episodic movement behaviors, which previous technologies did not enable.
- 5-HT released within A_{10} DA nerve terminals during movement and stereotypic behaviors was greater than that within A_9 DA nerve terminals and the latter, was greater than that 5-HT released within A_{10} somatodendrites during movement behaviors.
- The data suggest that 5-HT may control episodic and rhythmic movement behaviors in DA basal nuclei and in the brain stem nucleus, A_{10} somatodendrites. This control or modulation is different in basal nuclei compared with the brain stem nucleus, A_{10} somatodendrites.
- Superior temporal resolution is a crucial component of technologies that claim to study neurotransmitters and behavior within the same animal, in vivo, and in real time.

8. COCAINE DISRUPTS NORMAL RHYTHMIC, EPISODIC MODULATION OF MOVEMENT VIA 5-HT IN MOTOR CIRCUITS

8.1. Basal Nucleus, vlNAcc (A_{10})

Something happened to the rhythmic nature of 5-HT released in A_{10} NAcc, as 5-HT release relates to movement during cocaine psychomotor stimulant behaviors. Figure 11 shows the 5-HT response to cocaine, plotted with resulting Ambulations (top) and Fine Movement (bottom) during the psychomotor effects of cocaine, as movement occurred (same animal control in real time). This figure shows that the usual normal communication between basal 5-HT release in NAcc and movement behaviors (shown in Fig. 9) has been disrupted; i.e., temporal synchrony between 5-HT release and move-

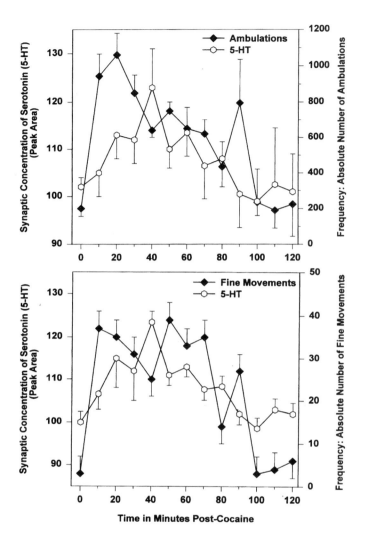

Fig. 11. Cocaine neurochemistry and behavior: Line graph depicting endogenous 5-HT release (open circles) at basal nucleus A_{10} terminals, vlNAcc, in real time, while the freely moving, male, Sprague-Dawley laboratory rat is actually behaving, during cocaine-induced behavior (intraperitoneal injection of cocaine: 2-h study). Serotonin, detected within seconds of release, is plotted with a line graph derived from simultaneous infrared photobeam monitoring of behavior (closed circles): (top) Locomotions (Ambulations); (bottom) Stereotypy (Fine Movements). Open-field behaviors were studied in units of frequency of events, which were recorded every 100 ms during normal/natural locomotor behavior. Data show that cocaine disrupted the normal episodic, rhythmic nature of locomotor and stereotypic movement that may be neuromodulated by 5-HT within the basal nucleus, A_{10} terminals. Data suggest that cocaine caused a neuroadaptive process in 5-HT mechanisms in DA basal nuclei.

ment behaviors is no longer seen (same animal control). Although 5-HT is still enhanced after cocaine, rhythmic control of movement by 5-HT is no longer observable in either Ambulatory (locomotor) or Fine Movement (stereotypic) behaviors. Although 5-HT is still enhanced after cocaine, the increase after cocaine, is significantly less than 5-HT released and observed during natural movement without cocaine. Cocaine-induced behaviors after habituation are still increased, but the behaviors occurred in a frequency similar to those frequencies usually observed in smaller, younger, animals *(37)*.

8.2. Somatodendrites, VTA (A_{10})

Something also happened to the rhythmic nature of 5-HT released in A_{10} somatodendrites during cocaine psychomotor-stimulant behavior. It is important to point out that although VTA is not a basal nucleus, these DA cell bodies are clearly a component of the mesocorticolimbic motor circuit. Figure 12 shows the 5-HT response to cocaine, plotted with resulting Ambulations (top) and Fine Movement (bottom) behaviors during the psychomotor effects of cocaine, as movement occurred (same animal control in real time). This figure shows that the previous normal/natural communication (shown in Fig. 10) between basal 5-HT release in A_{10} somatodendrites and movement behaviors has been disrupted. The data show that enhanced 5-HT release in VTA after cocaine is no longer synchronous with movement behaviors. Thus, Ambulations (locomotion) and Fine Movement behaviors of grooming and sniffing, are not related temporally to 5-HT release at A_{10} somatodendrites after cocaine. Serotonin release has increased when compared with 5-HT during habituation behavior but is again reduced from that 5-HT released during normal movement. Similar to cocaine effects in A_{10} terminal fields, 5-HT release and psychomotor stimulant behaviors are increased, but even in the first half hour, when both neurochemistry and behavior are enhanced, 5-HT, that may well have directed normal, rhythmic episodic movements, no longer seems to do so. Also, episodic movement is no longer observable.

From Figs. 11 and 12, a synopsis of important messages about cocaine-induced neuroadaptation in 5-HT release in NAcc and VTA with movement behaviors in the open-field paradigm, follows:

- General directional values for cocaine's effect on 5-HT and movement behaviors are confirmed.
- In vivo microvoltammetric studies enable the detection of subtle changes necessary to see alterations in normal/natural neurochemistry and behavior that existed before the administration of cocaine.
- Previous studies have not been able to detect these subtle changes nor have these previous studies been able to detect normal/natural episodic, rhythmic nature of locomotor (exploratory) movement or stereotypy, either in neurochemistry or behavior.
- 5-HT control or modulation of movement behaviors in A_{10} basal nucleus and in A_{10} somatodendrites during normal/natural movement behaviors, is subsequently disrupted by cocaine.
- 5-HT release in basal nuclei and VTA DA somatodendrites after cocaine is greater than those during habituation but less than those seen during normal/natural movement behaviors.
- Even in the first 30 min after cocaine, the episodic rhythmic nature of locomotor (exploratory) movement behavior and stereotypic behavior has been disrupted.

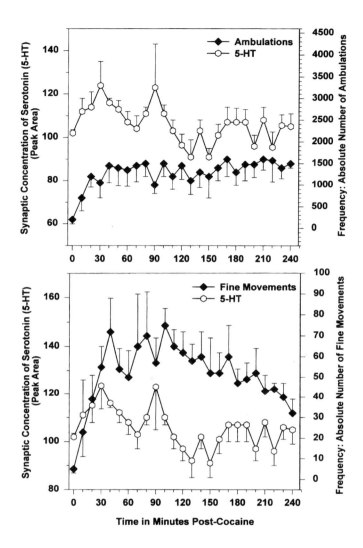

Fig. 12. Cocaine neurochemistry and behavior: Line graph depicting endogenous 5-HT release (open circles) at basal stem nucleus, DA A_{10} somatodendrites, VTA, in real time, while the freely moving, male, Sprague-Dawley laboratory rat is actually behaving during cocaine behavior (subcutaneous injection of cocaine: 4-h study). Serotonin, detected within seconds of release, is plotted with a line graph derived from simultaneous infrared photobeam monitoring of behavior (closed circles): (top) Locomotion (Ambulations); (bottom) Stereotypy (Fine Movements). Open-field behaviors were studied in units of frequency of events, which were recorded every 100 ms during normal/natural locomotor behavior. Data show that cocaine disrupted the normal episodic, rhythmic nature of locomotor movement, likely by disturbing 5-HT neuromodulation of behavior in DA motor circuits and causing neuroadaptation. Figures 8–12 adapted with permission from ref. *(44)*.

- The studies show that neuronal damage to basal nuclei and brain stem nuclei may have occurred after the administration of cocaine.
- Neuroadaptation cannot be determined by simply studying the general direction of the response of 5-HT to cocaine.
- Neuroadaptative responses by 5-HT in motor circuits is seen after a single injection of cocaine.
- Neuroadaptation may be a predisposition to cocaine neurotoxicity.
- At the risk of sounding repetitive, superior temporal resolution is a crucial component of technologies that claim to study neurotransmitters and behavior within the same animal and in real time.

9. CENTRAL PATTERN GENERATORS (CPGS)

9.1. What are cpgs?

A central pattern generator (cpg) is a neuronal network capable of generating a rhythmic pattern of motor activity either in the presence or absence of phasic sensory input from peripheral receptors. cpgs have been identified and analyzed in more than 50 rhythmic motor systems and cpgs can generate a variety of motor patterns. A universal characteristic of this wide variety of motor patterns is that they consist of rhythmic and alternating motions of the body or appendages. It is the rhythmicity of these behaviors that make these behaviors appear stereotypic and it is the repetitive quality of these behaviors that enables stereotypic behaviors to be controlled automatically. This automaticity or autoactivity means that there may be little or no need for intervention from higher brain centers, given the caveat that environment remains stable.

The simplest cpgs contain neurons that are able to burst spontaneously. Such endogenous bursters can drive other motor neurons and some motor neurons are themselves endogenous bursters. Importantly, bursters are common in cpgs that produce continuous rhythmic movement, such as locomotion. However, locomotion is an episodic rhythmic behavior and thus, further regulation by neurochemicals becomes necessary. Endogenous bursts (cell firing) of neurons involved in locomotion, must be regulated by neurotransmitters and neuromodulators, substances that can alter the cellular properties of neurons involved in cpgs. Brief depolarizations occur and lead to maintained depolarizations (plateau potentials) that can last for long periods of time. These maintained depolarizations far outlast the initial depolarization and it is these maintained depolarizations that are necessary for rhythmic movements. The generation of rhythmic motor activity by cpgs can be altered by amines and peptides *(186,187)*, thereby enabling a cpg to generate an even greater variety of repetitive motor patterns. Motor cpgs produce a complex temporal pattern of activation of different groups of motor functions and each pattern can be divided into a number of distinct phases even within a phase. cpgs are time-dependent *(188)*.

9.1.2. Serotonin Is Intrinsic to cpg Control of Rhythmic Movement in Invertebrates

Serotonin is an important neuromodulator for cpgs and can control the cpg underlying the escape swim response in the mollusc *Tritonia diomedea*. The dorsal swim interneurons (DSIs) are a bilaterally represented set of three 5-HT-ergic neurons that participate in the generation of the rhythmic-swim motor program. Serotonin from these cpg neurons are said to function as both fast neurotransmitter and as a slower neuromodulator. In its modulatory role, 5-HT enhances the release of neurotransmitter from another cpg neuron, C2, and also increases C2 excitability by decreasing spike frequency adaptation. Serotonin intrinsic to the cpg may neuromodulate behavioral sensitization and habituation and 5-HT intrinsic to the DSI, enhances synaptic potentials evoked by another neuron in the same circuit *(189,190)*. In another mollusc, the pteropod *Clione limacina,* the cpg for swimming, located in the pedal ganglia and formed by three groups of interneurons that are critical for rhythmic activity, was enhanced by 5-HT *(191)*. In the pond snail *Lymnaea stagnalis*, 5-HT is the main neurotransmitter in its stereotypic feeding circuit *(192)*. In the sea slug *Aplysia*, the cpg for biting is modulated both intrinsically and extrinsically. Intrinsic modulation has been reported to be mediated by cerebral peptide-2 (cp-2) containing CB1-2 interneurons and is mimicked by application of CP-2, whereas extrinsic modulation is mediated by the 5-HT-ergic metacerebral cell (MCC) neurons and is mimicked by application of 5-HT *(193)*.

9.1.3. Serotonin, Within 5-HT Somatodendrites, Is Intrinsic to cpg Control of Rhythmic Movement in Vertebrates

The 5-HT somatodendritic nuclei, the raphe, comprise the most expansive and complex anatomic and neurochemical system in CNS. Raphe nuclei almost exclusively reside along the midline in the rat and in the primate, fewer reside along the midline, but several exhibit a paramedian organization *(194)*. The rostral 5-HT raphe group and caudal linear nucleus sends 5-HT efferents to A_9 basal nuclei motor systems and the caudal 5-HT group, whereas the interfascicular aspect of the 5-HT-ergic dorsal raphe projects efferents to A_{10} basal ganglia (nuclei) regions *(195)*.

Electrophysiological studies have shown that the most prominent action of increased 5-HT cell firing, in 5-HT somatodendrites in treadmill locomotion for example, is to increase the flexor and extensor burst amplitude of 5-HT cell firing in DR somatodendrites for 5-HT, during locomotion *(196)*. Further evidence for 5-HT controlling motor output, is seen from studies in which 5-HT, directly injected into the motor nucleus of the trigeminal nerve, increased the amplitude of both the tonic electromyogram of the masseter muscle and the externally elicited jaw-closure (masseteric) reflex *(197–199)*. In fact, Jacobs and Azmitia have proposed that 5-HTs primary function in CNS neuronal circuitry, is to facilitate motor output *(195)*.

Serotonin neurons within 5-HT somatodendrites, depolarize with such extraordinary regularity that they exhibit automaticity, i.e., they can act by a cpg and produce plateau potentials. Thus, 5-HT neurons exhibit repetitive discharge characteristics. Increased 5-HT neuronal cell firing in somatodendritic raphe nuclei generally precedes the onset of movement or even increased muscle tone in arousal by several seconds and is maintained during sustained behavior *(200)*. Importantly, 5-HT cell firing in raphe nuclei is sometimes phase-locked to repetitive behavioral stereotypic responses. The regular firing of 5-HT somatodendrites in raphe nuclei is activated preferentially in associated with locomotion and chewing, stereotypic behaviors that are stimulated by cpgs *(182)*. Serotonin intrinsic cpgs have been reported to be responsible for inducing rhythmic motor activity in spinal cord of the turtle and the lamprey *(201,202)*. The evidence in the lamprey suggest that 5-HT may have a role in the generation of a family of related undulatory movements, including swimming, crawling, burrowing, actually by one single cpg.

9.2. cpgs *Within Basal Nuclei May Induce Rhythmic Movement by 5-HT: An Hypothesis*

To date, there have not been any reports or even suggestions of 5-HT modulation that is intrinsic to cpgs that operate rhythmic locomotion or stereotypy in basal nuclei. Yet, basal nuclei are known to be involved in the development of automaticity and to play a primary role in both movement preparation and execution, possibly via optimizing muscular activity patterns, once a motor decision has been made *(103)*. However, where the analysis of neurotransmitters in basal nuclei and brain-stem nuclei have been concerned, DA has been the major target of study. For example, it is known that the basic rhythm for locomotion is generated centrally in spinal networks and the transition from stance to swing is regulated by afferent signals from leg flexor and extensor muscles, ultimately influenced in intensity and pattern by descending signals from CNS neuronal circuitry *(188)* and again, the catecholamines have taken preference as targets for study. Landmark studies, performed about 30 yr ago, showed that injection of the catecholaminergic drugs L-DOPA and nialamide into spinal cord, generated spontaneous locomotor activity *(203–204)*.

Moreover, insofar as DA is concerned, electrophysiologic studies of this monoamine in the basal nucleus, DStr, have shown that DA neurons operate in bursts of action potentials, which increase bursting and change bursting patterns when 96% DA neurons are damaged *(205)*. Other electrophysiologic studies have shown that the excitotoxin, kainic acid, when injected into the basal nucleus, DStr, changed the pattern of the normal neuronal rhythm in the basal-stem nucleus, SN. Since SN usually exhibits a slow rhythmic firing of action potentials, damage to the neurons has been reported to cause a disorganized rhythm. This SN model has been used as an animal model to study the movement disorder, Huntington's Disease (HD) *(206)*. Therefore, there are empirical precedents that provide evidence for a clear association between DA, neuronal damage, and disorganized rhythms, at least from electrophysiologic studies.

However, now we are focusing on the proverbial "other end of the elephant," by looking into the matter of 5-HT, the biogenic amine that is emerging in importance in both cocaine movement dysfunction, schizophrenia, and other movement disorders. The unique technology presented here provides a way to enable the study of 5-HT release in basal nuclei and movement circuits and to do so at the same time as behavior, with the same animal control.

Based on the empirical evidence in this chapter, the hypotheses is submitted for the first time, that (1) 5-HT in basal nuclei may be responsible, at least in part, for the normal/natural episodic, rhythmicity known to exist with locomotor and stereotypic movements; and (2) a subtle neuroadaptation is caused by cocaine between 5-HT and cocaine-induced movements, movements that are so well-known as "psychotic behavior," via a single or multple cpg network. Interestingly, neuroadaptation, induced by cocaine, is highly time-dependent. There is an empirical precedent for this hypothesis. Neuromodulatory inputs can reconfigure cpg networks to produce specific motor-output patterns *(207)*.

Thus, the hypothesis is posited that cocaine may be acting through a 5-HT cpg neuronal network, a time-dependent network, and in this way, cocaine is causing a neuroadaptation to occur that may lead to cocaine neurotoxicity. This cocaine-5-HT driven neuroadaptation may reflect neuronal damage and may be a marker for cocaine neurotoxicity.

9.2.1. Normal/Natural Locomotion and Stereotypy Is Rhythmic

Locomotor (exploratory) activity and stereotypic behaviors are episodic and rhythmic. Most do not think of or at least write about these behaviors as such. Figures 8–10 depict the episodic, rhythmicity seen in normal/natural movement behaviors. Neuromodulation by the biogenic amine, 5-HT within basal nuclei and A_{10} brain stem nucleus, is depicted as these movements occur and as these movements are presumably either controlled, directed, modulated, or regulated by 5-HT.

9.2.2. Cocaine-Induced Locomotion and Stereotypy Is Not Rhythmic

Most researchers in the cocaine field of research conceptualize hyperactive locomotion and stereotypic behaviors as psychomotor-stimulant behavior. In addition, repetitive behaviors induced by cocaine have been generally thought of as "meaningless behaviors"; as behaviors that have no goals. It has been said that the term "stereotypy" applies to a behavioral act that is repeated again and again, but unlike a motivational act, it makes no sense because it does not achieve an adaptive outcome *(87)*. However, repetitive behaviors produced by cocaine may not be meaningless or nonadaptive. The hypothesis submitted here is that neuroadaptation from cocaine, possibly leading to habit-forming behavior, may be the unfortunate maladaptive outcome. Figures 11 and 12 show that cocaine disrupted the normal episodic rhythm of natural movement; cocaine caused normal rhythmic movement to be disorganized.

It is interesting that the concept of "rhythm" in normal open-field movement is virtually ignored or forgotten when one studies the literature on the mechanism of action of cocaine. Conceptually, when neuroscientists speak of cocaine-induced psychomotor-stimulant behavior, it seems as if movement does not occur until cocaine is administered or injected. What was observed in these studies, with the same animal control, was that there were actually greater enhancements in 5-HT during normal movement without cocaine than during cocaine-induced movement. In addition, cocaine-induced movement was not significantly increased over movement without cocaine.

9.2.3. Implications for Schizophrenia

The idea that schizophrenia may be associated with 5-HT-ergic abnormalities began with the observation that there was a structural similarity between the molecule 5-HT and the hallucinogenic drug lysergic acid diethylamide (LSD) *(208,209)*. Snyder *(210)* reported, however, that the psychosis induced by LSD in humans exhibited a vastly different symptomatology that than of schizophrenic-induced psychosis. A revival of interest in the relationship between 5-HT and schizophrenia occurred about 15 yr ago, when the atypical neuroleptic was found to have a high affinity for 5-HT_2 receptors *(211)*. Also, clozapine was found to be particularly effective in treating patients intractable to other neuroleptics and clozapine was very interestingly, found to produce less extrapyramidal side effects (EPS) (movement disorders) than did other previous neuroleptics *(212,213)*.

A mediation for 5-HT in either the disease of schizophrenia itself or in the movement disorders, known to be caused by the classical neuroleptics, remains under study; two excellent reviews are published *(214,215)*. Nonetheless, a current hypothesis, derived from human and animal studies, regarding this atypical neuroleptic, is that clozapine acts via its $5-HT_2$ antagonistic effect to alleviate movement disorders in psychosis. Furthermore, in treating the schizophrenic psychotic abnormality via its DAD_2 antagonistic-receptor action, the drug produces less EPS than its classical counterparts, via 5-HT *(78,79,83,216–218)* and possibly by its DAD_4 action *(219)*. Perhaps the present data can lend an explanatory note to a fairly recent study in which the classical DAD_2 receptor antagonist haloperidol was shown to induce the movement dysfunction, *catalepsy,* via a 5-HT-ergic mediation *(220)*.

10. CONCLUDING REMARKS

The hypothesis is posited, for the first time, that 5-HT within DA A_9 and A_{10} basal nuclei and the A_{10} brain-stem nucleus acts via a 5-HTregulated cpg, presumably originating from raphe somatodendrites. The basis of the hypothesis derives from empirical studies using in vivo microvoltammetry with BRODERICK PROBE® Microelectrodes. Animals exhibited repetitive, episodic, and rhythmic normal/natural movements, influenced by 5-HT within DA A_9 and A_{10} neural circuits without any drug treatment. Furthermore, cocaine disrupted such normal/natural episodic rhythmic movement by altering release of 5-HT, precisely within the DA basal nuclei, which are responsible for controlling voluntary movement. A further disruption of normal, episodic rhythmic movement by 5-HT after cocaine, occurred in the brain-stem nucleus, VTA, the cell bodies for the basal nucleus, NAcc. Thus, 5-HT neuroadaptation by cocaine, may be a predisposition or marker for cocaine-induced neuronal damage or neurotoxicity. Implications for the study of other movement disorders, like spinal-cord injury, through these empirical data, are noteworthy. This author's sister, Josephine Broderick Pearson was a spinal-cord injury victim; she became a talented and recognized artist, painting by mouth. It is hoped that these data will contribute to spinal-cord research as well as to other research involved with movement disorders.

ACKNOWLEDGMENTS

Partial support: NIH NIGMS Award #08168 for manuscript preparation. The author wishes to express appreciation to Ed Lineen, former research assistant, presently a medical student at NY Medical College, Valhalla, NY, for laboratory assistance and to Bridget Teresa O'Sullivan O.P., M.A., for assistance with word processing a vast amount of detailed references.

DEDICATION

This chapter is dedicated to the memory of the late Dr. Monty Piercey, cherished colleague and a true neuroscientist, who has greatly contributed to the study of brain mechanisms involved in cocaine addiction and schizophrenia. Dr. Piercey greatly contributed to pharmacotherapeutics in these research areas as well.

REFERENCES

1. Westerink, B. H., Damsma, G., Rollema, H., DeVries, J. B., and Horn, A. S. (1987) Scope and limitations of in vivo brain dialysis: a comparison of its application to various neurotransmitter systems. *Life Sci.* **41,** 1763–1776.
2. Koob, G. F. and Nestler, E. J. (1997) The neurobiology of drug addiction. *J. Neuropsychiat. Clin. Neurosci.* **9,** 482–497.
3. Olds, M. E. and Olds, J. (1969) Effects of lesions in the medial forebrain bundle on self-stimulation behavior. *Am. J. Physiol.* **217,** 1253–1254.
4. Olds, J. (1977) *Drives and Reinforcements: Behavioral Studies of Hypothalamic Function.* Raven Press, NY.
5. Montagu, K. A. (1957) Catechol compounds in rat tissues and in brains of different animals. *Nature* **180,** 244–245.
6. Weil-Malherbe, H. and Bone, A. D. (1957) Intracellular distribution of catecholamines in the brain. *Nature* **180,** 1050–1051.
7. Carlsson, A., Lindqvist, M., Magnusson, T., and Waldeck, B. (1958) On the presence of 3-hydroxytyramine in brain. *Science* **127,** 471.
8. Randrup, A. and Munkvad, I. (1965) Special antagonism of amphetamine-induced abnormal behavior. *Psychopharmacologia* **7,** 416–422.
9. Fog, R. I., Randrup, A., and Pakkenberg, H. (1967) Aminergic mechanisms in corpus striatum and amphetamine-induced stereotyped behavior. *Psychopharmacologia* **1,** 179–183.
10. Randrup, A. and Munkvad, I. (1967) Stereotyped activities produced by amphetamine in several animal species and man. *Psychopharmacologia* **11,** 300–310.
11. Ernst, A. M. and Smelik, P. G. (1966) Site of action of dopamine and apomorphine on compulsive gnawing behaviour in rats. *Experientia* **22,** 837–838.
12. Randrup, A., Munkvak, I., and Udsen, P. (1963) Adrenergic mechanisms and amphetamine-induced abnormal behaviour. *Acta Pharmacol. Toxicol.* **20,** 145–157.
13. Cools, A. R. and van Rossum, J. M. (1970) Caudal dopamine and sterotype behaviour of cats. *Arch. Int. Pharmacodyn.* **187,** 163–173.
14. Costall, B. and Naylor, R. J. (1973) The role of telencephalic dopaminergic systems in the mediation of apomorphine-stereotyped behaviour. *Eur. J. Pharmacol.* **24,** 8–24.
15. Pijnenburg, A. J. J., Honig, W. M. M., and van Rossum, J. M. (1975) Effects of antagonists upon locomotor stimulation induced by injection of dopamine and noradrenaline into the nucleus accumbens of nialamide-pretreated rats. *Psychopharmacologia* **41,** 175–180.
16. Wise, R. A. and Bozarth, M. A. (1987) A psychostimulant theory of addiction. *Psychol. Rev.* **94,** 469–492.
17. Gray, J. A. (1982) *The Neuropsychology of Anxiety: An Inquiry into the Functions of the Septohippocampal System.* Oxford University Press, NY.
18. Stein, L., Wise, C. D., and Belluzzi, J. D. (1977) Neuropharmacology of reward and punishment, in *Handbook of Psychopharmacology. Drugs, Neurotransmitters and Behavior,* vol. 8 (Iversen, L. L., Iversen, S. D., and Snyder, S.H., eds.), Plenum Press, NY, pp. 25–53.
19. Stein, L., Wise, C. D., and Berger, B. D. (1973) Antianxiety action of benzodiazepines: decrease in activity of serotonin neurons in the punishment system, in *The Benzodiazepines* (Garattini, E., Mussine, E., and Randall, L., eds.), Raven Press, NY, pp. 299–326.
20. Wise, C. D., Berger, B. W., and Stein, L. (1973) Evidence of alpha-noradrenergic reward receptors and serotonergic punishment receptors in the rat brain. *Biol. Psychiatry* **6,** 3–21.
21. Fuxe, K., Ogren, S. O., Agnati, L. F., Jonsson, G., and Gustafsson, J. A. (1978) Dihydroxytryptamine as a tool to study the functional role of central hydroxytryptamine neurons. *Ann. NY Acad. Sci.* **305,** 346–369.

22. Soubrie, P. (1986) Reconciling the role of central serotonin neurons in human and animal behavior. *Behav. Brain Sci.* **9**, 319–364.
23. Spoont, M. R. (1992) Modulatory role of serotonin in neuronal information processing: implications to human psychopathology. *Psychol. Bull.* **112**, 330–350.
24. Tye, N. C., Everitt, B. J., and Iversen, S. D. (1977) 5-Hydroxytryptamine and punishment. *Nature (Lond.)* **268**, 741–742.
25. Stein, L., Wise, C. D., and Belluzzi, J. D. (1975) Effects of benzodiazepines on central serotonergic mechanisms. *Adv. Biochem. Pharmacol.* **14**, 29–44.
26. Broderick, P. A. (1997) Alprazolam, diazepam, yohimbine, clonidine: in vivo CA_1 hippocampal norepinephrine and serotonin release profiles under chloral hydrate anesthesia. *Prog. Neuro-Psychopharmacol. Biol. Psychiat.* **21**, 1117–1140.
27. Broderick, P. A., Hope, O., and Jeannot, P. (1998) Mechanism of triazolo-benzodiazepine and benzodiazepine action in anxiety and depression: behavioral studies with concomitant in vivo CA_1 hippocampal norepinephrine and serotonin release detection in the freely moving animal. *Prog. Neuro-Psychopharmacol. Biol. Psychiat.* **22**, 353–386.
28. Broderick, P. A. and Piercey, M. F. (1990) Regulation of nerve impulse frequency and transmitter release by serotonergic autoreceptor agonists, in *Presynaptic Receptors and the Question of Autoregulation of Neurotransmitter Release*, vol. 604 (Kalsner, S. and Westfall, T. C., eds.), *Ann. NY Acad. Sci.* pp. 596–597.
29. Broderick, P. A. and Piercey, M. F. (1991) 5-HT_{1A} agonists uncouple noradrenergic somatodendrite impulse flow and terminal release. *Brain Res. Bull.* **27**, 693–696.
30. Hutson, P. H., Sarna, G. S., O'Connell, M. T., and Curzon, G. (1989) Hippocampal 5-HT synthesis and release in vivo is decreased by infusion of 8-OH-DPAT into the nucleus raphe dorsalis. *Neurosci. Lett.* **100**, 276–280.
31. Sharp, T., Bramwell, S., Clark, D., and Grahame-Smith, D. G. (1989) 5-HT_{1A} agonists reduce 5-hydroxytryptamine release in rat hippocampus in vivo as determined by brain microdialysis. *Br. J. Pharmacol.* **96**, 283–290.
32. Wright, I. K., Upton, N., and Marsden, C. A. (1992) Effect of established and putative anxiolytics on extracellular 5-HT and 5-HIAA in the ventral hippocampus of rats during behavior on the elevated x-maze. *Psychopharmacology* **109**, 338–346.
33. Schwarting, R. K., Thiel, C. M., Muller, C. P., and Huston, J. P. (1998) Relationship between anxiety and serotonin in the ventral striatum. *Neuro. Report* **9**, 1025–1029.
34. Loh, E. A., Fitch, T., Vickers, G., and Roberts, D. C. (1992) Clozapine increases breaking points in a progressive-ratio schedule reinforced by intravenous cocaine. *Pharmacol. Biochem. Behav.* **42**, 559–562.
35. Loh, E. A. and Roberts, D. C. (1990) Breakpoints on a progressive-ratio schedule reinforced by intravenous cocaine increase following depletion of forebrain serotonin. *Psychopharmacology* **101**, 262–266.
36. Porrino, L. J., Ritz, M. C., Goodman, N. L., Sharpe, L. B., Kuhar, M. J., and Goldberg, S. R. (1989) Differential effects of the pharmacological manipulation of serotonin systems on cocaine and amphetamine self-administration in rats. *Life Sci.* **45**, 1529–1535.
37. Broderick, P.A. (1992) Cocaine's colocalized effects on synaptic serotonin and dopamine in ventral tegmentum in a reinforcement paradigm. *Pharmacol. Biochem. Behav.* **42**, 889–898.
38. Broderick, P. A. (1992) Distinguishing effects of cocaine (IV) and (SC) on mesoaccumbens dopamine and serotonin release with chloral hydrate anesthesia. *Pharmacol. Biochem. Behav.* **43**, 929–937.
39. Broderick, P. A. (1993) In vivo electrochemical studies of gradient effects of (SC) cocaine on dopamine and serotonin release in dorsal striatum of conscious rats. *Pharmacol. Biochem. Behav.* **46**, 973–984.

40. Broderick, P. A., Kornak, E. P., Eng, F., and Wechsler, R. W. (1993) Real time detection of acute (IP) cocaine-enhanced dopamine and serotonin release in ventrolateral nucleus accumbens of the behaving Norway rat. *Pharmacol. Biochem. Behav.* **46,** 715–722.

41. Bradberry, C. W., Nobiletti, J. B., Elsworth, J. D., Murphy, B., Jatlow, P., and Roth, R. H. (1993) Cocaine and cocaethylene: microdialysis comparison of brain drug levels and effects on dopamine and serotonin. *J. Neurochem.* **60,** 1429–1435.

42. Parsons, L. H. and Justice, J. B., Jr. (1993) Serotonin and dopamine sensitization in the nucleus accumbens, ventral tegmental area and dorsal raphe nucleus following repeated cocaine administration. *J. Neurochem.* **61,** 1611–1619.

43. Tenaud, L. M., Baptista, T., Murzi, E., Hoebel, B. G., and Hernandez, L. (1996) Systemic and local cocaine increase extracellular serotonin in the nucleus accumbens. *Pharmacol. Biochem. Behav.* **53,** 747–752.

44. Broderick, P. A. and Phelix, C. F. (1997) I. Serotonin (5-HT) within dopamine reward circuits signals open-field behavior. II. Basis for 5-HT-DA interaction in cocaine dysfunctional behavior. *Neurosci. Biobehav. Rev.* **21,** 227–260.

45. Mills, K., Arsah, T. A., Ali, S. F., and Shockley, D. C. (1998) Calcium channel antagonist isradipine attenuates cocaine-induced motor activity in rats: correlation with brain monoamine levels. *Ann. NY Acad. Sci.* **844,** 201–207.

46. de Wit, H. and Wise, R. A. (1977) Blockade of cocaine reinforcement in rats with the dopamine receptor blocker pimozide but not with the noradrenergic blockers, phentolamine or phenoxybenzamine. *Can. J. Psychol.* **31,** 195–203.

47. Roberts, D. C. S. and Ranaldi, R. (1995) Effect of dopaminergic drugs on cocaine reinforcement, in *Clinical Neuropharmacology*, vol. 18 (Suppl. 1) (Carlsson, A. and Piercey, M. F., eds.), Raven Press, NY, pp. 584–595.

48. Reith, M. E., Li, M. Y., and Yan, Q. S. (1997) Extracellular dopamine, norepinephrine, and serotonin in the ventral tegmental area and nucleus accumbens of freely moving rats during intracerebral dialysis following systemic administration of cocaine and other uptake blockers. *Psychopharmacology (Berl.)* **134,** 309–317.

49. Koob, G. F. (1999) The role of the striato-pallidal and extended amygdala systems in drug addiction. *Ann. NY Acad. Sci.* **877,** 445–460.

50. Bardo, M. T. (1998) Neuropharmacological mechanisms of drug reward: beyond dopamine in the nucleus accumbens. *Crit. Rev. Neurobiol.* **12,** 37–67.

51. Leshner, A. I. and Koob, G. F. (1999) Drugs of abuse and the brain. *Proc. Assoc. Am. Phys.* **111,** 99–108.

52. Cornish, J. L. and Kalivas, P. W. (2000) Glutamate transmission in the nucleus accumbens mediates relapse in cocaine addiction. J. Neurosci. **20,** RC89.

53. Tandon, R. and De Quardo, J. R. (1996) Psychoses and epilepsy, in *Psychological Disturbances in Epilepsy* (Sackellares, J. C. and Berent, S., eds.), Butterworth-Heinemann, Boston, MA, pp. 171–189.

54. Young, D. and Scoville, W. B. (1938) Paranoid psychosis in narcolepsy and the possible dangers of benzedrine treatment. *Med. Clin. North Am.* **22,** 637–643.

55. Sherer, M. A., Kumor, K. M., Cone, E. J., and Jaffe, J. H. (1988) Suspiciousness induced by four-hour intravenous infusions of cocaine. Preliminary findings. *Arch. Gen. Psychiat.* **45,** 673–677.

56. Nambudin, D. E. and Young, R. C. (1991) A case of late-onset crack dependence and subsequent psychosis in the elderly. *J. Subst. Abuse Treat.* **8,** 253–255.

57. Mendoza, R., Miller, B. L., and Mena, I. (1992) Emergency room evaluation of cocaine-associated neuropsychiatric disorders. *Recent Dev. Alcohol* **10,** 73–87.

58. Taylor, W. A. and Staby, A. E. (1992) Acute treatment of alcohol and cocaine emergencies. *Recent Dev. Alcohol* **10,** 179–191.

59. Tueth, M. J. (1993) High incidence of psychosis in cocaine intoxication and preventing violence. *Am. J. Emerg. Med.* **11**, 676.

60. Miller, B. L., Mena, I., Giombetti, R., Villanueve-Meyer, J., and Djenderedjian, A. H. (1992) Neuropsychiatric effects of cocaine: SPECT Measurements. *J. Addict. Dis.* **11**, 47–58.

61. Rosse, R. B., Collins, J. P., Jr., Fay-McCarthy, M., Alim, T. M., Wyatt, R. J., and Deutsch, S. I. (1994) Phenomenologic comparison of the idiopathic psychosis of schizophrenia and drug-induced cocaine and phencyclidine psychoses: a retrospective study. *Clin. Neuropharmacol.* **17**, 359–369.

62. Mitchell, J. and Vierkant, A. D. (1991) Delusions and hallucinations of cocaine abusers and paranoid schizophrenics: a comparative study. *J. Psychol.* **125**, 301–310.

63. Brady, K. T., Lydiard, R. B., Malcolm, R., and Ballenger, J. C. (1991) Cocaine-induced psychosis. *J. Clin. Psychiatry* **52**, 509–512.

64. Satel, S. L. and Edell, W. S. (1991) Cocaine-induced paranoia and psychosis proneness. *Am. J. Psychiat.* **148**, 1708–1711.

65. Satel, S. L., Seibyl, J. P., and Charney, D. S. (1991) Prolonged cocaine psychosis implies underlying major psychopathology. *J. Clin. Psychiatry* **52**, 349–350.

66. Castaneda, R., Galanter, M., Lifshutz, H., and Franco, H. (1991) Effect of drugs of abuse on psychiatric symptoms among hospitalized schizophrenics. *Am. J. Drug Alcohol Abuse* **17**, 313–320.

67. Brady, K., Anton, R., Ballenger, J. C., Lydiard, R. B., Adinoff, B., and Selander, J. (1990) Cocaine abuse among schizophrenic patients. *Am. J. Psychiatry* **147**, 1164–1167.

68. Lysacker, P., Bell, M., Beam-Goulet, J., and Milstein, R. (1994) Relationship of positive and negative symptoms to cocaine abuse in schizophrenia. *J. Nerv. Ment. Dis.* **182**, 109–112.

69. Serper, M. R., Alpert, M., Richardson, N. A., and Dickson, S. (1995) Clinical effects of recent cocaine use on patients with acute schizophrenia. *Am. J. Psychiatry* **152**, 1464–1469.

70. Unnithan, S. B. and Cutting, J. C. (1992) The cocaine experience: refuting the concept of a model psychosis. *Psychopathology* **25**, 71–78.

71. Rosenthal, R. N. and Miner, C. R. (1997) Differential diagnosis of substance-induced psychosis and schizophrenia in patients with substance use disorders. *Schizophr. Bull.* **23**, 187–193.

72. Mendoza, R. and Miller, B. L. (1992) Neuropsychiatric disorders associated with cocaine use. *Hosp. Comm. Psychiat.* **43**, 677–678.

73. Ries, R. K. (1993) The dually diagnosed patient with psychotic symptoms. *J. Addict. Dis.* **12**, 103–122.

74. Schottenfield, R., Carroll, K., and Rounsaville, B. (1993) Comorbid psychiatric disorders and cocaine abuse. *NIDA Res. Monogr.* **135**, 31–47.

75. Broderick, P. A. and Piercey, M. F. (1998) Neurochemical and behavioral evidence supporting (+) —AJ 76 as a potential pharmacotherapy for cocaine abuse. *J. Neural. Transm.* **105**, 1307–1324.

76. Carlsson, A. and Piercey, M. F. (eds.) (1995) Dopamine receptor subtypes in neurological and psychiatric diseases, in *Clinical Neuropharmacology*, vol. 18, (Suppl. 1), Raven Press, NY, pp. 1–215.

77. Lieberman, J. A., Kinon, B. J., and Loebel, A. D. (1990) Dopaminergic mechanisms in idiopathic and drug-induced psychosis. *Schizophr. Bull.* **16**, 97–110.

78. Meltzer, H. Y. (1989) Clinical studies on the mechanism of action of clozapine: the dopamine-serotonin hypothesis of schizophrenia. *Psychopharmacology* **99**(Suppl.), pp. 18–27.

79. Broderick, P. A. and Piercey, M. F. (1998) Clozapine, haloperidol, and the D$_4$ antagonist, PNU–101387G: in vivo effects on mesocortical, mesolimbic, and nigrostriatal dopamine and serotonin release. *J. Neural. Transm.* **105**, 749–767.

80. Kelland, M. D. and Chiodo, L. A. (1996) Serotonergic modulation of midbrain dopamine systems, in *The Modulation of Dopaminergic Neurotransmission by Other Neurotransmitters* (Ashby, Jr., C. R., ed.), CRC Press Inc., Boca Raton, FL, pp. 87–117.

81. Svensson, T. H., Mathe, J. M., Nomikos, G. G., Schilstrom, B., Marcus, M., and Fagerquist, M. (1998) Interactions between catecholamines and serotonin: relevance to the pharmacology of schizophrenia. *Adv. Pharmacol.* **42**, 814–818.

82. Kosten, T. A. and Nestler, E. J. (1994) Clozapine attenutes cocaine conditioned place preference. *Life Sci.* **55**, 9–14.

83. Okonji, C., Hope, O., Lineen, E., Saleem, A., and Broderick, P. A. (1995) Neurochemical and behavioral effects of the simultaneous administration of acute (IP) cocaine and clozapine in the nucleus accumbens in the behaving, male Sprague-Dawley rat. NIH/NIGMS Symposium, Washington, D.C.

84. Fog, R. (1972) On stereotypy and catalepsy: studies on the effect of amphetamine and neuroleptics in rat. *Acta Neurol. Scand.* **48(Suppl. 50)**, 11–67.

85. Costall, B. and Naylor, R. J. (1975) The behavioral effects of dopamine applied intracerebrally to areas of mesolimbic system. *Eur. J. Pharmacol.* **32**, 87–92.

86. Costall, B. and Naylor, R. J. (1977) Mesolimbic and extrapyramidal sites for the mediation of stereotyped behaviour patterns and hyperactivity by amphetamine and apomorphine in the rat. *Adv. Behav. Biol.* **21**, 47–76.

87. Teitelbaum, P., Pellis, S. M., and De Vietti, T. L. (1990) Disintegration into stereotypy induced by drugs or brain damage: a microdescriptive behavioral analysis, in *Neurobiology of Stereotyped Behaviour* (Cooper, S. J. and Dourish, C. T., eds.), Oxford Univ. Press, NY, pp. 169–199.

88. Cooper, S. V. and Dourish, C. T. (eds.) (1990) *Neurobiology of Stereotyped Behaviour.* Oxford University Press, New York, NY.

89. Lucki, I. (1992) 5-HT$_1$ receptors and behaviors. *Neurosci. Biobehav. Rev.* **16**, 83–93.

90. Bouhuys, A. L. and Van den Hoofdakker, R. H. (1977) Effects of midbrain raphe destruction on sleep and locomotor activity in rats. *Physiol. Behav.* **19**, 535–541.

91. Kohler, C. and Lorens, S. A. (1978) Open field activity and avoidance behavior following serotonin depletion: a comparison of the effects of parachlorophenylalanine and electrolytic midbrain raphe lesions. *Pharmacol. Biochem. Behav.* **8**, 223–233.

92. Lorens, S. A., Guldberg, H. C., Hole, K., Kohler, C., and Srebro, B. (1976) Activity, avoidance learning and regional 5-hydroxytryptamine following intrabrain stem 5,7-dihydroxytryptamine and electrolytic midbrain raphe lesions in the rat. *Brain Res.* **108**, 97–113.

93. Schlosberg, A. J. and Harvey, J. A. (1979) Effects of L-dopa and L-5-hydroxytryptophan on locomotor activity of the rat after selective or combined destruction of central catecholamine and serotonin neurons. *J. Pharmacol. Exp. Therap.* **211**, 296–304.

94. Srebro, B. and Lorens, S. A. (1975) Behavioral effects of selective midbrain raphe lesions in the rat. *Brain Res.* **89**, 303–325.

95. Hillegaart, V., Wadenberg, M. L., and Ahlenius, S. (1989) Effects of 8-OH-DPAT on motor activity in the rat. *Pharmacol. Biochem. Behav.* **32**, 797–800.

96. Yeghiayan, S. K., Kelley, A. E., Kula, N. S., Campbell, A., and Baldessarini, R. J. (1997) Role of dopamine in behavioral effects of serotonin microinjected into rat striatum. *Pharmacol. Biochem. Behav.* **56**, 251–259.

97. Post, R. (1975) Cocaine psychoses: a continuum model. *Am. J. Psychol.* **132**, 225–231.

98. Roffman, J. H. and Raskin, L. A. (1997) Stereotyped behavior: effects of d-amphetamine and methylphenidate in the young rat. *Pharmacol. Biochem. Behav.* **58**, 1095–1102.

99. Segal, D. S. and Kuczenski, R. (1997) Behavioral alterations induced by an escalating dose-binge pattern of cocaine administration. *Behav. Brain Res.* **88,** 251–260.

100. Ryan, L., Martone, M., Linder, J., and Groves, P. (1988) Cocaine, in contrast to d-amphetamine, does not cause axonal terminal degeneration in neostriatum and agranular frontal cortex of Long-Evans rats. *Life Sci.* **43,** 1403–1409.

101. Seiden, L. S. and Kleven, M. S. (1988) Lack of toxic effects of cocaine on dopamine and serotonin neurons in rat brain, in *Mechanisms of Cocaine Abuse and Toxicity* (A NIDA Research Monograph (Clouet, D., Asghar, K., and Brown, R., eds.), DHHS Pub # (ADM) 88–1585, Rockville, MD, pp. 276–289.

102. Lindsay, K. W., Bone, I., Callander, R., and van Gijn, J. (1997) *Neurology and Neurosurgery Illustrated*. Churchill Livingstone, NY, pp. 348–350.

103. Brooks, D. J. (1996) Basal ganglia function during normal and parkinsonian movement, Pet activation studies, in *Advances in Neurology* (Battistin, L., Scarlato, G., Caraceni, T., and Ruggieri, S., eds.), Lippincott-Raven, Philadelphia, PA, pp. 433–441.

104. Frith, C. D., Friston, K. J., Liddle, P. F., and Frackowiak, R. S. J. (1991) Willed action and the prefrontal cortex in man: a study with PET. *Proc. R. Soc. Lond. Biol.* **244,** 241–246.

105. Thaler, D. E. and Passingham, R. E. (1989) The supplementary motor cortex and internally directed movement, in *Neural Mechanisms in Disorders of Movement* (Crossman, A. R. and Sambrook, M., eds.), Libby, London, pp. 175–181.

106. Posner, M. I. and Peterson, S. E. (1990) The attention system of the human brain. *Ann. Rev. Neurosci.* **13,** 25–42.

107. Rolls, E. T., Burton, M. J., and Mora, F. (1980) Neurophysiological analysis of brain-stimulation reward in the monkey. *Br. Res.* **194,** 339–357.

108. Lader, M. (1980) Brain organization and behavior, in *Introduction to Psychopharmacology,* A Scope Publication. The Upjohn Company, Kalamazoo, MI, pp. 30–42.

109. Bertler, A. and Rosengren, E. (1959) Occurrence and distribution of dopamine in brain and other tissues. *Experientia* **15,** 10–11.

110. Carlsson, A. (1959) The occurrence, distribution and physiological role of catecholamines in the nervous system. *Pharmacol. Rev.* **11,** 490–493.

111. Sano, I., Gamo, T., Kakimoto, Y., Taniguchi, K., Takesade, M., and Nishinuma, K. (1959) Distribution of catechol compounds in human brain. *Biochim. Biophys. Acta* **32,** 586–587.

112. Bertler, A. (1961) Occurrence and localization of catecholamines in the human brain. *Acta Physiol. Scand.* **51,** 97–107.

113. Carlsson, A., Falck, B., and Hillarp, N.-A. (1962) Cellular localization of brain monoamines. *Acta Physiol. Scand.* **56**(Suppl. 196), 1–27.

114. Dahlstrom, A. and Fuxe, K. (1964) Evidence for the existence of monoamine-containing neurons in the central nervous system. I. Demonstration of monoamines in the cell bodies of brain stem neurones. *Acta Physiol. Scand.* **62** (Suppl. 232), 1–55.

115. Fuxe, K. (1965) Evidence for the existence of monoamine neurons in the central nervous system. IV. Distribution of monoamine nerve terminals in the central nervous system. *Acta Physiol. Scand.* **64** (Suppl. 247), 41–85.

116. Falck, B., Hillarp, N.-A., Thieme, G., and Torp, A. (1962) Fluorescence of catecholamines and related compounds condensed with formaldehyde. *J. Histochem. Cytochem.* **10,** 348–354.

117. Anden, N. E., Dahlstrom, A., Fuxe, K., Larsson, K., Olson, L., and Ungerstedt, U. (1966) Ascending monoamine neurones to the telencephalon and diencephalon. *Acta Physiol. Scand.* **67,** 313–326.

118. Creese, I. and Iversen, S. D. (1975) The pharmacological and anatomical substrates of the amphetamine response in the rat. *Brain Res.* **83,** 419–436.

119. Kelly, P. H., Seviour, P., and Iversen, S. D. (1975) Amphetamine and apomorphine responses in the rat following 6-OHDA lesions of the nucleus accumbens septi and corpus striatum. *Brain Res.* **94,** 507–522.

120. Gawin, F. H. and Kleber, H. D. (1986) Abstinence symptomatology and psychiatric diagnosis in cocaine abusers. Clinical observations. *Arch. Gen. Psychiatry* **43,** 104–113.

121. Dackis, C. A. and Gold, M. S. (1985) New concepts in cocaine addiction: the dopamine depletion hypothesis. *Neurosci. Biobehav. Rev.* **9,** 1–9.

122. Parsons, L. H., Koob, G. F., and Weiss, F. (1996) Extracellular serotonin is decreased in the nucleus accumbens during withdrawal from cocaine self-administration. *Behav. Brain Res.* **73,** 225–228.

123. Broderick, P. A., Penn Erskine, C., Charleton, H., Green, S., and Okonji, C. (1997) A four week follow-up study of serotonin (5-HT) and dopamine (DA) release in nucleus accumbens of animals, behaving in an open-field paradigm. *Soc. Neurosci. Abstr.* **23,** 1867.

124. Parent, A., Descarries, L., and Baudet, A. (1981) Organization of ascending serotonin systems in the adult rat brain. A radio-autographic study after intraventricular administration of [^{3}H]–5-hydroxytryptamine. *Neuroscience* **6,** 115–138.

125. Taber-Pierce, E., Foote, W. E., and Hobson, J. A. (1976) The efferent connection of the nucleus raphe dorsalis. *Brain Res.* **107,** 137–144.

126. Steinbusch, H. W. M. (1981) Distribution of serotonin-immunoreactivity in the central nervous system of the rat-cell bodies and terminals. *Neuroscience* **6,** 557–618.

127. Herve, D., Pickel, V. M., Joh, T. H., and Beaudet, A. (1987) Serotonin axon terminals in the ventral tegmental area of the rat: fine structure and synaptic input to dopaminergic neurons. *Brain Res.* **435,** 71–83.

128. Van Bockstaele, E. J., Biswas, A., and Pickel, V. M. (1993) Topography of serotonin neurons in the dorsal raphe nucleus that send axon collaterals to the rat prefrontal cortex. *Brain Res.* **624,** 188–198.

129. Jacobs, B. L., Foote, S. L., and Bloom, F. E. (1978) Differential projections of neurons within the dorsal raphe nucleus of the rat: a horseradish peroxidase. (HRP) study. *Brain Res.* **147,** 149–153.

130. Azmitia, E. C. and Segal, M. (1978) An autoradiographic analysis of the differential ascending projections of the dorsal and median raphe nuclei in the rat. *J. Comp. Neurol.* **179,** 641–667.

131. O'Hearn, E. and Molliver, M. E. (1984) Organization of raphe cortical projections in rat: a quantitative retrograde study. *Brain Res. Bull.* **13,** 709–726.

132. Hillegaart, V. (1991) Functional topography of brain serotonergic pathways in the rat. *Acta Physiol. Scand.* **142(Suppl. 598),** 1–54.

133. Broderick, P. A. (1989) Cathodic electrochemical current arrangement with telemetric application. U.S. Patent # 4, 883, 057.

134. Broderick, P. A. (1995) Microelectrodes and their use in a cathodic electrochemical current arrangement with telemetric application. U.S. Patent # 5, 433, 710.

135. Broderick, P .A. (1997) Microelectrodes and their use in electrochemical current arrangements with telemetric application. European Patent # EP 0 487 647 B1.

136. Broderick, P. A. (1999) Microelectrodes and their use in an electrochemical arrangement with telemetric application. U.S. Patent # 5, 938, 903.

137. Broderick, P. A. (1999) Microelectrodes and their use in electrochemical current arrangements with telemetric application. Hong Kong, HK # 1007350.

138. Broderick, P. A. (1988) Distinguishing in vitro electrochemical signatures for norepinephrine and dopamine. *Neurosci. Lett.* **95,** 275–280.

139. Broderick, P. A. (1989) Characterizing stearate probes *in vitro* for the electrochemical detection of dopamine and serotonin. *Brain Res.* **495,** 115–121.

140. Broderick, P. A. (1990) State-of-the-art microelectrodes for in vivo voltammetry. *Electroanalysis* **2**, 241–251.

141. Broderick, P. A. (2000) Serotonin (5-HT) deficiency but high tryptophan (L-TP) concentrations within hippocampal subparcellations in patients with mesial temporal sclerosis (MTS). *Amer. Epilepsy Soc. Los Angeles, CA, Epilepsia* **(Suppl.)41**, 91.

142. Pacia, S. V., Broderick, P. A., Doyle, W. K., and Devinsky, O. (2000) Serotonin (5-HT) and tryptophan (L-TP) concentrations in temporal neocortex of patients with neocortical (NTLE) and mesial temporal lobe epilepsy (MTLE) determined by in situ microvoltammetry with microelectrodes. *Am. Clin. Neurophysiol. Soc;* Sept. 22, 23, 2000, Montreal, PQ, Canada.

143. Broderick, P. A., Pacia, S. V., Doyle, W. K., and Devinsky, O. (2000) Monoamine neurotransmitters in resected hippocampal subparcellations from neocortical and mesial temporal lobe epilepsy patients: in situ microvoltammetric studies. *Brain Res.* **878**, 49–63.

144. Allen, S. M. and Davis, W. M. (1999) Relationship of dopamine to serotonin in the neonatal 6-OHDA rat model of Lesch-Nyhan Syndrome. *Behav. Pharmacol.* **10**, 467–474.

145. Patten, J. (1980) *Neurological Differential Diagnosis.* Harold Starke Limited, London and Springer-Verlag Inc., NY, pp. 127–128.

146. Adams, R. N. and Marsden, C. A. (1982) Electrochemical detection methods for monoamine measurements in vitro and in vivo, in *Handbook of Psychopharmacology* (Iversen, L. L. and Snyder, S. H., eds.), Plenum Press, NY, pp. 1–74.

147. Kissinger, P. T., Preddy, C. R., Shoup, R. E., and Heineman, W. R. (1996) Fundamental concepts of analytical electrochemistry, in *Laboratory Techniques in Electroanalytical Chemistry* (Kissinger, P. T. and Heineman, W. R., eds.), Marcell Dekker Inc., NY, pp. 11–50.

148. Dayton, M. A., Brown, J. C., Stutts, K. J., and Wightman, R. M. (1980) Faradaic electrochemistry at microvoltammetric electrodes. *Anal. Chem.* **52**, 948–950.

149. Oldham, K. (1973) Semi-integral electroanalysis: analog implementation. *Anal. Chem.* **45**, 39–50.

150. Coury, L. A., Huber, E. W., and Heineman, W. P. (1989) Applications of modified electrodes in the voltammetric determination of catecholamine neurotransmitters. *Biotechnology* **11**, 1–37.

151. Stoecker, P. W. and Yacynyck, A. M. (1990) Chemically modified electrodes as biosensors. *Selective Electrode Rev.* **12**, 137–160.

152. Hope, O., Lineen, E., Okonji, C., Green, S., Saleem, A., Aulakh, C. S., and Broderick, P. A. (1995) Cocaine has remarkable nucleus accumbens effects *on line*, with behavior in the serotonin-deficient Fawn Hooded rat. NIH/NIGMS Symposium, Washington, D.C.

153. Broderick, P. A., Jean-Baptiste, P., Vuong, A. V., Pacia, S. V., Doyle, W. K., and Devinsky, O. (1999) Neurochemical signals from living neocortex of Mesial Temporal Lobe Epilepsy (MTLE) patients studied by Broderick Probe® lauric acid and stearic acid miniature sensors. *Epilepsia* (Suppl. 7)**40**, 78–79.

154. Pellegrino, L. J., Pellegrino, A. S., and Cushman, A. J. (1979) *A Stereotaxic Atlas of the Rat Brain.* Plenum Press, NY.

155. Zaborszky, L., Alheid, G.F., Beinfeld, M. C., Eiden, L. E., Heimer, L., and Palkovits, M. (1985) Cholecystokinin innervation of the ventral striatum: a morphological and radio immunological study. *Neuroscience* **14**, 427–453.

156. Voorn, P., Gerfen, C. R., and Groenewegen, H. J. (1989) Compartmental organization of the ventral striatum of the rat: immunohistochemical distribution of enkephalin, substance P, dopamine and calcium-binding protein. *J. Comp. Neurol.* **289**, 189–201.

157. Jongen-Relo, A. L., Groenewegen, H. J., and Voorn, P. (1993) Evidence for a multicompartmental histochemical organization of the nucleus accumbens in the rat. *J. Comp. Neurol.* **337**, 267–276.

158. Jongen-Relo, A. L., Voorn, P., and Groenewegen, H. J. (1994) Immunohistochemical characterization of the shell and core territories of the nucleus accumbens in the rat. *Eur. J. Neurosci.* **6,** 1255–1264.

159. Meredith, G. E., Pattiselanno, A., Groenewegen, H. J., and Haber, S. N. (1996) Shell and core in monkey and human nucleus accumbens identified with antibodies to calbindin-D28k. *J. Comp. Neurol.* **365,** 628–639.

160. Heimer, L., Zahm, D. S., Churchill, L., Kalivas, P. W., and Wohltmann, C. (1991) (a) Specificity in the projection patterns of accumbal core and shell in the rat. *Neuroscience* **41,** 89–125.

161. Heimer, L., Zahm, D. S., Churchill, L., Kalivas, P. W., and Wohltmann, C. (1991) (b) The ventral striato-pallidal parts of the basal ganglia in the rat. III Compartmentation of ventral striatal efferents. *Neuroscience* **34,** 707–731.

162. Meredith, G. E., Agolia, R., Arts, M. P. M., Groenewegen, H. J., and Zahm, D. S. (1992) Morphological differences between projection neurons of the core and shell in the nucleus accumbens of the rat. *Neuroscience* **50,** 149–162.

163. Hurd, Y. L., Svensson, P., and Ponten, M. (1999) The role of dopamine, dynorphin, and CART systems in the ventral striatum and amygdala in cocaine abuse. *Ann. NY Acad. Sci.* **877,** 499–506.

164. McDonald, A. J. (1991) Topographic organization of amygdaloid projections to the caudate putamen, nucleus accumbens and related striatal-like areas of the rat brain. *Neuroscience* **44,** 15–33.

165. Brog, J. S., Salyaponose, A., Deutch, A. Y., and Zahm, D. S. (1993) The patterns of afferent innervation of the core and shell of the "accumbens" part of the rat ventral striatum: immunohistochemical detection of retrogradely transported fluoro-gold. *J. Comp. Neurol.* **338,** 255–278.

166. Wright, C. I., Beijer, A. V. J., and Groenewegen, H. J. (1996) Basal amygdaloid complex afferents to the rat nucleus accumbens are compartmentally organized. *J. Neurosci.* **16,** 1877–1893.

167. Van Bockstaele, E. J. and Pickel, V. M. (1993) Ultrastructure of serotonin-immuno reactive terminals in the core and shell of the rat nucleus accumbens. Cellular substrates for interactions with catecholamine afferents. *J. Comp. Neurol.* **334,** 603–617.

168. Brown, P. and Molliver, M. E. (2000) Dual serotonin (5-HT) projections to the nucleus accumbens core and shell: relation of the 5-HT transporter to amphetamine-induced neurotoxicity. *J. Neurosc.* **20,** 1952–1963.

169. Pickel, V. M. and Chan, J. (1999) Ultrastructural localization of the serotonin transporter in limbic and motor compartments of the nucleus accumbens. *J. Neurosci.* **19,** 7356–7366.

170. Phelix, C. F., Rodriguez, V. R., Rodriguez, J. S., and Broderick, P. A. (2001) Comparative morphometric analysis of serotonin axons in the nucleus accumbens subterritories of albino rat, *Rattus Norvegicus,* and white-footed mouse, *Peromyscus Leucopus.* Soc. Neurosci. Abstr. 26, 1927; *J. Chem. Neuroanat.* In press.

171. Phelix, C. F., Russell, M. J., Kumar, P., and Broderick, P. A. (1995) Serotonin innervation of dopamine neurons in rat ventral tegmentum. *Soc. Neurosci. Abstr.* **21,** 1694.

172. Phelix, C. F. and Broderick, P. A. (1995) Light microscopic immunocytochemical evidence of converging serotonin and dopamine terminals in ventrolateral nucleus accumbens. *Brain Res. Bull.* **37,** 37–40.

173. Swanson, L. W. and Cowan, W. M. (1975) A note on the connections and development of the nucleus accumbens. *Brain Res.* **92,** 324–330.

174. Swanson, L. W. (1982) The projections of the ventral tegmental area and adjacent regions: a combined fluorescent retrograde tracer and immunofluorescence study in the rat. *Brain Res. Bull.* **9,** 321–353.

175. Domesick, V. B. (1988) Neuroanatomical organization of dopamine neurons in the ventral tegmental area. *NY Acad. Sci.* 537, 10–26.
176. Whishaw, I. Q., Fiorino, D., Mittleman, G., and Casteneda, E. (1992) Do forebrain structures compete for behavioral expression? Evidence from amphetamine-induced behavior, microdialysis and caudate-accumbens lesions in medial frontal cortex damaged ras. *Brain Res.* **576**, 1–11.
177. Oades, R. D. (1985) The role of noradrenaline in tuning and dopamine in switching between signals in the CNS. *Neurosci. Biobehav. Rev.* **9**, 261–282.
178. Vanden Bos, R., Charria Ortiz, G. A., Bergmans, A. C., and Cools, A. R. (1991) Evidence that dopamine in the nucleus accumbens is involved in the ability of rats to switch to cue directed behaviors. *Behav. Brain Res.* **42**, 107–114.
179. Van Bockstaele, E. J., Biswas, A., and Pickel, V. M. (1993) Topography of serotonin neurons in the dorsal raphe nucleus that send axon collaterals to the rat prefrontal cortex and nucleus accumbens. *Brain Res.* **624**, 188–198.
180. Geyer, M. A., Russo, P. V., and Masten, V. L. (1986) Multivariate assessment of locomotor behavior: pharmacological and behavioral analysis. Pharmacol. Biochem. Behav. **25**, 277–288
181. Lucki, I. (1998) The spectrum of behaviors influenced by serotonin. *Biol. Psychiatry* **44**, 151–162.
182. Jacobs, B. L. and Fornal, C. A. (1991) Activity of brain serotonergic neurons in the behaving animal. *Pharmacol. Rev.* **43**, 563–578.
183. Grace, A. and Bunney, B. S. (1985) Dopamine, in *Neurotransmitter Actions in the Vertebrate Nervous System* (Rogawski, M. A. and Barker, J. L., eds.), Plenum Press, NY, Chapter 9.
184. Llinas, R., Greenfield, S. A., and Jahnsen, H. (1984) Electrophysiology of pars compacta cells in the in vitro substantia nigra: a possible mechanism for dendritic release. *Brain Res.* 294, 127–132.
185. Trent, F. and Tepper, J. M. (1991) Dorsal raphe stimulation modifies striatal-evoked antidromic invasion of nigral dopaminergic neurons in vivo. *Exp. Brain Res.* **84**, 620–630.
186. Grillner, S., Wallen P., Dale, N., Brodìn, I., Buchanan, J., and Hill, R. (1987) Transmitter, membrane properties and network circuitry in the control of locomotion in the lamprey. *Trends Neurosci.* **10**, 34–41.
187. Rossignol, S. and Dubue, R. (1994) Spinal pattern generation. *Curr. Opin. Neurobiol.* **4**, 894–902.
188. Pearson, K. and Gordon, J. (2000) Locomotion, in *Principles of Neural Science*, 4th ed. (Kandel, E. R., Schwartz, J. H., and Jessell, T. M., eds.), The McGraw Hill Companies, Inc., NY, pp.738–755.
189. Katz, P. S. (1998) Neuromodulation intrinsic to the central pattern generator for escape swimming in Tritonia. *Ann. NY Acad. Sci.* **860**, 181–188.
190. Katz, P. S., Getting, P. A., and Frost, W. N. (1994) Dynamic neuromodulation of synaptic strength intrinsic to a central pattern generator circuit. *Nature* **367**, 729–731.
191. Arshavsky, Y. I., Deliagina, T. G., Orlovsky, G. N., Panchin, Y. V., Popova, L. B., and Sadreyev, R. I. (1998) Analysis of the central pattern generator for swimming in the mollusk, Clione. *Ann. NY Acad. Sci.* **860**, 51–69.
192. Sadamoto, H., Hatakeyama, D., Kojima, S., Fujito, Y., and Ito, E. (1998) Histochemical study on the relation between NO-generative neurons and central circuitry for feeding in the pond snail, *Lymnaea Stagnalis. Neurosi. Res.* **32**, 57–63.
193. Morgan, P. T., Perrins, R., Lloyd, P. E., and Weiss, K. R. (2000) Intrinsic and extrinsic modulaton of a single central pattern generating circuit. *J. Neurophysiol.* **84**, 1186–1193.
194. Azmitia, E. C. (1986) Re-engineering the brain serotonin system: localized application of neurotoxins and fetal neurons. *Adv. Neurol.* **43**, 493–507.

195. Jacobs, B. L. and Azmitia, E. C. (1992) Structure and function of the brain serotonin system. *Physiol. Rev.* **72,** 165–229.

196. Barbeau, H. and Rossignol, S. (1991) Mitigation and modulation of the locomotor pattern in the adult chronic spinal rat by noradrenergic and dopaminergic drugs. *Brain Res.* **546,** 250–260.

197. McCall, R. B. and Aghajanian, G. K. (1979) Serotonergic facilitation of facial motor neuron excitation. *Brain Res.* 169, 11–27.

198. McCall, R. B. and Aghajanian, G. K. (1980) Pharmacological characterization of serotonin receptors in the facial motor nucleus: a microiontophoretic study. *Eur. J. Pharmacol.* **65,** 175–183

199. Ribeiro-Do-Valle, L. E., Fornal, C. A., Litto, W. J., and Jacobs, B. L. (1989) Serotonergic dorsal raphe unit activity related to feeding/grooming behaviors in cats. *Soc. Neurosci. Abstr.* **15,** 1283.

200. Jacobs, B. L. (1986) Single unit activity of brain monoamine containing neurons in freely moving animals, in *Neurochemical Analysis of the Conscious Brain: Voltammetry and Push-Pull Perfusion* (Myers, R. D. and Knott, P. J., eds.), *Ann. NY Acad. Sci.* pp. 70–79.

201. Guertin, P.A. and Hounagaard, J. (1998) Chemical and electrical stimulation induce rhythmic motor activity in an in vitro preparation of the spinal cord from adult turtles. *Neurosci. Lett.* **245,** 5–8.

202. Harris-Warrick, R. M. and Cohen, A. H. (1985) Serotonin modulates the central pattern generator for locomotion in the isolated lamprey spinal cord. *J. Exp. Biol.* **116,** 27–46.

203. Jankowska, E., Jukes, M. G. M., Lund, S., and Lundberg, A. (1967) The effect of DOPA on the spinal cord. 5. Reciprocal organization of pathways transmitting excitatory action to alpha motoneurones of flexors and extensors. *Acta Physiol. Scand.* **70,** 369–388.

204. Jankowska, E., Jukes, M.G.M., Lund, S. and Lundberg, A. (1967) The effect of DOPA on the spinal cord. VI. Half-centre organization of interneurons transmitting effects from flexor reflex afferents. *Acta Physiol. Scand.* **70,** 389–402.

205. Hollermann, J. R. and Grace, A. A. (1990) The effects of dopamine-depleting brain lesions on the electrophysiological activity of rat substantia nigra dopamine neurons. *Brain Res.* **533,** 203–212.

206. Doudet, D., Gross, C., Seal, G., and Bioulac, B. (1984) Activity of nigral dopaminergic neurons after lesion of the neostriatum in rats. *Brain Res.* **302,** 45–55.

207. Kiehn, O. and Kjaerulff, O. (1996) Spatiotemporal characteristics of 5-HT and dopamine-induced rhythmic activity in the in vitro neonatal rat. *J. Neurophysiol.* **75,** 1472–1482.

208. Gaddum, J. H. (1954) Drug antagonistic to 5-hydroxytryptamine, in *Ciba Foundation Symposium on Hypertension* (Wolstenholme, G. W., ed.), Little, Brown, Boston, MA, pp. 75–77.

209. Wooley, D. W. and Shaw, E. (1954) A biological and pharmacological suggestion of certain mental disorders. *Proc. Natl. Acad. Sci. USA* **40,** 228–231.

210. Snyder, S. H. (1972) Catecholamines in the brain as mediator of amphetamine psychosis. *Arch. Gen. Psychiatry* **45,** 789–796.

211. Altar, C. A., Wasley, A. M., Neale, R. F., and Stone, G. A. (1986) Typical and atypical antipsychotic occupancy of D2 and S2 receptors: an autoradiographic analysis in rat brain. *Brain Res. Bull.* **16,** 517–525.

212. Kane, J., Honigfeld, G., Singer, J., and Meltzer, H. (1988) Clozapine for the treatment resistant schizophrenic. A double-blind comparison with chlorpromazine. *Arch. Gen. Psychiat.* **45,** 789–796.

213. Tamminga, C. A. and Gerlach, J. (1987) New neuroleptics and experimental antipsychotics in schizophrenia, in *Psychopharmacology: The Third Generation of Progress* (Meltzer, H. Y., ed.), Raven Press, NY, pp. 1129–1140.

214. Iqbal, N. and van Praag, H. M. (1995) The role of serotonin in schizophrenia. *Eur. Neuropsychopharmacol.* **5**(Suppl.), 11–23.
215. Abi, Dargham, A., Laruelle, M., Aghajanian, G. K., Charney, D., and Krystal, J. (1977) The role of serotonin in the pathophysiology and treatment of schizophrenia. *J. Neuropsychiatric Clin. Neurosci.* **9,** 1–17.
216. Wadenburg, M. L. (1996) Serotonergic mechanisms in neuroleptic-induced catalepsy in the rat. *Neurosci. Biobehav. Rev.* **20,** 325–329.
217. Kapur, S. and Remington, G. (1996) Serotonin-dopamine interaction and its relevance to schizophrenia. *Am. J. Psychiatry* **153(4),** 466–476.
218. Martin, P. (1998) 5-HT$_2$ Receptor Antagonism and Antipsychotic Drugs: A Behavioral and Neurochemical Study in a Rodent Hypoglutamatergia Model. PhD. Thesis, Goteborg University, Sweden, pp. 1–64.
219. Van Tol, H. H. M., Bunzow, J. R., Guan, H. C., Sunuahara, R. K., Seeman, P., Niznik, H. B., and Civello, O. (1991) Cloning of the gene for human dopamine D$_4$ receptor with high affinity for the antipsychotic clozapine. *Nature* **350,** 610–614.
220. Neal-Beliveau, B. S., Joyce, J. N., and Lucki, I. (1993) Serotonergic involvement in haloperidol-induced catalepsy. *J. Pharmacol. Exp. Ther.* **265,** 207–217.

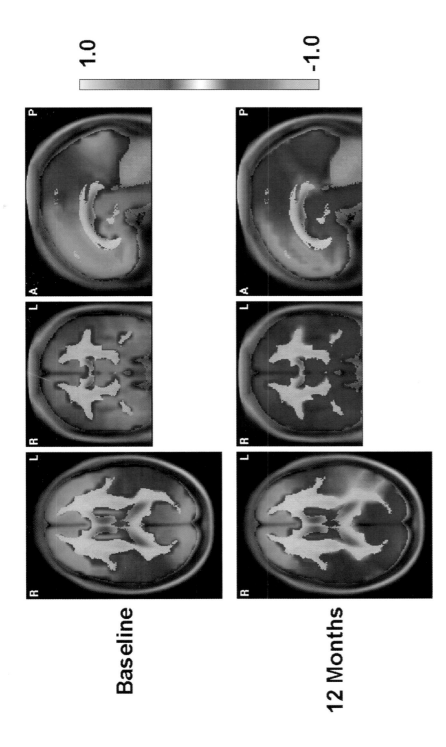

Baseline

12 Months

1.0

−1.0

Color Plate 1, Fig. 2 (*see* discussion in Chapter 5, p. 140). Group average (*n* = 13) QEEG VARETA 3D images at 1.95 Hz. Images are shown for transaxial, coronal, and sagittal sections at baseline (top row, 5–14 d after last reported use of cocaine) and in the same patients after 12 mo of sustained abstinence (bottom row). Color-coding is in standard deviation units of the distribution of source strengths in each voxel in the normal population, with white representing the center of the scale, shades of red to yellow showing increasing excess, and green showing increasing deficit. The Z scale range is ±1.0, the significance of which is evaluated by multiplying the Z value times the square root of the group size. Note that these images follow radiologic convention, i.e., the nose is up but laterality is reversed so right is left.

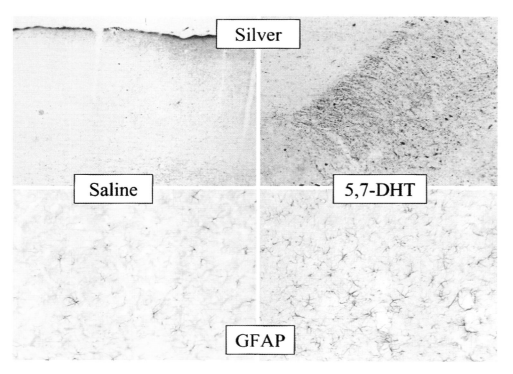

Color Plate 2, Fig. 3 (*see* full caption and discussion in Chapter 11, p. 283). The known serotonergic neurotoxicant, 5, 7-dihydroxytryptamine (5,7-DHT) causes a silver degeneration-staining pattern in cortex characterized by the presence of argyrophilic debris (upper right panel) and the induction of hypertrophied astrocytes characteristic of gliosis (lower right panel).

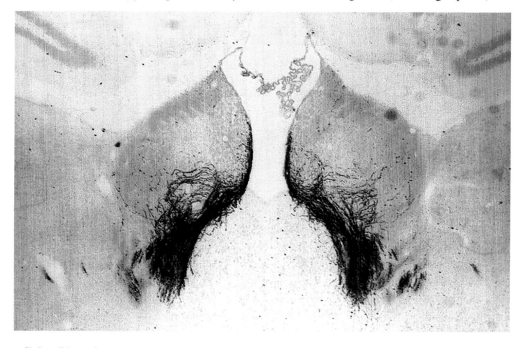

Color Plate 3, Fig. 6 (*see* discussion in Chapter 12, p. 317). Degeneration in FR induced by nicotine.

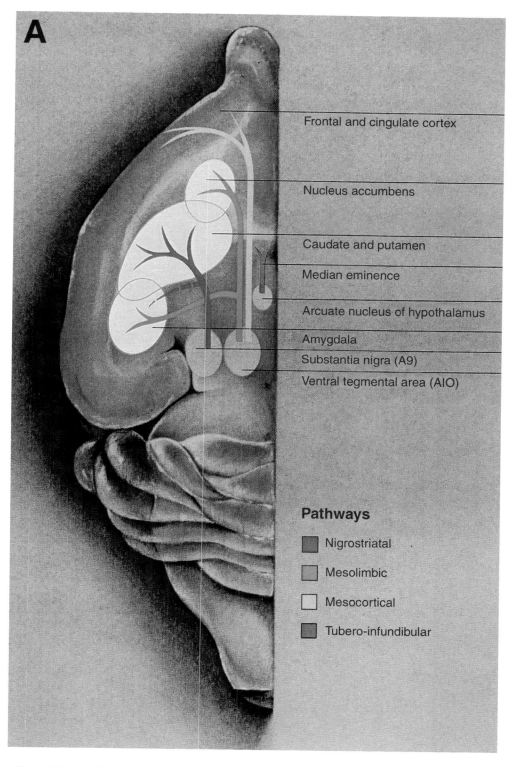

A

Frontal and cingulate cortex

Nucleus accumbens

Caudate and putamen

Median eminence

Arcuate nucleus of hypothalamus

Amygdala

Substantia nigra (A9)

Ventral tegmental area (AIO)

Pathways

Nigrostriatal

Mesolimbic

Mesocortical

Tubero-infundibular

Color Plate 4, Fig. 3A (*see* discussion in Chapter 13, p. 331). Schematic diagram of anatomic dopamine (DA) tracts in the rat brain, represented longitudinally. Adapted with permission from ref. *(108)*.

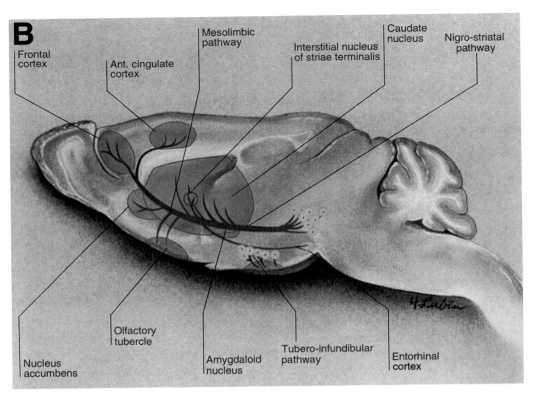

Color Plate 5, Fig. 3B (*see* discussion in Chapter 13, p. 332). Schematic diagram of anatomic dopamine (DA) tracts in the rat brain, represented sagittally. Adapted with permission from ref. *(108).*

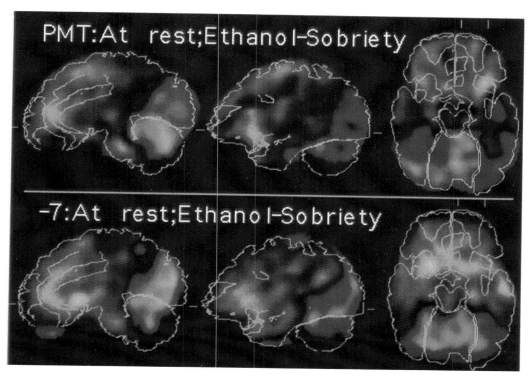

Color Plate 6, Fig. 2 (*see* full caption and discussion in Chapter 14, p. 376). Illustration of the region specific effects during the acute administration of ethanol. Adapted with permission from ref. *(40)*.

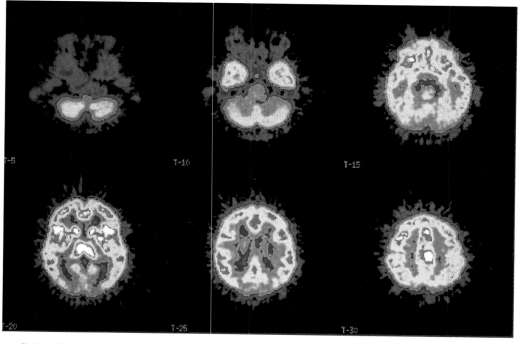

Color Plate 7, Fig. 1 (*see* discussion in Chapter 15, p. 401). Six transverse slices of a PET scan showing (11C)-Diprenorphine binding in the brain of a normal volunteer.

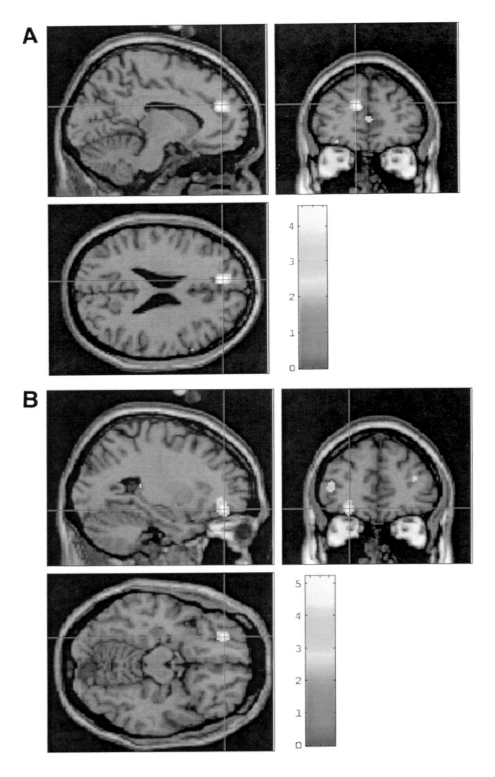

Color Plate 8, Fig. 2A,B (*see* discussion in Chapter 15, p. 408). (**A**) Areas of increased rCBF in response to opioid-related stimuli. (**B**) Area of increased rCBF correlated with subjective opioid craving.

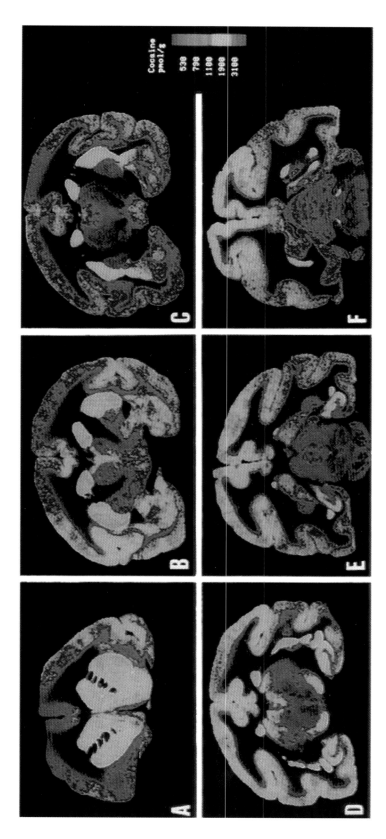

Color Plate 9, Fig. 1 (*see* discussion in Chapter 16, p. 416). Distribution of [3H] cocaine in coronal sections of a squirrel monkey brain. [3H] cocaine (0.1 mg/kg) was administered intravenously 15 min before sacrifice. Shown are 6 levels from anterior (**A**) at the level of the striatum to posterior (**F**) at the level of the locus coeruleus. Prominent labeling is seen throughout the striatum (**A–D**), cortex (**A–F**), ventral midbrain (**D–E**), hippocampus (**D–E**), and locus coeruleus (**F**). Adapted with permission from ref. (*47*).

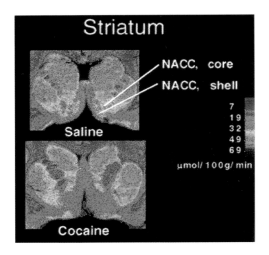

Color Plate 10, Fig. 2 (*see* full caption and discussion in Chapter 16, p. 421). Effects of the acute intravenous administration of cocaine at a dose of 1.0 mg/kg (top panel) and saline (bottom panel) on rates of local cerebral glucose utilization in the ventral striatum. From ref. *(32)*, Copyright 1996, by the Society for Neuroscience.

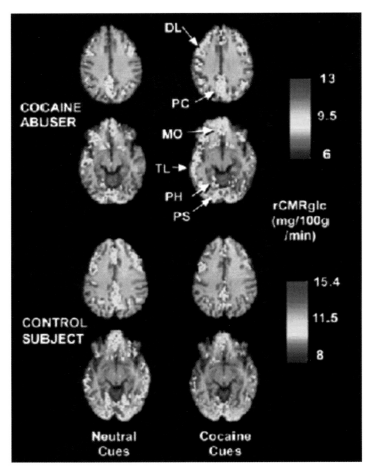

Color Plate 11, Fig. 3 (*see* full caption and discussion in Chapter 16, p. 428). Effects of neutral and cocaine cues on rates of local cerebral glucose utilization in cocaine using (upper panels) and control (lower panels) subjects. Shown are horizontal sections at two dorsoventral levels. Arrows indicate regions in which glucose utilization was increased in the cocaine group. From ref. *(110)*, Copyright 1996, National Academy of Sciences, USA.

III
IMAGING

14

Impact of Intoxication

Structural and Functional Modifications in the Brain Induced by Ethanol Exposure

David J. Lyons, Cory S. Freedland, and Linda J. Porrino

1. ROLE OF IMAGING IN ALCOHOL RESEARCH

During the past three decades, methods have been developed that provide accurate measures of brain structure and function in vivo. These methods are powerful tools for studying the effects of a wide variety of pharmacological, physiological, and psychological stimuli, and they have given us new insights into the way the brain works.

The use of imaging methods is one part of a multidisciplinary effort to understand alcoholism and alcohol-related brain damage, which also includes neuropsychological evaluation, neuropathological examination, and animal experimentation *(1)*. The localization of brain lesions, atrophy and functional brain activity is the contribution made by the mapping of brain. Charness *(1)* points out that 50–70% of detoxified alcoholics are neuropsychologically impaired around the period of detoxification *(2)* and although many will approach full recovery over time, about 10% will remain severely impaired *(3,4)*. Imaging methods such as those described in this chapter are ideal strategies with which to achieve a better understanding of the loci in which alcohol injures brain, alters functional activity, and produces cognitive impairment. It is also possible to use imaging methods to resolve the functional anatomy associated with tolerance, physiological and psychological dependence, withdrawal, and the recovery of specific physiological functions and behaviors. The purpose of this chapter is to familiarize the reader with some of the most relevant findings.

2. NEUROIMAGING

Computed tomography (CT) and magnetic resonance imaging (MRI) specifically depict the structure of brain, allowing the anatomy of the brain to be visualized in great detail. As in vivo techniques, they are particularly important tools for the clinical evaluation of lesions and diseases that alter brain structure. Structural-imaging methods have also been applied to research questions and have provided insights into the abnormalities that accompany neurodegenerative diseases as well as the deleterious effects of

From: Handbook of Neurotoxicology, Vol. 2
Edited by: E. J. Massaro © Humana Press Inc., Totowa, NJ

chronic alcohol exposure. A description of the brain morphology does not relay all needed information, however. It cannot tell us whether structural abnormalities also result in abnormal brain function. The role of brain activity is addressed by functional-imaging methods that permit the visualization of dynamic neurochemical processes within the brain *(5,6,6a)*.

The aim of functional studies is to identify local changes in neuronal firing. A fundamental concept pertaining to these methods is the link between neuronal firing, cellular metabolism, and localized changes in blood flow. The greatest energy demand placed on neurons is the maintenance of ionic gradients. The flux of ions across the membrane during an action potential places heavy demand on ATP-dependent ion transporters. Under normal physiological conditions, glucose is virtually the exclusive substrate for energy metabolism in brain, which places glucose in a unique position to serve as a functional marker. Although there are a number of energy-requiring processes in brain that contribute to basal rates of glucose utilization, e.g., transmitter synthesis, release, and reuptake, and protein synthesis, it has been estimated that 80% of the energy generated in brain is used to maintain and restore ionic gradients *(7)*. It is important to appreciate that the changes in rates of glucose utilization that are evoked by an experimental manipulation are thought to result mainly from increases or decreases in electrical activity or synaptic activity in the central nervous system (CNS). These processes form the foundation for the measurement of local cerebral glucose utilization (LCGU; *5,8*)

To function properly, the brain must be continuously supplied with nutrients. In contrast to other organs, the brain cannot store sufficient nutrients and therefore depends on a constant supply delivered by the blood. Brain regions that are more active require more nutrients, and regional rates of blood flow within the brain are modulated to keep pace with the changing demands. These characteristics form the basis for the measurement of regional cerebral blood flow (rCBF; *6,9*). In fact, local changes in blood flow far exceed demand, providing a strong signal. The amplification of energy demand into greater changes in blood flow do present difficulties in interpretation in that the coupling of neuronal activity to blood flow is less precise than to glucose utilization. The particular advantage of rCBF over cerebral metabolic methods is the short time window during which blood flow is determined. Unlike the measurement of glucose utilization, a scan of rCBF can be completed within a few minutes such that several scans can be conducted under a variety of conditions in a single subject visit. It is also important to recognize that although blood-flow changes result from fluctuations in energy demand, they change as a consequence of the direct effects of alcohol and other drugs on cerebral vasculature as well *(10)*. Proper interpretation of studies of rCBF must keep in mind that findings are likely to be the result of a combination of modifications in perfusion as well as function.

The generation of 3-dimensional tomographic images of the living brain can be accomplished in several ways *(11)*. Positron emission tomography (PET) and single-photon emission tomography (SPECT) produce images after the injection of a radiolabeled tracer into the patient followed by the localization of tracer in brain tissue with the aid of sensitive detectors positioned around the subject. Another means for visualizing structure and function is MRI, which is most commonly used to evaluate tissue structural morphology. More recently, however, functional MRI (fMRI) has been employed magnetic-resonance technology to determine changes in blood flow and blood oxygenation.

This chapter will focus on what imaging the brain has told us about the neurobiological consequences of alcohol use and alcoholism. These methods have opened the black box containing the brain and allowed us to investigate ethanol exposure in living creatures, including humans. By identifying specific regions of brain that are particularly sensitive to the acute and/or chronic effects of ethanol, we have begun to piece together the relationship between alcohol drinking and altered brain structure and function.

3. NEUROPHARMACOLOGY OF ETHANOL

Ethanol is a notoriously dirty drug, a pharmacologically complex agent that is believed to act on a host of receptor systems in brain *(12)*. In the recent past, the best explanation of ethanol's effects included the notion of changes in membrane fluidity. Although ethanol is a polar molecule, it can associate with the cellular membrane. Due to the polar nature of ethanol, its interaction at the membrane is largely restricted to the polar-head region of the lipid bilayer, rather than intercalating deep within lipophilic regions *(13)*. Nonetheless, ethanol-related changes in membrane fluidity can alter protein-membrane and protein-ligand interactions *(14)*. Like early descriptions of the mechanism of action of gaseous anesthetics, it was postulated that disruptions in neuronal firing and receptor activity induced by ethanol were secondary to alterations in membrane properties.

Although still indirect, ethanol may also disrupt normal ligand-protein interactions as a result of its ability to alter the solvation of membrane proteins or polar groups on membrane phospholipids *(15)*. By virtue of its dipole and ability to form hydrogen bonds, ethanol can perturb the aqueous environment surrounding membrane components and alter normal cellular interactions with ligands and ions. Importantly, however, these mechanisms appear to fall short of explaining ethanol drinking, because the concentrations needed to induce membrane changes (>100 mM) far exceed those necessary to produce mild to moderate levels of intoxication (5–30 mM; *12*). It is still possible that local concentrations may achieve high enough concentrations, yet this possibility remains to be demonstrated. Interestingly, recent proton MR spectroscopy studies have found that the ability to detect ethanol in brain by this method is altered by repeated ethanol exposure. In individuals without significant ethanol exposure, the levels of detection after the acute intake of ethanol is less than 30% of actual levels in venous blood and brain *(16–20)*. The reason for these low levels of detection is poorly understood; however, it appears that an interaction between ethanol and membranes in the CNS is a key feature of this phenomenon. It turns out that several hours after a single dose of ethanol or following repeated exposure, the levels of ethanol detection in brain rise significantly *(18,20)*. A change in membrane composition currently is the best explanation for these findings *(18)*. The implication of these results is that there appears to be an adaptive response to ethanol exposure in human brain cellular membranes, which may in turn play a role in tolerance, dependence and withdrawal. Consequently, the role of alcohol's action on membranes remains acutely relevant.

During the past decade, it has become generally accepted that ethanol can act on various neuroreceptors at physiologically relevant concentrations *(12,21–25)*. In addi-

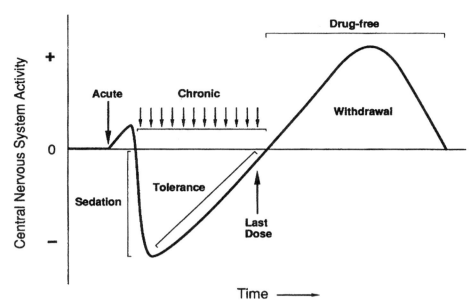

Fig. 1. Time-line describing the hypothetical change in CNS activity during various stages of ethanol exposure. Adapted with permission from ref. *(119)*. Soon after intake, ethanol can be stimulating, then later it becomes sedating. After repeated exposure, tolerance and physical dependence can develop. Upon the cessation of exposure, withdrawal may ensue followed by a period of return to baseline.

tion, studies of site-directed mutagenesis have identified specific sites on these proteins that are necessary to yield alcohol effects via a variety of receptors, particularly ion channels: acetylcholine *(26–28)*, serotonin 5-HT3 *(27–28)*, GABA$_A$, glycine *(29)*, and N-methyl-D-aspartate (NMDA) *(30)*. When it was believed that ethanol acted solely by perturbing membranes, theoretically ethanol could influence the activity of virtually all receptors. Now that it is known that ethanol interacts with specific receptor proteins, the numbers of types of receptors within the potential influence of ethanol has been greatly reduced. Similarly, the variety of neural circuits that might participate in the effects of ethanol are more limited as well. Nonetheless, the large number of receptors known to be sensitive to ethanol makes it clear that the task of understanding the sundry circuits affected by ethanol and their varied interactions is likely to be extremely complex.

4. ETHANOL ALTERS ACTIVITY WITHIN INTERDEPENDENT NEURAL CIRCUITS

Ethanol is a substance that has complex physiological, behavioral, and biochemical actions. It is known that the physiological and behavioral responses to ethanol are not the result of a single action in a single brain region, but is the product of multiple processes at a number of distinct anatomical sites. Consequently, the effects of ethanol administration on brain as a whole vary dramatically depending upon a number of factors. Figure 1 contains a time-line describing the hypothetical change in CNS activity during various stages of ethanol exposure. Presumably, various neural circuits interact in unique ways under each of these conditions: initial response, chronic exposure, and withdrawal. The diversity of ethanol's neurochemical effects make accurate predictions of its actions at the circuit or systems level in the CNS extremely difficult. In order to characterize the neuroanatomical substrates of the effects of ethanol under various conditions of dose, time, and repeated exposure, therefore, it is necessary to measure these neural events directly. Imaging methods provide the means to accomplish this task by examining the entire CNS simultaneously.

5. FUNCTIONAL EFFECTS OF ACUTE ETHANOL ADMINISTRATION

The potency of ethanol differs across neurotransmitter systems *(31)*, and the behavioral effect of ethanol is highly dose-dependent. At low doses, alcohol can act as a stimulant, activating spontaneous locomotor activity in rodents, while at higher doses, alcohol produces sedation, motor incoordination, and anesthesia. In humans, increased verbal activity, behavioral disinhibition, reduced anxiety and euphoria can accompany low doses, whereas the ingestion of higher doses can result in motor and sensory impairments. Determining the substrates of varying doses of alcohol, therefore, has been an important focus of a number of imaging studies in both rodents and humans.

Mild to moderate levels of intoxication, like those accompanying intake of 2–4 standard drinks (0.5–1.0 g/kg), have been shown to increase CBF in a region-specific manner *(32–37)*. Whereas prefrontal and temporal cortices were often activated *(34,36,37)*, the frontal cortex was sensitive to the lowest doses (0.5–0.7 g/kg). To elicit effects in temporal cortex, slightly higher doses were required (1.0–1.5 g/kg). Since the dose-response relationship appears to be different in these cortices, each region may play a unique role in the response to ethanol within the CNS and on behavior. These studies are important because they demonstrate that alcohol in low doses can increase functional activity in a region-specific manner, implicating these cortices in the positive mood-altering effects of ethanol intake.

High doses of ethanol (> 1.5 g/kg), similar to intake of greater than 6 standard drinks, decreases CBF and LCGU globally in humans *(37–39)*. The effect is a much more homogenous reduction in activity throughout the brain. One potentially important exception is the cerebellum, in which reduced functional activity was found after more moderate doses (1.0 g/kg). The unique response in cerebellar cortex suggests that, like prefrontal and temporal cortex, it may exhibit a unique pharmacological response to ethanol. To date, then, findings from functional-imaging studies agree with reports of the biphasic effects of ethanol on behavior. It also appears thus far that portions of prefrontal and temporal cortex may play a role in the activating effects of ethanol following low doses, and the cerebellum may be critically involved in motor incoordination. One of the significant limitations of this work is that functional imaging in humans cannot resolve relatively small subcortical sites. Ingvar and colleagues *(40)* made attempts to overcome this limitation by scanning subjects repeatedly, under conditions of sobriety or intoxication. As shown in Fig. 2, these investigators found at blood ethanol levels in the moderate range (0.07%) that rCBF was increased in ventral prefrontal regions, including the anterior insula, anterior cingulate, gyrus rectus, and temporal cortex, while decreases were found in cerebellum and occipital cortex. These authors conclude that the regions in which blood flow was elevated ethanol are those involved in the cerebral-reward system, part of the brain responsible for regulating mood and motivation *(40)*. Furthermore, they argue that the pattern is similar to that seen in people craving cocaine *(41)* and alcohol *(42)*.

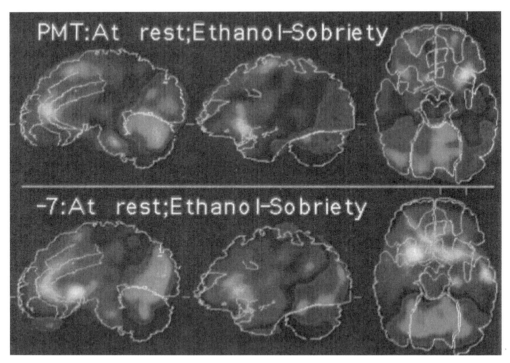

Fig. 2. Illustration of the region specific effects during the acute administration of ethanol. Adapted with permission from ref. *(40)*. Images represent column contrasts between alcohol (0.07% blood ethanol level) and sober conditions at rest. Relative CBF increases are represented in red-yellow and decreases are in blue. The anatomic orientation of the slices are as follows: Left, midline sagittal; middle, sagittal section off midline; Right, horizontal at the level of basal forebrain. Note the convergence of increased blood flow in inferior frontal regions and basal forebrain, and the decreased blood flow in posterior cerebral cortex and cerebellum. (*See* color plate 6 appearing in the insert following p. 368.)

Human studies pose specific experimental challenges, largely because of the subject sample. Animals studies, on the other hand, permit the careful manipulation of experimental factors that may go unchecked in human studies. In animal work, effects can be attributed directly to alcohol without any confounds of past history of alcohol use or use of other common psychoactive substances, e.g., nicotine, caffeine, over-the-counter drugs, etc. Furthermore, autoradiographic methods of imaging have the power to resolve subcortical sites and can therefore contribute significantly to our understanding of the functional anatomy pertaining to alcohol exposure. Although there have not been a large number of studies, the results to date closely parallel the effects noted in humans. When low doses are administered, alcohol can increase functional activity in forebrain regions, whereas when higher doses are administered, functional activity is reduced.

A few animal studies have examined the brain regions affected by different alcohol doses in detail *(43–47)*. Eckardt and coworkers *(43)* found that ethanol at high doses decreased rates of cerebral metabolism in most affected sites (auditory system, cerebellum, vestibular nucleus, and median raphe nucleus), yet the lowest dose increased LCGU in at least two sites: the dentate gyrus of the hippocampus and the superior olivary nucleus. In a study by Williams-Hemby and Porrino *(45)*, three doses of ethanol (0.25, 0.5, and 1.0 g/kg, ip) were administered to alcohol-naive rats, and brain mapping was conducted during the period associated with the peak of the blood ethanol curve. The patterns of LCGU among brain structures depended on the alcohol dose. The 0.25 g/kg dose of alcohol increased neural activity, most prominently in brain structures of the mesocorticolimbic system. The 1.0 g/kg alcohol dose, in contrast, caused a distinctly different pattern of decreased activity in the thalamus, hippocampus, and locus coeruleus. First, these data demonstrate the dose-dependent nature of the functional response to acute ethanol. Second, the brain structures in which changes in functional activity were detected are consistent with the observed behavioral changes induced by alcohol. The low-alcohol dose led to a widespread increase in brain activity in areas, which may correspond to the behaviorally arousing and rewarding effects, whereas the moderate-alcohol dose suppressed brain function, potentially related to the suppressive and sedating effects on behavior.

In a second study by Williams-Hemby and Porrino *(46)*, it was reported that when 0.25, 1.0, or 2.0 g/kg of ethanol was administered; all doses tested increased rates of cerebral metabolism in various structures, most prominently in the mesocorticolimbic system. In contrast to the first study, this study determined functional activity immediately after administration during the period when blood levels where rapidly rising. After the administration of ethanol by either intraperitoneal injection or lavage, levels of blood alcohol quickly rise to a peak within about 15 min. These data suggest then that the period along the rising phase of the blood ethanol curve may be accompanied by a specific pattern of brain activity, one that is very similar to the pattern that is sustained for longer periods by a low dose.

Several additional imaging studies have examined higher doses of ethanol, which lead to motor-behavior impairment. Like the human work, these animal studies indicate that the cerebellum is a site where functional activity is frequently reduced. Other regions where high-dose alcohol diminished functional activity include auditory structures, the hippocampus and portions of the thalamus *(48–53)*. At present, high-dose ethanol appears to alter function in a number of brain regions, but aside from the auditory system, a clear picture of a role for specific circuits is difficult to discern. Like global changes seen in humans after high doses, the effects in this dose range within animal brain are characterized by widespread changes.

6. TIME-COURSE OF ACUTE ETHANOL EFFECTS

Another important factor that is involved in determining the behavioral response to alcohol is the time since ingestion. Here too the effects of alcohol have been shown to be biphasic. Alcohol's effects on behavior and brain functioning depend not only on the amount consumed but also on the time that has elapsed since alcohol ingestion. Following high doses (1.5–6.0 g/kg in rodents) responsiveness is often decreased and may be replaced several hours later by a rebound phenomenon of hyper-responsiveness. This has been shown to occur on various measures including, seizure activity, pain thresholds, and motor activity *(54)*. In contrast, following low to moderate doses of ethanol there may be a brief period of behavioral stimulation and euphoria, which is replaced later with sedation *(55–60)*. This early period of euphoria is particularly interesting because it may be responsible for the positive reinforcement associated with ethanol intake that is critical for ethanol-seeking behavior.

Acute tolerance to the effects of ethanol is another important time-dependent phenomena. This form of tolerance occurs during the course of a single exposure to ethanol, and is classically described as a greater effect on the ascending limb of the blood alcohol curve than the one found on the descending limb at the same blood alcohol concentration *(61–64)*. Acute tolerance to the effects of ethanol has been clearly demonstrated in a number of motor, sensory, and cognitive tasks *(62,65)*, and has also been demonstrated to occur in neurons within the CNS *(33,54,56,66–71)*.

One of the first studies to address the time-dependent nature of alcohol's effects was conducted by Hadji-Dimo et al. *(72)* in cats. A biphasic response was found by these investigators who demonstrated that following the administration of ethanol there was an initial increase in CBF and EEG frequency index, which was later replaced with decreases in these measures. Alterations in brain blood flow that appear to be consistent with acute tolerance have also been reported. For example, Friedman et al. *(48)* examined CBF in awake dogs and found that 30 min after the initiation of repeated ethanol infusion, blood flow was decreased in cortex, cerebellum, brain stem, and white matter, whereas only a small but significant change in CBF could be found in the cerebellum at 90 min. This occurred despite the fact that ethanol blood levels were considerably higher at 90 min.

To investigate whether functional changes in brain activity reflect these behavioral observations, Lyons et al. *(73)* first demonstrated that a 0.8 g/kg dose of ethanol (ip) increased rCBF in various sites in rat brain 5 min after administration. These changes were no longer detectable, however, at 15 min after administration, despite significant blood alcohol levels at both times. Moreover, this early activation and later disappearance of rCBF changes were seen even when blood alcohol levels were held constant across time. This time measuring local cerebral glucose utilization, these investigators *(74)* compared functional activity immediately after administration, largely along the ascending limb of the blood ethanol curve, and at 45 min at a point on the descending limb. Functional activity was increased in the mesocorticolimbic system early after administration and decreased later in the hippocampus and septum, compared to water treatment. Time differences and the vasodilatory effects of ethanol are likely to explain the discrepancy in findings at the later time-points in these studies. Given that the rewarding aspects of alcohol intake appear to predominate early and that the ventral striatum is known to play a role in reward and reinforcement, the selective effects of ethanol found in the mesocorticolimbic suggest that this system plays a role in the processing of ethanol's reinforcing effects much like it does for other drugs of abuse *(75,76)*. The mechanisms underlying the emergence of multiple phases of functional activity during the with-session time-course of ethanol exposure are not known. It is likely, however, that it is at least partially due to the variety of receptor systems affected by ethanol.

7. BEHAVIORAL CONTEXT

One important determinant of the response to a pharmacological agent such as alcohol is the behavioral context of the presentation. There are a number of studies that have shown that the pharmacological effects of a drug are distinctly different depending on whether the drug is voluntarily self-administered or passively administered by the experimenter. For example, Dworkin and colleagues *(77)* have shown that if animals are chronically administered cocaine passively at a rate and in a pattern identical to that followed by rats self-administering the drug, cocaine can have lethal effects. This, despite the fact that the self-administering rats find the effects sufficiently reinforcing for responding to be maintained at a high rate. This distinction between self-administration and passive administration has also been seen with alcohol. Alcohol that is voluntarily ingested by rats decreases thresholds for electrical brain-stimulation reward, while similar amounts of alcohol passively administered have no effect on thresholds *(78)*. It is of importance therefore, to consider the neural correlates of alcohol when it is consumed voluntarily. It is these effects that have the most relevance to models of human alcohol consumption.

Porrino and colleagues *(79,80)* have recently used metabolic mapping methods to identify the neural substrates of the effects of voluntarily consumed alcohol. In this study rats were trained to ingest alcohol using a modification of the sucrose-fading method developed by Samson et al. *(81)*. Once alcohol consumption stabilized, the deoxyglucose method was applied to rats immediately following a drinking session in which they drank 0.5 g/kg of alcohol, a dose equivalent to one or two drinks. Rates of cerebral glucose utilization were significantly increased throughout portions of the mesocorticolimbic system including the nucleus accumbens, medial prefrontal cortex, and basolateral amygdala when compared to those of controls drinking either water or sucrose *(79,80)*. This pattern of activation is considerably different from that obtained following the passive ip administration of an identical dose of ethanol. This again emphasizes the importance of the context of administration. When ingested voluntarily, the effects of alcohol appear to be restricted to brain regions that are critical to the mediation of positive reinforcement *(82)*. This is in clear contrast to its effects when administered passively, where effects are evident predominantly in the hippocampus and in sensory systems *(45)*. This distinction between the effects of self-administered alcohol and those of alcohol administered by an experimenter are present regardless of the dose of alcohol consumed during the experiment. Activation in the mesolimbic system appears to be a consistent feature of the effects of self-administered alcohol. Although a number of factors differ in these comparisons, the rate of administration and the behavioral history for instance, the context of administration appears to be more important than the pharmacological effects in determining the nature of the pattern of brain activation produced by alcohol.

Thus, although only a relatively few studies have fully utilized functional imaging methods to study the effects of alcohol to date, the results show that the neuroanatomical substrates of the effects of alcohol are the result of the interaction of both dose and time since ingestion. Because of their ability to examine the entire brain simultaneously, imaging methods may be invaluable tools for a closer examination of the neurobiological basis of the effects of alcohol.

8. STRUCTURAL ALTERATIONS IN ALCOHOLISM

Ethanol appears to induce structural brain damage via a number of means (for review, *see* ref. *1*). Our understanding of the biochemical mechanisms involved remains poor, however. The ability to discern the neurotoxic effects of ethanol is made more difficult by the fact that severe chronic alcoholism is often accompanied by malnutrition and vitamin deficiencies, when nearly all calories are acquired from alcohol alone. The comorbid presentation of alcoholism and diseases with known relationship to nutritional status hamper efforts to pinpoint the role of alcohol exposure in producing neurological deficits. The variety of neurological disease states that frequently coexist along side severe alcoholism are great: Wernicke's encephalopathy, Korsakoff's disease, Marchiafava-Bignami syndrome, hepatocerebral degeneration, pellagra, central pontine myelinolysis, cerebellar atrophy, and head trauma *(1)*.

Neuroradiological techniques, such as MRI and CT, have been useful in characterizing the structural changes in brain associated with chronic alcoholism. Many of these studies have attempted to demonstrate a link between brain dysmorphology and the neurological and neuropsychological deficits observed in this population, e.g, Korsakoff's syndrome, amnesia, and seizures. While no causal relationships between structural change and pathology have been clearly elucidated, a number of structural deficits in specific populations of alcoholics have been reported.

MRI studies of chronic alcoholics have demonstrated the presence of structural abnormalities in a number of brain regions. Sullivan et al. *(83)* compared the brains of alcoholics with and without a history of seizures. Significant structural abnormalities in brain were identified in both groups of alcoholics when compared to controls. Alcoholics in general presented with gray-matter volume deficits in the temporal lobe, frontal-parietal cortex, and anterior hippocampus, and white-matter volume deficits were observed in both groups of alcoholics in the frontal-parietal cortex. Alcoholics with a history of seizures exhibited additional deficits in white matter volume within temporal cortex. In addition, both groups showed marked increases in both temporal and frontal-parietal sulcal cerebrospinal fluid (CSF) volumes *(83)*.

Similar findings have been reported by Pfefferbaum et al. *(84)* who demonstrated both white- and gray-matter volume deficits in frontal cortex as well as volume enlargement of the cortical sulci, lateral, and third ventricles in alcoholics. It has also been demonstrated that alcoholics show bilateral mammillary-body volume deficits *(85,86)*, frontal cortical gray-matter volume loss *(84)*, as well as tissue-volume loss in both the cerebellar hemispheres and vermis *(86)*. In the study by Sullivan et al. *(85)*, the severity of mammillary-body volume deficit was related to the severity of memory and cognitive dysfunction in this group of alcoholics. Studies utilizing CT have produced largely similar results. For example, Shimamura and colleagues *(87)* reported cortical atrophy in frontal sulcal and perisylvian areas as well as decreases in left posterior white matter in brains of chronic alcoholics *(87)*.

It has been suggested by several investigators that some of the structural deficits observed in the brains of alcoholics may be attenuated following a protracted period of abstinence *(88–90)*. The amount of deficit reversal appears to be related to the length of abstinence. In a study by Pfefferbaum and colleagues *(91)*, MRI was utilized to visualize the brains of alcoholics following a 3–4-wk period of abstinence. Over time, alcoholics exhibited global increases in CSF volume and total cortical CSF as well as marked decreases in intracranial tissue volume and total cortical gray and white matter. Region of interest analysis also revealed significant increases in CSF volume, in prefrontal, frontal, fronto-temporal, temporo-parietal, parietal, parieto-occipital, and subcortical regions. Alcoholics presented with decreased gray-matter volume in all of these cortices compared to controls. Significant enlargement of both the lateral and third ventricles were also observed *(91)*.

In contrast, longer periods of abstinence have been shown to result in partial reversal of the CSF and white-matter volume deficits associated with alcoholism. Shear et al. *(90)* demonstrated significant decreases in CSF volume and increases in white-matter volume in alcoholics who had abstained for 3 mo when compared to alcoholics with shorter histories of abstinence. In a comprehensive, longitudinal study, Pfefferbaum and coworkers *(92)* examined the temporal course of abstinence-related normalization of brain volumes using MRI. In this study, alcoholics were compared to controls following 2 wk, 1 mo, and 3 mo of abstinence. A significant portion of the alcoholic group relapsed before the third scan and was used as a comparison group for the alcoholics who remained abstinent. Following 2 wk of abstinence, alcoholics exhibited increased sulcal CSF volumes and decreased in gray- and white-matter volumes vs controls in a number of brain regions including anterior and posterior cortical areas and thalamus. In addition, alcoholics had significantly increased lateral and third ventricle volumes. The same pattern of deficits emerged when subjects received their second MRI following 1 mo of abstinence. Following 3 mo of abstinence, alcoholics showed improvement in cortical gray matter, sulcal, and lateral ventricular volumes. Importantly, subjects who relapsed showed larger decreases in white matter and increased third ventricular volumes than subjects who abstained *(92)*.

In summary, chronic alcoholism results in significant dysmorphic changes in brain, decreasing gray- and white-matter volumes while increasing sulcal and ventricular volumes. Some of these changes, such as cortical gray-matter volume deficits, appear to partially reverse in alcoholics who abstain for at least 3 mo, however this reversal is far from complete and significant structural abnormalities are still present in the brain of abstinent alcoholics.

9. FUNCTIONAL ADAPTATION TO LONG-TERM ALCOHOL EXPOSURE

Animal models of chronic alcohol exposure are useful because they eliminate confounding factors that are difficult to control in a population of chronic drinkers. These factors are varied and include, for example, ethanol-intake history, nutrition, and co-morbid psychiatric disorders. Using animals instead, direct evidence can be obtained regarding the long-term pharmacologic consequences specifically attributable to ethanol exposure. In addition, the spatial resolution of autoradiographic techniques currently surpasses that of in vivo imaging and makes more careful study of neuroanatomical circuits possible. Since defining circuitry is one of the primary goals of this research approach, imaging of animals is capable of providing much more detailed anatomical descriptions of the functional consequences of chronic alcohol intake.

Rodent studies of chronic alcohol exposure have either evaluated high-doses for short periods of time, usually on the order of days *(93,94)*, or low doses in the diet or drinking water for periods of a few weeks *(50,92,95)*, or a period of months to years *(96,97)*. Short-term experiments using the intra-arterial Xenon method or the deoxyglucose method found that rats became tolerant after 3–4 d of nearly continuous intoxication to the effects of ethanol on CBF and cerebral metabolic rates for oxygen utilization, i.e., fewer structures were affected by an acute dose of ethanol and to a lesser degree *(43,94)*. Repeated ethanol dosing also blunted the hypercapnic response, suggesting that cerebrovascular reactivity is compromised following repeated ethanol exposure *(94)*. Similar findings of tolerance to ethanol-induced changes in function after prolonged ethanol exposure have been reported after 3 or 8 wk of daily ethanol intake in the diet *(50,53)*. Together, these data show that relatively short-term chronic treatment on the order of a few days to a few weeks can lead to functional adaptation in brain.

Three studies have examined the functional consequences of ethanol administered via the diet for periods of 2 mo or more, and each study found evidence of altered function in portions of the Papez circuit, which is a circular network within the limbic system that comprises the mammillary bodies, anterior thalamus, cingulate cortex, and the hippocampus. Pietrzak et al. *(98)* evaluated rats, within a few hours of removing access to ethanol that had consumed ethanol for 7 mo and found increased rates of cerebral metabolism, possibly due to withdrawal. Unlike other studies of withdrawal following much shorter chronic regimens, however, this study found the greatest changes in LCGU in the cingulate cortex-mammillary body-anterior thalamus pathway, as well as amygdala and septum. In another study, after at least 70 d of daily intake under schedule-induced polydipsia, rates of LCGU in rats immediately following a session of ethanol intake were found to be depressed in the hippocampal complex, habenula, anterior ventral thalamus, and mammillary bodies and increased in the nucleus accumbens *(97)*. In the third study, Bontempi et al. *(96)* showed that residual functional deficits persist after alcohol exposure has stopped by determining functional activity 7 wk after the termination of ethanol intake. These researchers also controlled for the residual effects of withdrawal by removing the concentration of ethanol in a stepwise fashion to prevent overt withdrawal symptoms. It was found that 6 mo of ethanol intake in these mice had little effect on the uptake of deoxyglucose, whereas 12 mo of exposure decreased uptake in the lateral mammillary body and anterior thalamus and 18 mo of exposure affected all of the mammillary body, more of the thalamus and portions of the hippocampus. Overall, these findings are strikingly consistent with findings in humans with the Wernicke-Korsakoff Syndrome. Future use of this animal model may be effective for studying the mechanism responsible for the diencephalic pathology found in the Papez circuit in some alcoholics. In addition, it should be pointed out that there is an absence of data on alcohol-induced changes on frontal-lobe function in the rodent, leaving us without an animal model for the frontal-lobe pathology frequently found in human drinkers. A model of cortical neurodegeneration has been advanced in which a few days of very high-dose ethanol leads to neuronal death in temporal cortex *(99,100)*. Frontal damage is largely absent under these conditions, however. The establishment of an animal model of frontal lobe damage for use in imaging is still needed.

10. LONG-TERM ETHANOL INTAKE IN HUMANS: RELATIONSHIP TO TASK PERFORMANCE

It is well-established that heavy alcohol consumption reduces cortical volume *(101,102)*. Large ventricles and wide cortical and cerebellar sulci can be present, and subcortical atrophy of hippocampus and mammillary bodies have been reported, even in non-Korsakoff alcoholics. It is also important that although atrophy can be seen throughout the brains of heavy drinkers, the changes in prefrontal cortex may be more pronounced *(101)*. This cortical atrophy is not necessarily permanent; ventricular size and sulcal width have been shown to at least partially recover during abstinence. Efforts thus far to link specific structural changes in brain with changes in cognitive function of alcoholics have met with only limited success *(102,103)*. One hope of studying the functional consequences of chronic alcohol intake is, therefore, to identify functional deficits in specific brain regions that are responsible for this cognitive impairment in a way that structural imaging has not.

The smaller tissue volume in some alcoholics poses a particular problem for imaging studies, because apparent decreases in functional activity may simply be the result of normal activity in less tissue. Nonetheless, there is good evidence that functional activity is diminished in the frontal and temporal lobes and cerebellum of alcoholics *(81,104–111)*. Using SPECT technology, Melgaard et al. *(112)* found that the magnitude of the decreased rCBF in the medial prefrontal cortex of alcoholics was greater than that found in periventricular regions, where cortical atrophy appears to be greatest. These authors reasoned, therefore, that the changes in prefrontal cortex were likely to be functional. Furthermore, alcoholics without atrophy also had diminished rCBF in frontal cortex. Erbas et al. *(113)* compared rCBF and atrophy determined by CT in alcoholics. Here rCBF was normalized to whole-slice CBF, which partially compensated for cortical atrophy (to the degree that atrophy is equally distributed throughout the slice). In alcoholics, frontal rCBF was lower and significant cortical atrophy was evident; however, rCBF and cortical atrophy were not significantly correlated in this study, which suggests that these variables may function independently at least to some degree. Furthermore, since reduced rCBF is found in alcoholics without atrophy *(81,113,114)*, these structural and functional forms of alcoholic pathology can be differentiated.

A few studies compared neuropsychological function and rCBF and both found that hypoperfusion was significantly correlated with poor task performance in alcoholics who otherwise appeared to be unimpaired *(112,114)*. Nicolas et al. *(114)* reported that 18 of 29 alcoholics without detectable atrophy were found to have frontal hypoperfusion. Furthermore, 17 of the 18 alcoholics with frontal hypoperfusion (but not atrophy) presented with cognitive impairment, whereas only one of 11 alcoholics without atrophy or altered frontal perfusion was neuropsychologically impaired. These data demonstrate that rCBF is a sensitive measure of function in alcoholics and that it was a better predictor of performance than the degree of atrophy. Furthermore, in alcoholics who abstained from alcohol for 2 mo, those without atrophy had normal frontal perfusion. Those with atrophy improved but did not return to normal levels, which suggests that the prognosis for cognitive recovery may be better in nonatrophic alcoholics. It appears then, that regardless of the degree to which these structural and functional methods may be independent, they both retain an important relationship with cognitive impairment. Gansler et al. *(115)* investigated whether longer-term abstinence would result in improved rCBF. In this study hypoperfusion was evident within the inferofrontal region in alcoholics with fewer than 4 yr of abstinence, when compared to controls or alcoholics with greater than 4 yr of abstinence. These data imply that years of abstinence may be necessary to achieve normalized brain function. The number of alcohol detoxifications appears to important as well. Alcoholics with greater that two detoxifications had more significant alterations in medial temporal, inferior frontal and paralimbic regions, compared to alcoholics with only one detoxification *(111)*.

Reduced LCGU in the frontal cortex of alcoholics has also been correlated with poor performance on tests of frontal-lobe function, including the Symbol Digit Modalities written test *(108)* and the Wisconsin Card Sorting Test *(104)*. Wang et al. *(108)* also found that frontal LCGU in alcoholics was positively correlated with performance on the Weschler Memory Scale. Eckardt and coworkers *(116)* reported that the recognition of whether a word had been provided by the subject or the experimenter during test sessions 2 d earlier was impaired in their alcoholic population and that performance on this task further correlated with reduced metabolism in left prefrontal, temporal, and posterior orbitofrontal cortex. Here again, strong evidence has been provided, this time assessing cerebral metabolism, that poor cognitive performance and regional functional deficits concentrated in the frontal lobe is found in alcoholics. At this point, however, we do not know how long this relationship lasts in the sober, recovering alcoholic because functional activity can recover during abstinence *(112)*. These changes in function may in fact be the consequence of recent drinking, since altered functional activity has been correlated with the amount of recent alcohol intake *(114)*, the number of days since last use *(39)*, and the severity of alcoholism *(112)*. Future work is needed, therefore, to differentiate between these relatively short-lived residual changes in brain function associated with recent ethanol use and more permanent functional deficits.

In summary, functional deficits in CBF and metabolism have been clearly demonstrated in chronic alcoholics and the majority of this work indicates that dysfunction can be found in the frontal lobes. These deficits are at least partially independent of cortical atrophy and are apparent in alcoholics with demonstrable cognitive impairment and in those that appear neurologically intact. Furthermore, abstaining from alcohol leads to improvements in functional activity in these populations, although whether all alcoholics can attain complete recovery remains to be determined.

Two studies by Rogers and coworkers emphasize the importance of understanding the neurobiological consequences of the habit of drinking alcohol. Using the 13 Xenon inhalation technique in a large study of 218 social drinkers, these investigators first found that global rates of CBF were negatively correlated with the average level of alcohol consumption over the past 5 yr *(117)* the greater the alcohol intake, the lower the level of CBF. This study provided a solid foundation for the assertion that alcohol intake has long-term effects on human brain function even in the unimpaired social drinker. It also begs the question of whether there are concomitant changes in cognitive ability as well. In a second study, this time of severe chronic alcoholics, these investigators found that global CBF improved between the first test after initial detoxification (postwithdrawal) and a retest 3–13 wk into a period of continued abstinence *(118)*. In contrast to the first experiment, these results demonstrated the dramatic recovery in cerebral perfusion that can occur during abstinence. Together, this work indicates that alcohol-related changes in brain function are likely to exist in a sizeable portion of the current population, and that these changes are clearly not limited to populations of alcoholics. Yet, the degree to which brain function is altered by alcohol intake is also highly fluid, showing remarkable improvement when abstinence is sustained, even in those among us who are likely to be the most impaired. Nonetheless, recovery of function is often not complete, which means that there are in fact permanent consequences of ethanol use on brain activity. At this point, it is not clear to what degree these deficits in functional activity contribute to long-term behavioral impairment and who is at risk for these persistent deficits.

11. WITHDRAWAL

Physical symptoms of ethanol withdrawal include anxiety, hallucinations, seizures, irritability, nausea, vomiting, insomnia, tremor, hypothermia, hyperventilation, and tachycardia (*see* ref. *119*). The study of withdrawal is important for at least two reasons. First, in the severe chronic alcoholic withdrawal can be severe and require medical intervention. A clearer understanding of the functional basis of withdrawal and current treatments that alleviate it will likely lead to more rational treatment strategies. Second, it is not known whether withdrawal leads to residual deficits in brain function. Since cognitive deficits occur in alcoholics, the role withdrawal plays, if any, in the establishment of alcohol-related impairment needs to be determined. The studies reviewed below are the initial attempts to investigate the functional consequences of withdrawal, and they describe the regional changes in the brains of humans and animals during the early stages of abstinence from alcohol.

The functional consequences of withdrawal in humans appear to be regionally heterogeneous, leading to increased activity in some areas and decreases in others. Eisenberg *(120)* first reported a change in functional activity in humans suffering from delirium tremens and found general reductions in CBF. Berglund and Risberg *(121)* and Caspari et al. *(122)* later found increased functional activity in portions of the temporal cortex in at least some of their withdrawing subjects, while at the same time decreased activity was found in other portions of temporal cortex or in parietal cortical regions. The increased temporal lobe activity was associated with greater levels of agitation *(121)*. As might be expected, increased functional activity was also found in the temporal and occipital lobes of patients experiencing auditory and visual hallucinations in the context of alcoholic withdrawal *(121)*. In an interesting case study, a highly circumscribed region of decreased rCBF was found at the junction of the frontal, temporal, and parietal lobes in the left hemisphere of a patient undergoing withdrawal associated with chronic alcohol and diazepam abuse *(35)*. A recent report described hypoperfusion on the day of admission to detoxification in predominantly frontal and temporal regions *(123)*. Frontal hypoperfusion showed signs of recovery, whereas temporal-lobe changes may be longer lasting. Although more work is needed these data suggest that increased functional activity predominately in or around the temporal lobe can be found in withdrawing patients, and this change may be most closely identified with agitation and auditory hallucinations. Decreased functional activity in other nearby regions is also a feature of withdrawal, and the extent of these decreases has been correlated with the length of the preceding binge *(121)*. Given that chronic alcohol exposure diminishes functional activity in and of itself, the decreased functional activity found during withdrawal may be more related to factors associated with the length of chronic abuse rather than to the magnitude of the acute episode of withdrawal.

There are reports in animals that withdrawal leads to marked increases in functional activity as assessed using global *(124)* or local *(51,125)* measures. Global increases have also been found in animal-subjects that did not display overt withdrawal symptoms in following voluntary consumption of ethanol for a minimum of 70 d (2.2 " 1.0 g/kg ethanol for 14 d prior to the experimental procedure) *(97)*.

Other studies have found localized changes in function in withdrawing animals. Campbell et al. *(126)* reported distinct patterns of increased glucose uptake in withdrawing animals that had received 8–11 g/kg of ethanol over 3–4 d. These functional CNS increases were localized to frontal-sensorimotor cortex, globus pallidus, several thalamic nuclei, parts of the cerebellum, genu of corpus callosum, and internal capsule. Eckardt et al. *(93)* using a similar procedure, also reported a variety of changes in glucose utilization in a study of withdrawing animals; this time a group of intoxicated ethanol-dependent animals was included. Besides a major trend of decreased glucose utilization in both acute and chronic treatment groups and a corresponding increase in glucose utilization in withdrawing animals, some cortical structures showed a decrease in glucose utilization during intoxication with no corresponding change when undergoing withdrawal. This suggests that certain brain structures are less likely to exhibit increased functional activity than others, despite their sensitivity to the acute effects of enthanol. These structures included parts of the cerebellum and various limbic regions. Yet another group of brain structures showed increased glucose utilization during withdrawal without the characteristic decrease during intoxication. These structures included sensorimotor areas, sensory systems, cingulate cortex, and the habenula. Future work that investigates functional changes in animals that are treated with a range of doses for varying time periods may provide a clearer picture of the discrete patterns of regional change in the CNS during ethanol abstinence.

12. WERNICKE-KORSAKOFF SYNDROME

In developed countries, poor nutrition in the context of severe chronic alcoholism is the leading cause of the Wernicke-Korsakoff Syndrome *(127)*. The disease, also known as the Alcohol Amnestic Disorder or Korsakoff's Disease (KD) is a devastating short-term memory disorder. The primary clinical symptom is profound recent memory loss and ensuing anterograde amnesia. Korsakoff's disease is often preceded by acute Wernicke's encephalopathy, which is a clinical state consisting of ataxia, incoordination, ocular disturbances, and mental confusion resulting from a nutritional thiamine deficiency. Lesions have been identified in these patients with KD in midline brain structures including the mammillary bodies and portions of the thalamus, as well in the hippocampus and other structures *(128)*. This mesial amnestic syndrome can be differentiated from other syndromes of recent memory loss *(129)*. An overview of the imaging literature relevant to KD will be presented.

Global decreases *(130–133)* or no change *(134,135)* in functional activity were found in patients presenting with Wernicke's encephalopathy and/or during the initial presentation of Korsakoff's disease. In one study *(133)*, rCBF in frontal cortex was significantly correlated with performance on neuropsychological tests of frontal-lobe function. Several studies have also examined patients during the long-term course of KD. In a series of experiments, Eckardt and coworkers *(136,137)* found diminished rCBF in left cerebellar, left parietal, and right anterior temporal regions. In addition, the anterior and posterior portions of the cingulate gyrus and the precuneate region in the parietal lobe had diminished glucose utilization in Korsakoff patients. The majority of amnestic patients in this study had abstained from alcohol use for a year or more, indicating that the diminished functional activity in these regions may in fact be permanent. Fazio and coworkers *(138)* evaluated 11 so-called "pure" amnestics (patients with marked memory loss without other changes in cognitive function), two of whom had Korsakoff's disease, and found absolute values of LCGU were bilaterally decreased in the cingulate gyrus, basal forebrain, hippocampus, and the thalamus when compared to normal controls. These investigators interpreted these results as implicating the Papez circuit in the generation of memories, which is clearly consistent with known neuropathology found in KD. Moffoot et al. *(139)* tested the effect of clonidine to alter rCBF in 19 patients with Korsakoff's psychosis, based on the hypothesis that this population manifests a noradrenergic impairment *(139,140)*. Clonidine treatment significantly improved verbal fluency in the Korsakoff patients, although the saline-treated group also improved making interpretation of this study difficult *(141)*.

In summary, patients with KD are subject to disturbances in functional activity in midline brain structures as expected based on the known histopathology of the disease. Since these functional deficits can be detected in living brain, imaging provides a means for more careful examination of the interaction between the functional and behavioral deficits associated with KD and for understanding the neurobiological basis of memory formation in general. There is also a recent case report that describes a patient who was first evaluated during the early stages of Wernicke-Korsakoff's syndrome when she was exhibiting the feature of confabulation, i.e., providing fabricated descriptions of the recent past that she believed to be true *(142)*. She was then tested 4 mo later when confabulation had ceased, but the amnestic disorder remained. Initially rCBF was low in ventral and medial prefrontal regions corresponding to orbitofrontal and cingulate cortices. After 4 mo, blood flow had improved in these regions, while rCBF in mesial subcortical sites in thalamus remained relatively poor, implicating these frontal sites in confabulation and mesial sites again in amnesia.

13. SUMMARY AND CONCLUSIONS

Parallel to behavior and subjective experience, moderately intoxicating doses of ethanol produce increases in functional activity in regions that support mood and motivation, while higher doses produce decreases in metabolism first in cerebellum and the medial temporal lobe and then more globally as the dose increases. Alcoholics have lower levels of functional activity throughout the brain, and these differences are most pronounced in frontotemporal regions and the cerebellum. Cerebral atrophy in gray and white matter is present in alcoholics, yet after extended periods of sobriety these dysmorphic features abate, although not completely. There is some evidence of a concordance between structural and functional abnormalities. Functional deficits appear to proceed structural changes, however, suggesting that measures of function may have clinical utility and the presence of cortical atrophy indicates a more advanced state of the disease. In fact, patients with the presence of atrophy are less likely to show recovery. In severely impaired patients with KD, a mesial localization of brain dysfunction is partially supported; however, cortical sites including the cingulate may also play in important role.

ACKNOWLEDGMENTS

This work was supported by National Institute on Alcoholism and Alcohol Abuse Grants AA123356 (DL), AA09291(LJP) and AA11997. We thank Leigh Williams for her assistance in the preparation of this manuscript.

REFERENCES

1. Charness, M. E. (1993) Brain lesions in alcoholics. *Alcohol Clin. Exp. Res.* **17**, 2–11.
2. Martin, P. R., Adinoff, B., Weingartner, H., Mukherjee, A. B., and Eckardt, M. J. (1986) Alcoholic organic brain disease: nosology and pathophysiologic mechanisms. *Prog. Neuropsychopharmacol. Biol. Psychiatry* **10**, 147–164.
3. Carlen, P. L., Wilkinson, D. A., Wortzman, G., and Holgate, R. (1984) Partially reversible cerebral atrophy and functional improvement in recently abstinent alcoholics. *Can. J. Neurol. Sci.* **11**, 441–446.
4. Muuronen, A., Bergman, H., Hindmarsh, T., and Telakivi, T. (1989) Influence of improved drinking habits on brain atrophy and cognitive performance in alcoholic patients: a 5-year follow-up study. *Alcohol Clin. Exp. Res.* **13**, 137–141.
5. Sokoloff, L. (1984) Modeling metabolic processes in the brain in vivo. *Ann. Neurol.* **15(Suppl.),** S1–11.
6. Sokoloff, L. and Porrino, L. J. (1986) Some fundamental considerations in the application of the deoxyglucose method in pharmacological studies, in *Pharmacology of Cerebral Ischemia* (Kriegelstein, I., ed.), Amsterdam, pp. 65–76.
6a. Lyons, D. and Porrino, L. J. (1997) Dopamine depletion in the rostral nucleus accumbens alters the cerebral metabolic response to cocaine in the rat. *Brain Res.* **753**, 69–79.
7. Kurumaji, A., Dewar, D., and McCulloch, J. (1993) Metabolic mapping with deoxyglucose autoradiography as an approach for assessing drug action in the central nervous system, in *Imaging Drug Action in the Brain* (London, E. D., ed.), CRC Press, Boca Raton, pp. 219–245.
8. Sokoloff, L., Reivich, M., Kennedy, C., Des Rosiers, M. H., Patlak, C. S., Pettigrew, K. D., et al. (1977) The 2-[14C]deoxyglucose method for the measurement of local cerebral glucose utilization: theory, procedure, and normal values for conscious and unanesthized albino rat. *J. Neurochem.* **28**, 897–916.
9. Sakurada, O., Kennedy, C., Jehle, J., Brown, J. D., Carbin, G. L., and Sokoloff, L. (1978) Measurement of laocal cerebral blood flow with iodo[^{14}C]antipyrine. *Am. J. Physiol.* **234**, H59–H66.
10. Altura, B. M. and Altura, B. T. (1987) Peripheral and cerebrovascular actions of ethanol, acetaldehyde, and acetate: relationship to divalent cations. [Review] [98 refs]. *Alcohol. Clin. Exp. Res.* **11**, 99–111.
11. Lyons, D., Whitlow, C. T., Smith, H., and Porrino, L. J. (1998b) Brain imaging: gunctional consequences of ethanol in the central nervous system, in *Recent Developments in Alcoholism: The Consequences of Alcoholism* (Galanter, M., ed.), Plenum Press, New York, pp. 253–284.
12. Harris, R. A. (1999) Ethanol actions on multiple ion channels: which are important? *Alcohol Clin. Exp. Res.* **23**, 1563–1570.
13. Barry, J. A. and Gawrisch, K. (1994) Direct NMR evidence for ethanol binding to the lipid-water interface of phospholipid bilayers. *Biochemistry* **33**, 8082–8088.
14. Wang, D. C., Taraschi, T. F., Rubin, E., and Janes, N. (1993a) Configurational entropy is the driving force of ethanol action on membrane architecture. *Biochim. Biophys. Acta* **1145**, 141–148.
15. Yurttas, L., Dale, B. E., and Klemm, W. R. (1992) FTIR evidence for alcohol binding and dehydration in phospholipid and ganglioside micelles. *Alcohol Clin. Exp. Res.* **16**, 863–869.

16. Mendelson, J. H., Woods, B. T., Chiu, T. M., Mello, N. K., Lukas, S. E., Teoh, S. .K, et al. (1990) In vivo proton magnetic resonance spectroscopy of alcohol in human brain. *Alcohol* **7,** 443–447.

17. Rose, S. E., Crozier, S., Brereton, I. M., Moxon, L. N., Galloway, G. J., Bore, P., and Doddrell, D. M. (1992) Measurement of the T2 relaxation time of ethanol and cerebral metabolites, in vivo. *Magn. Reson. Med.* **23,** 333–345.

18. Chiu, T. M., Mendelson, J. H., Woods, B. T., Teoh, S. K., Levisohn, L., and Mello, N. K. (1994) In vivo proton magnetic resonance spectroscopy detection of human alcohol tolerance. *Magn. Reson. Med.* **32,** 511–516.

19. Kaufman, M. J., Chiu, T. M., Mendelson, J. H., Woods, B. T., Mello, N. K., Lukas, S. E., et al. (1994) In vivo proton magnetic resonance spectroscopy of alcohol in rhesus monkey brain. *Magn. Reson. Imaging* **12,** 1245–1253.

20. Kaufman, M. J., Chiu, T. M., Mendelson, J. H., Woods, B. T., Teoh, S. K., Eros-Sarnyai, M., et al. (1996) Brain alcohol detectability increase with repeated administration in humans: a proton spectroscopy study. *Magn. Reson. Med.* **35,** 435–440.

21. Franks, N. P. and Lieb, W. R. (1982) Molecular mechanisms of general anaesthesia. *Nature* **300,** 487–493.

22. Franks, N. P. and Lieb, W. R. (1991) Stereospecific effects of inhalational general anesthetic optical isomers on nerve ion channels. *Science* **254,** 427–430.

23. Franks, N. P. and Lieb, W. R. (1994) Molecular and cellular mechanisms of general anaesthesia. *Nature* **367,** 607–614.

24. Lovinger, D. M., White, G., and Weight, F. F. (1989) Ethanol inhibits NMDA-activated ion current in hippocampal neurons. *Science* **243,** 1721–1724.

25. Dickinson, R., Franks, N. P., and Lieb, W. R. (1993) Thermodynamics of anesthetic/protein interactions. Temperature studies on firefly luciferase. *Biophys. J.* **64,** 1264–1271.

26. Forman, S. A., Miller, K. W., and Yellen, G. (1995) A discrete site for general anesthetics on a postsynaptic receptor. *Mol. Pharmacol.* **48,** 574–581.

27. Yu, D., Zhang, L., Eisele, J. L., Bertrand, D., Changeux, J. P., and Weight, F. F. (1996) Ethanol inhibition of nicotinic acetylcholine type alpha 7 receptors involves the amino-terminal domain of the receptor. *Mol. Pharmacol.* **50,** 1010–1016.

28. Zhang, L., Oz, M., Stewart, R. R., Peoples, R. W., and Weight, F. F. (1997) Volatile general anaesthetic actions on recombinant nACh alpha 7, 5-HT3 and chimeric nACh alpha 7–5-HT3 receptors expressed in Xenopus oocytes. *Br. J. Pharmacol.* **120,** 353–355.

29. Mihic, S. J., Ye, Q., Wick, M. J., Koltchine, V. V., Krasowski, M. D., Finn, S. E., et al. (1997) Sites of alcohol and volatile anaesthetic action on GABA(A) and glycine receptors. *Nature* **389,** 385–389.

30. Wright, J. M., Peoples, R. W., and Weight, F. F. (1996) Single-channel and whole-cell analysis of ethanol inhibition of NMDA-activated currents in cultured mouse cortical and hippocampal neurons. *Brain Res.* **738,** 249–256.

31. Grant, K. A. and Lovinger, D. M. (1995) Cellular and behavioral neurobiology of alcohol: receptor-mediated neuronal processes. *Clin. Neurosci.* **3,** 155–164.

32. Mathew, R. J. and Wilson, W. H. (1986) Regional cerebral blood flow changes associated with ethanol intoxication. *Stroke* **17,** 1156–1159.

33. Mullin, M. J., Dalton, T. K., Hunt W. A., Harris, R. A., and Majchrowicz, E. (1987) Actions of ethanol on voltage-sensitive sodium channels: effects of acute and chronic ethanol treatment. *J. Pharmacol. Exp. Ther.* **242,** 541–547.

34. Sano, M., Wendt, P. E., Wirsen, A., Stenberg, G., Risberg, J., and Ingvar, D. H. (1993) Acute effects of alcohol on regional cerebral blood flow in man. *J. Studies Alcohol* **54,** 369–376.

35. Schwartz, J. A., Speed, N. M., Gross, M. D., Lucey, M. R., Bazakis, A. M., Hariharan, M., and Beresford, T. P. (1993) Acute effects of alcohol administration on regional cerebral blood flow: the role of acetate. *Alcohol Clin. Exp. Res.* **17,** 1119–1123.

36. Tiihonen, J., Kuikka, J., Hakola, P., Paanila, J., Airaksinen, J., Eronen, M., and Hallikainen, T. (1994) Acute ethanol-induced changes in cerebral blood flow. *Am. J. Psychiatry* **151,** 1505–1508.

37. Volkow, N. D., Mullani, N., Gould, L., Adler, S. S., Guynn, R. W., Overall, J. E., and Dewey, S. (1988) Effects of acute alcohol intoxication on cerebral blood flow measured with PET. *Psychiatry Res.* **24,** 201–209.

38. De Wit, H., Metz, J., Wagner, N., and Cooper, M. (1990) Behavioral and subjective effects of ethanol: relationship to cerebral metabolism using PET. *Alcohol Clin. Exp. Res.* **14,** 482–489.

39. Volkow, N. D., Hitzemann, R., Wolf, A. P., Logan, J., Fowler, J. S., Christman, D., et al. (1990) Acute effects of ethanol on regional brain glucose metabolism and transport. *Psychiatry Res.* **35,** 39–48.

40. Ingvar, M., Ghatan, P. H., Wirsen-Meurling, A., Risberg, J., Von, H. G., Stone-Elander, S., and Ingvar, D. H. (1998) Alcohol activates the cerebral reward system in man. *J. Stud. Alcohol* **59,** 258–269.

41. Childress, A. R., Mozley, P. D., McElgin, W., Fitzgerald, J., Reivich, M., and O'Brien, C. P. (1999) Limbic activation during cue-induced cocaine craving. *Am. J. Psychiatry* **156,** 11–18.

42. Modell, J. G. and Mountz, J. M. (1995) Focal cerebral blood flow change during craving for alcohol measured by SPECT. *J. Neuropsychiatry* **7,** 15–22.

43. Eckardt, M. J., Campbell, G. A., Marietta, C. A., Majchrowicz, E., and Weight, F. F. (1988) Acute ethanol administration selectively alters localized cerebral glucose metabolism. *Brain Res.* **444,** 53–58.

44. Hoffman, W. E., Miletich, D. J., and Albrecht, R. F. (1986) Dose and time dependent cerebrovascular and metabolic effects of ethanol. *Alcohol* **3,** 23–26.

45. Williams-Hemby, L. and Porrino, L. J. (1994) Low and moderate doses of ethanol produce distinct patterns of cerebral metabolic changes in rats. *Alcohol Clin. Exp. Res.* **18,** 982–988.

46. Williams-Hemby, L. and Porrino, L. J. (1997a) I. Functional consequences of intragastrically administered ethanol in rats as measured by the 2-[14C]deoxyglucose method. *Alcohol. Clin. Exp. Res.* **21,** 1573–1580.

47. Williams-Hemby, L. and Porrino, L. J. (1997b) II. Functional consequences of intragastrically administered ethanol in rats as measured by the 2-[14C]deoxyglucose method: the contribution of dopamine. *Alcohol. Clin. Exp. Res.* **21,** 1581–1591.

48. Friedman, H. S., Lowery, R., Archer, M., Shaughnessy, E., and Scoarza, J. (1984) The effects of ethanol on brain blood flow in awake dogs. *J. Cardiovasc. Pharmacol.* **6,** 344–348.

49. Goldman, H., Sapirstein, L. A., Murphy, S., and Moore, J. (1973) Alcohol and regional blood flow in brains of rats. *Proc. Soc. Exp. Biol. Med.* **144,** 983–988.

50. Grunwald, F., Schrock, H., Biersack, H. J., and Kuschinsky, W. (1993) Changes in local cerebral glucose utilization in the awake rat during acute and chronic administration of ethanol. *J. Nuclear Med.* **34,** 793–798.

51. Hemmingsen, R., Barry, D. I., Hertz, M. M., and Klinken, L. (1979) Cerebral blood flow and oxygen consumption during ethanol withdrawal in the rat. *Brain Res.* **173,** 259–269.

52. Ligeti, L., Hines, K., Dora, E., Sinnwell, T., Huang, M., and McLaughlin, A. C. (1991) Cerebral blood flow and metabolic rate in the conscious freely moving rat: the effects of hypercapnia, and acute ethanol administration. *Alcohol Clin. Exp. Res.* **15,** 766–770.

53. Vina, J. R., Salus, J. E., DeJoseph, M. R., Pallardo, F., Towfighi, J., and Hawkins, R. A. (1991) Brain energy consumption in ethanol-treated, Long-Evans rats. *J. Nutr.* **121,** 879–886.

54. Pohorecky, L. A. and Newman, B. (1977) Effect of ethanol on dopamine synthesis in rat striatal synaptosomes. *Drug Alcohol Depend.* **2,** 329–334.

55. Lewis, M. J. and June, H. L. (1990) Neurobehavioral studies of ethanol reward and activation. *Alcohol* **7,** 213–219.

56. Lukas, S. E., Mendelson, J. H., Benedikt, R. A., and Jones, B. (1986) EEG alpha activity increases during transient episodes of ethanol-induced euphoria. *Pharmacol. Biochem. Behav.* **25,** 889–895.

57. Lukas, S. E., Mendelson, J. H., Amass, L., Benedikt, R. A., Henry, Jr., J. A., Kouri, E. M. (1991) Electrophysiological correlates of ethanol reinforcement, in *Alcohol Reinforcement* (Koob, G., Lewis, M., Meyer, R., and Paul, S., eds.), Birkhauser Boston Inc., Cambridge, pp. 605–606.

58. Risinger, F. O. and Cunningham, C. L. (1992) Ethanol produces rapid biphasic hedonic effects. *Ann. NY Acad. Sci.* **654,** 506–508.

59. Ekman, G. M., Frankenhaeuser, M., Goldberg, L., Hagdahl, R., and Myrsten, A.-L. (1964) Subjective and objective effects of alcohol as functions of dosage and time. *Psychopharmacology* **6,** 399–409.

60. Portans, I., White, J. M., and Staiger, P. K. (1989) Acute tolerance to alcohol: changes in subjective effects among social drinkers. *Psychopharmacology* **97,** 365–369.

61. Kalant, H., LeBlanc, A. E., and Gibbins, R. J. (1971) Tolerance to, and dependence on, some non-opiate psychotropic drugs. [Review]. *Pharmacol. Rev.* **23,** 135–191.

62. Le, A. D. and Mayer, J. M. (1996) Aspects of alcohol tolerance in humans and experimental animals, in *Pharmacological Dffects of Dthanol on the Nervous system* (Deitrich, R. A. and Erwin, V. G., eds.), CRC Press, Boca Raton, pp. 251–268.

63. Mellanby, E. (1919) Alcohol: Its absorption into and disappearance from blood under different conditions. Great Britain Medical Research Council, Special report series No. 31. 1919. Her Majesty's Statistics Office, London.

64. Pohorecky, L. A. (1977) Biphasic action of ethanol. *Biobehav. Rev.* **1,** 231–240.

65. Goldberg, L. (1943) Quantitative studies on alcohol tolerance in man. *Acta. Physiol. Scand.* **5,** 1–26.

66. Campanelli, C., Le, A. D., Khanna, J. M., and Kalant, H. (1988) Effect of raphe lesions on the development of acute tolerance to ethanol and pentobarbital. *Psychopharmacology (Berl.)* **96,** 454–457.

67. Durand, D., Corrigall, W. A., Kujtan, P., and Carlen, P. L. (1981) Effect of low concentrations of ethanol on CA1 hippocampal neurons in vitro. *Can. J. Physiol. Pharmacol.* **59,** 979–984.

68. Givens, B. S. and Breese, G. R. (1990) Electrophysiological evidence that ethanol alters function of medial septal area without affecting lateral septal function. *J. Pharm. Exp. Ther.* **253,** 95–103.

69. Grover, C. A., Frye, G. D., and Griffith, W. H. (1994) Acute tolerance to ethanol inhibition of NMDA-mediated EPSPs in the CA1 region of the rat hippocampus. *Brain Res.* **642,** 70–76.

70. Noldy, N. E. and Carlen, P. L. (1990) Acute, withdrawal, and chronic alcohol effects in man: event-related potential and quantitative EEG techniques. *Ann. Med.* **22,** 333–339.

71. Sinclair, J. G., Lo, G. F., and Tien, A. F. (1980) The effects of ethanol on cerebellar Purkinje cells in naive and alcohol-dependent rats. *Can. J. Physiol. Pharmacol.* **58,** 429–432.

72. Hadji-Dimo, A. A., Ekberg, R., and Ingvar, D. H. (1968) Effects of ethanol on EEG and cortical blood flow in the cat. *Q. J. Studies Alcohol* **29,** 828–838.

73. Lyons, D., Miller, M. D., Hedgecock-Rowe, A. A., Crane, A. M., and Porrino, L. J. (1998c) Time-dependent effects of acute ethanol administration on regional cerebral blood flow in the rat. *Alcohol* **16,** 213–219.

74. Lyons, D., Whitlow, C. T., and Porrino, L. J. (1998a) Multiphasic Consequences of the acute administration of ethanol on cerebral glucose metabolism in the rat. *Pharmacol. Biochem. Behav.* **61,** 201–206.

75. Hammer, Jr., R. P. and Cooke, E. S. (1994) Gradual tolerance of metabolic activity is produced in mesolimbic regions by chronic cocaine treatment, while subsequent cocaine challenge activates extrapyramidal regions of rat brain. *J. Neurosci.* **14,** 4289–4298.

76. Kornetsky, C., Huston-Lyons, D., and Porrino, L. J. (1991) The role of the olfactory tubercle in the effects of cocaine, morphine and brain-stimulation reward. *Brain Res.* **541,** 75–81.

77. Dworkin, S. I., Goeders, N. E., Grabowski, J., and Smith, J. E. (1987) The effects of 12-hour limited access to cocaine: reduction in drug intake and mortality. *NIDA Res. Monogr.* **76,** 221–225.

78. Moolten, M. and Kornetsky, C. (1990) Oral self-administration of ethanol and not experimenter-administered ethanol facilitates rewarding electrical brain stimulation. *Alcohol* **7,** 221–225.

79. Porrino, L. J., Whitlow, C. T., and Samson, H. H. (1998a) Effects of the self-administration of ethanol and ethanol/sucrose on rates of local cerebral glucose utilization in rats. *Brain Res.* **791,** 18–26.

80. Porrino, L. J., Williams-Hemby, L., Whitlow, C., Bowen, C., and Samson, H. H. (1998b) Metabolic mapping of the effects of oral alcohol self-administration in rats. *Alcohol Clin. Exp. Res.* **22,** 176–182.

81. Samson, Y, Baron, J., Feline, A., Bories, J., and Crouzel, C. (1986b) Local cerebral glucose utilisation in chronic alcoholics: a positron tomography study. *J. Neurol. Neurosurg. Psychiatry* **49,** 1165–1170.

82. Koob, G. F. and Bloom, F. E. (1988) Cellular and molecular mechanisms of drug dependence. *Science* **242,** 715–723.

83. Sullivan, E. V., Marsh, L., Mathalon, D. H., Lim, K. O., and Pfefferbaum, A. (1996) Relationship between alcohol withdrawal seizures and temporal lobe white matter volume deficits. *Alcohol Clin. Exp. Res.* **20,** 348–354.

84. Pfefferbaum, A., Sullivan, E. V., Mathalon, D. H., and Lim, K. O. (1997) Frontal lobe volume loss observed with magnetic resonance imaging in older chronic alcoholics. *Alcohol Clin. Exp. Res.* **21,** 521–529.

85. Sullivan, E. V., Lane, B., Deshmukh, A., Rosenbloom, M. J., Desmond, J. E., Lim, K. O., and Pfefferbaum, A. (1999) In vivo mammillary body volume deficits in amnesic and nonamnesic alcoholics. *Alcohol Clin. Exp. Res.* **23,** 1629–1636.

86. Shear, P. K., Sullivan, E. V., Lane, B., and Pfefferbaum, A. (1996) Mammillary body and cerebellar shrinkage in chronic alcoholics with and without amnesia. *Alcohol Clin. Exp. Res.* **20,** 1489–1495.

87. Shimamura, A. P., Jernigan, T. L., and Squire, L. R. (1988) Korsakoff's syndrome: radiological (CT) findings and neuropsychological correlates. *J. Neurosci.* **8,** 4400–4410.

88. Schroth, G., Naegele, T., Klose, U., Mann, K, and Petersen, D. (1988) Reversible brain shrinkage in abstinent alcoholics, measured by MRI. *Neuroradiology* **30,** 385–389.

89. Zipursky, R. B., Lim, K. C., and Pfefferbaum, A. (1989) MRI study of brain changes with short-term abstinence from alcohol. *Alcohol Clin. Exp. Res.* **13,** 664–666.

90. Shear, P. K., Jernigan, T. L., and Butters, N. (1994) Volumetric magnetic resonance imaging quantification of longitudinal brain changes in abstinent alcoholics [published erratum appears in *Alcohol Clin. Exp. Res.* 1994 Jun;**18(3),** 766]. *Alcohol Clin. Exp. Res.* **18,** 172–176.

91. Pfefferbaum, A., Lim, K. O., Zipursky, R. B., Mathalon, D. H., Rosenbloom, M. J., Lane, B., et al. (1992) Brain gray and white matter volume loss accelerates with aging in chronic alcoholics: a quantitative MRI study. *Alcohol Clin. Exp. Res.* **16,** 1078–1089.

92. Pfefferbaum, A., Sullivan, E. V., Mathalon, D. H., Shear, P. K., Rosenbloom, M. J., and Lim, K. O. (1995) Longitudinal changes in magnetic resonance imaging brain volumes in abstinent and relapsed alcoholics. *Alcohol Clin. Exp. Res.* **19,** 1177–1191.

93. Eckardt, M. J., Campbell, G. A., Marietta, C. A., Majchrowicz, E., Rawlings, R. R., and Weight, F. F. (1992) Ethanol dependence and withdrawal selectively alter localized cerebral glucose utilization. *Brain Res.* **584,** 244–250.

94. Hemmingsen, R. and Barry, D. I. (1979) Adaptive changes in cerebral blood flow and oxygen consumption during ethanol intoxication in thr rat. *Acta Physiol. Scand.* **106,** 249–255.

95. Denays, R., Chao, S. L., Mathur-Devre, R., Jeghers, O., Fruhling, J., Noel, P., and Ham, H. R. (1993) Metabolic changes in the rat brain after acute and chronic ethanol intoxication: a 31P NMR spectroscopy study. Magn. Resonance Med. **29,** 719–723.

96. Bontempi, B., Beracochea, D., Jaffard, R.,and Destrade, C. (1996) Reduction of regional brain glucose metabolism following different durations of chronic ethanol consumption in mice: a selective effect on diencephalic structures. *Neuroscience* **72,** 1141–1153.

97. Williams-Hemby, L., Grant, K. A., Gatto, G. J., and Porrino, L. J. (1996) Metabolic mapping of the effects of chronic voluntary ethanol consumption in rats. *Pharmacol. Biochem. Behav.* **54,** 415–423.

98. Pietrzak, E. R., Wilce, P. A., and Shanley, B. C. (1989) The effect of chronic ethanol consumption on [14C]deoxyglucose uptake in rat brain in vivo. *Neurosci. Lett.* **100,** 181–187.

99. Collins, M. A., Corso, T. D., and Neafsey, E. J. (1996) Neuronal degeneration in rat cerebrocortical and olfactory regions during subchronic "binge" intoxication with ethanol: possible explanation for olfactory deficits in alcoholics. *Alcohol Clin. Exp. Res.* **20,** 284–292.

100. Collins, M. A., Zou, J. Y., and Neafsey, E. J. (1998) Brain damage due to episodic alcohol exposure in vivo and in vitro: furosemide neuroprotection implicates edema-based mechanism. *FASEB J.* **12,** 221–230.

101. Courville, C. B. (1955) Effects of alcohol in the nervous system in man. San Lucas Press, Los Angeles.

102. Rosenbloom, M. J., Pfefferbaum, A., and Sullivan, E. V. (1995) Structural brain alterations associated with alcoholism. *Alcohol Health Res. World* **19,** 266–272.

103. Parsons, O. (1987) Neuropsychological consequences of alcohol abuse: many questions —some answers, in *Neuropsychology of Alcoholism: Implications for Diagnosis and Treatment* (Parsons, O., Butters, N., and Nathan, P., eds.), Guilford Press, New York, pp. 153–175.

104. Adams, K. M., Gilman, S., Koeppe, R. A., Kluin, K. J., Brunberg, J. A., Dede, D., et al. (1993) Neuropsychological deficits are correlated with frontal hypometabolism in positron emission tomography of older alcoholics patients. *Alcohol Clin. Exp. Res.* **17,** 205–210.

105. Sachs, H., Russell, J. A., Christman, D. R., and Cook, D. (1987) Alteration of regional cerebral glucose metabolic rate in non-Korasakoff chronic alcoholism. *Arch. J.* **44,** 1242–1251.

106. Volkow, N. D., Hitzemann, R., Wang, G. J., Fowler, J. S., Burr, G., Pascani, K., et al. (1992) Decreased brain metabolism in neurologically intact healthy alcoholics. *Am. J. Psychiatry* **149,** 1016–1022.

107. Wang, G., Volkow, N. D., Hitzemann, R., Oster, Z. H., Roque, C., and Cestaro, V. (1992) Brain imaging of an alcoholic with MRI, SPECT, and PET. *Am. J. Imaging* **3,** 194–198.

108. Wang, G., Volkow, N. D., Roque, C. T., Cestaro, V. L., Hitzemann, R. J., Cantos, E. L., et al. (1993b) Functional importance of ventricular enlargement and cortical atrophy in healthy subjects and aloholics as assessed with PET, MR Imaging, and Neuropsychologic testing. *Radiology* **186,** 59–65.

109. Wik, G., Borg, S., Sjogren, I., Wiessel, F. A., Blomqvist, G., Borg, J., et al. (1988) PET determination of regional cerebral glucose metabolism in alcohol-dependent men and healthy controls using 11C-glucose. *Acta Psychiatrica Scand.* **78,** 234–241.

110. Harris, G. J., Oscar-Berman, M., Gansler, A, Streeter, C., Lewis, R. F., Ahmed, I., and Achong, D. (1999) Hypoperfusion of the cerebellum and aging effects on cerebral cortex

blood flow in abstinent alcoholics: a SPECT study. *Alcohol Clin. Exp. Res.* **23,** 1219–1227.

111. George, M. S., Teneback, C. C., Malcolm, R. J., Moore, J., Stallings, L. E., Spicer, K. M., et al. (1999) Multiple previous alcohol detoxifications are associated with decreased medial temporal and paralimbic function in the postwithdrawal period. *Alcohol Clin. Exp. Res.* **23,** 1077–1084.

112. Melgaard, B., Henriksen, L., Ahlgren, P., Danielsen, U. T., Sorensen, H., and Paulson, O. B. (1990) Regional cerebral blood flow in chronic alcoholics measured by single photon emission computerized tomography. *Acta Neurol. Scand.* **82,** 87–93.

113. Erbas, B., Bekdik, C., Erbengi, G., Enunlu, T., Aytac, S., Kumbasar, H., and Dogan, Y. (1992) Regional cerebral blood flow changes in chronic alcoholism using Tc–99m HMPAO SPECT comparison with CT parameters. *Clin. Nuclear Med.* **17,** 123–127.

114. Nicolas, J. M., Catafau, A. M., Estruch, R., Lomena, F., Salamero, M., Herranz, R., et al. (1993) Regional cerebral blood flow-SPECT in chronic alcoholism: relation to neuropsychological testing. *J. Nuclear Med.* **34,** 1452–1459.

115. Gansler, D. A., Harris, G. J., Oscar-Berman, M., Streeter, C., Lewis, R. F., Ahmed, I., and Achong, D. (2000) Hypoperfusion of inferior frontal brain regions in abstinent alcoholics: a pilot SPECT study. *J. Stud. Alcohol* **61(1),** 32.

116. Weingartner, H. J., Andreason, P. J., Hommer, D. W., Sirocco, K. Y., Rio, D. E., Ruttimann, U. E., et al. (1996) Monitoring the source of memory in detoxified alcoholics. *Biol. Psychiatry* **40,** 43–53.

117. Rogers, R. L., Meyer, J. S., and Shaw, T. J. (1983) Reductions in regional cerebral blood flow associated with chronic consumption of alcohol. *J. Am. Geriatr. Soc.* **31,** 540–543.

118. Ishikawa, Y., Meyer, J. S., Tanahashi, N., Hata, T., Velez, M., Fann, W., et al. (1986) Abstinence improves cerebral perfusion and brain volume in alcoholic neurotoxicity without Wernicke-Korsakoff syndrome. *J. Cereb. Blood Flow Metab.* **6,** 86–94.

119. Metten, P. and Crabbe, J. C. (1996) Dependence and withdrawl, in *Pharmacological Effects of Ethanol on the Nervous System* (Deitrich, R. A. and Erwin, V. G., eds.), CRC Press, Boca Raton, pp. 269–290.

120. Eisenberg, S. (1968) Cerebral blood flow and metabolism in patients with delirium tremens. *Clin. Res.* **16,** 17.

121. Berglund, M. and Risberg, J. (1981) Regional cerebral blood flow during alcohol withdrawal. *Arch. Gen. Psychiatry* **38,** 351–355.

122. Caspari, D., Trabert, W., Heinz, G., Lion, N., Henkes, H., and Huber, G. (1993) The pattern of regional cerebral blood flow during alcohol withdrawal: a single photon emission tomography study with 99mTc-HMPAO. *Acta Psychiatrica Scand.* **87,** 414–417.

123. Tutus, A., Kugu, N., Sofuoglu, S., Nardali, M., Simsek, A., Karaaslan, F., Gonul, A. S. (1998) Transient frontal hypoperfusion in Tc-99m hexamethylpropyleneamineoxime single photon emission computed tomography imaging during alcohol withdrawal. *Biol. Psychiatry* **43,** 923–928.

124. Newman, L. M., Hoffman, W. E., Miletich, D. J., and Albrecht, R. F. (1985) Regional blood flow and cerebral metabolic changes during alcohol withdrawal and following midazolam therapy. *Anesthesiology* **63,** 395–400.

125. Eckardt, M. J., Campbell, G. A., Marietta, C. A., Majchrowicz, E., Wixon, H. N., and Weight, F. F. (1986) Cerebral 2-deoxyglucose uptake in rats during ethanol withdrawal and postwithdrawal. *Brain Res.* **366,** 1–9.

126. Campbell, G. A., Eckardt, M. J., Majchrowicz, E., Marrietta, C. A., and Weight, F. F. (1982) Ethanol-withdrawal syndrome associated with both general and localized increases in glucose uptake in rat brain. *Brain Res.* **237,** 517–522.

127. Meyer, J. S., Tanahashi, N., Ishikawa, Y., Hata, T., Velez, M., Fann, W, E., et al. (1985) Cerebral atrophy and hypoperfusion improves during treatment of Wernicke-Korsakoff syndrome. *J. Cereb. Blood Flow Metab.* **5,** 376–385.

128. Victor, M., Adams, R. D., and Collins, G. H. (1971) The Wernicke-Korsakoff syndrome. A clinical and pathological study of 245 patients, 82 with post-mortem examinations. *Contemp. Neurol.* **7,** 1–206.

129. Walsh, K. W. (1985) *Understanding Brain Damage: A Primer of Neuropsychological Evaluation.* Churchill Livingstone, New York.

130. Headlund, S., Kohler, V., and Nylin, G. (1964) Cerebral circulation in dementia. *Acta Psychiatrica Scand.* **40,** 77–106.

131. Kruger, G., Haubitz, I., Weinhardt, F., and Hoyer, S. (1980) Brain oxidative metabolism and blood flow in alcoholic syndromes. Subst. *Alcohol Actions/Misuse* **1,** 295–307.

132. Shimojyo, S., Scheinberg, P., and Reinmuth, O. (1967) Cerebral blood flow and metabolism in the Wernicke-Korsakoff syndrome. *J. Clin. Invest.* **46,** 849–854.

133. Hunter, R., McLuskie, R., Wyper, D., Patterson, J., Christie, J. E., Brooks, D. N., et al. (1989) The pattern of function-related regional cerebral blood flow investigated by single photon emission tomography with 99mTc-HMPAO in patients with presenile Alzheimer's disease and Korsakoff's psychosis. *Psychol. Med.* **19,** 847–855.

134. Berglund, M. and Ingvar, D. H. (1976) Cerebral blood flow and its regional distribution in alcoholism and in Kosakoff's psychosis. J. Studies Alcohol **37,** 586–597.

135. Simard, D., Olesen, J., Paulson, O. B., Lassen, N. A., and Skinhoj, E. (1971) Regional cerebral blood flow and its regulation in dementia. *Brain* **94,** 273–288.

136. Martin, P. R., Rio, D., Adinoff, B., Johnson, J. L., Bisserbe, J. C., Rawlings, R. R., et al. (1992) Regional cerebral glucose utilization in chronic organic mental disorders associated with alcoholism. *J. Neuropsychiatry Clin. Neurosci.* **4,** 159–167.

137. Joyce, E. M., Rio, D. E., Ruttimann, U. E., Rohrbaugh, J. W., Martin, P. R., Rawlings, R. R., and Eckardt, M. J. (1994) Decreased cingulate and precuneate glucose utilization in alcoholic Korsakoff's syndrome. *Psychiatry Res.* **54,** 225–239.

138. Fazio, F., Perani, D., Gilardi, M. C., Colombo, F., Cappa, S. F., Vallar, G., et al. (1992) Metabolic impairment in human amnesia: a PET study of memory networks. *J. Cereb. Blood Flow Metab.* **12,** 353–358.

139. Moffoot, A., O'Carroll, R. E., Murray, C., Dougall, N., Ebmeier, K., and Goodwin, G. M. (1994) Clonidine infusion increases uptake of 99mTc-Exametazime in anterior cingulate cortex in Korsakoff's psychosis. *Psychol. Med.* **24,** 53–61.

140. McEntee W. J. and Mair R. G. (1990) The Korsakoff syndrome: a neurochemical perspective [published erratum appears in *Trends Neurosci* 1990 Nov;**13(11),** 446]. *Trends Neurosci.* **13,** 340–344.

141. O'Carroll, R. (1993) Neuropsychological and neuroimaging aspects of latent hepatic encephalopathy (LHE). [Review] [16 refs]. *Alcohol Alcohol* **(Suppl.)2,** 191–195.

142. Benson, D. F., Djenderedjian, A., Miller, B. L., Pachana, N. A., Chang, L., Itti, L., and Mena, I. (1996) Neural basis of confabulation. *Neurology* **46,** 1239–1243.

15

Structural and Functional Neuroimaging of the Effects of Opioids

David Nutt and Mark Daglish

1. INTRODUCTION

This chapter is concerned with the effects of opioids on the human brain. When examining the effects of abused drugs, one of the main difficulties is to separate any effects caused by the drug itself from the effects of the impurities invariably present in illicit drugs and from the effects of the mode of delivery. The only common exception to this problem is alcohol. In specific relation to opioid drugs, one is usually trying to examine the effects of "street" heroin or prescribed, purer, substitutes. In this chapter, we will examine the effects of the impurities of "street" heroin and its mode of delivery only briefly when talking about possible chronic structural effects of opioids. In particular, we will briefly examine the effects on the brain of injecting impure "street" heroin.

The major part of this chapter will be given over to an examination of the functional effects of opioids. This will be subdivided into a study of the acute effects of opioids and then a study of the chronic effects, as far as they can be separated into these somewhat arbitrary categories. Finally, we will discuss the progress in the field of functional neuroimaging in looking at cognitive circuits of opioid dependence, in particular those of craving and reward.

2. CHRONIC STRUCTURAL EFFECTS OF OPIOIDS

2.1. Introduction

Somewhat surprisingly, there have been few studies that have systematically looked for changes in brain structure following chronic heroin use. Even more surprisingly those studies that have been done have tended to find little or no evidence of chronic structural changes. Before it can be used, "street" heroin, with all its impurities, is usually so insoluble as to require cooking up in a solution of either citric acid, dissolved vitamin C tablets, or as a last resort, lemon juice or vinegar. The resultant mixture is then filtered through cotton wool or the filter from a cigarette before being injected directly into a vein. It is not uncommon for crystalline debris and filter fibers to be found in the lungs of intravenous heroin users at autopsy (1), which results from

From: Handbook of Neurotoxicology, Vol. 2
Edited by: E. J. Massaro © Humana Press Inc., Totowa, NJ

this practice. While the capillary bed of the lungs acts as a filter for most of this debris, some of it must get through into the systemic circulation and thence to the brain. It is hard to imagine that this does not cause long-term damage.

Aside from the effects of injecting, the other widespread potential cause for structural changes in the brain in heroin users is HIV infection. It is beyond the scope of this chapter to discuss the effects of HIV, AIDS, and AIDS-related conditions on the brain. For those interested in this area Handelsman *(2)* studied structural magnetic resonance imaging (MRI) changes in drug users with and without HIV infection.

2.2. Structural Neuroimaging in Opioid Dependence

There are problems when attempting to study long-term structural changes in the brain in heroin users. The biggest problem that clouds the interpretation of most studies is the tendency for heroin users to use other drugs that may also have neurotoxic effects. Other chapters in this section will deal with the effects of cocaine, amphetamines, and MDMA (Ecstasy) for example, although studies of these drugs' effects are confounded by heroin use in many cases. The few systematic studies of structural changes have tended to find evidence of only subtle changes, if anything, which are always open to the criticism that they are premorbid and perhaps an indication of a predisposition to drug-dependency problems.

The largest systematic study of MRI brain scans in drug users is by Aasly et al. *(3)*. Their cohort of drug users encompassed users of cannabis, cocaine, solvents, and amphetamines in addition to opioid users and all were heavy alcohol users. The only reported differences in the MRI scans of the drug users compared to a control cohort were atrophy of the cerebellum and a trend toward larger lateral ventricles. Importantly, these changes were thought to be related to the effects of alcohol rather than the effects of any of the other abused drugs in this cohort.

Amass et al. *(4)* undertook a study of MRI regional T1 and T2 times in a cohort of opioid- and/or cocaine-dependent subjects. They found no significant changes in any of the brain regions studied compared to matched controls. From this they conclude that the MRI technology available at that time was inadequate to demonstrate the microstructural changes in the brain resulting from chronic opioid use.

The only significant change in brain structure associated with opioid and cocaine use yet demonstrated by MRI is an increase in pituitary volume *(5)*. This study showed a 190 mm^3 (35%) mean increase in pituitary volume in the drug dependent-group compared to a control group. These changes were found in the absence of measurable changes in blood hormone levels. The authors suggested that these volumetric changes were most likely to be related to anterior pituitary lactotroph hyperplasia in response to opioid and cocaine use.

Although not strictly a structural-imaging technique, perfusion scans using either PET or SPET can be used to demonstrate possible structural changes in the brain, especially when performed in a resting state. Gerra et al. *(6)* used resting SPET HMPAO scans to examine for hypoperfusion defects in abstinent opioid users. They demonstrated a number of regions of significant hypoperfusion compared with healthy control subjects as well as a trend for a global decrease in cerebral blood flow (CBF) in the abstinent dependent group. However, these changes were not related to the substance-abuse history, but rather to other comorbid diagnoses of depression or antisocial per-

Table 1
Distribution of Opioid-Receptor Subtypes in the Human Brain

Brain region	Mean total specific ligand binding (fmol/mg protein)	Component (%)		
Thalamus	202	74	11	15
Temporal cortex	149	44	6	50
Claustrum	115	32	8	61
Caudate nucleus	112	49	3	48
Substantia nigra	63	40	16	13
Putamen	58	43	22	34
Globus pallidus (lat)	14	43	29	29
Globus pallidus (med)	7	43	57	<1

Adapted from Cross et al. *(9)*.

sonality disorder. Specifically, significant hypoperfusion in the right frontal and left temporal cortices was associated with comorbid depression and hypoperfusion in the right frontal lobe was also associated with "antisocial tendencies."

The case-report literature is littered with reports of the potential neurotoxic effects of the use of "street" opioids. Two main types of neurological insult are reported most commonly, a spongiform leukoencephalopathy *(7)* and hypoxic injury related to the respiratory depression of opioid overdose *(8)*. The spongiform leukoencephalopathy reported is characterized by edema of white matter in either the cerebrum or cerebellum, sometimes also effecting gray matter. At the microscopic level, there is swelling and vacuolation of the myelin sheaths but sparing of the axons. The leukoencephalopathy tends to occur sporadically and it has therefore been suggested that it may be related to a neurotoxic contaminant rather than the heroin itself. There are also reports of ischaemic infarcts, which may be related to embolic phenomena, either thrombo-embolic, infective micro-emboli associated with the increased risk of endocarditis in intravenous drug abuse, or foreign bodies from injection of insoluble contaminants.

3. FUNCTIONAL NEUROIMAGING OF ACUTE EFFECTS OF OPIOIDS

3.1. Introduction

This section examines the contribution of functional neuroimaging to the study of the acute effects of opioids. We will not, therefore, discuss the myriad other measures of the acute effects of opioids like changes in pupil size or galvanic skin responses, except where they relate to changes in functional neuroimaging. This section is split into studies examining the effects of opioids on normal subjects and the effects in subjects now, or previously, opioid-dependent. Each subsection is further divided based on the different modalities of functional neuroimaging, like PET and fMRI.

The opioid-receptor system is characterized by three basic forms of the receptor mu (μ), delta (δ), and kappa (κ). There are further subdivisions of these subtypes, but this level of detail is not required here. Fully demonstrating the distribution of the different opioid receptor subtypes is not yet possible in humans in vivo, because of the lack of sufficient selective tracers, but has been demonstrated using autoradiographic techniques in vitro. Cross et al. *(9)* demonstrated the different anatomical distribution of

Table 2
Available Radiotracers for the Opioid System for SPECT and PET

Ligand	Imaging type	Receptor profile	Species
^{11}C-Diprenorphine	PET	μ, δ, κ -opioid antagonist	Human and animal
^{123}I-Diprenorphine	SPET	μ, δ, κ -opioid antagonist	Animal
^{11}C-Carfentanil	PET	μ -opioid agonist	Human and animal
^{11}C-Methylnaltrindole	PET	δ -opioid antagonist	Human and animal
^{123}I-Naltrindole	SPET	δ -opioid antagonist	Animal
^{18}F-Cyclofoxy	PET	μ, κ -opioid antagonist	Human and animal
^{123}I-Cyclofoxy	SPET	μ, κ -opioid antagonist	Animal
^{11}C-Buprenorphine	PET	μ -opioid partial agonist and opioid κ -antagonist	Animal

the three subtypes in the human brain and highlighted the major differences between the pattern in humans and other mammals. Table 1 summarizes the distribution patterns found in this study.

The various subtypes of the opioid receptor are thought to mediate different components of the actions of opioids, both external and endogenous. In particular the μ receptor is thought to mediate the analgesic and euphoric effects of opioids, as well as the addictive properties.

3.2. Functional Neuroimaging of the Opioid System in Normal Volunteers

The basic mechanisms of PET and SPECT have been described in the first chapter in this section. From this it should be apparent that in order to examine the characteristics of the opioid system in the central nervous system (CNS), the primary pre-requisite is the availability of suitable neuroimaging tracers. There are two main PET ligands that are used to label this system, each with its own advantages and disadvantages. To date there are no SPECT ligands for the opioid system that have been used in humans, but there are agents in development in animals, which show promise (*see* Table 2).

PET studies of the opioid system in normal volunteers have confirmed the postmortem study findings that opioid receptors are extremely widespread in the human brain. Using ^{11}C-Diprenorphine, which labels all the opioid-receptor subtypes, it is possible to demonstrate the normal distribution of opioid receptors in healthy volunteers *(10)*. The main areas of concentration of opioid receptors are found in the thalamus; caudate nucleus; and temporal, frontal, and parietal cortices (*see* Fig. 1 of normal diprenorphine scan). There is very little binding of tracer in the occipital cortex as would be expected from the low levels of opioid receptor in this area. ^{11}C-carfentanil can be used as a more selective μ-opioid-receptor tracer to show the distribution of this subtype alone. The distribution is as expected from postmortem studies with the largest signal present in the thalamus. There is relatively less binding in the cingulate and frontal cortex compared to ^{11}C-diprenorphine as further evidence of the increased numbers of δ- and κ-opioid receptors in these areas *(11)*. More recently, a relatively new PET ligand, ^{11}C-methylnaltrindole, has been used to demonstrate the distribution of the δ-opioid receptor in vivo in humans *(12)*. As predicted from the in vitro studies, there was a high level of tracer binding in the putamen and caudate; intermediate binding in the frontal,

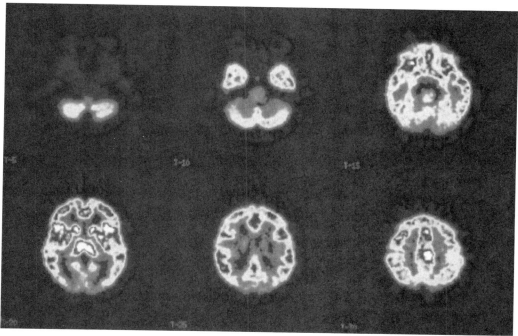

Fig. 1. Six transverse slices of a PET scan showing (11C)-Diprenorphine binding in the brain of a normal volunteer. (*See* color plate 7 appearing in the insert following p. 368.)

parietal, occipital and cingulate cortices; and lower binding in the thalamus and _cerebellum.

The opioid system is not a static entity. The number and distribution of opioid-binding sites has been shown to vary with age, gender *(13)*, and, for women, phase of the menstrual cycle *(14)*. The density of binding sites for many receptor systems changes with age, but the opioid system is unusual in that the density generally increases with age. A further complication is that the age-related changes are not uniform throughout the brain and they are gender-dependent. Age- and gender-related effects were shown in prefrontal, anterior cingulate, temporal, and parietal cortices. Age-related effects were also found in the putamen and gender-related effects in the caudate nucleus and the cerebellum. Age-by-gender interaction effects were also found in the amygdala and thalamus. It is therefore important that comparisons of opioid-receptor measures between groups ensure adequate matching of these confounding factors.

The next section of this chapter deals with the effects of acute doses of opioid drugs on the brain in healthy volunteers. However, there are other nondrug interventions that have shown measurable effects with functional neuroimaging of the opioid system. This system has long been implicated in the perception of pain and a site of action for potent analgesics. Chronic pain and the removal of chronic pain have been shown to alter the pattern and density of available binding sites for opioid PET ligands. Jones et al. *(15)* showed that in patients with chronic arthritis the levels of ^{11}C-diprenorphine binding decreased when the patient was in pain and increased when scanned during pain-free periods. They suggest that this was an effect of endogenous opioids being released to a greater degree during pain, thereby decreasing the number of available binding sites for the tracer. A similar increase in ^{11}C-diprenorphine binding was seen in patients with trigeminal neuralgia following surgical intervention to terminate their pain when they were scanned before and after the procedure *(16)*.

3.3. Functional Neuroimaging of Acute Effects of Opiates in Normal Volunteers

Before it is possible to fully understand the effects of opioid drugs in dependent users, it is necessary to understand what these drugs are doing in the normal healthy volunteer. The most thorough neuroimaging study of the acute pharmacokinetics of commonly used opioids was carried out on the rhesus monkey. Hartvig et al. *(17)* gave rhesus monkeys a range of ^{11}C-labeled opioids and imaged the distribution and kinetics using PET. The drugs used in this study were heroin, morphine, codeine, and pethidine. Because of the low spatial resolution obtainable from PET scanning at that time, the results were only differentiated into whole brain, nose, extra-cranial soft tissue, and pituitary regions. One of the most striking results from this study is the large difference in kinetics between the whole brain and the pituitary. Following intravenous administration, the peak level of morphine in the pituitary was reached after 5 min compared with 10 min for the whole brain. The level of uptake into the pituitary region was also almost double that in the rest of the brain. These studies also showed that elimination half-lives for these opioids were not the same in brain, extra-cranial soft tissue, or plasma. Morphine elimination half-life from the brain is substantially longer than from other tissues. Conversely, pethidine showed rapid uptake and elimination from brain with much longer plasma half-life. The authors suggested that this may be the result of differences in the lipophilic characteristics of the drugs studied; for example, pethidine has higher lipid solubility than morphine, which explains its faster brain uptake, but not the slower plasma elimination. This is a clear example of functional neuroimaging helping to explain clinical anomalies like the shorter duration of analgesic action of pethidine compared to morphine despite its much longer plasma half-life.

There is a single study of the acute effects of opioid drugs in healthy volunteers using functional neuroimaging. Firestone et al. *(18)* gave fentanyl to a healthy cohort and measured regional cerebral blood flow (rCBF) using H215O PET. The same group also used the same paradigm to study the acute effects of fentanyl on acute pain in a healthy population *(19)*. Fentanyl was shown to consistently increase rCBF in the anterior cingulate cortex, irrespective of whether the subject was in pain or resting. In the first study, in the resting state, fentanyl also produced increases in rCBF in the prefrontal and orbito-frontal cortices and caudate nucleus. Fentanyl also caused decreases in rCBF in frontal, temporal, and cerebellar regions. Interestingly the effect of fentanyl on rCBF changes induced by pain was to augment the increase in rCBF in the supplementary motor area and left inferior frontal cortex. Jones et al. *(20)* also studied the effects on rCBF of an analgesic dose of morphine in a single patient with chronic pain. In this case morphine induced increases in rCBF in similar areas, specifically the anterior cingulate, prefrontal cortex, caudate, and putamen. Increased rCBF was also seen in the insular cortex contralateral to the site of the pain and ipsilateral temporal cortex.

3.4. Functional Imaging of Acute Doses in Addicts

One of the most obvious ways to study the effects of drugs of abuse is to give known doses of drug to users and measure the effects. This idea has been tried with opioid users being given opioid drugs while imaging the resultant effects in the brain. Unfortunately there are many practical problems and constraints that have to be dealt with resulting from the process of functional neuroimaging. One of the largest problems is the nature of the scanner environment. Much work has been done that shows that the "set and setting" in which a drug is taken heavily influences the subjective effects of the drug. Animal work also suggests that there are differences in effect dependant on whether the drug is administered or self-administered. Another major problem relates to the stage of dependence the subject population is at during the study. If the subjects are actively dependent, then their recent drug use will impinge heavily on any neuroimaging results, as opioids can take many days to fully washout from the brain. If the subjects are in treatment, then they are likely to be maintained on long-acting substitute opioids like methadone, which take even longer to washout. If the subjects are opioid-free, then this is almost certainly going to be as a result of detoxification with permanent abstinence as the long-term goal, in which case the ethics of administration of an opioid require very careful scrutiny. Inevitably a compromise between scientific rigor and practical and ethical considerations has to be achieved. Therefore the results of all neuroimaging studies using this type of paradigm need to be interpreted in the light of such a compromise.

Bearing in mind what we noted earlier, the studies of the effects of acute opioid doses have generally either looked at the effects in users who were currently abstinent or who were currently actively dependent. Schlaepfer et al. *(21)* studied the effects of two opioids with different receptor profiles on rCBF using HMPAO SPET. The opioids studied were hydromorphone, which is a δ agonist, and butorphanol, which is a δ agonist. This study allows us to see the differential effects of opioid action on different receptor subtypes on both subjective mental state and rCBF simultaneously. Butorphanol produced subjective results of "bad effects" and "LSD-like effects" with a diffuse pattern of activation of rCBF, especially in the anterior temporal lobes. Hydromorphone produced euphoriant effects and increased rCBF in the anterior cingulate, thalamus, and amygdala regions. The effects of acute doses of morphine on regional cerebral metabolic rate of glucose (rCMRglu) were studied by London et al. *(22)*. As has been demonstrated in several paradigms, morphine induced a global decrease in cerebral activity as measured by CMRglu using [18-F] deoxyglucose ([18F]-FDG) with PET scanning. These changes were widespread throughout the brain, with many regions showing significant reductions in the frontal, parietal, and temporal cortices. Anterior cingulate region, caudate nucleus, and amygdala also showed significant reductions. Of all these regions, only four showed any significant correlation with the subjective measures of morphine effects that were taken during the scan. Both the paracentral lobule and left cerebellar cortex showed positive correlations with the subjective responses, and two regions in the occipital cortex showed negative correlations. There is an obvious discrepancy between these studies with one showing increases in rCBF and the other showing decreases in rCMRglu. These may be explained by the differences in the method of correction for global changes between the two studies, as regions that show a smaller reduction in rCBF than the decrease in the whole brain will appear as increases in rCBF when the global changes are partialled out of the statistical model. However, there are other possible explanations for the differences related to timing of the acute drug dose with the injection of radiotracer, or differences between glucose metabolism and blood flow, for example.

In a similar study, Sell et al. *(23)* used fMRI to examine the acute effects of heroin injection in users maintained on methadone and heroin. They only examined the effects of the drug on responses to photic stimulation. The effect of the heroin on the visual cortex was to decrease the blood oxygen level dependent (BOLD) response to the photic stimulation. This is consistent with the reported effects of morphine to reduce global cerebral metabolism, but not consistent with the reported lack of effect in the visual cortex in the same study *(22)*. In a later study, Sell et al. *(24)* used PET to study rCBF changes in response to heroin and heroin-related cues. In this study heroin caused increases in rCBF in the brain stem, the periaqueductal gray matter (PAG) and the ventral tegmental area (VTA). The heroin also appeared to alter the relationship between the level of rCBF in the anterior cingulate and basal forebrain regions. The authors suggest that this could be interpreted as heroin altering the manner in which these brain areas respond to the presentation of drug-related stimuli via its effects on midbrain activation.

The effects of buprenorphine, an opioid μ partial agonist and κ antagonist, were studied by Walsh et al. *(25)*. This study used (18F)-FDG to examine rCMRglu in polydrug abusers using a placebo-controlled, double-blind design. Buprenorphine produced a global decrease in cerebral metabolism, as is consistent with the effects of other opioids reported earlier. The regions most affected were medial thalamus, orbitofrontal cortex, and hippocampus. However, there were very few regions that did not show some reduction in rCMRglu in response to the buprenorphine injection. Surprisingly, given the results from other studies (e.g., ref. *22*) the amygdala was one of these regions that did not show a response. However, while this may reveal a difference in the effects of morphine and buprenorphine, or the experimental setting, it may well represent differences in the statistical methods of analysis and the effects of use of different statistical thresholds used to guard against false-positive results.

4. FUNCTIONAL NEUROIMAGING OF CHRONIC EFFECTS OF OPIOIDS

4.1. Effects of Chronic Opioid Exposure

Having examined the acute effects of opioid drugs on the brain, the next logical step is to attempt to examine the chronic effects of these drugs. It should be remembered that opioid-dependent individuals are often using opioids for many years in doses that are far higher than can be tolerated by nondependent individuals. In fact, very few studies have looked at the effects of current long-term use of opioid drugs. Most studies have looked at the short-term effects of treatment with substitute opioids on drug-dependent patients.

The technique of phosphorus magnetic resonance spectroscopy (^{31}P-MRS) can be used to derive measures of bioenergetic status, and markers of cell-membrane integrity and turnover. Kaufman et al. *(26)* used this technique to study the effects of substitute methadone on heroin-dependent patients. The study showed that there were disturbances in bioenergetic status (decreased levels of phosphocreatine) and phospholipid levels (elevated phosphomonoesters and phosphodiesters) in the methadone-treated group compared to a control group. It was also shown that the methadone group who were most affected were those who had received treatment for the shortest time. The authors interpret this as possible evidence that methadone treatment helps to normalize the abnormalities produced by heroin use and dependence. It is worth noting that the pattern of abnormalities found quite closely resembled that found in chronic ischaemia. Given the findings in other studies of areas of hypoperfusion in heroin users, they argue that this is a possible cause of the ^{31}P-MRS abnormalities. It may also be evidence of subclinical degrees of neuronal cell loss as has also been suggested in the structural studies described at the start of this chapter.

One study that partially confirms the finding of hypoperfusion deficits following chronic heroin use is that of Danos et al. *(27)*. This study used HMPAO SPECT scans of rCBF to measure the effects of heroin withdrawal and methadone substitution on a cohort of heroin-dependent subjects. This group showed an increased number of hypoperfusion areas in comparison with a control group. For those subjects who were also on methadone, the degree of hypoperfusion was inversely related to the methadone dose. In other words, those on higher methadone doses had smaller decreases in perfusion. This is obviously in direct contrast to the acute studies, which showed a decrease in rCBF in response to opiates, as described in the previous section. Krystal et al. *(28)* also showed a reduction in rCBF in a population receiving chronic methadone treatment. Specifically the methadone group showed significantly less rCBF compared to controls in the parietal and frontal cortices. They also showed significantly increased rCBF compared to controls in the thalamus bilaterally.

There are two studies, by the same group, on the effects of the opioid partial agonist buprenorphine on rCBF using SPECT *(29,30)*. In both cases, the studies looked at its effects on abstinent heroin and cocaine users, and the hypoperfusion defects that have been found following prolonged cocaine use. Taking the results from both studies, the data suggest that treatment with buprenorphine led to an improvement in the hypoperfusion deficits associated with chronic use of cocaine and heroin. Interestingly, the placebo group in this study had worsening hypoperfusion deficits following detoxification, while those on 6 mg/d buprenorphine showed no change and those on 12 mg/d buprenorphine showed improvements. Unfortunately these differences did not persist beyond the end of the treatment period after the buprenorphine had been withdrawn.

Recent work in our unit has begun to look at the effects of methadone treatment on opioid receptor availability using the PET tracer ^{11}C-Diprenorphine *(31)*. In these studies we have been examining the effects of current methadone treatment and also the changes during detoxification. Early results show that, as expected, methadone produces a significant decrease in mean global volume of distribution (VD) for the tracer (an index of free-receptor density) compared to a control group. However, there appears to be no clear relationship between plasma methadone levels and changes in mean global VD. It is possible, although too early to be definite, that this lack of a clear dose-response effect may be related to innate differences between the subjects that may be an explanation for why some individuals require higher doses of methadone than do others.

In another study that looked at changes in receptor availability, Wang *(32)* used ^{11}C-raclopride to study the D_2-Dopamine receptor system in opioid-dependent subjects. The study also used a naloxone challenge to study the effects of opioid withdrawal on dopamine release and the results of this part of the study are discussed further below. Interestingly the baseline comparison of opioid-dependent subjects against controls following a placebo injection revealed lower resting ^{11}C-raclopride binding in the opioid-dependent group. The authors hypothesize that these baseline differences may be due to the effects of chronic release of dopamine in response to heroin administration in the dependent group. Alternatively they suggest that as the similar differences found in cocaine users do not diminish even after prolonged abstinence, these may represent differences that were present prior to the onset of drug use.

4.2. Effects of Withdrawal from Opioids

Studies of the effects of opioid withdrawal naturally fall into two distinct categories; the effects of abstinence and the effects of antagonist-precipitated withdrawal. In this section, we will examine the published studies in this order.

Abstinence from opioids will provoke a withdrawal syndrome in dependent opioid users. The severity and time-scale of the withdrawal syndrome varies depending on the level of dependence and the specific opioid abused. Attempts have been made to investigate the underlying neurochemical changes that mediate the observable and subjective effects of opioid withdrawal. Changes in rCBF in early and late withdrawal from heroin were studied by Rose et al. *(33)*. Ten heroin-dependent subjects undergoing inpatient detoxification were studied using HMPAO SPECT. Visual interpretation of rCBF scans at 1 and 3 wk, following opioid withdrawal showed focal perfusion deficits in 9 out 10 subjects. All subjects showed improvements in these lesions at 3 wk of abstinence. The perfusion deficits were scattered throughout the cortex, with sparing of the cerebellum, although this area was used to normalize the scans for global changes. The frontal cortex was most frequently affected, with 8 of the 9 abnormal scans showing lesions in this area. Six of the 9 subjects showed lesions in the parietal and temporal cortices. One subject had large abnormalities in the parietal and occipital regions. The majority of these perfusion defects were < 1 cm in size, but 5 subjects had lesions that were larger than 1 cm. All subjects in this study had normal structural brain scans (either CT or MRI). The etiology of these perfusion defects is unclear. They are unlikely to be related to injection of insoluble foreign bodies or contaminants of the heroin as 4 of the 9 subjects that had abnormal scans had no history of intravenous drug use. Similar findings have been described in cocaine abusers, where the changes had possibly been thought to result from the vasoconstrictive properties of cocaine *(29)*. However, heroin does not typically produce cerebral vasoconstriction. It is also difficult to ascribe the reported changes in rCBF to heroin withdrawal as the scans took place after the withdrawal signs and symptoms had subsided.

Early results from our own work suggest that there may be changes in the opioid-receptor system in patients in early abstinence from methadone (unpublished). Using the technique of ^{11}C-diprenorphine PET scanning, we have studied opioid receptor availability in patients who have just completed detoxification from methadone compared with a control population. Only 6 subjects in each group have been scanned to date, but there is a nonsignificant trend for global ^{11}C-diprenorphine binding to be increased in the opioid-withdrawal group compared to matched controls. This may represent an increase in the density of opioid receptors or a decrease in the levels of endogenous opioids.

It is well-known that administration of an opioid antagonist (e.g., naloxone or naltrexone) to an opioid-dependent individual will precipitate the opioid-withdrawal syndrome by displacing the agonist (e.g., heroin or methadone) from the receptors. HMPAO SPECT has been used to study the effects of naltrexone-precipitated withdrawal from buprenorphine on rCBF *(34)*. They showed no significant changes in rCBF in response to the withdrawals compared to the placebo condition, but did show that rCBF in the anterior cingulate region was inversely associated with the severity of the opioid withdrawal induced. Krystal et al. *(28)*, in the study previously mentioned, also looked at rCBF changes in response to naloxone-precipitated withdrawals in subjects maintained on methadone. There was a significant reduction in global CBF in the methadone group, with no reduction in the control group. Surprisingly, the control group showed significant increases in rCBF in the right parietal and temporal cortices in response to naloxone, where the methadone group showed no regional changes at all.

The effects of naloxone-precipitated withdrawals on the dopamine system have also been studied by Wang et al. *(32)* in the study previously mentioned. In the opioid-dependent group studied naloxone did not significantly change ^{11}C-raclopride binding compared with placebo. However, the subgroup who received the higher dose of naloxone, when analyzed separately, did show a decrease in ^{11}C-raclopride binding. This is not what would be expected, as this result would tend to suggest an increase in synaptic dopamine levels in withdrawal where animal studies have found a decrease using microdialysis techniques *(35)*. The explanation for this difference is not obvious. It may be that the results represent true inter-species differences in opioid-withdrawal effects, or may reflect the difference in the experience of withdrawal from a self-administered drug on which you are dependent and an experimentally administered drug over which you have no control. Lastly, it is not always possible to exclude the effects of changes in blood flow (and hence tracer delivery and washout) from changes in radiotracer binding-sites in PET scans.

5. THE OPIOID REWARD SYSTEM: CORRELATION OF NEUROIMAGING FINDINGS IN HUMANS AND ANIMAL MODELS

5.1. Introduction

There is one major area of the effects of opioids on the brain that we have left untouched, the neural circuits potentially implicated in the processes of reward, dependence, or addiction. In this final section of the chapter, we will briefly discuss the few human neuroimaging studies that have attempted to examine this area and their possible relation to animal models of opioid dependence.

5.2. The Reward Pathway and Opioid Dependence

For many years, it has been known that animals will self-administer opioid drugs into certain specific regions of the brain. The two main regions for which the best evidence has accumulated are the VTA and the nucleus accumbens (NAcc) *(36)*. These regions, along with the PAG and the medial forebrain bundle (MFB) are part of a dopaminergic pathway called the mesocortical-limbic system. This pathway has been implicated as a general reward pathway for diverse stimuli (e.g., sex and food) as well as drugs of abuse *(37)*. It is thought that opioids exert their addictive properties by "hijacking" this natural reward pathway by causing excessive release of dopamine

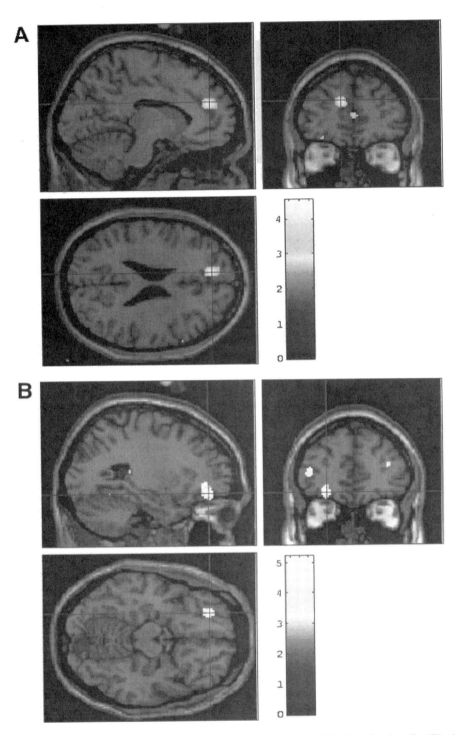

Fig. 2. (A) Areas of increased rCBF in response to opioid-related stimuli. **(B)** Area of increased rCBF correlated with subjective opioid craving. (*See* color plate 8 appearing in the insert following p. 368.)

within the pathway that is not subject to the same homeostatic regulation as the natural rewards *(38)*.

There is evidence from animal studies that opioids do release dopamine in this pathway. Using microdialysis techniques it has been possible to measure extra-cellular dopamine levels in distinct anatomical regions in response to opioid drugs *(39,40)*. For example, opioid micro-injections into the VTA stimulate the release of dopamine in the NAcc in rats *(41)*, and systemic opioids have similar effects *(39)*. Further evidence of the role of dopamine in the rewarding effects of opioids is provided by the ability of dopamine antagonists to partially block the ability of opioids to act as unconditioned stimuli in animal studies (e.g., *see* ref. *42*).

It is now gradually becoming possible to try to tie together the animal and human work on the brain circuits of addiction. The human neuroimaging studies of the acute effects of opioid drugs can now be compared to the animal data. The study of Sell et al. *(24)* showed that acute doses of heroin activated the PAG and VTA, as would be expected from the animal models. Unfortunately, current PET imaging techniques do not possess sufficient spatial resolution for it to be possible to image the NAcc. It is possible to look at effects in the striatum as a whole, and the areas of the cortex that receive projections from this region; for example, the study of London et al. *(22)* showed the effects of morphine in the caudate.

5.3. Imaging of Opioid Craving

Craving is a clinically relevant concept in the treatment of opioid dependence. This persistent desire for the drug and a sense of compulsion to use have long been recognized as important elements of the dependence syndrome and triggers for relapse to drug use. Craving has also been the subject of several neuroimaging studies, however, all of these studies have looked at cocaine craving. Our own work has looked at the effects on rCBF of autobiographical memories of opiate craving *(43)*. This showed increased rCBF in the left anterior cingulate in response to the stimuli and activity in the left orbito-frontal cortex that correlated with the degree of subjective craving for opioids (*see* Fig. 2: maps of activation in these areas). This is consistent with previous studies of cocaine craving *(44,45)*, suggesting that similar processes might be involved in craving for both classes of drug.

6. CONCLUSION

Opioid drugs have a relatively straightforward pharmacology, in that they bind to opioid receptors with only three specific subtypes. Despite this, they appear to have many and varied effects upon the brain, as we hope has been shown to some degree by this chapter. In comparison to cocaine, there has been much less research on their effects on brain function in general, including the mechanisms of opioid dependence. We hope that we have also shown that the techniques of neuroimaging, and functional neuroimaging with SPECT, PET, and fMRI, are particularly well-suited to expanding the current knowledge in this field.

REFERENCES

1. Gross, M. (1978) Autopsy findings in drug addicts. *Pathol. Ann.* **13**, 35–67.
2. Handelsman, L., Song, I. S., Losonczy, M., et al. (1993) Magnetic resonance abnormalities in HIV infection: a study in the drug-user risk group. *Psychiatry Res.* **47**, 175–186.

3. Aasly, J., Storsaeter, O., Nilsen, G., Smevik, O., and Rinck, P. (1993) Minor structural brain changes in young drug abusers. A magnetic resonance study. *Acta Neurol. Scand.* **87,** 210–214.

4. Amass, L., Nardin, R., Mendelson, J. H., Teoh, S. K., and Woods, B. T. (1992) Quantitative magnetic resonance imaging in heroin- and cocaine-dependent men: a preliminary study. *Psychiatry Res.* **45,** 15–23.

5. Siew, K. T., Mendelson, J. H., Woods, B. T., et al. (1993) Pituitary volume in men with concurrent heroin and cocaine dependence. *J. Clin. Endocrinol. Metab.* **76,** 1529–1532.

6. Gerra, G., Calbiani, B., Zaimovic, A., et al. (1998) Regional cerebral blood flow and comorbid diagnosis in abstinent opioid addicts. *Psychiatry Res. Neuroimaging* **83,** 117–126.

7. Celius, E. G. and Andersson, S. (1996) Leucoencephalopathy after inhalation of heroin: a case report. *J. Neurol. Neurosurg. Psychiatry* **60,** 694–695.

8. Vila, N. and Chamorro, A. (1997) Ballistic movements due to ischemic infarcts after intravenous heroin overdose: report of two cases. *Clin. Neurol. Neurosurg.* **99,** 259–262.

9. Cross, A. J., Hille, C., and Slater, P. (1987) Subtraction autoradiography of opiate receptor subtypes in human brain. *Brain Res.* **418,** 343–348.

10. Jones, A. K., Luthra, S. K., Maziere, B., et al. (1988) Regional cerebral opioid receptor studies with (11C)diprenorphine in normal volunteers. *J. Neurosci. Methods* **23,** 121–129.

11. Frost, J. J., Mayberg, H. S., Sadzot, B., et al. (1990) Comparison of (11C)diprenorphine and (11C)carfentanil binding to opiate receptors in humans by positron emission tomography. *J. Cereb. Blood Flow Metab.* **10,** 484–492.

12. Smith, J. S., Zubieta, J. K., Price, J. C., et al. (1999) Quantification of delta-opioid receptors in human brain with N1'-((11C)methyl) naltrindole and positron emission tomography. *J. Cereb. Blood Flow Metab.* **19,** 956–966.

13. Zubieta, J. K., Dannals, R. F., and Frost, J. J. (1999) Gender and age influences on human brain mu-opioid receptor binding measured by PET. *Am. J. Psychiatry* **156,** 842–848.

14. Smith, Y. R., Zubieta, J. K., del Carmen, M. G., et al. (1998) Brain opioid receptor measurements by positron emission tomography in normal cycling women: relationship to luteinizing hormone pulsatility and gonadal steroid hormones. *J. Clin. Endocrinol. Metab.* **83,** 4498–4505.

15. Jones, A. K. P., Cunningham, V. J., Ha-Kawa, S., et al. (1994) Changes in central opioid receptor binding in relation to inflammation and pain in patients with rheumatoid arthritis. *Br. J. Rheumatol.* **33,** 909–916.

16. Jones, A. K., Kitchen, N. D., Watabe, H., et al. (1999) Measurement of changes in opioid receptor binding in vivo during trigeminal neuralgic pain using (11C) diprenorphine and positron emission tomography. *J. Cereb. Blood Flow Metab.* **19,** 803–808.

17. Hartvig, P., Bergstrom, K., Lindberg, B., et al. (1984) Kinetics of 11C-labeled opiates in the brain of rhesus monkeys. *J. Pharmacol. Exp. Ther.* **230,** 250–255.

18. Firestone, L. L., Gyulai, F. E., Mintun, M. A., Adler, A. J., Urso, K., and Winter, P. M. (1996) Human brain activity response to fentanyl imaged by positron emission tomography. *Anesthesia Analgesia* **82,** 1247–1251.

19. Adler, L. J., Gyulai, F. E., Diehl, D. J., Mintun, M. A., Winter, P. M., and Firestone, L. L. (1997) Regional brain activity changes associated with fentanyl analgesia elucidated by positron emission tomography. *Anesthesia Analgesia* **84,** 120–126.

20. Jones, A. K. P., Friston, K. F., Qi, L. Y., et al. (1991) Sites of action of morphine in the brain. *Lancet* **338,** 825–825.

21. Schlaepfer, T. E., Strain, E. C., Greenberg, B. D., et al. (1998) Site of opioid action in the human brain: mu and kappa agonists' subjective and cerebral blood flow effects. *Am. J. Psychiatry* **155,** 470–473.

22. London, E. D., Broussolle, E. P., Links, J. M., et al. (1990) Morphine-induced metabolic changes in human brain. Studies with positron emission tomography and (fluorine 18)fluorodeoxyglucose. *Arch. Gen. Psychiatry* **47,** 73–81.

23. Sell, L. A., Simmons, A., Lemmens, G. M., Williams, S. C., Brammer, M., and Strang, J. (1997) Functional magnetic resonance imaging of the acute effect of intravenous heroin administration on visual activation in long-term heroin addicts: results from a feasibility study. *Drug Alcohol Depend.* **49,** 55–60.

24. Sell, L. A., Morris, J., Bearn, J., Frackowiak, R. S., Friston, K. J., and Dolan, R. J. (1999) Activation of reward circuitry in human opiate addicts. *Eur. J. Neurosci.* **11,** 1042–1048.

25. Walsh, S. L., Gilson, S. F., Jasinski, D. R., et al. (1994) Buprenorphine reduces cerebral glucose metabolism in polydrug abusers. *Neuropsychopharmacology* **10,** 157–170.

26. Kaufman, M. J., Pollack, M. H., Villafuerte, R. A., et al. (1999) Cerebral phosphorus metabolite abnormalities in opiate-dependent polydrug abusers in methadone maintenance. *Psychiatry Res.* **90,** 143–152.

27. Danos, P., Kasper, S., Grunwald, F., et al. (1998) Pathological regional cerebral blood flow in opiate-dependent patients during withdrawal: a HMPAO-SPECT study. *Neuropsychobiology* **37,** 194–199.

28. Krystal, J. H., Woods, S. W., Kosten, T. R., et al. (1995) Opiate dependence and withdrawal: preliminary assessment using single photon emission computerized tomography (SPECT). *Am. J. Drug Alcohol Abuse* **21,** 47–63.

29. Holman, B. L., Mendelson, J., Garada, B., et al. (1993) Regional cerebral blood flow improves with treatment in chronic cocaine polydrug users. *J. Nuclear Med.* **34,** 723–727.

30. Levin, E. D. and Rose, J. E. (1995) Acute and chronic nicotinic interactions with dopamine systems and working memory performance. *Ann. NY Acad. Sci.* **757,** 245–252.

31. Melichar, J., Law, F. D., Daglish, M. R. C., Myles, J. S., and Nutt, D. J. (1999) Pharmacokinetics and pharmacodynamics of methadone dependent individuals investigated using PET neuroimaging (11C-Diprenorphine) and the hydromorphone challenge test. *J. Psychopharmacol.* **13,** A24.

32. Wang, G. J., Volkow, N. D., Fowler, J. S, et al. (1997) Dopamine D2 receptor availability in opiate-dependent subjects before and after naloxone-precipitated withdrawal. *Neuropsychopharmacology* **16,** 174–182.

33. Rose, J. S., Branchey, M., Buydens-Branchey, L., et al. (1996) Cerebral perfusion in early and late opiate withdrawal: a technetium-99m-HMPAO SPECT study. *Psychiatry Res. Neuroimag.* **67,** 39–47.

34. van Dyck, C. H., Rosen, M. I., Thomas, H. M., et al. (1994) SPECT regional cerebral blood flow alterations in naltrexone-precipitated withdrawal from buprenorphine. *Psychiatry Res.* **55,** 181–191.

35. Acquas, E., Carboni, E., and Di Chiara, G. (1991) Profound depression of mesolimbic dopamine release after morphine withdrawal in dependent rats. *Eur. J. Pharmacol.* **193,** 133–134.

36. Wise, R. A. and Hoffman, D. C. (1992) Localization of drug reward mechanisms by intracranial injections. *Synapse* **10,** 247–263.

37. Nutt, D. J. (1996) Addiction: brain mechanisms and their treatment implications. *Lancet* **347,** 31–36.

38. Robinson, T. E. and Berridge, K. C. The neural basis of drug craving: an incentive-sensitization theory of addiction. *Brain Res. Brain Res. Rev.* **18,** 247–291.

39. Cadoni, C. and Di Chiara, G. (1999) Reciprocal changes in dopamine responsiveness in the nucleus accumbens shell and core and in the dorsal caudate-putamen in rats sensitized to morphine. *Neuroscience* **90,** 447–455.

40. Wise, R. A., Leone, P., Rivest, R., and Leeb, K. (1995) Elevations of nucleus accumbens dopamine and DOPAC levels during intravenous heroin self-administration. *Synapse* **21,** 140–148.

41. Devine, D. P., Leone, P., Pocock, D., Wise, R. A. (1993) Differential involvement of ventral tegmental mu, delta and kappa opioid receptors in modulation of basal mesolimbic dopamine release: in vivo microdialysis studies. *J. Pharmacol. Exp. Ther.* **266,** 1236–1246.

42. Longoni, R., Cadoni, C., Mulas, A., Di Chiara, G., and Spina, L. (1998) Dopamine-dependent behavioural stimulation by non-peptide delta opioids BW373U86 and SNC 80: 2. Place-preference and brain microdialysis studies in rats. *Behav. Pharmacol.* **9,** 9–14.
43. Daglish, M. R. C., Weinstein, A., Malizia, A. L., Wilson, S., Melichar, J. K., Britten, S., Brewer, C., Lingford-Hughes, A., et al. (2001) Changes in regional cerebral blood flow elicited by craving memories in abstinent opiate-dependent subjects. *Am. J. Psychiatry* **158,** 1680–1686.
44. Childress, A. R., Mozley, P. D., McElgin, W., Fitzgerald, J., Reivich, M., and O'Brien, C. P. (1999) Limbic activation during cue-induced cocaine craving. *Am. J. Psychiatry* **156,** 11–18.
45. Wang, G. J., Volkow, N. D., Fowler, J. S., et al. (1999) Regional brain metabolic activation during craving elicited by recall of previous drug experiences. *Life Sci.* **64,** 775–784.

16

Structural and Functional Neuroimaging of the Effects of Cocaine in Human and Nonhuman Primates

Linda J. Porrino, David J. Lyons, Sharon R. Letchworth, Cory S. Freedland, and Michael A. Nader

1. INTRODUCTION

Cocaine abuse throughout the world continues to be a major public-health concern. Drug abuse has enormous psychological, medical, economic, and social costs. Dependence on cocaine has been associated with increased rates of incarceration, high rates of infection with HIV, impaired job performance, and significant family dysfunction. Intense research efforts over the past few decades have resulted in a greatly increased understanding of the neurobiological basis of cocaine's effects and the adaptations that occur as a result of its chronic use and abuse.

Cocaine has complex actions in the central nervous system (CNS), but the primary neurochemical action of cocaine in brain is the blockade of the reuptake of dopamine *(1,2)*, norepinephrine *(2,3)*, and serotonin *(4)*. Behaviorally, cocaine has a variety of actions in humans, as well as in animal models, including reinforcing effects *(5,6)*, discriminative stimulus effects *(7,8)*, and locomotor-activating properties *(9–11)*. Cocaine also has important effects on the cardiovascular system *(12)* and in the liver *(13)*.

2. COCAINE USE AND ABUSE

Cocaine is thought to exert its powerful reinforcing effects via interactions with brain dopamine systems, in particular the dopaminergic pathway extending from the ventral tegmental area (VTA) to the nucleus accumbens (NAcc) that has come to be known as the brain reward circuit. The evidence that this system is central to the reinforcing properties of abused drugs is substantial. Disruption of dopaminergic activity as a result of 6-hydroxydopamine (6-OHDA) lesions of the nucleus accumbens, for example, significantly diminishes cocaine self-administration in rats in a variety of paradigms *(14–20)*. These effects on responding have been shown to be specific to drug intake. When responding maintained by cocaine is either reduced or abolished, responding maintained by other reinforcers such as food is not necessarily reduced in

From: Handbook of Neurotoxicology, Vol. 2
Edited by: E. J. Massaro © Humana Press Inc., Totowa, NJ

parallel *(21)*. Microinjections of dopamine antagonists directly into the NAcc also alters the patterns of responding maintained by cocaine infusions in rats in an analogous manner *(22–25)*, as does depletion of dopamine in the VTA, the main source of the dopaminergic innervation of the NAcc *(26)*. Further evidence of the involvement of the mesolimbic dopamine pathway in cocaine self-administration has been reported in in vivo microdialysis studies, in which increases in extracellular levels of dopamine within the NAcc accompany each cocaine infusion during a self-administration session *(27,28)*. In electrophysiological studies, NAcc neurons of rodents have been characterized both by increased firing rates immediately before cocaine-reinforced responses, as well as by changes in neuronal-firing patterns immediately following the presentation of the reinforcer *(29–31)*. The importance of dopamine in the NAcc as a substrate of cocaine's actions is also evident in studies of nonhuman *(32,33)* and human *(34)* primates. The firing patterns of NAcc neurons in monkeys show parallel changes in anticipation of, or following, cocaine as well as the presentation of other reinforcers such as juice *(35–37)*. These reports, then, along with a vast number of others, have shown that activity in the dopaminergic mesolimbic system is associated with the reinforcing effects of cocaine and other drugs of abuse.

Cocaine's reinforcing effects are thought to derive from its ability to produce pleasurable sensations and it is this euphoria that is responsible for its abuse. This is, however, only one aspect of cocaine use and abuse. It has long been recognized that drug use undergoes a progression through a number of temporal stages that advance from initial experimentation through casual use and finally to addiction. The longitudinal course of cocaine abuse has been described in terms of clearly definable clinical phases (e.g., *38–41*). Reports by cocaine users portray their initial experience with cocaine as highly pleasurable. Cocaine induces intense feelings of euphoria and well-being, along with an intensification of emotions and sexual feelings (e.g., *39,42*). In those individuals who continue to use the drug, use patterns shift from casual occasional use to high-dose, long-duration binges accompanied by intense feelings of pleasure and a decreased sensitivity to the negative effects of the drug *(39,40)*. With continued high-intensity use and binging, reports of panic attacks, paranoia, and intense anxiety states become more frequent *(41)* as abusers become sensitized to the effects of cocaine.

Cocaine abstinence has also been characterized as containing a series of clinically defined phases. Gawin and Kleber *(38)*, based on their naturalistic study of abstinent cocaine abusers, have proposed a three-stage model of abstinence. Immediately after a cocaine binge, there is a "crash," lasting from 1–4 d, which is accompanied by intense craving, agitation, depression, and anxiety. The second phase, withdrawal, lasts from 1–10 wk and is characterized by anhedonia and a lack of energy and motivation. The final phase or extinction is marked by a significant decrease in craving and lowered probability of relapse, but during this phase the presence of conditioned cues can still readily induce feelings of craving.

Underlying this course of cocaine addiction and abstinence are changes within the CNS as brain systems adapt to, and compensate for, cocaine use and the cessation of its effects. Identifying these systems and various neuroadaptations that accompany cocaine use and abuse is a complex issue. It is highly unlikely that these effects are within a single brain region or the result of changes in a single neurotransmitter system. It is more likely that alterations in brain structure and function are the result of multiple processes at a number of anatomical sites. In order to determine the neural substrates of the actions of cocaine, it is necessary to identify neural events in circuits and pathways throughout the brain, not just a single location. This requires either that we investigate small portions of the brain one at a time as with electrophysiological methods or that we use methods capable of surveying the entire brain simultaneously. Neuroimaging methods, both in vivo and in vitro, allow us to visualize structural and functional changes that have occurred as a result of acute or chronic exposure to cocaine. In this chapter we will review neuroimaging studies in both human and nonhuman primates, designed to characterize these changes.

3. DISTRIBUTION OF COCAINE BINDING SITES IN BRAIN

Given the fact that cocaine binds with relatively equivalent affinity at the dopamine, norepinephrine, and serotonin transporters *(43,44)* it might be expected that cocaine-binding sites in brain would be widespread. This question has been addressed in non-human and human primates and the methods employed demonstrate the variety of imaging methods available as tools to those investigating the effects of cocaine.

In an early landmark study, Fowler and colleagues *(45)* used positron emission to-mography (PET) with [^{11}C] cocaine as a ligand to show that cocaine preferentially binds in human brain to the striatum and predominantly to dopamine transporters. More recently, this group of investigators has shown that the highest activity for [^{11}C] cocaine was in striatal area, but that moderate activity was also evident in thalamus, posterior cingulate, amygdala, hippocampus, and temporal pole, suggesting a far more wide-spread distribution of cocaine in brain. This is consistent with the results of studies in postmortem human tissue *(46)* in which in vitro receptor autoradiography with [^{3}H] cocaine was used to demonstrate a very similar regional distribution of high-affinity specific binding of cocaine. In addition, in this study appreciable binding was also reported in substantia nigra (SN), dorsal raphe (DR), and hypothalamus.

The distribution of cocaine-binding sites in nonhuman primates was addressed with ex vivo autoradiographic methods in which [^{3}H] cocaine was infused intravenously (*see* Fig. 1). Both tracer and physiologically relevant doses, the latter in the range of doses self-administered by nonhuman primates via this route as shown in laboratory studies *(47),* were administered, and the accumulation of the labeled cocaine measured throughout the brain. The distribution of label was very similar following the adminis-tration of both doses with high levels noted in the caudate, putamen, and NAcc. Mod-erate amounts of cocaine were evident in hippocampus, stria terminalis, locus coeruleus, amygdala, and SN. Cocaine binding was not restricted to dopaminergic areas, however, but distributed throughout those areas innervated by norepinephrine and serotonin as well. This is particularly clear when the distribution of [^{3}H] cocaine is compared to the distribution of the dopamine-uptake agent mazindol, which clearly had a very different topography from that of cocaine. This study, when considered in conjunction with studies in humans discussed earlier, emphasize that cocaine's effects are not likely to be restricted solely to the dopaminergic system and cannot be fully understood without consideration of the effects throughout the entire brain.

Beyond the regional distribution of cocaine, imaging methods have been useful in determining pharmacokinetic properties of cocaine and its distribution in the other parts of the body outside the brain. PET studies have shown that cocaine is taken up in heart,

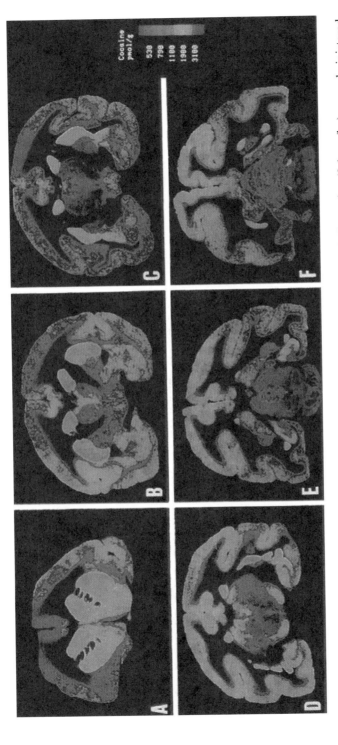

Fig. 1. Distribution of [3H] cocaine in coronal sections of a squirrel monkey brain. [3H] cocaine (0.1 mg/kg) was administered intravenously 15 min before sacrifice. Shown are 6 levels from anterior (**A**) at the level of the striatum to posterior (**F**) at the level of the locus coeruleus. Prominent labeling is seen throughout the striatum (**A–D**), cortex (**A–F**), ventral midbrain (**D**), hippocampus (**D–E**), and locus coeruleus (**F**). Adapted with permission from ref. *(47)*. (*See* color plate 9 appearing in the insert following p. 368.)

kidneys, liver, bladder and adrenals, with uptake in the heart actually faster than that in brain *(48)*. The uptake in the adrenals, among the highest of all organs, could be in part responsible for the release of catecholamines peripherally, and the high levels of uptake in heart responsible for the high degree of cardiotoxicity associated with cocaine.

Uptake in brain is very rapid with the peak usually occurring only 4–6 min after intravenous administration of tracer amounts of [^{11}C]cocaine. It also clears from the brain rapidly, with the half-life in the striatum estimated to be only 20 min. The rapid time course of cocaine's binding and clearance correlate closely with its subjective effects in humans *(45,49)*.

3.1. Acute Effects of Cocaine

PET studies have been very influential in examining the effects of cocaine on dopamine directly in humans. There are two main strategies that examine different aspects of the dopamine system following acute cocaine administration. The first of these involves measurements of dopamine levels using [^{11}C] raclopride, which has been shown to be sensitive to concentrations of synaptic dopamine *(50,51)*. Increased concentrations of dopamine such as those produced by a stimulant drug like cocaine displace the bound ligand, thereby reducing levels of tracer actually measured. By comparing baseline and challenged conditions, the degree and time-course of dopamine increase can be inferred. Schlaepfer and colleagues used this strategy to measure dopamine levels following the intravenous administration of cocaine *(52)*. They showed that binding was decreased in the striatum, indicating higher concentrations of synaptic dopamine, at a time that corresponded to the peak physiological effects of cocaine.

Volkow and colleagues *(49)* have used a similar approach to study the effects of methylphenidate, a psychostimulant that has effects similar to cocaine at dopamine and serotonin transporters, but has a longer duration of action. Their study, like the one mentioned previously, showed dopamine concentrations increased as a result of psychostimulant administration, the time-course of which followed its subjective effects on mood. Furthermore, they showed that the intensity of the "high," as assessed by their subjects on an analog-rating scale, significantly correlated with the levels of released dopamine in the striatum. The use of [^{11}C] raclopride to measure dopamine concentrations clearly demonstrates that the increases in dopamine levels associated with the administration of psychostimulants follow the physiological and subjective effects of the drug. It is dopamine, then, that appears to be critical for the experience of the euphorigenic effects of cocaine.

The second strategy involves the direct measurement of dopamine-transporter occupancy. Similar to the previous approach, this has been a particularly powerful procedure when combined with behavioral reports. The subjective effects of a drug like cocaine can be related to its effects on dopamine-transporter occupancy simultaneously in the same human subjects. This is an important strategy because this is the type of question that can only be addressed in human subjects. Volkow and her co-workers have shown, in an elegant series of studies, that the administration of cocaine dose-dependently blocks dopamine transporter occupancy with the onset and duration of the "high" produced by cocaine paralleling its effects on transporter occupancy *(53)*. They further showed that a minimum of approx 50% of dopamine transporters needed to be occupied for subjects to report significant subjective effects of cocaine on mood ratings.

In their earlier studies, this group had used another ligand for the dopamine trans-porter, [^{11}C] threo-methylphenidate, and measured the effects of methylphenidate on dopamine-transporter occupancy. These studies, while important and displaying some-what similar results, were limited by the fact that methylphenidate does not occupy the transporter in the same way as cocaine, nor does it have exactly the same potencies for aminergic-uptake carriers as cocaine. By utilizing [^{11}C] cocaine and administering cocaine, they were able to visualize the effects of cocaine directly at the sites that cocaine occupies in the brain.

PET studies in humans have the obvious advantage of measuring the effects of cocaine directly in the species of interest. The use of animal models can be limited by issues of species differences and the inability to measure the subjective effects of drugs like cocaine. Verbal reports give a direct measure of cocaine's subjective effects that can only be inferred in studies using animal models. Studies in humans, however, are limited by the fact that the resolution that can be achieved with PET is often not suffi-cient to analyze the effects of cocaine in the ventral striatum. This is the brain region most closely associated with the rewarding effects of cocaine (*see* earlier discussion), but it is the changes in dopamine systems that occur in the dorsal striatum that are generally measured in PET studies. Even though both the dorsal and ventral striatum are included in the measurement, the dorsal striatum is larger and has a greater dopam-ine content. However, with the increasing resolution brought about by advances in PET technology, it will soon be possible to measure effects in the NAcc. It will no longer be necessary to make inferences about the ventral striatum based on measurements in the caudate and putamen.

3.2. Acute Effects of Cocaine on CBF and Metabolism

A variety of imaging methods have been used to investigate the neural basis of the subjective and physiological effects of cocaine in the living human brain. In the major-ity of these studies, PET is used to measure CBF and/or cerebral metabolism. In addi-tion, recent studies have made use of fMRI to assess the effects of cocaine in humans. All of these studies have evaluated the effects of cocaine in drug using populations. Thus, the effects of cocaine are measured in a very specific cohort. These individuals are chronic drug users, frequently heavy users of cocaine and other drugs as well. They generally found drug exposure to be a strong reinforcer and have difficulty controlling their drug use despite negative consequences. In addition, the chronic exposure to drugs induces significant neuroadaptations in brain. The assessments of the functional effects of cocaine in humans, therefore, need to be viewed in this light. There are limitations and qualifications that must be kept in mind when considering this literature.

In polydrug abusers, the acute administration of cocaine decreases cerebral glucose metabolism in a global fashion *(54,55)*. London and coworkers *(54)* reported that rates of cerebral metabolism were significantly decreased in 26 of 29 measured regions after the intravenous administration of 40 mg of cocaine. Changes in rates of metabolism were correlated with subjective report of "rush" and "high." There was, however, some variation in the degree of reduction of cerebral metabolism (5–26%) detected, indicat-ing some regional variation. A subsequent report similarly described only global decreases in cerebral metabolism after the administration of cocaine *(55)*. In another study, the monoamine oxidase B inhibitor, selegiline, which reduces the subjective response to cocaine, was evaluated for its ability to alter the effects of cocaine on regional cerebral metabolism in cocaine-dependent subjects *(56)*. The findings in three regions were reported: amygdala, hippocampus, and thalamus. Selegiline treatment specifically blocked the effect of cocaine in the amygdala. In hippocampus, selegiline treatment reduced metabolism in both the control condition and following the acute administration of cocaine. No effect was found in the thalamus. These data suggest that the alteration of cerebral metabolism in limbic sites may underlie the subjective "high," and modulation of monoamine oxidase activity may influence this function.

Several studies of regional cerebral blood flow (rCBF) have found evidence of region-specific changes following cocaine administration that are likely to be related to changes in function. Localized reductions in blood flow were found in frontal cortex and the basal ganglia after intravenous cocaine, and these changes were negatively correlated with subjective effects *(57)*. Dose-dependent changes in blood flow following cocaine use were reported in prefrontal, parietal, and temporal cortices and the basal ganglia *(58)*. These effects of cocaine appeared to be most concentrated in dopamine-rich prefrontal cortex and basal ganglia *(58)*. Not all studies, however, have found localized changes *(59)*.

To function properly, the brain must be continuously supplied with nutrients. In contrast to other organs, the brain cannot store sufficient nutrients and therefore depends on a constant supply delivered by the blood. Brain regions that are more active require more nutrients, and regional rates of blood flow within the brain are modulated to keep pace with the changing demands. These characteristics form the basis for the measurement of rCBF *(60,61)*. It is also important to recognize that although blood-flow changes result from fluctuations in energy demand, blood flow also changes as a consequence of the direct effects of cocaine and other drugs on cerebral hemodynamics, as well. Proper interpretation of studies of rCBF must therefore take into account that findings are likely to be due to a combination of modifications in perfusion as well as function.

There is strong evidence that cocaine use can produce cerebral ischemia, stroke, and seizures *(62,63)*, although the precise mechanisms for producing this pathology is poorly understood. One hypothesis is that cocaine induces transient vasospasm. Using transcranial doppler sonography to measure various hemodynamic parameters in cocaine users, Herning and colleagues *(64)* found that the acute administration of cocaine resulted in a short-lived (2-min) period of acute vasoconstriction, which may play an important role in the generation of neurovascular deficits in users. The L-type calcium-channel blocker, isradipine, has been shown to reduce brain ischemia in rodents, and the ability of isradipine to reverse the acute effects of cocaine on rCBF in users has been investigated *(65)*. Cocaine reduced blood flow in a number of regions in this study, and although isradipine alone was not tested, isradipine plus cocaine resulted in higher rates of blood flow in most regions compared to placebo. These data suggest that isradipine may have clinical utility for reversing cocaine-induced ischemia.

Functional magnetic resonance imaging (fMRI) is also used to assess changes in blood flow and oxygenation as well as to investigate the acute effects of cocaine. Like PET studies of blood flow, fMRI signal changes are likely to result from alterations in perfusion and function. In one study of cocaine, the acute administration of cocaine induced localized decreases in fMRI signal in amygdala, medial prefrontal cortex, and the temporal pole *(34)*. These decreases in signal intensity found in the amygdala and limbic-related prefrontal and temporal cortex are easily reconciled with the previous data previously mentioned. This study also found, however, increased signal intensity in a variety of other regions of brain, including the ventral striatum/subcallosal cingulate, ventral tegmentum, and several other cortical regions. The fact that this method measures blood oxygenation levels, rather than blood flow, may partially explain discrepancies between this study and others.

The potential for this method is still great, despite current limitations in interpreting the data. It has been recently shown, for example, that changes in fMRI signal associated with visual stimulation can be detected even during the acute administration of cocaine, which demonstrates that cocaine-induced cerebrovascular changes do not completely prevent the detection of functional changes *(66)*. This provides some validation for previous studies of the effects of cocaine alone on fMRI signal, because it can now be argued that cocaine-induced changes may be attributed to changes in function, as well as perfusion. Another study has shown, however, that the fMRI signal induced by visual stimulation, although detectable, is subtly altered by cocaine administration *(67)*. This study demonstrated that within individual structures, i.e., visual and motor cortex, cocaine altered the spatial-coincidence coefficient, which measures "functional connectivity" within a brain region by assessing the degree to which all the voxels within a brain region change as a group. Thus, it appears that functional changes in a brain region resulting from visual stimulation may be detected by fMRI, while at the same time the concerted function within that region is partially disrupted by cocaine.

The use of nonhuman primates provides one avenue to investigate the effects of cocaine in subjects without a prior history of cocaine abuse. In this way, it is possible to distinguish the pharmacological effects of cocaine from the effects of varying drug histories and psychopathology. Nonhuman primate models have been used to assess both the behavioral and neurobiological basis of the effects of cocaine. One strategy has been the use of the autoradiographic 2-[^{14}C] deoxyglucose method *(68)*. In these studies rates of local cerebral glucose utilization were determined in male macaques after the administration of either cocaine (1.0 mg/kg, i.v.) or saline *(32)*. Rather than global decreases in cerebral metabolism as observed in human drug users, discrete decreases in rates of glucose utilization were found in anatomically linked limbic sites. These regions included the dorsal and ventral striatum *(see Fig. 2)*, the medial and orbitofrontal prefrontal cortex, the hippocampus, and the anterior thalamus. Changes in the striatum are not surprising, given the high concentrations of dopamine transporter *(see Fig. 1)* *(47)* located there, and the well-established role for striatal circuits in the effects of cocaine in the rodent *(69)*. Although a clear understanding of the functions supported by the medial and orbitofrontal cortex remains elusive, this region of brain appears to play an important role in mood and stimulus-reward associations *(70–72)*. Such a role is plainly consistent with the known effects of cocaine on mood and reinforcement. It is also important to recognize that the cocaine stimulus in this study was novel, since these animals had no history of cocaine exposure. New learning associated with the novel stimulus, therefore, is likely to explain the functional changes noted in hippocampus and anterior thalamus. There are several potential sources for the differences between this nonhuman primate study in which localized changes in glucose metabolism were found and human studies in which global changes were

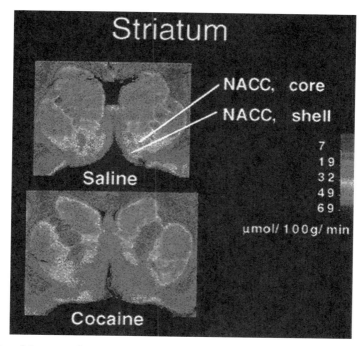

Fig. 2. Effects of the acute intravenous administration of cocaine at a dose of 1.0 mg/kg (top panel) and saline (bottom panel) on rates of local cerebral glucose utilization in the ventral striatum. Shown are color-coded transformations of autoradiograms of coronal sections of cynomolgus monkeys. Each color represents a range of rates of glucose utilization. NACC, nucleus accumbens. From ref. *(32)*, Copyright 1996, by the Society for Neuroscience. (*See* color plate 10 appearing in the insert following p. 368.)

reported. The most important difference may be the absence of any prior exposure to cocaine in the monkeys, as well as the absence of any other prior drug use. It is important to recognize that the information that can be obtained from studies in nonhuman primates and human cocaine addicts is decidedly different. Human studies are more directed towards the mechanisms underlying addiciton while studies in nonhuman primate models of substance abuse have the capacity to address the basic neurobiological mechanisms underlying the effects of cocaine.

4. ASSESSING THE EFFECTS OF CHRONIC COCAINE ADMINISTRATION

The studies reviewed previously have focused largely on the basic actions of cocaine when it was administered acutely. Changes in dopamine-transporter occupancy or effects on brain functional activity, whether assessed in drug-naive or chronic drug abusers, represent the direct mechanisms of cocaine's actions. It is also essential to recognize that chronic cocaine use produces fundamental long-term changes in brain structure and function. Once again, because such changes can occur throughout the brain, imaging studies have made central contributions, whether carried out in humans or nonhuman primates.

4.1. Effects on Dopamine Systems

Since cocaine binds directly to DAT, researchers have hypothesized that DAT may be altered by repeated exposure to cocaine. To that end, alterations in the density of DAT binding sites have been examined within the brains of human cocaine addicts using in vivo imaging methods as well as in vitro ligand binding in postmortem tissue. Increases in human DAT density have been reported using radiolabeled cocaine analogs, such as [³H]WIN 35,428, to label DAT (73–76; but *see* ref. 77). For example, Little et al. (76) reported 40–45% increases in striatal [³H] WIN 35,428 binding sites in tissue sections from human cocaine users and 50% increases in binding sites in caudate-putamen homogenates. The greatest increases in [³H]WIN 35,428 sites to date were reported by Staley et al. (73) for cocaine-overdose victims, with the largest changes found in the ventral caudate, ventromedial putamen, and NAcc. These studies noted that the affinity of [³H] WIN 35,428 for DAT was not different in the cocaine-user population as compared to controls (73,74,76).

Studies using the cocaine analog [¹²⁵I] RTI–55 (β-CIT) to label DAT have also reported increases in DAT binding sites. For example, Little and colleagues used [¹²⁵I] RTI–55 in postmortem tissue sections from a small population of cocaine users and found a statistical trend with 23–35% increases in striatal DAT sites. Malison et al. (77a) used in vivo SPECT imaging with [¹²⁵I] β-CIT and measured 20% increases in striatal DAT binding sites in human cocaine users. In contrast, studies using markers structurally unrelated to cocaine exhibited binding site decreases in the striatum ([³H] mazindol) (78) and prefrontal cortex ([³H]GBR 12,935) (79).

It is exceedingly difficult to examine the temporal development of changes in DAT binding sites in human cocaine abusers. Accurate data is usually not available on duration or extent of drug use, especially when postmortem tissue is involved. This is an important question, however, and has been addressed in nonhuman primate models. In a study carried out in our laboratories, the effects of initial (5 d), chronic (3.3 mo), and long-term (1.5 yr) exposure to cocaine self-administration on DAT binding sites were assessed in rhesus monkeys (80). [³H]WIN 35,428 autoradiography was conducted to examine changes in DAT binding site levels in subregions of the caudate, putamen, and NAcc. This study demonstrated a progression of changes in DAT binding-site density over time. In the initial stages of cocaine self-administration (5 d), DAT binding sites were moderately reduced. In contrast, prolonged stages of cocaine self-administration (3.3 mo and 1.5 yr) resulted in large increases in DAT density in the ventral striatum, which includes the ventral caudate, ventral putamen, and NAcc. Moreover, effects of cocaine dose on DAT density were observed so that after chronic exposure, higher cocaine doses yielded larger increases in the density of DAT binding sites. These findings are of particular importance because only one previous study of human cocaine users has observed any relationship between the severity of cocaine use and increases in DAT levels (76). Using a nonhuman primate model, it is clear that with longer periods of cocaine exposure and at higher doses, greater increases were observed and more striatal regions exhibited these changes. Furthermore, these data are similar to those from studies of human cocaine abusers described earlier (73,76) that used radiolabeled cocaine analogs to measure dopamine transporter in which increased densities of DAT binding sites were observed. However, many subjects used in studies of human cocaine abuse have years of cocaine experience. These data from cocaine self-administering monkeys, however, indicate that the increases associated with prolonged cocaine exposure begin to occur on the order of months rather than years.

4.2. Dopamine D₁- and D₂-Like Receptors

Studies of the effects of chronic cocaine on dopaminergic receptors have been carried out in both human drug abusers and in nonhuman primate models of cocaine abuse. Here, too, there is complementary information to be gleaned from both species. In humans the earliest work was carried out by Volkow and her colleagues measuring dopamine D_2-receptor availability in chronic cocaine users with [^{18}F] N-methylspiroperidol and PET *(81,82)*. Cocaine abusers had significantly lower levels of dopamine D_2 receptors when compared to drug-naive subjects. These investigators also showed that in these drug abusers, a decreased dopamine D_2-receptor availability was associated with decreased glucose utilization in the orbitofrontal cortex as well as self-ratings of dysphoria *(82)*. These authors point to the importance of dopaminergic function in the negative subjective feelings that accompany withdrawal. Another important feature of these studies was the retest of some subjects after completion of a drug-treatment program. The downregulation observed within a 1-wk period of abstinence persisted for up to 4 mo of cocaine abstinence, suggesting a very long-term effect of cocaine use that is not readily reversed even with prolonged abstinence. One problem, however, is that it is difficult to distinguish effects of chronic cocaine use from effects due to withdrawal from cocaine itself. Moreover, the possibility that these abusers already had decreased receptor populations prior to any cocaine experience cannot be disregarded.

Postmortem studies of dopamine-receptor systems, however, have not been consistent with the in vivo PET studies. Staley and Mash *(83)* failed to show any alterations in the dopamine D_2-receptor system of cocaine overdose victims and studies of levels of dopamine D_1- and D_2-receptor mRNA in postmortem brain tissue from cocaine-abusing subjects also failed to demonstrate any alterations in these markers *(84)*. Staley and Mash *(83)*, however, did show dramatic changes in dopamine D_3 receptors. In these studies D_3 receptors were upregulated specifically throughout the ventral striatum. The absence of changes in dopamine D_2 receptors in these postmortem reports may be from the differences in the populations of cocaine abusers studied. Abusers who die of overdoses may represent a particular subset of those addicted to cocaine that may be more vulnerable to the toxic effects of the drug. Differences in the kinds of ligands and other procedural differences may have resulted in the discrepancies as well.

Because it can be difficult to evaluate the effects of chronic drug exposure in a human addict population, studies in nonhuman primate models of substance abuse can provide important information without the confounds inherent in human studies as discussed earlier. The first nonhuman primate study to examine the effects of chronic cocaine administration on D_1 and D_2 receptor density was by Farfel et al. *(85)*. In that study, cocaine was administered four times per day for 2 wk. After a two-week abstinence period, the monkeys were euthanized and their brains were prepared for receptor autoradiography. The density of D_1 receptors in the caudate was reduced by over 50% compared to tissue from control monkeys, while D_2-receptor density in the caudate was not significantly different between cocaine- and saline-treated monkeys. Other structures examined, in particular the prefrontal cortex, SN, and NAcc, did not show changes in D_1- or D_2-receptor density as a consequence of cocaine administration, consistent with the human postmortem studies *(83,84)*. Farfel and colleagues suggested that the changes seen in D_1 in the caudate might be related to the phenomena of behavioral sensitization, which may lead to continued drug-taking.

More recent studies in nonhuman primates have extended the work of Farfel et al. *(85)* to include: (1) self-administration of cocaine rather than experimenter administered; (2) extended periods of cocaine exposure; and (3) minimizing the withdrawal period following cocaine treatment and prior to tissue procurement. There is a growing body of research suggesting that the effects of cocaine (and other drugs of abuse) are different depending on whether the drug is self-administered by the animal or experimenter-administered (e.g., *86*). While it is certainly labor-intensive to prepare and maintain an animal with an indwelling intravenous catheter, studying reinforcing doses of cocaine enhances the validity and reliability of the animal model. Perhaps the most important variable that operates when the drug is passively administered may be the stress associated with the injection and/or the unexpected dose that is received. Since stress clearly modifies the DA-receptor density and function (e.g., *87*), control of this variable by allowing the animal to self-administer the drug is an important experimental manipulation.

Long treatment regimens of nearly 2 yr and higher cocaine doses than those reported by Farfel et al. *(85)* have been studied in monkeys that had an extensive history of self-administering cocaine *(88,89)*. Monkeys used in these studies had self-administered cocaine daily (5–7 d/wk), resulting in lifetime cocaine intakes of as much as 600 mg/kg. There were significant reductions in both D_1- and D_2-receptor densities in all regions of the striatum including the caudate, putamen, and both the shell and core of the NAcc *(88,89)*. Thus, these findings convincingly indicate that daily, stable rates of cocaine self-administration can produce profound reductions in D_1- and D_2-like receptor densities. The differences between these data and those in previous autoradiographic studies can be attributed to differences in durations of treatment as well the fact that cocaine was self-administered in this study. This serves to emphasize the importance of the paradigms used to study the effects of cocaine and the relevance of the models to substance abuse issues.

In a second series of studies from these laboratories *(90)*, issues of dose and treatment duration were addressed by studying separate groups of monkeys self-administering two doses of cocaine (0.03 or 0.3 mg/kg/infusion resulting in daily intakes of 0.9 or 9 mg/kg) for two different durations of drug exposure (5 d or 3.3 mo). At the end of self-administration for 5 or 100 sessions, receptor autoradiographic studies were conducted to assess D_2-like receptors in both groups of monkeys and a control group of monkeys that responded in daily experimental sessions under a food-reinforcement schedule. After 3.3 mo of self-administration (total intake 90 or 900 mg/kg), both cocaine groups showed profound and significant reductions in D_2-receptor densities throughout the striatum, as compared to control monkey tissue. Importantly, there were no differences between the 0.3 and 0.03 mg/kg/injection cocaine groups. That is, approx 100 sessions of "cocaine seeking" seemed to have a greater impact than the dose of cocaine self-administered. When shorter periods of cocaine self-administration were studied (5 sessions totally 4.5 and 45 mg/kg cocaine), no effect on D_2 receptors, relative to controls, was observed *(90)*. These findings suggest that environmental modulation, in terms of stimuli associated with cocaine-seeking, may be as important to dopamine-receptor changes as direct pharmacological consequences of cocaine exposure. Volkow et al. *(82)* made an extremely interesting observation in their study of cocaine abusers: they found that D_2-receptor density was significantly correlated with years of cocaine use, but not with the doses of cocaine used. While the assumption is that the cocaine-related reductions in D_2-receptor binding potential were primarily consequences of cocaine-induced neuropharmacological changes, the correlational data reported by Volkow et al. *(82)* suggest that the entire behavioral repertoire, not just the pharmacology of cocaine, significantly impacted D_2-receptor numbers.

In another series of studies, Nader and his colleagues *(91)* used the D_2-selective ligand [^{18}F] fluoroclebopride (FCP), which has been thoroughly studied by our group (e.g., *92,93*) to examine the effects of cocaine self-administration on dopamine D_2 receptors in rhesus monkeys. In these PET studies they found that within 1 wk of initiating cocaine self-administration, D_2-receptor binding potential was reduced by approx 15% and that the reductions persisted at approx 20% for the duration of the maintenance phase (1 yr). These findings are similar to the effects reported in human cocaine abusers *(82)* and suggest that the changes in D_2 receptor numbers are a result of cocaine, not a pre-existing condition. Overall, these findings suggest that D_2 receptors are intimately involved in cocaine's reinforcing effects and that they may certainly be involved in mediating the high rates of relapse, since recovery of receptor number during abstinence is slow.

4.3. Consequences of Chronic Cocaine Use on CBF and Metabolism

Beyond the changes in dopamine systems that have been shown to occur with chronic cocaine exposure, there is now growing evidence that long-term cocaine use leads to adaptation on a functional level in the brains of users. Volkow and colleagues *(82,94–97)* have reported, for example, changes in both resting levels of cerebral metabolism and blood flow, as well as altered responses to pharmacologic challenge in cocaine abusers. The time-course of recovery is also an issue of critical interest, from the stages of acute drug withdrawal to longer periods of abstinence.

In recently abstinent cocaine users during the first week of treatment, increases in cerebral metabolism have been reported in the basal ganglia and orbitofrontal cortex *(95)*. At 2–4 wk, in contrast, no differences were found between users and normal controls *(95)*. Significant correlations were found between the number of days since last use and rates of metabolism in basal ganglia and orbitofrontal cortex, as well as between craving scores and metabolism in the orbitofrontal region. In a study of CBF done at 72 h after admission to inpatient treatment, cocaine users exhibited spotty derangements of perfusion throughout the brain, with the most profound reductions in prefrontal cortex and cerebellum *(94)*. Regional cortical decreases and smaller local derangements in regional cerebral blood flow have now been found by several groups *(98–101)*. Taken together, the initial phases of abstinence are accompanied by elevated cerebral metabolism, likely a response to acute drug withdrawal. Furthermore, CBF is disrupted throughout the brain, though profound reductions in flow may be concentrated in certain chiefly anterior regions. It is not clear what the neurologic ramifications of these findings are; however, it is tempting to speculate that users may be particularly vulnerable to cerebrovascular accidents at this stage.

At later stages of abstinence a different pattern of cerebral metabolic activity appears to dominate, while the presentation of disrupted rCBF remains unchanged. Volkow and colleagues *(102)* studied cocaine abusers 1–6 wk into abstinence and then 3 mo later. Rather than the high rates seen during the first week of abstinence, lower rates of cerebral metabolism (compared to normals) were found in frontal cortex, and these differences persisted through the 3-mo follow-up. The further examination of dopamine D_2 receptors within the basal ganglia in these subjects revealed decreased D_2 availability that was strongly correlated with the reduced rates of metabolism found in the orbitofrontal cortex *(82)*. Similarly, the pattern of functional activity in rhesus monkeys was most different in the medial and orbitofrontal regions of the frontal lobe when compared to the effects of acute cocaine in animals with no prior cocaine exposure to animals that had self-administered cocaine for approx 1.5 yr *(103)*. As a whole, these data suggest that chronic cocaine use alters dopaminergic systems, and these changes are translated into disrupted functional activity in prefrontal cortex that can persist for at least 3 mo into abstinence.

A few studies have examined the short-term recovery of rCBF in cocaine abusers. It appears that the regular user and the recently abstinent individuals present with irregularities in cerebral blood characterized by a combination of reduced flow largely in frontal cortex superimposed on randomly distributed, smaller foci of poor perfusion *(56,94,99,101,104)*. Recovery has been reported for some subjects at 10 d *(94)* and 21 d of abstinence *(101)*, although poor perfusion persisted in other subjects. These data suggest that at least partial spontaneous recovery is possible, though some individuals may be at risk for long-term perfusion deficits.

5. CRAVING

One other aspect of cocaine use and abuse that has received considerable attention in imaging studies is craving. Drug craving is a hallmark feature of drug addiction and has been implicated in drug use as well as relapse to drug taking following a period of abstinence. Cocaine craving can be elicited by internal cues (dysphoria, desire to avoid or decrease withdrawal severity), pharmacological drug cues, and drug-related environmental stimuli *(105,106)*. As such, identifying the neurobiological substrates that underlie craving may be critical in the development of effective therapies for the treatment of cocaine dependence. Numerous investigators have applied noninvasive neuroimaging techniques in an effort to describe the neural substrates involved in craving. The majority of these studies have utilized external cues to elicit craving in cocaine abusers. These cues include drug-related videos (portraying the acquisition, preparation, and/or administration of drug), drug paraphernalia, and even cocaine itself.

In a study by Childress et al. *(107)*, nondrug and cocaine-related videos were used to elicit craving in cocaine abusers. These investigators utilized $[^{15}O]$-labeled water to characterize the effects of cue-induced craving on rCBF. Compared with the nondrug video, cocaine abusers exhibited increased relative rCBF in amygdala and anterior cingulate following presentation of cocaine-related videos. Significant decreases in rCBF were observed in the caudate and lenticular nucleus, however. Interestingly, absolute rCBF was not different in these regions when responses of cocaine abusers and control subjects to the cocaine-related video were compared, reflecting decreased baseline rCBF values in these regions of the brains of cocaine abusers *(107)*. Similarly Maas et al. *(108)* demonstrated significant activation of anterior cingulate and dorsolateral prefrontal cortex in crack-cocaine abusers presented with drug-related audiovisual stimuli when compared to control subjects. In addition, increases in craving score were correlated with increased activation of these brain regions *(108)*.

Other studies have relied on combinations of internal and external representations of drug preparation and administration. Wang et al. *(109)* utilized structured interviews and drug paraphernalia to elicit craving in a population of cocaine users. PET scans with [^{18}F] fluorodeoxyglucose were employed to measure glucose utilization following neutral stimuli interviews and those designed to elicit cocaine craving. Whole-brain metabolism did not differ across interview conditions, however, significant increases in functional activity were observed for orbitofrontal and left insular cortices following the cocaine theme interview. Interestingly, only 7 of 13 subjects reported feelings of craving following the interview. In these subjects, the increases in metabolism in right insular cortex were significantly correlated with self-reports of craving.

The most aggressive strategy employed to date to elicit drug craving was reported by Grant et al. *(110)*. In this study, cocaine abusers were presented with drug-related paraphernalia, a video of cocaine self-administration (smoking and inhalation), and cocaine itself. Subjects were told that they would be able to self-administer (by inhalation) the cocaine at the conclusion of the experiment. Cocaine abusers exhibited increased cerebral glucose utilization in dorsolateral prefrontal, medial orbitofrontal, retrosplenial, peristriate, temporal, and temporal/parietal cortices following exposure to the drug-related stimuli compared with the neutral stimulus condition (*see* Fig. 3). Significant correlations between subjective reports of craving and changes in metabolism were demonstrated for dorsolateral prefrontal cortex, medial temporal lobe, amygdala, and cerebellum.

In summary, cue-induced craving results in activation of a number of brain structures including portions of frontal cortex (dorsolateral, anterior cingulate), amygdala, and cerebellum. These findings suggest that craving involves multiple neurobiological substrates representing various aspects of this process, including the degree of motivation for drug and the salience of the reinforcing stimuli. Further research is clearly needed to determine the specific circuits involved with each aspect of this complex behavior. This is essential for the development of therapeutic strategies for the treatment of cocaine addictions.

6. SUMMARY AND CONCLUSIONS

Neuroimaging studies have been essential for our growing understanding of the neurobiological basis of cocaine use and abuse. Studies in humans and in animal models have provided complementary information about the euphorigenic properties of cocaine that lead to its abuse, the neuroadaptations that result from continued use, the potential for recovery with continued abstinence, and the basis for one of the most difficult elements of cocaine addiction: drug craving. One important element that must always be kept in mind when evaluating human studies is the nature of the populations under study. Although it is frequently not possible to know exact drug histories, the degree of polydrug abuse, co-morbid psychiatric conditions, and age of onset of drug use, are all important factors that can significantly influence the outcomes of studies with humans. Similarly, in studies with animals, it is important to recognize what aspects of cocaine

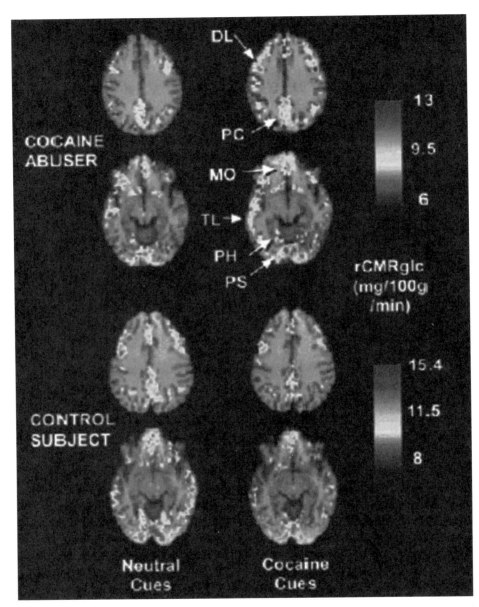

Fig. 3. Effects of neutral and cocaine cues on rates of local cerebral glucose utilization in cocaine using (upper panels) and control (lower panels) subjects. Shown are horizontal sections at two dorsoventral levels. Arrows indicate regions in which glucose utilization was increased in the cocaine group. DL, dorsolateral prefrontal cortex; PC, precuneus; PS, peristriate cortex; MO, medial orbitofrontal cortex; TL, temporal lobe; PH, parahippocampal gyrus. From ref. *(110)*, Copyright 1996, National Acacemy of Sciences, U.S.A. (*See* color plate 11 in the insert following p. 368.)

use and abuse are specifically being modeled in the paradigms chosen for investigation. Both strategies are critical if we are to develop effective means to combat substance abuse in the future.

ACKNOWLEDGMENTS

This work was supported by National Institute on Drug Abuse Grants DA09085 (LJP), DA 10230 (LJP), DA06634, DA08648 (MAN), DA10584 (MAN), and DA 05940 (CSF). We thank Stephanie Hart for her assistance in the preparation of this manuscript.

REFERENCES

1. Heikkila, R. E., Cabbot, F.S., Manzino, L., and Duvoisin, R. C. (1979) Rotational behavior induced by cocaine analogs in rats with unilateral 6-hydroxydopamine lesions of the substantia nigra: dependence upon dopamine uptake inhibition. *J. Pharmacol. Exp.* Ther. **211**, 189.
2. Moore, K. E., Chiueh, C. C., and Zeldes, G. (1977) Release of neurotransmitters from the brain in vivo by amphetamine, methylphenidate and cocaine, in *Cocaine and Other Stimulants* (Ellinwood, E. H. and Kilbey, M. M., eds.), Plenum Press, New York, pp. 143–160.
3. Hertting, G., Axelrod, J., and Whitby, L. G. (1961) Effect of drugs on the uptake and metabolism of 3H-norepinephrine. *J. Pharmacol. Exp. Ther.* **134**, 146.
4. Ross, S. F. and Renyi, A.L. (1967) Inhibition of the uptake of tritiated catecholamines by antidepressants and related agents. *Eur. J. Pharmacol.* **2**, 181.
5. Goldberg, S. R. and Kelleher, R. T. (1976) Behavior controlled by scheduled injections of cocaine in squirrel and rhesus monkeys. *J. Exp. Anal. Behav.* **25**, 93.
6. Pickens, R. and Thompson, T. (1968) Cocaine reinforced behavior in rats. Effects of reinforcement magnitude and fixed ratio size. *J. Pharmacol. Exp. Ther.* **161**, 122.
7. Colpaert, F. C., Niemegeers, J. E., Janssen, P. A. J. (1978) Neuroleptic interference with cocaine cue. Internal stimulus control of behavior and psychosis. *Psychopharmacology* **58**, 347.
8. Kilbey, M. M. and Ellinwood, E. H. (1979) Discriminative stimulus properties of psychomotor stimulants in cats. *Psychopharmacology* **63**, 151.
9. Post, R. M. and Contel, N. R. (1983) Human and animal studies of cocaine: implications for the development of behavioral pathology, in *Stimulants: Neurochemical, Behavioral and Clinical Perspectives* (Creese, I., ed.), Raven Press, New York, pp. 169–203.
10. Post, R. M. and Rose, H. (1976) Increasing effects of repetitive cocaine adminstration in the rat. *Nature* **260**, 731–732.
11. Scheel-Kruger, J. (1971) Comparative studies of various amphetamine analogues demonstrating different interactions with the metabolism of the catecholamines in the brain. *Eur. J. Pharmacol.* **14**, 47.
12. Fischman, M. W., Schuster, C. R., Rosnekov, L., Shick, J. F. E., Krasnegor, N. A., Fennell, W., and Freedman, D. X. (1976) Cardiovascular and subjective effects of intravenous cocaine administration in humans. *Arch. Gen. Psychiatry* **33**, 983.
13. Shuster, L., Quimby, F., Bates, A., and Thompson, M. L. (1977) Liver damage from cocaine in mice. *Life Sci.* **20**, 1035.
14. Roberts, D. C. S., Corcoran, M. E., and Fibiger, H. C. (1977) On the role of ascending catecholaminergic systems in intravenous self-administration of cocaine. *Pharmacol. Biochem. Behav.* **6**, 615–620.
15. Roberts, D. C. S., Koob, G. F., Klonoff, P., and Fibiger, H. C. (1980) Extinction and recovery of cocaine self-administration following 6-hydroxydopamine lesions of the nucleus accumbens. *Pharmacol. Biochem. Behav.* **12**, 781–787.

16. Pettit, H. O., Ettenberg, A., Bloom, F. E., Koob, G. F. (1984) Destruction of dopamine in the nucleus accumbens selectively attenuates cocaine but not heroin self-administration in rats. *Psychopharmacology* **84,** 167–173.
17. Roberts, D. C. (1989) Breaking points on a progressive ratio schedule reinforced by intravenous apomorphine increase daily following 6—hydroxydopamine lesions of the nucleus accumbens. *Pharmacol. Biochem. Behav.* **32,** 43–47.
18. Koob, G. F., Le, H. T., and Creese, I. (1987) The D1 dopamine receptor antagonist SCH 23390 increases cocaine self-administration in the rat. *Neurosci. Lett.* **79,** 315–320.
19. Caine, S. B. and Koob, G. F. (1994a) Effects of dopamine D-1 and D-2 antagonists on cocaine self-administration under different schedules of reinforcement in the rat. *J. Pharmacol. Exp. Ther.* **270,** 209–218.
20. Gerrits, M. A. and Van Ree, J. M. (1996) Effect of nucleus accumbens dopamine depletion on motivational aspects involved in initiation of cocaine and heroin self-administration in rats. *Brain Res.* **713,** 114–124.
21. Caine, S. B. and Koob, G. F. (1994b) Effects of mesolimbic dopamine depletion on responding maintained by cocaine and food. *J. Exp. Anal. Behav.* **61,** 213–221.
22. Phillips, A. G., Broekkamp, C. L., and Fibiger, H. C. (1983) Strategies for studying the neurochemical substrates of drug reinforcement in rodents. *Prog. Neuropsychopharm. Biol. Psychiatry* **7,** 585–590.
23. McGregor, A. and Roberts, D. C. (1993) Dopaminergic antagonism within the nucleus accumbens or the amygdala produces differential effects on intravenous cocaine self-administration under fixed and progressive ratio schedules of reinforcement. *Brain Res.* **624,** 245–252.
24. Phillips, G. D., Howes, S. R., Whitelaw, R. B., Robbins, T. W., and Everitt, B. J. (1994) Isolation rearing impairs the reinforcing efficacy of intravenous cocaine or intra-accumbens d-amphetamine: impaired response to intra-accumbens D1 and D2/D3 dopamine receptor antagonists. *Psychopharmacology* **115,** 419–429.
25. Caine, S. B., Heinrichs, S. C., Coffin, V. L., and Koob, G. F. (1995) Effects of the dopamine D-1 antagonist SCH 23390 microinjected into the accumbens, amygdala or striatum on cocaine self-administration in the rat. *Brain Res.* **692,** 47–56.
26. Roberts, D. C. S. and Koob, G. F. (1982) Disruption of cocaine self-administration following 6-hydroxydopamine lesions of the ventral tegmental area in rats. *Pharmacol. Biochem. Behav.* **17,** 901–904.
27. Pettit, H. O. and Justice, J. B., Jr. (1991) Effect of dose on cocaine self-administration behavior and dopamine levels in the nucleus accumbens. *Brain Res.* **539,** 94–102.
28. Maisonneuve, I. M. and Kreek, M. J. (1994) Acute tolerance to the dopamine response induced by a binge pattern of cocaine administration in male rats: an in vivo microdialysis study. *J. Pharmacol. Exp. Ther.* **268,** 916–921.
29. Carelli, R. M. and Deadwyler, S. A. (1994) A comparison of nucleus accumbens neuronal firing patterns during cocaine self-administration and water reinforcement in rats. *J. Neurosci.* **14,** 7735–7746.
30. Carelli, R. M. and Deadwyler, S. A. (1996a) Dual factors controlling activity of nucleus accumbens cell-firing during cocaine self-administration. *Synapse* **24,** 308–311.
31. Carelli, R. M. and Deadwyler, S. A. (1996b) Dose-dependent transitions in nucleus accumbens cell firing and behavioral responding during cocaine self-administration sessions in rats. *J. Pharmacol. Exp. Ther.* **277,** 385–393.
32. Lyons, D., Friedman, D. P., Nader, M. A., and Porrino, L. J. (1996) Cocaine alters cerebral metabolism within the ventral striatum and limbic cortex of monkeys. *J. Neurosci.* **16,** 1230–1238.
33. Bradberry, C. W., Barrett-Larimore, R. L., Jatlow, P., and Rubino, S. R. (2000) Impact of self-administered cocaine and cocaine cues on extracellular dopamine in mesolimbic and sensorimotor striatum in rhesus monkeys. *J. Neurosci.* **20,** 3874–3883.

34. Breiter, H. C., Gollub, R. L., Weisskoff, R. M., Kennedy, D. N., Makris, Berke, J. D., et al. (1997) Acute effects of cocaine on human brain activity and emotion. *Neuron* **19,** 591–611.

35. Apicella, P., Ljungberg, T., Scarnati, E., and Schultz, W. (1991) Responses to reward in monkey dorsal and ventral striatum. *Exp. Brain Res.* **85,** 491–500.

36. Schultz, W., Apicella, P., Scarnati, E., and Ljungberg, T. (1992) Neuronal activity in monkey ventral striatum related to the expectation of reward. *J. Neurosci.* **12(12),** 4595–4610.

37. Bowman, E. M., Aigner, T. G., and Richmond, B. J. (1996) Neural signals in the monkey ventral striatum related to motivation for juice and cocaine rewards. *J. Neurophysiol.* **75,** 1061–1073.

38. Gawin, F. and Klebler, H. D. (1986) Abstinence symptomatalogy and psychiatric diagnosis in cocaine abusers. *Arch. Gen. Psychiatry* **43,** 107–113.

39. Gawin, F. (1991) Cocaine addiction:psychology and neurophysiology. *Science* **251,** 1580–1589.

40. Gawin, F. (1992) Psychology, neuropsysiology, and treatment, in *Biological Basis of Substance Abuse* (Korenman, S. and Barchas, J., eds.), pp. 425–442.

41. Post, R. and Weiss, S. (1988) Psychomotor stimulant vs. local anesthetic effects of cocaine: role of behavioral sensitization and kindling, in *Mechanisms of Cocaine Abuse and Toxicity* (Clout, D., Asghar, K., and Brown, R., eds.), National Institute on Drug Abuse Monograph 88, DHHS Pub. No. (ADM) 88-1588. Washington, DC, pp. 217–238.

42. Johanson, C. and Fischman, M. (1989) The pharmacology of cocaine related to its abuse. *Pharmacol. Rev.* **41,** 3–52.

43. Reith, M. E. A., Meisler, B. E., Sershen, H., and Lajtha, A. (1986) Structural requirements for cocaine congeners to interact with dopamine and serotonin uptake sites in mouse brain and to induce stereotyped behavior. *Biochem. Pharm.* **35,** 1123–1129.

44. Ritz, M. C., Lamb, R. J., Goldberg, S. R., and Kuhar, M. J. (1987) Cocaine receptor on dopamine transporter are related to self-administration of cocaine. Science **237,** 1219–1223.

45. Fowler, J. S., Volkow, N. D., Wolf, A. P., Dewey, D., Schlyer, D., and MacGregor, R. R. (1989) Mapping cocaine binding sites in human and baboon brain in vivo. *Synapse* **4,** 371–377.

46. Biegon, A., Dillon, K., Volkow, N. D., Hitzemann, R. J., Fowler, J. S., and Wolf, A. P. (1992) Quantitative autoradiography of cocaine binding sites in human brain postmortem. *Synapse* **10,** 126–130.

47. Madras, B. K. and Kaufman, M. J. (1994) Cocaine accumulates in dopamine-rich regions of primate brain after i.v. administration: comparison with mazindol distribution. *Synapse* **18,** 261–275.

48. Volkow, N. D., Fowler, J. S., Wolf, A. P., Wang, G. J., Logan, J., MacGregor, R., et al. (1992a) Distribution and kinetics of Carbon–11-Cocaine in the human body measured with PET. *J. Nuclear Med.* **33,** 521–525.

49. Volkow, N. D., Wang, G. J., Fowler, J. S., Logan, J., Gatley, S. J., Wong, C., et al. (1999) Reinforcing effects of psychostimulants in humans are associated with increases in brain dopamine and occupancy of D2 receptors. *J. Pharmacol. Exp. Ther.* **291,** 409–415.

50. Volkow, N. D., Wang, G. J., Fowler, J. S., Logan, J., Schlyer, D., Hitzemann, R., et al. (1994) Imaging endogenous dopamine competition with [11C]raclopride in the human brain. *Synapse* **16,** 255–262.

51. Farde, L., Hall, H., Ehrin, E., and Sedvall, G. (1986) Quantitative analyses of D2-dopamine receptor binding in the living human brain by positron emission tomography. *Science* **231,** 258–260.

52. Schlaeper, T. E., Pearlson, G. D., Wong, D. F., and Dannals, R. F. (1997) PET studies of the competition between intravenous cocaine and [11C]raclopride at dopamine receptors in human subjects. *Am. J. Psychiatry* **154,** 1209–1213.

53. Volkow, N. D., Wang, G. J., Fischman, M. W., Foltin, R. W., Fowler, J. S., Abumrad, N. N., et al. (1997) Relationship between subjective effects of cocaine and dopamine transporter occupancy. *Nature* **386,** 827–830.

54. London, E. D., Cascella, N. G., Wong, D. F., Phillips, R. L., Dannals, R. F., Links, J. M., et al. (1990) Cocaine-induced reduction of glucose utilization in human brain. *Arch. Gen. Psychiatry* **47,** 567–574.

55. Morgan, M. J., Cascella, N. G., Stapleton, J. M., Phillips, R. L., Yung, B. C., Wong, D. F., et al. (1993) Sensitivity to subjective effects of cocaine in drug abusers: relationship to cerebral ventricle size. *Am. J. Psychiatry* **150,** 1712–1717.

56. Bartzokis, G., Beckson, M., Newton, T., Mandelkern, M., Mintz, J., Foster, J. A., et al. (1999) Selegiline effect on cocaine-induced changes in medial temporal lobe metabolism and subjective ratings of euphoria. *Neuropsychopharmacology* **20,** 582–590.

57. Pearlson, G. D., Jeffery, P. J., Harris, G. J., Ross, C. A., Fischman, M. W., and Camargo, E. E. (1993) Correlation of acute cocaine-induced changes in local cerebral blood flow with subjective effects. *Am. J. Psychiatry* **150,** 495–497.

58. Johnson, B., Lamki, L., Fang, B., Barron, B., Wagner, L., Wells, L., et al. (1998) Demonstration of dose-dependent global and regional cocaine-induced reductions in brain blood flow using a novel approach to quantitative single photon emission computerized tomography. *Neuropsychopharmacology* **18,** 377–384.

59. Wallace, D. R., Mactutus, C. F., and Booze, R. M. (1996) Repeated intravenous cocaine administration: locomotor activity and dopamine D2/D3 receptors. *Synapse* **23,** 152–163.

60. Sakurada, O., Kennedy, C., Jehle, J., Brown, J. D., Carbin, G. L., and Sokoloff, L. (1978) Measurement of local cerebral blood flow with iodo[14C]antipyrine. *Am. J. Physiol.* **234,** H59–H66.

61. Sokoloff, L. (1986) Cerebral circulation, energy metabolism, and protein synthesis: general characteristics and principles of measurement, in *Positron Emission Tomography and Autoradiography: Principles and Applications for the Brain and Heart* (Phelps, M., Mazziotta, J., and Shelbert, H., eds.), Raven Press, New York, pp. 1–71.

62. Kosten, T. R. (1998) Pharmacotherapy of cerebral ischemia in cocaine dependence. *Drug Alcohol Depend.* **49,** 133–44 (Review).

63. Brown, E., Prager, J., Lee, H. Y., and Ramsey, R. G. (1992) CNS complications of cocaine abuse: prevalence, pathophysiology, and neuroradiology. *AJR Am. J. Roentgenol.* **159,** 137–147 (Review).

64. Herning, R. I., Better, W., Nelson, R., Gorelick, D., and Cadet, J. L. (1999) The regulation of cerebral blood flow during intravenous cocaine administration in cocaine abusers. *Ann. NY Acad. Sci.* **890,** 489–494.

65. Johnson, B., Barron, B., Fang, B., Lamki, L., Wagner, L., Wells, L., et al. (1998) Isradipine prevents global and regional cocaine-induced changes in brain blood flow: a preliminary study. *Psychopharmacology* **136,** 335–341.

66. Gollub, R. L., Breiter, H. C., Kantor, H., Kennedy, D., Gastfriend, D., Mathew, R. T., et al. (1998) Cocaine decreases cortical cerebral blood flow but does not obscure regional activation in functional magnetic resonance imaging in human subjects. *J. Cereb. Blood Flow Metab.* **18,** 724–734.

67. Li, S. J., Biswal, B., Li, Z., Risinger, R., Rainey, C., Cho, J. K., Salmeron, B. J., and Stein, E. A. (2000) Cocaine administration decreases functional connectivity in human primary visual and motor cortex as detected by functional MRI. *Magn. Reson. Med.* **43,** 45–51.

68. Sokoloff, L., Reivich, M., Kennedy, C., Des Rosiers, M. H., Patlak, C. S., Pettigrew, K. D., et al. (1977) The 2-[14C]deoxyglucose method for the measurement of local cerebral glucose utilization: theory, procedure, and normal values for conscious and unanesthized albino rat. *J. Neurochem.* **28,** 897–916.

69. Koob, G. F. and Bloom, F. E. (1988) Cellular and molecular mechanisms of drug dependence. *Science* **242,** 715–723.

70. Schultz, W., Tremblay, L., and Hollerman, J. R. (2000) Reward processing in primate orbitofrontal cortex and basal ganglia. *Cereb. Cortex* **10,** 272–283.

71. Rolls, E. T. (2000) The orbitofrontal cortex and reward. *Cereb. Cortex* **10,** 284–294.

72. Bechara, A., Damasio, H., and Damasio, A. R. (2000) Emotion, decision making and the orbitofrontal cortex. *Cereb. Cortex* **10,** 295–307.

73. Staley, J. K., Hearn, W. L., Ruttenberg, A. J., Wetli, C. V., and Mash, D. C. (1994) High affinity cocaine recognition sites on the dopamine transporter are elevated in fatal cocaine overdose victims. *J. Pharmacol. Exp. Ther.* **271,** 1678–1685.

74. Little, K. Y., Kirkman, J. A., Carroll, F. I., Clark, T. B., and Duncan, G. E. (1993) Cocaine use increases [3H]WIN35428 binding sites in human striatum. *Brain Res.* **628,** 17–25.

75. Little, K. Y., McLaughlin, D. P., Lian, Z., McFinton, P. R., Dalak, G. W., Cook, E., et al. (1998) Brain dopamine transporter messenger RNA and binding sites in cocaine users: A postmortem study. *Arch. Am. Gen. Psych.* **55,** 793–799.

76. Little, K. Y., Zhang, L., Desmond, T., Frey, K. A., Dalack, G. W., and Cassin, B. J. (1999) Striatal dopaminergic abnormalities in human cocaine users. *Am. J. Psychiatry* **156,** 238–245.

77. Wilson, J. M., Levey, A. I., Bergeron, C., Kalasinsky, K., Ang, L., Peretti, F., et al. (1996) Striatal dopamine, dopamine transporter, and vesicular monoamine transporter in chronic cocaine users. *Ann. Neurol.* **40,** 428–439.

77a. Malison, R. T., Best, S., van Dyck, C. H., McCance, E. F., Wallace, E. A., Laruelle, M., et al. (1998) Elevated striatal dopamine transporters during abstinence as measured by 123Iß-CIT SPECT. *Am. J. Psychiatry* **155,** 832–834.

78. Hurd, Y. L. and Herkenham, M. (1993) Molecular alterations in the neostriatum of human cocaine addicts. *Synapse* **13,** 357–369.

79. Hitri, A., Karoum, F., and Wyatt, R. J. (1995) Questions about the dopamine terminals in human frontal cortex. *J. Neurochem.* **64,** 1901–1902.

80. Letchworth, S. R., Nader, M. A., Smith, H. R., Friedman, D. P., and Porrino, L. J. (2000) Progression of changes in dopamine transporter binding site density as a result of cocaine self-administration in rhesus monkeys. *J. Neurosci.* **21,** 2799–2807.

81. Volkow, N. D., Fowler, J. S., Wolf, A. P., Schlyer, D. S., Shiue, C.-Y., Alpert, R., et al. (1990) Effects of chronic cocaine abuse on postsynaptic dopamine receptors. *Am. J. Psychiatry* **147,** 719–724.

82. Volkow, N. D., Fowler, J. S., Wang, G.-J., Hitzemann, R., Logan, J., Schlyer, D. J., et al. (1993) Decreased dopamine D2 receptor availability is associated with reduced frontal metabolism in cocaine abusers. *Synapse* **14,** 169–177.

83. Staley, J. K. and Mash, D. C. (1996) Adaptive increase in D3 dopamine receptors in the brain reward circuits of human cocaine fatalities. *J. Neurosci.* **16,** 6100–6106.

84. Meador-Woodruff, J. H., Little, K. Y., Damask, S. P., Mansour, A., and Watson, S. J. (1993) Effects of cocaine on dopamine receptor gene expression: a study in the postmortem human brain. *Biol. Psychiatry* **34,** 348–355.

85. Farfel, G. M., Kleven, M. S., Woolverton, W. L., Seiden, L. S., and Perry, B. D. (1992) Effects of repeated injections of cocaine on catecholamine receptor binding sites, dopamine transporter binding sites and behavior in rhesus monkey. *Brain Res.* **578,** 235–243.

86. Dworkin, S. I., Mirkis, S., Smith, J. E. (1995) Response-dependent versus response-independent presentation of cocaine: differences in the lethal effects of the drug. *Psychopharmacology* **117,** 262–266.

87. Morgan, D., Grant, K. A., Mach, R. H., Gage, H. D., Ehrenkaufer, R. L., Kaplan, J. R., et al. (Submitted) Brain imaging in monkeys: effects of social dominance on dopamine D2 receptors. *Proc. Natl. Acad. Sci. USA.*

88. Moore, R. J., Vinsant, S. L., Nader, M. A., Porrino, L. J., and Friedman, D. P. (1998a) The effect of cocaine self-administration on striatal dopamine D1 receptors in rhesus monkeys. *Synapse* **28,** 1–9.

89. Moore, R. J., Vinsant, S. L., Nader, M. A., Porrino, L. J., and Friedman, D. P. (1998b) Effect of cocaine self-administration on dopamine D2 receptors in rhesus monkeys. *Synapse* **30,** 88–96.

90. Nader, M. A., Daunais, J., Moore T, Nader, S. H., Moore, R., Lyons, D., Friedman, D. P., and Porrino, L. J. (2000a) Effects of long-term cocaine self-administration on mesolimbic and nigrostriatal dopamine systems in rhesus monkeys. In preparation.

91. Nader, M. A., Mach, R. H., Nader, S. H., Moore, T., Gage, H. D., and Buchheimer, N. (2000b) Manuscript in preparation.

92. Mach, R. H., Nader, M. A., Ehrenkaufer, R. L. E., Line, S. W., Smith, C. R., Luedtke, R. R., et al. (1996) A comparison of two fluorine–18 labeled benzamide derivatives that bind reversibly to dopamine D2 receptors: in vitro binding studies and positron emission tomography. *Synapse* **24,** 322–333.

93. Mach, R. H., Nader, M. A., Ehrenkaufer, R. L. E., Line, S. W., Smith, C. R., Gage, H. D., and Morton, T. E. (1997) The use of positron emission tomography to study the dynamics of psychostimulant-induced dopamine release. *Pharmacol. Biochem. Behav.* **57,** 477–486.

94. Volkow, N. D., Mullani, N., Gould, K. L., Adler, S., and Krajewski, K. (1988) Cerebral blood flow in chronic cocaine users: a study with positron emission tomography. *Br. J. Psychiatry* **152,** 641–648.

95. Volkow, N. D., Fowler, J. S., Wolf, A. P., Hitzemann, R., Dewey, S., Bendriem, B., et al. (1991) Changes in brain glucose metabolism in cocaine dependence and withdrawal. *Am. J. Psychiatry* **148,** 621–626.

96. Volkow, N. D., Wang, G. J., Fowler, J. S., Hitzemann, R., Gatley, S. J., Dewey, S. S., and Pappas, N. (1998) Enhanced sensitivity to benzodiazepines in active cocaine-abusing subjects: a PET study. *Am. J. Psychiatry* **155,** 200–206.

97. Volkow, N. D., Wang, G. J., Fowler, J. S., Franceschi, D., Thanos, P. K., Wong, C., et al. (2000) Cocaine abusers show a blunted response to alcohol intoxication in limbic brain regions. *Pharmacol. Lett.* **66,** 161–167.

98. Tumeh, S. S., Nagel, J. S., English, R. J., Moore, M., and Holman, B. L. (1990) Cerebral abnormalities in cocaine abusers: demonstration by SPECT perfusion brain scintigraphy. *Radiology* **176,** 821–824.

99. Weber, D. A., Franceschi, D., Ivanovic, M., Atkins, H. L., Cabahug, C., Wong, C. T. C., and Susskind, H. (1993) SPECT and planar brain imaging in crack abuse: Iodine-123-iodoamphetamine uptake and localization. *J. Nucl. Med.* **4,** 899–907.

100. Holman, B. L., Mendelson, J., Garada, B., Teoh, S. K., Hallgring, E., Johnson, K. A., and Mello, N. K (1993) Regional cerebral blood flow improves with treatment in chronic cocaine polydrug users. *J. Nuclear Med.* **34,** 723–727.

101. Kosten, T. R., Cheeves, C., Palumbo, J., Seibyl, J. P., Price, L. H., and Woods, S. W. (1998) Regional cerebral blood flow during acute and chronic abstinence from combined cocaine-alcohol abuse. *Drug Alcohol Depend.* **50,** 187–195.

102. Volkow, N. D., Hitzemann, R., Wang, G. J., Fowler, J. S., Wolf, A. P., Dewey, S. L., and Handlesman, L. (1992b) Long-term frontal brain metabolic changes in cocaine abusers. *Synapse* **11,** 184–190.

103. Porrino, L. J. and Lyons, D. (2000) Orbital and medial prefrontal cortex and psychomotor stimulants abuse: studies in animal models. *Cereb. Cortex* **10,** 326–333.

104. Bartzokis, G., Beckson, M., Lu, P. H., Edwards, N., Rapoport, R., Wiseman, E., and Bridge, P. (2000) Age-related brain volume reductions in amphetamine and cocaine addicts and normal controls: implications for addiction research. *Psychiatry Res.* **98,** 93–102.

105. Wallace, B. C. (1989) Psychological and environmental determinants of relapse in crack cocaine smokers. *J. Subst. Abuse Treat.* **6,** 95–106.

106. Gawin, F. H. and Khalsa-Denison, M. E. (1996) Is craving mood-driven or self-propelled? Sensitization and "street" stimulant addiction. *NIDA Res. Monogr.* **163,** 224–250.

107. Childress, A. R., Mozley, P. D., McElgin, W., Fitzgerald, J., Reivich, M., and O'Brien, C. P. (1999) Limbic activation during cue-induced cocaine craving. *Am. J. Psychiatry* **156(1),** 11–18.

108. Mass, L. C., Lukas, S. E., Kaufman, M. J., Weiss, R. D., Daniels, S. L., Rogers, V. W., et al. (1998) Functional magnetic resonance imaging of human brain ativation during cue-induced cocaine craving. *Am. J. Psychiatry* **155,** 124–126.

109. Wang, G. J., Volkow, N. D., Fowler, J. S., Cervany, P, Hitzemann, R. J., Pappas, N. R., et al. (1999) Regional brain metabolic activation during craving elicited by recall of previous drug experiences. *Life Sci.* **64,** 775–784.

110. Grant, S., London, E. D., Newlin, D. B., Villemagne, V. L., Liu, X., Contoreggi, C., et al. (1996) Activation of memory circuits during cue-elicited cocaine craving. *Proc. Natl. Acad. Sci. USA* **93,** 12,040–12,045.

17

Functional Neuroimaging of Cannabinoid Effects

Godfrey D. Pearson

1. BACKGROUND

Marijuana continues to be the most frequently abused illicit drug in America, despite modest declines from the height of its use in the mid-1970s. Approximately 70% of adults between the ages of 27 and 32 have used marijuana recreationally during their lifetime. Hollister *(1)* and Dornbush *(2)*, respectively, showed that delta 9-tetrahydro-cannabinol (THC), is the principal psycho-pharmacologically active component of marijuana, and its effects are dose and blood level dependent *(3)*.

Marijuana has multiple and complex effects on mood, cognition, and behavior *(4–6)*. Different routes of administration (oral ingestion, intravenous injection, and smoking) of marijuana produce different behavioral and subjective effects *(7,8)*. Acute impairment (and metabolism) patterns are also influenced by casual vs heavy regular use *(9–11)*. Following acute doses sufficient to produce a moderate level of intoxication/euphoria, THC impairs multiple aspects of cognitive and psychomotor performance (e.g., *see* ref. *12*; for a critical overview, *see* ref. *13*). Marijuana is now being considered for use as a therapeutic agent for symptoms associated with AIDS, cancer, glaucoma, and multiple sclerosis (MS) (*see* review of ref. *14*). The American Medical Association (AMA) is urging federal funding of research to determine the validity of marijuana as an effective medical treatment and to further evaluate the abuse potential of this drug. Already, an oral form of synthetically derived THC, dronabinol (Marinol), is available by prescription as an appetite enhancer for cachectic patients.

There is a need to clarify the relationship between the neurobiology and cognitive/behavioral effects produced by THC and other cannabinoids as these drugs become more widely used both legally and illegally. Neuroimaging techniques continue to play an important role in this enterprise.

2. NEUROBIOLOGY OF CANNABINOIDS AND THEIR RECEPTORS

As recently reviewed *(15,16)*, Devane *(17,18)* identified and characterized the cannabinoid receptor in the central nervous system (CNS) and later described a naturally occurring cannabinoid ligand, "anandamide," with pharmacologic properties similar to delta-9-THC. Subsequent research found a peripheral cannabinoid receptor *(19)* and

From: Handbook of Neurotoxicology, Vol. 2
Edited by: E. J. Massaro © Humana Press Inc., Totowa, NJ

Table 1
Review of Prior Studies of Effects of Marijuana on Cerebral Blood Flow and Metabolism

Brain region	Marijuana effect	References
Generalized effects	↑Overall cortical rCBF	(39,43,46)
Cerebellum	↑rCGM	(36,47[a])
	↑rCBF (L side)	(44)[a]
	↓rCGM or rCBF at baseline in chronic users	(36,48)
	Mixed effects on rCBF	(46)
Prefrontal cortex	↑rCGM	(36)[b]
	↑rCBF	(44[a],49)
Orbito-frontal cortex	↑rCGM	(36)[b]
R Inferior frontal cortex	↓rCBF	(44)[a]
Anterior cingulate	↑rCBF	(44[a],49)
Insula	↑rCBF	(49)
Basal ganglia	↑rCGM	(36[b],49)
Hippocampus/amygdala	↓rCBF	(44)
L Inferior temporal cortex	↑rCBF	(44)[a]

[a]Correlated with THC blood level.
[b]Effects seen in marijuana abusers only.
rCGM, regional cerebral glucose metabolism; rCBF, regional cerebral blood flow.

additional subtypes of endogenous cannabinoid ligands *(20)*. The central receptor, termed CB1, is widely expressed in the brain *(21)* with high concentrations in the molecular layers of the cerebellum *(18,22,23)*. Herkenham *(22,23)* found also recorded numerous anandamide receptors in hippocampus, globus pallidus, and substantia nigra (SN) pars reticulata.

The putative endogenous ligands anandamide and 2-AG can be identified in the brain and their neurophysiology is an area of active exploration. Cannabinoids probably influence traditional neurotransmitter systems (Dewey 1986, Pertwee 1988, 1992) and cannabinoid receptors occur in regions associated with mediating brain reward.

3. BRAIN CHANGES: ANIMALS

In laboratory animals, administered THC has varied effects on cerebral metabolism or blood flow, including decreased regional cerebral blood flow (rCBF) in hippocampus, prefrontal cortex and nucleus accumbens (NAcc), but not most cortical regions or cerebellum *(27,28)*.

In contrast, THC is reported to lead to biphasic, dose-related increases in 2-deoxy D-glucose uptake in many limbic and cortical regions at low doses but decreased metabolism in these regions at higher doses, with particular hippocampal-dose sensitivity *(29)*. Scallet (30), and Landfield et al. *(31)* studied the long-term effects of cannabinoids on mammalian brain structure. The latter results raise the possibility that chronic THC exposure may alter hippocampal anatomical structure by interaction with, or mimicry of, adrenal steroid activity. Recent structural-imaging studies *(32)* suggest that early adolescent human use can lead to structural brain changes.

Following the IV administration of radiolabeled THC or analogs, significant regional uptake occurs in basal ganglia, thalamus, and cerebellum of baboon brain, with subsequent rapid clearance *(33)*. Similar preliminary data exist for mouse and human *(34,35)* although optimal ligands for human in vivo imaging still await development.

4. BRAIN CHANGES: HUMANS

As summarized in Table 1, functional brain scanning has been used to study effects on rCBF and metabolism of both chronic marijuana use *(31,36)* and acute changes during temporary THC intoxication *(33,36–45)*.

In initial human studies, Mathew et al. *(39)* reported that acute cannabis exposure in inexperienced users produced global CBF decreases, whereas in experienced users CBF increased in both hemispheres, especially in frontal and left temporal regions. CBF decreases in inexperienced subjects were interpreted as an accompaniment of the increased anxiety that they experienced following cannabis administration, whereas the increased CBF in experienced users was attributed to pharmacological effects of cannabis. This increased blood flow correlated with their intoxication levels (Mathew 1992) *(see* below). A potential confound with marijuana and related compounds is their ability to relax vascular smooth muscle and cause vasodilatation, which could possibly be misinterpreted as a primary functional cerebral change. However, there is no evidence for disproportionate local effects in this regard *(49)*.

However, Volkow and Fowler *(50)* found that very infrequent (about once yearly) users of marijuana had increased metabolic activity in the cerebellum and pre-frontal cortex following drug administration. In particular, these subjects' subjective sense of intoxication correlated with the degree of increased metabolism in the cerebellar cortex. Chronic users showed less marked regional metabolic changes and fewer subjective effects following drug, likely reflecting tolerance. Volkow *(36)* reported that marijuana abusers at baseline (i.e., prior to experimental drug administration) showed lower relative cerebellar metabolism than normal subjects. This can sensibly be interpreted as a "rebound" effect from chronic drug-induced metabolic increases, and is consistent with other reports of decreased cerebellar rCBF or rCGM at baseline in chronic users *(47,48)*. Volkow *(36)* reported that THC tended to increase relative cerebellar metabolism in both frequent and infrequent users, but only frequent marijuana abusers showed increases in orbitofrontal cortex, prefrontal cortex, and basal ganglia.

As shown in Table 2, some research has documented correlational relationships between the regional brain changes and the subjective effects provoked by the drug. In turn associations are recorded between plasma levels of drug or metabolite and either regional brain or subjective changes.

For example, Volkow *(47)* reported correlations between increased metabolic activity in the cerebellum, the subjective sense of THC intoxication, and plasma THC concentrations, and Mathew et al. *(46,49)* reported cerebellar changes were correlated with altered time sense after marijuana administration. Mathew and Wilson *(43)* reported a significant bilateral increase in CBF especially in the frontal regions and in cerebral blood velocity. The CBF increase was not related to plasma levels of THC, changes in general or extracranial circulation, or respiration. On the other hand, behavioral changes showed significant correlations with CBF. Changes in CBF in frontal and temporal regions particularly on the right side, were most heavily correlated with a pattern of

Table 2
Review of Studies of Effects of Marijuana Where Regionally Altered Cerebral Blood Flow or Metabolism Correlated with Subjective Effects

Brain region	Intoxication	Time alteration	Depersonalization
Cerebellum	*(36,44)*	*(46,49)*↓	
Prefrontal cortex	*(49)*↑(R)	*(44)*↑(L), *(49)* (R)	*(51)*↑(R) *(49)*
Orbito-frontal cortex			
R inferior frontal cortex	*(44)*↓		
Anterior cingulate	*(49)*↑	*(44)*↑(R)	*(51)*↑
Insula	*(49)*↑		
Basal ganglia			
Hippocampus/amygdala	*(44)*↓	*(49)*↓	
R temporal cortex		*(44)*↑, *(49)*	*(49)*
L occipital cortex	*(44)*↑		

L, left; R, right.

depersonalization, confusion, and temporal disintegration. Mathew et al. *(46)* linked decreased cerebellar blood flow after intravenous THC infusion with altered time sense. Other reports from this group *(51)* found THC-induced increased right frontal and anterior cingulate flow to be associated with depersonalization and Mathew et al. *(49)* reported a correlational relationship between lower hippocampal blood flow and subjective intoxication.

The Mathew et al. *(46,49)* studies cited earlier demonstrated these rCBF changes following intravenous THC in large numbers of well-characterized subjects with rCBF measures taken at several time points, although each subject was tested in only one condition and not used as his or her own control.

Pearlson et al. *(45)* examined effects of orally administered THC in 2 doses and placebo in a double-blind, randomized fashion in six marijuana-naïve healthy volunteers in three separate sessions. All possible dose-order combinations were used. Performance on several cognitive tasks was assessed, and 2.5 h after drug administration (capturing maximal clinical effects), five oxygen-15 PET scans were performed to assess rCBF. Three stimulus conditions pertained on each study day: "baseline" (low sensory stimulation), passive tone listening, and tone-activated time estimation. Subjective assessments of drug effect were also obtained. All subjects reported dose-related intoxication. CBF patterns following THC accorded with prior reports of cerebellar and prefrontal increases as well as limbic decreases. Time estimation in the drug-free state activated frontal, cerebellar, and limbic regions, as previously hypothesized. THC affected time estimation adversely. CBF patterns during time estimation on drug differed from those provoked by both drug-free time estimation and from THC alone, strongly suggesting a task-by-drug interaction. Activation patterns correlated with degree of analog self-rated intoxication in the left and right medial frontal regions, left occipital areas, and both anterior and posterior left cerebellum. Regions in which reduced rCBF activation correlated with subjective intoxication were amygdala and hippocampus, right inferior and medial frontal gyri, right anterior and posterior cingulate. These findings are in general agreement with those of those of Mathew et al. *(46,49,51)*, where activation correlated with subjective intoxication in portions of cerebellum and prefrontal cortex.

Thus, as summarized in Table 1, THC administration in humans in various forms and by various routes is most associated with reports of increased cerebellar metabolism *(36,47)*, and of metabolic increases in pre- and orbito-frontal regions and basal ganglia. There are generally similar increases (or in some cases, e.g., ref. *46*, reports of mixed effects) on rCBF. The rCBF increases include global *(39–43,46)*, and regional changes, especially in the cerebellum *(45)*, although not always reaching significance *(46,49)*, right hemisphere, portions of the frontal lobes and anterior cingulate *(46,49)*. Other sites of reported change include basal ganglia *(36,45,49)*, as well as amygdala/hippocampal and inferior frontal rCBF decreases *(45)*.

Based on the aforementioned evidence, and localization of cannabinoid receptors, is reasonable to hypothesize also that cerebral activation changes that are (1) from THC administration, (2) correlated with THC blood levels, and (3) associated with THC-induced intoxication share commonalities of cerebral location, related to known sites of numerous brain cannabinoid receptors.

Tentatively, some of these regional effects may also correlate with behavioral effects of cannabinoids (e.g., cerebellum/coordination, frontal lobe/disinhibition, hippocampus/memory).

Effects of THC on cognition, subjective sensations, and CBF and metabolism are clearly complex and not entirely consistent among prior investigations. (For general comments on relevant research design, *see* Friston et al. *[52]*). In part this is due to various nonoptimal or noncomparable design aspects to some of the aforementioned studies, including relatively low subject numbers, recruitment of subjects with very varied experience with the drug (ranging from very frequent use to none) (*see* relevant comments, ref. *10*), and use of various THC routes of administration (oral, smoked, or intravenous) (*see* ref. *53*) that do not necessarily represent naturalistic use. Other design differences between studies include variation in administered drug doses, the fact that some investigations used subjects as their own controls while others did not, as well as wide differences in data analytic designs. Potential problems with the latter include restriction of regions of interest to a few, often nonautomated (e.g., hand-traced) predetermined areas, and in most studies an absence of pixel-by-pixel comparisons to determine brain-wide correlations. Measures of altered cognitive or self-report variables have not always been objective, (e.g., only nonquantitative, subjective self-reports). Finally, it is clear that there is a likely dose-dependency to many metabolic or blood-flow effects in animal models, that is probably also true in humans, although few studies have explored dose-response relationships thoroughly.

ACKNOWLEDGMENTS

This work was supported by a grant from the Outpatient General Clinical Research Center (RR 00722) to GP. Data discussed in this chapter were presented in part at the 1999 American College of Neuropsychopharmacology meeting in Puerto Rico.

REFERENCES

1. Hollister, L. E. (1971) Actions of various marijuana derivatives in man. *Pharmacol. Rev.* **23**, 349–357.
2. Dornbush, R. L., Fink, M., and Freedman, A. M. (1971) Marijuana, memory, and perception. *Am. J. Psychiatry* **128**, 194–197.
3. Ford, R. D., Balster, R. L., Dewey, W. L., and Beckner, J. S. (1977) Delta 9-THC and 11-OH-delta 9-THC: behavioral effects and relationship to plasma and brain levels. *Life Sci.* **20**, 1993–2003.
4. Cone, E. J., Johnson, R. E., Moore, J. D., and Roache, J. D. (1986): Acute effects of smoking marijuana on hormones, subjective effects and performance in male human subjects. *Pharmacol. Biochem. Behav.* **24**, 1749–1754.
5. Stillman, R., Galanter, M., Lemberger, L., Fox, S., Weingartner, H., and Wyatt, R. J. (1976) Tetrahydrocannabinol (THC): metabolism and subjective effects. *Life Sci.* **19**, 569–576.
6. Kelly, T. H., Foltin, R. W., Emurian, C. S., and Fischman, M. W. (1990): Multidimensional behavioral effects of marijuana. *Prog. Neuropsychopharmacol. Biol. Psychiatry* **4**, 885–902.
7. Cohen, S. (1981): Adverse effects of marijuana: selected issues. *Ann. NY Acad. Sci.* **362**, 119–124.
8. Chesher, G. B., Bird, K. D., Jackson, D. M., Perrignon, A., and Starmer, G. A. (1990) The effects of orally administered delta 9-tetrahydrocannabinol in man on mood and performance measures: a dose-response study. *Pharmacol. Biochem. Behav.* **35**, 861–864.
9. Casswell, S. and Marks, D. (1973) Cannabis induced impairment of performance of a divided attention task. *Nature* **241**, 60–61.
10. Kelly, P. and Jones, R. T. (1992) Metabolism of tetrahydrocannabinol in frequent and infrequent marijuana users. *J. Anal. Toxicol.* **16**, 228–235.
11. Perez-Reyes, M. (1990): Marijuana smoking: factors that influence the bioavailability of tetrahydrocannabinol. *NIDA Res. Monogr.* **99**, 42–62.
12. Clark, L. D., Hughes, R., and Nakashima, E. N. (1970) Behavioral effects of marijuana: experimental studies. *Arch. Gen. Psychiatry* **23**, 193–198.
13. Chait, L. D. and Pierri, J. (1992) Effects of smoked marijuana on human performance: a critical review, in *Marijuana/Cannabinoids: Neurobiology and Neurophysiology* (Murphy, L. and Bartke, S., eds.), CRC Press, Boca Raton, pp. 387–423.
14. Watson, S. J., Benson, J. A., Jr., and Joy, J. E. (2000) Marijuana and medicine: assessing the science base. *Arch. Gen. Psychiatry* **57**, 547–552.
15. Musty, R. E., Reggio, P., and Consroe, P. (1995) A review of recent advances in cannabinoid research and the 1994 International Symposium on Cannabis and the Cannabinoids. *Life Sci.* **56**, 1933–1940.
16. Adams, I. B. and Martin, B. R. (1996) Cannabis: pharmacology and toxicology in animals and humans. *Addiction* **91**, 1585–1614.
17. Devane, W. A., Dysarz, F. A., Johnson, M. R., Melvin, L. S., and Howlett, A. C. (1988). Determination and characterization of a cannabinoid receptor in rat brain. *Mol. Pharmacol.* **34**, 605–613.
18. Devane, W. A., Hanus, L., Breuer, A., Pertwee, R. G., Stevenson, L. A., Griffen, G., et al. (1992) Isolation and structure of a brain constituent that binds to the cannabinoid receptor. *Science* **258**, 1946–1949.
19. Munro, S., Thomas, K. L., and Abu-Shaar, M. (1993). Molecular characterization of peripheral receptor for cannabinoids. *Nature* **365**, 61–64.
20. Mechoulam, R., Ben-Schabat, S., Hanus, L., Ligumsky, M., Kaminiski, N. E., Schatz, A. R., et ak, (1995) Identification of an endogeneous 2-monoglyceride, present in canine gut, that binds to cannabinoid receptors. *Biochem. Pharmacol.* **50**, 83–90.
21. Onaivi, E. S., Chakrabarti, A., and Chaudhuri, G. (1996) Cannabinoid receptor genes. *Prog. Neurobiol.* **48**, 275–305.

22. Herkenham, M., Lynn, A. B., Little, M. D., Ross-Johnson, M., Melvin, L. S., DeCosta, B. R., and Rice, K. C. (1990) Cannabinoid receptor localization in brain. *Proc. Natl. Acad. Sci. USA* **87,** 1932–1936.

23. Herkenham, M. (1995) Localization of cannabinoid receptors in brain and periphery, in *Cannabinoid Receptors* (Pertwee, R. G., ed.), Academic Press Orlando, FL, pp. 145–166.

24. Dewey, W. L. (1986) Cannabinoid pharmacology. *Pharmacol. Rev.* **38,** 151–178.

25. Pertwee, R. G. (1988) The central neuropharmacology of psychotropic cannabinoids. *Pharmacol. Ther.* **36,** 189–261.

26. Pertwee, R. (1992) In vivo interactions between psychotropic cannabinoids and other drugs involving central and peripheral neurochemical mediators, in *Marihuana/Cannabinoids: Neurobiology and Neurophysiology* (Murphy, L. and Bartke, A., eds.), CRC Press, Boca Raton, FL, pp. 165–218.

27. Bloom, A. S., Tershner, S., Fuller, S. A., and Stein, E. A. (1997) Cannabinoid-induced alterations in regional cerebral blood flow in the rat. *Pharmol. Biochem. Behav.* **57,** 625–631.

28. Goldman, H., Dagirmanjian, R., Drew, W. G., and Murphy, S. (1975) D9-tetrahydrocannabinol alters flow of blood to subcortical areas of the conscious rat brain. *Life Sci.* **17,** 477–482.

29. Margulies, J. E. and Hammer, R. P., Jr. (1991) Delta 9-tetrahydrocannabinol alters cerebral metabolism in a biphasic, dose-dependent manner in rat brain. *Eur. J. Pharmacol.* **202,** 373–378.

30. Scallet, A. C., Uemura, E., Andrews, A., Ali, S. F., McMillan, D. E., Paule, M. G., et al. (1987) Morphometric studies of the rat hippocampus following chronic delta-9-tetrahydrocannabinol (THC). *Brain Res.* **436,** 193–198.

31. Landfield, P. W., Cadwallader, L. B., and Vinsant, S. (1988) Quantitative changes in hippocampal structure following long-term exposure to delta-9-tetrahydrocannabinol: Possible mediation by glucocorticoid systems. *Brain Res.* **443,** 47–62.

32. Wilson, W., Mathew, R., Turkington, T., Hawk, T., Coleman, R. E., and Provenzale, J. (2000) Brain morphological changes and early marijuana use: a magnetic resonance and positron emission tomography study. *J. Addict. Dis.* **19,** 1–22.

33. Charalambous, A., Marciniak, G., Shiue, C. Y., Dewey, S. L., Schlyer, D. J., Wolf, A. P., and Makriyannis, A. (1991) PET studies in the primate brain and biodistribution in mice using (-)-5'-18F-Delta 8-THC. *Pharmacol. Biochem. Behav.* **40,** 503–507.

34. Gatley, S. J., Gifford, A. N., Volkow, N. D., Lan, R., and Makriyannis, A. (1996) 123I-Labeled AM251: a radioiodinated ligand which binds in vivo to mouse brain cannabinoid CB1 receptors. *Eur. J. Pharmacol.* **307,** 331–338.

35. Gatley, S. J., Lan, R., Volkow, N. D., Pappas, N., King, P., Wong, C. T., et al. (1998) Imaging the brain marijuana receptor: Development of a radioligand that binds to cannabinoid CB1 receptors in vivo. *J. Neurochem.* **70,** 417–423.

36. Volkow, N. D., Gillespie, H., Mullani, N., Tancredi, L., Grant, C., Valentine, A., and Hollister, L. (1996): Brain glucose metabolism in chronic marijuana users at baseline and during marijuana intoxication. *Psychiatry Res.* **67,** 29–38.

37. Mathew, R. J., Wilson, W. H., and Tant, S. R. (1989) Acute changes in cerebral blood flow associated with marijuana smoking. *Acta Psychiatrica Scand.* **79,** 118–128.

38. Mathew, R. J. and Wilson, W. H. (1991). Substance abuse and cerebral blood flow. *Am. J. Psychiatry* **148,** 292–305.

39. Mathew, R. J., Wilson, W. H., Humphreys, D. F., Lowe, J. V., and Wiethe, K. E. (1992a) Regional cerebral blood flow after marijuana smoking. *J. Cereb. Blood Flow Metab.* **12,** 750–758.

40. Mathew, R. J., Wilson, W. H., and Melges, F. T. (1992b) Temporal disintegration and its psychological and physiological correlates: changes in the experience of time after marijuana smoking. *Ann. Clin. Psychiatry* **4,** 235–245.

41. Mathew, R. J., Wilson, W. H., Humphreys, D., Lowe, J. V., and Wiethe, K. E. (1992c) Middle cerebral artery velocity during upright posture after marijuana smoking. *Acta Psychiatrica Scand.* **86,** 173–178.

42. Mathew, R. J., Wilson, W. H., Humphreys, D. F., Lowe, J. V., and Wiethe, K. E. (1992d): Changes in middle cerebral artery velocity after marijuana. *Biol. Psychiatry* **32,** 164–169.

43. Mathew, R. J. and Wilson, W. H. (1993) Acute changes in cerebral blood flow after smoking marijuana. *Life Sci.* **52,** 757–767.

44. Pearlson, G. D., Calhoun, V. D., Grygorcewicz, M., McGinty, V., and Kraut, M. (1999). Driving while intoxicated: An fMRI study with THC. American College of Neuropsychopharmacology. 38th Annual Meeting, Research Abstract 63, 122, Vanderbilt University School of Medicine, Nashville, TN.

45. Pearlson, G. D., Calhoun, V. D., Grygorcewicz, M., Schlaepfer, T. E., Nicastri, S., Stephane, M., et al. (2000) Effects of oral delta 9-tetrahydrocannabinol (THC), (Marinol) on time estimation, subjective intoxication and PET measures of regional cerebral bloodflow. *Neuropsychopharmacology*, in press.

46. Mathew, R. J., Wilson, W. H., Turkington, T. G., and Coleman, R. E. (1998) Cerebellar activity and disturbed time sense after THC. *Brain Res.* **797,** 183–189.

47. Volkow, N. D., Gillespie, H., Mullani, N., Tancredi, L., Grant, C., Ivanovic, M., and Hollister, L. (1991b) Cerebellar metabolic activation by delta-9-tetrahydro-cannabinol in human brain: a study with positron emission tomography and 18F-2-fluoro-2-deoxyglucose. *Psychiatry Res.* **40,** 69–78.

48. Block, R. I., O'Leary, D. S., Hichwa, R. D., Augustinack, J. C., Ponto, L. L., Ghoneim, M. M., et al. (2000) Cerebellar hypoactivity in frequent marijuana users. *NeuroReport* **11,** 749–753.

49. Mathew, R. J., Wilson, W. H., Coleman, R. E., Turkington, T. G., and DeGrado, T. R. (1997) Marijuana intoxication and brain activation in marijuana smokers. *Life Sci.* **60,** 2075–2089.

50. Volkow, N. D. and Fowler, J. S. (1993). Use of positron emission tomography to study drugs of abuse, in *Cannabis: Physiopathology, Epidemiology, Detection* (Nahas, C. G. and Latour, C., eds.), CRC Press, Boca Raton, FL, pp. 21–43.

51. Mathew, R. J., Wilson, W. H., Chiu, N. Y., Turkington, T. G., Degrado, T. R., and Coleman, R. E. (1999) Cerebral blood flow and depersonalization after tetrahydrocannabinol administration. *Acta Psychiatrica Scand.* **100,** 67–75.

52. Friston, K. J., Grasby, P. M., Bench, C. J., Frith, C. D., Cowen, P. J., Liddle, P. F., et al. (1992) Measuring the neuromodulatory effects of drugs in man with positron emission tomography. *Neurosci. Lett.* **141,** 106–110.

53. Mattes, R. D., Shaw, L. M., Edling-Owens, J., Engelman, K., and El Sohly, M. A. (1993) Bypassing the first-pass effect for the therapeutic use of cannabinoids. *Pharmacol. Biochem. Behav.* **44,** 745–747.

18

Neuroimaging of MDMA-Induced Neurotoxicity

Una D. McCann, Zsolt Szabo, and George A. Ricaurte

1. INTRODUCTION

(±) 3,4-Methylenedioxymethamphetamine (MDMA, "Ecstasy") is an increasingly popular drug of abuse in the United States, Europe, and Australia *(1–3)*. MDMA is a synthetic amphetamine analog that bears structural similarity to both the psychomotor stimulant, amphetamine, and the hallucinogen, mescaline. MDMA users report that in addition to having some stimulant and hallucinogenic effects, MDMA has unique qualities distinct from both of these drug classes *(4)*. Although it has been suggested that MDMA has potential therapeutic effects that may be useful in psychotherapy *(5)*, it is primarily used illicitly, in the setting of the "club" scene at dance parties known as "raves." In this venue, some MDMA users report using as much as 10 doses of MDMA in any given night *(6)*. In the present chapter, we will first briefly review the pharmacology of MDMA and evidence that it produces selective neurotoxicity toward brain serotonin (5-HT) neurons. We will then focus the discussion on recent efforts to detect MDMA-induced 5-HT injury using neuroimaging techniques and directions for future research endeavors.

2. PHARMACOLOGY

2.1. Neurochemistry

The most pronounced acute biochemical effect of MDMA is calcium-independent release of 5-HT from brain-serotonin neurons *(7,8)*, via vesicular and plasma membrane monoamine transporters *(9)*. MDMA also induces release of dopamine (DA) *(10–12)*. Like other amphetamines, and in contrast to classic hallucinogens, MDMA's acute neurochemical actions are primarily indirect, rather than mediated directly at postsynaptic 5-HT receptors *(13)*.

Although MDMA's primary effects are believed to be indirect, it does bind to a number of postsynaptic receptor sites *(14,15)*. Racemic MDMA's affinity is greatest for the serotonin transporter (SERT), followed in turn by the 5-HT2A receptor, the a-2 adrenergic receptor, the 5-HT2 receptor, the histamine H1 receptor, and the muscarinic M1 receptor. Binding potency at other 5-HT and adrenergic receptors, DA receptors, opioid receptors, and benzodiazepine receptors is 10 mM or higher *(14)*.

From: Handbook of Neurotoxicology, Vol. 2
Edited by: E. J. Massaro © Humana Press Inc., Totowa, NJ

2.2. Behavioral Effects

In animals, MDMA administration leads to typical signs of sympathomimetic stimulation *(16–18)*, although some behavioral studies suggest that MDMA can be distinguished from typical stimulants *(19,20)*. Consistent with observable behavioral effects, in drug-discrimination studies, MDMA substitutes for *d*-amphetamine in rats *(21)*, pigeons *(22)*, and monkeys trained to discriminate *d*-amphetamine from saline *(23)*. Despite structural similarities to mescaline, MDMA does not substitute for the potent hallucinogen, 4-methyl 2,5, dimethoxyamphetamine (DOB), in animals trained to discriminate DOB from saline *(24,25)*. In contrast, MDMA stimulus generalization was found with two derivatives of potent hallucinogens, the alpha-ethyl derivative of DOM, as well as the alpha ethyl derivative alpha-methyl-tryptamine, indicating that MDMA-like stimulus effects can be associated with an indolylalkylamine *(26)*. In addition to the large body of evidence that brain serotonin systems are important in the discriminative stimulus effects of MDMA *(7,27–31)*, there is also evidence that dopamine systems play a role, although less important that those of serotonin *(32)*. Self-administration studies in nonhuman primates indicate that baboons and monkeys self-administer MDMA *(33,34)*, consistent with clinical data indicating its abuse liability. This notion is further supported by the finding that in another animal model of drug-abuse liability, intracranial self-stimulation, MDMA consistently lowers the threshold for rewarding electrical stimulation delivered via electrodes stereotaxically implanted in the medial forebrain-bundle region *(35)*.

In humans, knowledge regarding the behavioral effects of MDMA in humans has come from both retrospective reports *(36,37)* and prospective controlled research settings *(38–40)*. As would be predicted by animal data, these sources indicate that MDMA has stimulant effects, in addition to effects that are most commonly associated with hallucinogens. Stimulant effects of MDMA are typically noted shortly after drug ingestion, and include increased heart rate, increased blood pressure, dry mouth, decreased appetite, increased alertness, elevated mood, and jaw clenching. Like other amphetamines, MDMA leads to enhanced mood and a sense of well-being. Most MDMA users do not report hallucinations, but often report increased emotional sensitiveness, depersonalization, derealization, and altered time perception.

2.3. MDMA-Induced Serotonin Neurotoxicity

In addition to its acute pharmacological effects, MDMA is known to be a selective and potent brain 5-HT neurotoxin. In particular, over the last 15 yr, a considerable body of data has been collected demonstrating that animals treated with MDMA develop significant, long-lasting reductions of various markers unique to brain-serotonin axons and axon terminals, with sparing of the cell body. Serotonergic markers reduced following MDMA administration include 5-HT, 5-hydroxyindoleacetic acid (5-HIAA), tryptophan hydroxylase (TPH), and the serotonin transporter (SERT) *(41–49)*. MDMA's neurotoxic effects are highly selective, exclusively damaging brain 5-HT neurons except when administered at extremely high dosages, when damage toward brain DA neurons can also be seen *(42)*. Interestingly, in the mouse, MDMA damages both 5-HT and DA neurons at moderate dosages, and is thus the only species in which MDMA-induced neurotoxicity is not selective for brain 5-HT neurons *(50)*.

Loss of brain serotonin markers persists for at least 7 yr in nonhuman primates and although some recovery appears to take place, regrowth of 5-HT axons appears to be aberrant *(51–53)*. Notably, dosages of MDMA that lead to brain 5-HT neuronal damage in animals overlap those used by humans for recreational purposes, once interspecies adjustments that account for body mass and surface area are made *(54,55)*. This has led a number of researchers to probe for evidence of MDMA-induced neurotoxicity in human MDMA users.

Early studies attempting to determine whether MDMA is neurotoxic in humans used a variety of indirect measures of brain-serotonin function, since direct methods for assessing the status of brain serotonin axon terminals in living humans have only recently been developed. Indirect measures utilized to probe for evidence of MDMA-induced brain serotonin injury in humans have included measurement of cerebrospinal fluid 5-hydroxyindoleacetic acid (CSF 5-HIAA), pharmacological/neuroendocrine challenges with drugs that act upon the brain-serotonin system, and measurement of behaviors believed to be mediated by brain 5-HT (e.g., cognitive functioning, sleep, impulsivity).

Of the various indirect measures that can be used to evaluate the status of brain serotonin neuronal functioning, only one has been validated as a measure of MDMA-induced 5-HT injury. In particular, studies in nonhuman primates have demonstrated that CSF 5-HIAA levels reflect MDMA-induced neurotoxic lesions, although underestimate the degree of damage *(47)*. The two controlled studies comparing CSF 5-HIAA levels in MDMA users and control subjects *(56,56a)* both found significant reductions in MDMA users, similar to those seen in monkeys with documented MDMA-induced 5-HT neuronal injury.

Studies probing for functional consequences of MDMA-induced neurotoxicity have also suggested long-lasting impairments in behaviors mediated by brain-serotonin systems. For example, several research groups have found MDMA users to have cognitive deficits, particularly on memory tasks *(56a,57–61)*. Neuroendocrine abnormalities in MDMA users following pharmacological challenges with 5-HT selective drugs have been found in some *(62,62a,63)* but not all *(56,64)* studies. Abnormalities in sleep architecture *(65,66)* and impulse regulation *(56,62,66,67)* in MDMA users are also suggestive of altered brain 5-HT function, although future efforts are needed to determine which, if any, of these functional abnormalities are direct consequences of MDMA-induced damage.

2.4. Neuroimaging of Brain-Serotonin Neurons

The fact that MDMA-induced neurotoxicity is associated with the loss of several markers unique to brain 5-HT axons and axon terminals makes it ideally suited for assessment using modern neuroimaging techniques. The ability for PET to detect drug-induced neurotoxicity was first demonstrated in 1985, when Calne and colleagues *(68)* demonstrated dopaminergic deficits in heroin addicts who unwittingly experimented with heroin contaminated with MPTP, a potent dopaminergic neurotoxin *(69)*. This, and subsequent successes in labeling several selective components of dopaminergic neurons with radiotracers suitable for neuroimaging generated significant interest in a similar development of single-photon emmission computed tomography (SPECT) or positron emission tomography (PET) radioligands selective for the brain-serotonergic system.

For a number of reasons, development of radioligands capable of binding selectively to brain serotonin terminals proved much more difficult than similar efforts directed toward dopaminergic neurons. The earliest successes were seen in the development of SPECT ligands. Mathis and colleagues reported that [^{123}I] iodonitroquipazine bound selectively to the SERT, and was useful for visualizing 5-HT neurons by SPECT *(70,71)*. At approximately the same time, the cocaine analog, CIT or RTI-55, labeled with ^{123}I, was also evaluated as a SPECT radiotracer for SERT *(72–75)*. For PET, a great deal of effort was spent attempting to develop SERT radioligands labeled with positron emitters such as [^{11}C] or [^{18}F] *(76–82a)*. However, these efforts failed because of low target-to-nontarget ratios in vivo, or, insufficient selectivity for the SERT.

In 1995, the first successful effort in labeling the SERT using PET was reported in nonhuman primates and healthy humans *(83,84)*. [^{11}C] McN-5652, a highly potent 5-HT uptake blocker with a Ki of 0.6 nM vs [^{3}H] 5-HT *(85–87)* was found to possess high target-to-nontarget ratios, high selectivity, and high specificity in binding to the SERT *(88)*. PET studies in nonhuman primates and humans replicated previous in vitro and in vivo findings indicating that the enantiomers of McN5652 display greatly different potencies towards the SERT (Ki = 0.4 and 58.4 nM for the (+) and (–) isomers, respectively). In particular, PET studies indicated that (+) enantiomer labels central SERT sites, whereas the (–) enantiomer does not. The stereoselectivity of [^{11}C] McN-5652 was put to good use in several subsequent PET studies, where (–) [^{11}C] McN5652 binding was used to estimate nonspecific binding of the ligand *(89,90)*.

3. NEUROIMAGING STUDIES IN MDMA USERS

PET, SPECT, and magnetic resonance spectroscopy (MRS) techniques have all been utilized to probe for evidence of CNS dysfunction in human MDMA users *(91–94)*. Studies in each of these categories will be described, in turn, below.

3.1. Positron Emission Tomography (PET)

As alluded to above, [^{11}C] McN-5652 is a recently developed PET radioligand capable of selectively labeling the SERT. The fact that (+) [^{11}C] McN-5652 labels the SERT, however, does not indicate that it has the requisite sensitivity for detecting MDMA-induced brain-serotonin neurotoxicity. As such, before studies were undertaken in human MDMA users, studies were first conducted in the nonhuman primate in an effort to validate this method *(95)*. In particular, following baseline scans with (+) [^{11}C] McN-5652, (–) [^{11}C]McN-5652, and [^{11}C] RTI-55, a cocaine derivative that labels both 5-HT and dopamine transporters, a baboon was treated with a neurotoxic regimen of MDMA. PET studies at 13, 19, and 40 d post-MDMA revealed significant decreases in (+) [^{11}C] McN-5652 binding, but no differences in binding of (–) [^{11}C] McN5652 or [^{11}C]RTI-55. Data obtained from PET studies correlated well with regional 5-HT axonal marker concentrations in the CNS measured after sacrifice of the animal, although decreases in (+) [^{11}C] McN-5652 binding tended to underestimate the extent of 5-HT damage found directly by neurochemical assay postmortem *(96)*. Findings from this study indicated that PET with (+) [^{11}C] McN-5652 was a suitable method for directly assessing MDMA-induced 5-HT neurotoxicity.

Once validated as a measure of MDMA-induced neurotoxicity in nonhuman primates, (+) [^{11}C] McN 5652 was used to probe for evidence of similar damage in human MDMA users. Fourteen MDMA users (who had used MDMA at least 25 times) and 15 control subjects (who had never previously used MDMA) underwent PET scans with (+) [^{11}C] McN 5652 and (–) [^{11}C] McN 5652 (with the difference in binding between the two isomers indicating specific binding). All subjects refrained from illicit drug use for at least 3 wk prior to scanning, with some subjects abstaining for several months. MDMA users were found to have global and regional reductions in (+) [^{11}C] McN 5652 binding, similar to those previously seen in MDMA-treated baboons. Notably, the magnitude of the decrease in (+) [^{11}C] McN 5652 binding directly correlated with the extent of previous MDMA use. These data strongly suggested that, as has been found in all other animal species, MDMA is a 5-HT neurotoxin in humans.

The one other PET study conducted in MDMA users utilized 2-18[F]-flouro-2-deoxy-D-glucose (FDG), in an effort to detect central nervous system (CNS) functional abnormalities following MDMA use *(93)*. Cumulative MDMA dosages in MDMA users were estimated to be between 12 and 840 single tablets of MDMA. Subjects reported that they were abstinent from MDMA for at least 2 mo. This study was not intended to detect 5-HT neurotoxicity per se, but rather, the possibility that 5-HT neurotoxicity might lead to persistent alterations in cerebral glucose utilization. Seven ecstasy users and seven age-matched controls who had never used MDMA underwent PET scans while resting, and metabolism in a small number of preselected regions of interest were compared. Glucose metabolic uptake differences were observed in the amygdala, hippocampus, and Brodmann's area 11 in the frontal cortex. No correlations were found between alterations in metabolism and extent of MDMA use or a variety of psychopathological measures. Although it is not known whether similar changes in brain metabolism are seen in animals with MDMA-induced 5-HT neurotoxicity, these results can be viewed as complementary to the previously described PET study with (+) [^{11}C]-McN562, possibly indicating persistent effects on neuronal activity resulting from brain 5-HT neurotoxicity. Future studies in nonhuman primates would be most helpful in sorting out specific effects of MDMA from nonspecific effects on regional glucose metabolism (e.g., preexisting abnormalities in glucose metabolism, effects of previous exposure to other drugs of abuse, etc.).

3.2. Single Photon Emission Computed Tomography (SPECT)

As reviewed earlier, the cocaine analog, [^{123}I] 2b-carboxy-methoxy-3b-(4-iodophenyl)tropane ([^{123}I] β-CIT) is a SPECT ligand that binds to both the SERT and dopamine transporter. Semple and colleagues *(92)* used this ligand to scan 10 MDMA users (who had a lifetime history of using at least 50 tablets of MDMA) and 10 matched controls that had never used MDMA. Results indicated a reduction in cortical βb-CIT binding, particularly prominent in primary sensory-motor cortex. Reductions in binding were correlated inversely correlated with time since last MDMA use (i.e., the more recent the MDMA use, the lower the binding of β-CIT), with no correlations between β-CIT binding and a variety of neuropsychological measures.

As with PET FDG studies, it would be extremely helpful to determine the sensitivity of SPECT with β-CIT for detecting MDMA-induced neurotoxic injury in nonhuman primates. Our experience with (+) [^{11}C] McN-5652 and PET indicates that this method, like CSF measurements of CSF 5-HIAA, tends to underestimate the extent of damage measured postmortem. Given that reductions of β-CIT were of a smaller degree than those found using (+) [^{11}C] McN-5652, it is possible that this method also lacks adequate sensitivity to detect smaller MDMA-induced 5-HT lesions.

A second SPECT study compared regional blood flow (rCBF) in 21 MDMA users and 21 age- and gender-matched control subjects using technetium-99m-d,l-hexamethyl-propylene amine oxime (99Tcm-HMPAO) *(97)*. SPECT scans were co-registered with magnetic resonance imaging (MRI) scans to facilitate comparisons between regions of interest. Ten MDMA subjects had a second SPECT scan approx 3 wk after receiving 2 dosages of MDMA, and 2 MDMA subjects had a third SPECT scan 2–3 mo after receiving MDMA. At baseline, no differences between global or rCBF patterns were noted. Approximately 3 wk after receiving MDMA, some regional decreases in blood flow were seen in visual cortex, caudate, superior parietal, and dorsolateral frontal regions when compared to baseline scans in the same individuals. Two to three months later, the two individuals who underwent a third SPECT scan were found to have increases, rather than decreases, in rCBF. In the absence of preclinical studies in nonhuman primates with documented MDMA-induced 5-HT injury, the potential interpretations of these data are numerous. However, it is possible that processes associated with MDMA-induced neuronal injury are associated with changes in CBF that vary over time.

3.3. Magnetic Resonance Spectroscopy (MRS)

In a study of 22 MDMA users and 37 normal volunteers, Chang and colleagues *(94)* used ^{1}H MRS to explore the possibility that this technique might detect alterations in neuronal markers that could be related to previous MDMA use. They measured N-acetylaspartate, (NA, a neuronal marker), myo-inositol (MI, a possible glial marker), and creatinine (CR) concentrations in regular MDMA users who had used MDMA at least six times, and control subjects who had never used MDMA. MDMA users refrained from MDMA use for at least 2 wk. Findings from the study indicated that NA levels were similar to those found in controls, but that MI and MI/CR ratios were reduced in MDMA users.

There have been no studies conducted in animals to determine whether MDMA-induced brain 5-HT neurotoxicity is associated with alterations in ^{1}H MRS patterns. However, differences in ^{1}H MRS patterns observed between MDMA users and controls are consistent with the view that MDMA leads to persistent alterations in CNS neurochemistry.

4. SUMMARY AND CONCLUSIONS

Neuroimaging techniques hold great promise for exploring the effects of MDMA and related neurotoxic amphetamine analogs on brain structure and function in living humans. In particular, PET and SPECT studies using radioligands selective for elements of brain-serotonin axons and axon terminals hold tremendous promise for characterizing the effects of MDMA on brain-serotonin neurons over time, and the interaction between MDMA and the aging brain (i.e., are older people more susceptible to MDMA-induced neurotoxicity than younger people?). Currently available radioligands may not have the requisite sensitivity to detect smaller MDMA-induced lesions, and continued efforts to develop sensitive, quantitative methods to evaluate the status of brain 5-HT axons and axon terminals are needed. As previously done with [^{11}C] McN 5652, potential new radioligands should first be tested in animals to validate the method and to compare the relative sensitivity of the agent to previously available compounds.

Functional neuroimaging techniques also have tremendous potential for better delineating the consequences of MDMA-induced neurotoxicity, once it has occurred. FDG, O-15, and fMRI techniques could all be brought to bear to address this question. In particular, studies conducted in the setting of pharmacological challenges known to differentially effect MDMA users (e.g., m-CPP) or while subjects are engaging in cognitive tasks that that have been demonstrated to be altered in MDMA users could all be useful in delineating the neuroanatomical substrates associated with previously demonstrated behavioral and neuroendocrine abnormalities in MDMA users. Notably, animal studies should be conducted in parallel to studies in humans (with the possible exception of cognitive studies) in order to eliminate potential confounds (e.g., alterations secondary to pre-existing conditions or previous exposure to other drugs of abuse).

^{1}H MRS and MRS studies directed at measuring chemicals associated with brain-serotonergic neurons (e.g., 5-HT) can potentially provide yet another complementary method for assessing the status of brain-serotonin neurons in living humans. The interpretation of data using these methods, like other neuroimaging techniques, can be strengthened considerably by laying the groundwork with preclinical studies in animals where direct, postmortem neurochemical and neuroanatomical studies can be conducted.

In conclusion, neuroimaging techniques have made it possible for the first time to assess the status of brain-serotonin neurons in living humans. None of the currently available methods are perfect, and continued efforts to develop more sensitive and selective methods are necessary. Despite limitations of currently available methods, PET using [^{11}C] McN 5652 has been validated in nonhuman primates as a measure of MDMA-induced 5-HT neuronal injury. This method, which underestimates the extent of brain-serotonin injury, indicates that MDMA can lead to neurotoxic injury in humans, and that more severe lesions are seen in individuals with greater MDMA exposure. Studies in larger cohorts of MDMA users with a wider range of exposure levels will be useful in better defining the risks of MDMA toward brain 5-HT neurons, and may help define populations at higher risk (e.g., older individuals). Longitudinal studies, similar to those that have been conducted in vivo in primates could potentially shed light on the fate of damaged brain 5-HT neurons with aging. Finally, functional neuroimaging studies, in concert with detailed neuropsychological and neuropsychiatric assessments, have potential for significantly increasing our understanding the role of brain-serotonin neuronal function in both normal behavior and neuropsychiatric disease states.

ACKNOWLEDGMENT

This work was supported by PHS grants DA05707, DA05938, DA00206, and AG14400.

REFERENCES

1. National Institute on Drug Abuse (1999) Epidemiologic trends in drug abuse: Vol. II: Proceedings of the International Epidemiology Work Group on Drug Abuse, US DHHS, NIH Pub. No. 00–4530, 1999.
2. Christophersen, A. S. (2000) Amphetamine designer drugs: an overview and epidemiology. *Toxicol Lett.* **112–113,** 127–131.
3. Topp, L., Hando, J., Dillon, P., Roche, A., and Solowij, N. (1999) Ecstasy use in Australia: patterns of use and associated harm. *Drug Alcohol Depend.* **55(1–2),** 105–115.
4. Eisner, B. (1989) Ecstasy: The MDMA Story. Ronin Publishing Inc., Berkeley, CA.
5. Greer, G. R. and Tolbert, R. (1998) A method of conducting therapeutic sessions with MDMA. *J. Psychoactive Drugs* **30(4),** 371–379.
6. McCann, U. D., Mertl, M. M., and Ricaurte, G. A. (1998a) Methylenedioxymethamphetamine (MDMA, "Ecstasy"), in *Sourcebook on Substance Abuse: Etiology, Methodology, and Intervention* (Tarter, R. E., Ammerman, R. T., and Ott, P. J., eds.), Allyn and Bacon, New York, pp. 567–577.
7. Johnson, M.P., Hoffman, A. H., and Nichols, D. E. (1986) Effects of the enantiomers of MDA, MDMA and related analogues on [3H]-serotonin and [3H]-dopamine release from superfused rat brain slices. *Eur. J. Pharmacol.* **132,** 269–276.
8. McKenna, D. J. and Peroutka, S. J. (1990) Neurochemistry and neurotoxicity of 3,4-methylenedioxymethamphetamine (MDMA, "ecstasy"). *J. Neurochem.* **54(1),** 14–22.
9. Rudnick, G. and Wall, S. C. (1992) The molecular mechanism of "ecstasy" [3,4-methylenedioxymethamphetamine (MDMA)]: serotonin transporters are targets for MDMA-induced serotonin release. *Proc. Natl. Acad. Sci. USA* **89,** 1817–1821.
10. Yamamoto, B. K. and Spanos, L. J. (1988) The acute effects of methylenedioxymethamphetamine on dopamine release in the awake-behaving rat. *Eur. J. Pharmacol.* **148,** 195–203.
11. Hiramatsu, M. and Cho, A. K. (1990) Enantiomeric differences in the effects of 3,4-methylenedioxymethamphetamine on extracellular monoamines and metabolites in the striatum of freely-moving rats. *Neuropharmacology* **29,** 269–275.
12. Nash, J. F., Meltzer, H. Y., and Gudelsky, G.A. (1990) Effect of 3,4-methylenedioxymethamphetamine on 3,4-dihydroxyphenyalanine accumulation in the striatum and nucleus accumbens. *J. Neurochem.* **54,** 1062–1067.
13. Titeler, M., Lyon, R. A., and Glennon, R. A. (1988) Radioligand binding evidence implicates the brain 5-HT2 receptor as a site of action for LSD and central phenylisopropylamine hallucinogens. *Psychopharmacology* **94,** 213–216.
14. Battaglia, G., Brooks, B. P., Kulsakdinum, C., and DeSouza, E. B. (1988a) Pharmacologic profile of MDMA (3,4-methylenedioxymethamphetamine) at various brain recognition sites. *Eur. J. Pharmacol.* **149,** 159–163.
15. Pierce, P. A. and Peroutka, S. J. (1988) Ring-substituted amphetamine interactions with neurotransmitter receptor binding sites in human cortex. *Neurosci Lett.* **95(1–3),** 208–212.
16. Gordon, C. J., Watkinson, W. P., O'Callaghan, J. P., and Miller, D. B. (1991) Effects of 3,4-methylenedioxymethamphetamine on autonomic thermoregulatory responses of the rat. *Pharmacol. Biochem. Behav.* **38(2),** 339–344.
17. Hardman, H. F., Haavik, C. O., and Seevers, M. H. (1973) Relationship of the structure of mescaline and seven analogs to toxicity and behavior in five species of laboratory animals. *Toxicol. Appl. Pharmacol.* **25,** 299–309.

18. Frith, C. H., Chang, L. W., Lattin, D. L., Walls, R. C., Hamm, J., and Doblin, R. (1987) Toxicity of methylenedioxymethamphetamine (MDMA) in the dog and the rat. *Fundam. Appl. Toxicol.* **9(1),** 110–119.

19. Gold, L. H., Koob, G. F., and Geyer, M. A. (1988) Stimulant and hallucinogenuc profiles of 3,4-methylenedioxymethamphetamine and N-ethyl–3,4-methylenedioxyamphetamine in rats. *J. Pharmacol. Exp. Ther.* **247,** 547–555.

20. Spanos, L.J. and Yamamoto, B. K. (1989) Acute and subchronic effects of methylenedioxymethamphetamine (+-MDMA) on locomotion and serotonin syndrome in the rat. *Pharmacol. Biochem. Behav.* **32,** 835–840.

21. Glennon, R. A. and Young, R. Y. (1984) Further investigations of the discriminative stimulus properties of MDA. *Pharmacol. Biochem. Behav.* **20,** 501–505.

22. Evans, S. M. and Johanson, C. E. (1986) Discriminative stimulus properties of (+/−)-3,4-methylenedioxymethamphetamine and (+/−)–3,4-methylenedioxyamphetamine in pigeons. *Drug Alcohol Depend.* **18(2),** 159–164.

23. Kamien, J. B., Johanson, C. E., Schuster, C. R., and Woolverton, W. L. (1986) The effects of (+)-methylenedioxymethamphetamine and (+)-methylenedioxyamphetamine in monkeys trained to discriminate (+)-amphetamine from saline. *Drug Alcohol Depend.* **18,** 139–147.

24. Glennon, R. A., Young, R., Rosecrans, J. A., and Anderson, G. M. (1982) Discriminative stimulus properties of MDA and related agents. *Biol. Psychiatry* **17,** 807–814.

25. Nichols, D. E. (1986) Differences between the mechanism of action of MDMA, MBDB, and the classic hallucinogens. Identification of a new therapeutic class, entactogens. *J. Psychoactive Drugs* **18,** 305–313.

26. Glennon, R. A. (1993) MDMA-like stimulus effects of alpha-ethyltryptamine and the alpha-ethyl homolog of DOM. *Pharmacol. Biochem. Behav.* **46(2),** 459–462.

27. Schechter, M. D. (1998) MDMA-like stimulus effects of hallucinogens in male Fawn-Hooded rats. *Pharmacol. Biochem. Behav.* **59(2),** 265–270.

28. Schechter, M. D. (1997) Drug-drug discrimination: stimulus properties of drugs of abuse upon a serotonergic-dopaminergic continuum. *Pharmacol. Biochem. Behav.* **56(1),** 89–96.

29. Schechter, M. D. (1997) Serotonergic mediation of fenfluramine discriminative stimuli in fawn-hooded rats. *Life Sci.* **60(6),** PL83–PL90.

30. Schechter, M. D. (1997) Drug-drug discrimination: stimulus properties of drugs of abuse upon a serotonergic-dopaminergic continuum. *Pharmacol. Biochem. Behav.* **56(1),** 89–96.

31. Steele, T. D., Nichols, D. E., and Yim, G. K. W. (1987) Stereochemical effects of 3,4-methylenedioxymethamphetamine (MDMA) and related amphetamine derivatives on inhibition of uptake of [3H]-monoamines into synaptosomes from different regions of rat brain. *Biochem. Pharmacol.* **36,** 2297–2303.

32. Schechter, M. D. (1988) Serotonergic-dopaminergic mediation of 3,4-methylenedioxymethamphetamine (MDMA, "ecstasy"). *Pharmacol. Biochem. Behav.* **31(4),** 817–824.

33. Lamb, R. J. and Griffiths, R. R. (1987) Self-injection of 3,4-methylenedioxymethamphetamine (MDMA) in the baboon. *Psychopharmacology* **91,** 268–272.

34. Beardsley, P. M., Balster, R. L., and Harris, L. S. (1986) Self-administration of methylenedioxymethamphetamine (MDMA) by rhesus monkeys. *Drug Alcohol Depend.* **18,** 149–157.

35. Hubner, C. B., Bird, M., Rassnick, S., and Kornetsky, C. (1988) The threshold lowering effects of MDMA (ecstasy) on brain-stimulation reward. *Psychopharmacology* **95(1),** 49–51.

36. Downing, J. (1986) The psychological and physiological effects of MDMA on normal volunteers. *J. Psychoactive Drugs* **18,** 335–340.

37. McCann, U. D. and Ricaurte, G. A. (1993) Reinforcing Subjective Effects of (+) 3,4-methylenedioxymethamphetamine (MDMA; "Ecstasy") may be separable from its neurotoxic actions: clinical evidence. *J. Clin. Psychopharmacol.* **13(3),** 214–217.

38. Grob, C. S., Poland, R. E., Chang, L., and Ernst, T. (1996) Psychobiologic effects of 3,4-methylenedioxymethamphetamine in humans: methodological considerations and preliminary observations. *Behav. Brain Res.* **73**, 103–107.

39. Vollenweider, F. X., Gamma, A., Liechti, M., and Huber, T. (1998) Psychological and cardiovascular effects and short-term sequelae of MDMA ("Ecstasy") in MDMA-naïve healthy volunteers. *Neuropsychopharmacology* **19**, 241–251.

40. Mas, M., Farre, M., de la Torre, R., Roset, P. N., Ortuno, J., Segura, J., and Cami, J. (1999) Cardiovascular and neuroendocrine effects and pharmacokinetics of 3, 4-methylenedioxymethamphetamine in humans. *J. Pharmacol. Exp. Ther.* **290(1)**, 136–145.

41. Schmidt, C. J. (1987) Neurotoxicity of the psychedelic amphetamine, methylenedioxymethamphetamine. *J. Pharmacol. Exp. Ther.* **240**, 1–7.

42. Commins, D. L., Vosmer, G., Virus, R., Woolverton, W., Schuster, C., and Seiden, L. (1987) Biochemical and histological evidence that methylenedioxymethylamphetamine (MDMA) is toxic to neurons in the rat brain. *J. Pharmacol. Exp. Ther.* **241**, 338–345.

43. Battaglia, G., Yeh, S. Y., O'Hearn, E., Molliver, M. E., Kuhar, M. J., and DeSouza, E. B. (1987) 3,4-Methylenedioxymethamphetamine and 3,4-methylenedioxy-amphetamine destroy serotonin terminals in rat brain: quantification of neurodegeneration by measurement of [3H]paroxetine-labeled serotonin uptake sites. *J. Pharmacol. Exp. Ther.* **242**, 911–916.

44. O'Hearn, E. G., Battaglia, G., De Souza, E. B., Kuhar, M. J., and Molliver, M. E. (1988) Methylenedioxyamphetamine (MDA) and methylenedioxymethamphetamine (MDMA) cause selective ablation of serotonergic axon terminals in forebrain: immunocytochemical evidence for neurotoxicity. *J. Neurosci.* **8**, 2788–2803.

45. Slikker, W., Ali, S. F., Scallet, C., Frith, C. H., Newport, G. D., and Bailey, J. R. (1988) Neurochemical and neurohistological alterations in the rat and monkey produced by orally administered methylenedioxymethamphetamine (MDMA). *Toxicol. Appl. Pharmacol.* **94**, 448–457.

46. Ricaurte, G. A., DeLanney, L. E., Irwin, I., and Langston, J. W. (1988a) Toxic effects of MDMA on central serotonergic neurons in the primate: importance of route and frequency of drug administration. *Brain Res.* **446**, 165–168.

47. Ricaurte, G. A., Delanney, L. E., Wiener, S. G., Irwin, I., and Langston, J. W. (1988b) 5-Hydroxyindoleacetic acid in cerebrospinal fluid reflects serotonergic damage induced by 3,4-methylenedioxymethamphetamine in CNS of non-human primates. *Brain Res.* **474**, 359–363.

48. Insel, T. R., Battaglia, G., Johannessen, J. N., Marra, S., and De Souza, E. B. (1989) 3,4-Methylenedioxymethamphetamine ("ecstasy") selectively destroys brain serotonin terminals in rhesus monkeys. *J. Pharmacol. Exp. Ther.* **249**, 713–720.

49. Molliver, M. E., Berger, U. V., Mamounas, L. A., Molliver, D. C., O'Hearn, E. G., and Wilson, M. A. (1990) Neurotoxicity of MDMA and related compounds: anatomic studies. *Ann. NY Acad. Sci.* **600**, 640–664.

50. Logan, B. J., Laverty, R., Sanderson, W. D., and Yee, Y. B. (1988) Differences between rats and mice in MDMA (methylenedioxymethylamphetamine) neurotoxicity. *Eur. J. Pharmacol.* **152(3)**, 227–234.

51. Ricaurte, G. A., Katz, J. L., and Martello, M. B. (1992) Lasting effects of (A)3,4-methylenedioxymethamphetamine on central serotonergic neurons in non-human primates. *J. Pharmacol. Exp. Ther.* **261**, 616–622.

52. Fischer, C. A., Hatzidimitriou, G., Katz, J. L., and Ricaurte, G. A. (1995) Reorganization of ascending serotonin axon projections in animals previously exposed to the recreational drug 3,4-methylenedioxymethamphetamine. *J. Neurosci.* **15**, 5476–5485.

53. Hatzidimitriou, G., McCann, U. D., and Ricaurte, G. A. (1999) Altered serotonin innervation patterns in the forebrain of monkeys treated with MDMA seven years previously: factors influencing abnormal recovery. *J. Neurosci.* **191(12)**, 5096–5107.

54. Mordenti, J. and Chappell, W. (1989) The use of interspecies scaling in toxicokinetics, in *Toxicokinetics in New Drug Development* (Yacobi, A., Kelly, J., and Batra, V. (eds.), Pergamon Press, New York, pp. 42–96.

55. Chappell, W. and Mordenti, J. (1991) Extrapolation of toxicological and pharmacological data from animals to humans, in *Advances in Drug Research*, vol. 20 (Testa, B., ed.), Academic Press, San Diego, CA, pp. 1–116.

56. McCann, U. D., Ridenour, A, Shaham, Y., and Ricaurte, G. A. (1994) Brain serotonergic neurotoxicity after MDMA ("ecstasy"): a controlled study in humans. *Neuropsychopharmacology* **10**, 129–138.

56a. McCann, U. D. and Mertl, M. M., Eligulashvili, V., and Ricaurte, G. A. (1999a) Cognitive performance in (±) 3,4-methylenedioxymethamphetamine (MDMA, "ecstasy") users: a controlled study. *Psychopharmacology* **143**, 417–425.

57. Krystal, J. H., Price, L. H., Opsahl, C., Ricaurte, G. A., and Heninger, G. R. (1992) Chronic 3,4-methylenedioxymethamphetamine (MDMA) use: effects on mood and neuropsychological function. *Am. J. Drug Alcohol Abuse* **18**, 331–341.

58. Parrot, A. C., Lees, A., Granham, N. J., Jones, M., and Wesnes, K. (1998) Cognitive performance in recreational users of MDMA or "ecstasy": evidence for memory deficits. *J. Psychopharmacol.* **12(1)**, 79–83.

59. Parrott, A. C. and Lasky, J. (1998) Ecstasy (MDMA) effects upon mood and cognition: before, during and after a Saturday night dance. *Psychopharmacology* **139(3)**, 261–268.

60. Bolla, K. I., McCann, U. D., and Ricaurte, G. A. (1998) Impaired memory function in abstinent MDMA ("Ecstasy") users. *Neurology* **51(6)**, 1532–1537.

61. Morgan, M. M. (1999) Memory deficits associated with recreational use of "ecstasy" (MDMA). *Psychopharmacology* **141**, 30–36.

62. Gerra, G., Zaimovic, A., Giucastro, G., Maestri, D., Monica, C., Sartori, R, et al. (1998) Serotonergic function after (+/-)3,4-methylene-dioxymethamphetamine ('Ecstasy') in humans. *Intl. Clin. Psychopharmacol.* **13(1)**, 1–9.

62a. Gerra, G., Zaimovic, A., Ferri, M., Zambelli, U., Timpano, M., Neri, E, et al. (2000) Long-lasting effects of (+/–)3,4-methylenedioxymethamphetamine (ecstasy) on serotonin system function in humans. *Biol. Psychiatry* **15;47(2)**, 127–136.

63. McCann, U. D., Eligulashvili, V., Mertl, M., Murphy, D. L., and Ricaurte, G. A. (1999b) Altered neuroendocrine and behavioral responses to m-chlorophenylpiperazine in 3,4-methylenedioxymethamphetamine (MDMA) users. *Psychopharmacology (Berl.)* **147(1)**, 56–65.

64. Price, L. H., Charney, D. S., Delgado, P. L., Goodman, W. K., Krystal, J. H., Woods, S. W., Heninger, G. R. (1990) Clinical studies of 5-HT function using I.V. L-Tryptophan. *Prog. Neuro. Psychopharmacol. Biol. Psychiatry* **14**, 459–472.

65. Allen, R. P., McCann, U. D., and Ricaurte, G. A. (1993) Persistent effects of (+/–)3,4-methylenedioxymethamphetamine (MDMA, "ecstasy") on human sleep. *Sleep* **16(6)**, 560–564.

66. McCann, U. D. and Ricaurte, G. A. Experimental studies on MDMA and its potential to damage brain serotonin neurons. *Neurotoxicity Res.*, in press.

67. Morgan, M. J. (1998) Recreational use of "ecstasy" (MDMA) is associated with elevated impulsivity. *Neuropsychopharmacology* **19(4)**, 252–264.

68. Calne, D. B., Langston, J. W., Martin, W., Stoessel, A., Ruth, T., Adam, M., and Schulzer, M. (1985) Positron emission tomography after MPTP: observations relating to the cause of Parkinson's disease. *Nature* **317**, 246–248.

69. Langston, J. W. (1985) MPTP and Parkinson's disease. *Trends Neurosci.* **8**, 79–83.

70. Mathis, C. A., Biegon, A., Taylor, S., Enas, J., Hanrahan, S., and Jagust, W. (1992) [I–125]5-Iodo–6-nitroquipazine: synthesis and evaluation of a potent and selective presynaptic serotonin ligand. *J. Nucl. Med.* **33**, 890.

71. Jagust, W. J., Eberling, J. L., Roberts, J. A., Brennan, K. M., Hanrahan, S. M., Vonbrocklin, H., et al. (1993) In vivo imaging of the 5-hydroxytryptamine reuptake sites in primate brain using single photon emission tomography and [123I]5-iodo-6-nitroquipazine. *Eur. J. Pharm.* **242**, 189–193.

72. Neumeyer, J. L., Wang, S., and Milius, R. A. (1991) [^{123}I]-2ψ-Carbomethoxy-3ψ-(4-iodophenyl)tropane: high affinity SPECT radiotracer of monoamine reuptake sites in brain. *J. Med. Chem.* **34**, 3144–3146.

73. Innis, R., Baldwin, R., Sybirska, E., Zea, Y., Laruelle, M., Al-Tikriti, M., et al. (1991) Single photon emission computed tomography imaging of monoamine reuptake sites in primate brain with [123I]CIT. *Eur. J. Pharmacol.* **200**, 369–370.

74. Scheffel, U., Dannals, R. F., Cline, E. J., Ricaurte, G. A., Carroll, F. I., Abraham, P., et al. (1992) [123/125I]RTI–55, an in vivo label for the serotonin transporter. *Synapse* **11**, 134–139.

75. Laruelle, M., Wallace, E., Seibyl, J., Baldwin, R., Zea-Ponmce, Y., Zoghbi, A., et al. (1994) Graphical, Kinetic, and Equilibrium Analyses of In Vivo [123I]b-CIT Binding to Dopamine Transporters in Healthy Human Subjects. *J. Cereb. Blood Flow Metab.* **14**, 982–994.

76. Maziere, M., Berger, G., and Comar, D. (1978) 11C-Chlorimipramine: synthesis and analysis. *J. Radioanal. Chem.* **45**, 453–457.

77. Hashimoto, K., Inoue, O., Suzuki, K., Yamasaki, T., and Kojima, M. (1987) Synthesis and evaluation of [11C]cyanoimipramine. *Nucl. Med. Biol.* **14**, 587–592.

78. Kilbourn, M. R., Carey, J. E., Koeppe, R. A., Haka, M. S., Hutchins, G. D., Sherman, P. S., and Kuhl, D. E. (1989) Biodistribution, dosimetry, metabolism and monkey PET studies of [18F]GBR 13119: imaging the dopamine uptake system in vivo. *Int. J. Radiat. Appl. Inst.* [B], **16(6)**, 569–576.

79. Scheffel, U., Dannals, R. F., Suehiro, M., Wilson, A. A., Ravert, H. T., Stathis, M., Wagner, H. N., Jr. (1990b) Evaluation of 11C-citalopram and 11C-fluoxetine as in vivo ligands for the serotonin uptake site. *J. Nucl. Med.* **31**, 883–884.

80. Hume, S. P., Pascali, C., and Pike, V. W. (1991) Citalopram: labeling with carbon-11 and evaluation in rat as a potential radioligand for in vivo PET studies of 5-HT re-uptake sites. *Nucl. Med. Biol.* **18**, 339–351.

81. Lasne, M. C., Pike, V. W., and Turton, D. R. (1989) The radiosynthesis of N-methyl-carbon–11-sertraline. *Appl. Radiat. Isot.* **40**, 147–152.

82. Suehiro, M., Wilson, A. A., Scheffel, U., Dannals, R. F., Ravert, H. T., and Wagner, H. N,. Jr. (1991) Radiosynthesis and evaluation of N-(3-[18F]fluoropropyl)paroxetine as a radiotracer for in vivo labeling of serotonin uptake sites by PET. *Nucl. Med. Biol.* **18**, 791–796.

82a. Suehiro, M., Scheffel, U., Dannals, R. F., Wilson, A. A., Ravert, H. T., and Wagner, H. N., Jr. (1992) A new radiotracer for in vivo labeling of serotonin uptake sites by PET, cis-N,N[11C]dimethyl-3-(2'-4'-dichlorophenyl)-indanamine, cis-[11C]DDPI. *Nucl. Med. Biol.* **19**, 549–553.

83. Szabo, Z., Kao, P., Scheffel, U., Suehiro, M., Mathews, W., Ravert, H., et al. (1995a) Positron emission tomography of serotonin transporter sites in human brain with [11C]McN5652. *Synapse* **20**, 37–43.

84. Szabo, Z., Scheffel, U., Suehiro, M., Dannals, R., Kim, S., Ravert, H., et al. (1995b) Positron emmision tomography of serotonin transporter sites in baboon brain with [11C]McN5652. *J. Cereb. Blood Flow* **15(5)**, 798–805.

85. Maryanoff, B. E., McComsey, D. F., Gardocki, J. F., Shank, R. P., Costanzo, M. J., Nortey, S. O., et al. (1987) Pyrroloisoquinoline antidepressants. 2. In-depth exploration of structure-activity relationships. *J. Med. Chem.* **30**, 1433–1454.

86. Maryanoff, B. E., Vaught, J. L., Shank, R. P., McComsey, D. F., Costanzo, M. J., and Nortey, S. O. (1990) Pyrroloisoquinoline antidepressants. 3. A focus on serotonin. *J. Med. Chem.* **33**, 2793–2797.

87. Shank, R. P., Vaught, J. L., Pelley, K. A., Setler, P. E., McComsey, D. F., and Maryanoff, B. E. (1988) McN-5652: a highly potent inhibitor of serotonin uptake. *J. Pharm. Exp. Ther.* **247**, 1032–1038.

88. Dannals, R. F., Scheffel, U., Suehiro, M., and Ricaurte, G. (1994) Radioligand development for studying serotonin uptake sites with positron emission tomography. *Med. Chem. Res.*, 228–244.

89. Meltzer, C. C., Smith, G., DeKosky, S. T., Pollock, B. G., Mathis, C. A., Moore, R. Y., et al. (1998) Serotonin in aging, late-life depression, and Alzheimer's disease: the emerging role of functional imaging. *Neuropsychopharmacology* **18(6)**, 407–430.

90. Szabo, Z., Scheffel, U., Mathews, W. B., Ravert, H. T., Szabo, K., Kraut, M., et al. (1999) Kinetic analysis of [11C]McN5652: A serotonin transporter radioligand. *J. Cereb. Blood Flow* **19**, 967–981.

91. McCann, U. D., Szabo, Z., Scheffel, U., Dannals, R. F., and Ricaurte, G. A. (1998b) Positron emission tomographic evidence of toxic effect of MDMA ("Ecstasy") on brain serotonin neurons in human beings. *Lancet* **352(9138)**, 1433–1437.

92. Semple, D. M., Ebmeier, K. P., Glabus, M. F., O'Carroll, R. E., and Johnstone, E. C. (1999) Reduced in vivo binding to the serotonin transporter in the cerebral cortex of MDMA ('ecstasy') users. *Br. J. Psychiatry* **175**, 63–69.

93. Obrocki, J., Buchert, R., Vaterlein, O., Thomasius, R., Beyer, W., and Schiemann, T. (1999) Ecstasy: long-term effects on the human central nervous system revealed by positron emission tomography. *Br. J. Psychiatry* **175**, 186–188.

94. Chang, L., Ernst, T., Grob, C. S., and Poland, R. E. (1999) Cerebral (1)H MRS alterations in recreational 3, 4-methylenedioxymethamphetamine (MDMA, "ecstasy") users. *J. Magn. Reson. Imag.* **10(4)**, 521–526.

95. Scheffel, U., Szabo, Z., Mathews, W. B., Finley, P. A., Dannals, R. F., Ravert, H. T., et al. (1998) In vivo detection of short- and long-term MDMA neurotoxicity. A positron emission tomography study in the living baboon brain. *Synapse* **29**, 183–192.

96. Kerenyi, L. L., Szabo, Z., Scheffel, U., Matthews, W. B., Ravert, H. T., Szabo, K., et al. (1999) Assessment of serotonergic inervation with [C-11] McN5652/PET. *Soc. Nuc. Med.* **40**, 115.

97. Chang, L., Grob, C. S., Ernst, T., Itti, L., Mishkin, F. S., Jose-Melchor, R., and Poland, R. E. (2000) Effect of ecstasy [3,4-methylenedioxymethamphetamine (MDMA)] on cerebral blood flow: a co-registered SPECT and MRI study. *Psychiatry Res.* **98(1)**, 15–28.

IV
NEUROBEHAVIORAL
ASSESSMENT METHODS

19

Tier 1 Neurological Assessment in Regulated Animal Safety Studies

Joseph F. Ross

1. INTRODUCTION

Explicit, systematic testing for neurotoxicity in regulated animal safety studies is a relatively new phenomenon—newer even than genetic toxicology testing. Just 20 years ago, the typical evaluation for neuropathological effects included a few sagittal sections of an immersion-fixed brain. The functional testing of subjects included through-the-cage wall observations for spontaneous behavioral and neurological effects (e.g., convulsions, narcosis) and "hand-held" observation taken during routine clinical observations. This functional testing was neither explicit nor systematic, and the observations were typically recorded "by exception" (i.e., only significant abnormalities were recorded).

During the late 1970s and early 1980s, there arose significant scientific and political pressure to improve the morphological and functional assessment of the nervous system *(1)*. However, within the neurotoxicology community there was considerable disagreement about the best way to conduct this testing. At least in part, the controversy arose because the nervous system has enormous morphological and functional complexity.

In human medical practice, the potential dysfunction of the nervous system is addressed by a cadre of professionals, including neurologists, psychologists, and psychiatrists (*see* Chapter 20 by Albers). These professionals possess years of training in their disciplines and are required to pass several rigorous proficiency examinations before they can claim membership in their profession. They also have an enormous array of diagnostic technology at their disposal. For many reasons, the same level of expertise and technology is not available to evaluate the nervous system during toxicity studies in animals. However, the challenge for neurologists and toxicologists is similar: to detect and characterize changes in nervous system function. Faced with this dilemma, the scientific and regulatory communities participated in many symposia and workshops to discuss the functional endpoints that should be included in routine and specialized neurotoxicity studies (*see* ref. *2* for a list of relevant symposia and conferences). The results of these meetings are now reflected by a variety of regulatory guidelines that require explicit and systematic evaluation of morphological and functional

From: Handbook of Neurotoxicology, Vol. 2
Edited by: E. J. Massaro © Humana Press Inc., Totowa, NJ

endpoints in safety studies conducted with animals *(3)*. Although some specialized neurotoxicity studies are conducted, the vast majority of these evaluations are performed as part of standard acute- and subchronic-toxicity studies conducted using rats. These studies are conducted to detect and provide initial characterization of potential neurotoxic effects of chemicals.

The current requirements for testing are exemplified by the language in the Organization for Economic Cooperation and Development (OECD) guidelines for a 13-wk oral dosing study (OECD #408):

> "These observations should be made outside the home cage, preferably in a standard arena and at similar times on each occasion. They should be carefully recorded, preferably using scoring systems, explicitly defined by the testing laboratory."

> "Signs noted should include, but not be limited to, changes in skin, fur, eyes, mucous membranes, occurrence of secretions and excretions and autonomic activity (e.g., lacrimation, piloerection, pupil size, unusual respiratory pattern). Changes in gait, posture, and response to handling as well as the presence of clonic or tonic movements, stereotypes (e.g., excessive grooming, repetitive circling) or bizarre behavior (e.g., self-mutilation, walking backwards) should also be recorded."

> "Towards the end of the exposure period and in any case not earlier than in week 11, sensory reactivity to stimuli of different types (e.g., auditory, visual and proprioceptive stimuli), assessment of grip strength and motor activity assessment should be conducted."

The language of the US Environmental Protection Agency (EPA) guidelines for subchronic studies (EPA 870.3100) is almost identical. The guidelines for acute toxicity studies (EPA 870.1100; OECD 401) contain similar language, except that locomotor activity is not measured, and there are fewer specifications for conducting the tests and recording the observations.

While the current testing guidelines require explicit and systematic evaluation of neurological function, they also provide the laboratory personnel significant flexibility in how the neurological endpoints are measured. Because of this flexibility, different laboratories use different tests and combinations of tests to evaluate nervous-system function. The primary purpose of this chapter is to describe, compare, and critically evaluate some of the more common observations and procedures that are used or can be used to meet these requirements. Although there are many tests available for measuring neurological function in experimental neuroscience, only a small proportion of these tests are appropriate as part of a battery used to evaluate the large number of animals typically used in safety studies. This chapter will discuss these endpoints from the perspective of their relationship to a neurological examination conducted in a human or veterinary clinic. There are several reasons for this approach. Specifically, tests with strong links to endpoints used in a human and veterinary neurological examination enable the toxicologist to exploit the enormous literature describing the anatomical basis of the test, proper conduct of the test, and interpretation of the test results in the context of other neurological tests and other clinical and anatomical pathology endpoints. This linkage is particularly valuable when the data are evaluated, since it is generally agreed that the clinical observation results need to be integrated with effects demonstrated in anatomical and clinical pathology (e.g., ref. *4*).

2. FUNCTIONAL TESTS COMMONLY USED IN REGULATED SAFETY STUDIES

2.1. Clinical Observations

2.1.1. Introduction

Clinical observations are typically organized into endpoints that are collected as the rat is observed in its home cage, as it is removed from the cage and held in the tester's hand, or observed as it wanders freely in an open field arena. Strictly speaking, the ubiquitous involvement of the nervous system in organ-system function means that it is difficult to exclude *a priori* a neurological explanation for observations of dysfunction in many organ systems. For example, the neurotoxicant capsaicin produces a variety of transient and persistent neurotoxic effects that manifest as alterations in respiratory, cardiovascular, thermoregulatory, and integumentary systems, depending on the dose level and route of administration *(5)*. Conversely, while changes in posture and gait may often result from nervous-system dysfunction, they may also result from primary disease in the musculoskeletal system. Nonetheless, a certain subset of clinical observations is generally considered to be analogous to a human or veterinary neurological examination, and are particularly pertinent to the assessment of neurotoxicity. Some endpoints (e.g., surface-righting reaction, auditory startle reaction [ASR]) are recorded subjectively, using categorical (present/absent) or ordinal (e.g., absent, minimal, moderate, severe) scales. For these endpoints, the subject's data are based on the opinion of the tester, much as a veterinary neurologist evaluates a patient. For a quantitative procedure (e.g., forelimb/hindlimb gripstrength, tail flick) the subject's response is detected by a transducer (e.g., strain gauge, photocell) and a value recorded.

Many tests available to human and veterinary neurologists cannot be conducted in laboratory rats. The small size of the rat obviates the use of some reflexes (e.g., the patella reflex). Rats do not follow verbal instructions nor give verbal reports, and these limitations make sensory testing much more difficult than in humans, who can indicate verbally that they perceive a visual, auditory or tactile stimulus. Some tests that can be conducted in rats in experimental neuroscience and psychology cannot be used in the context of standard safety studies. Specifically, it is difficult to use tests that require prolonged training or food/water deprivation or involve significant stress (e.g., tests that involve electric shock), because these procedures might compromise the conduct and/or interpretation of the study. Nonetheless, it is still possible to organize the available tests into a limited neurological examination that includes spinal and cranial nerve reflexes, examination of postural reactions, a sensory evaluation, and observation of spontaneous behavior (e.g. posture, gait). Detailed descriptions and pictures of the tests as they are conducted in rats and domestic animals are available *(6–8)*.

2.1.2. Reflexes and Postural Reactions

A reflex is an involuntary and relatively stereotyped response to a specific sensory stimulus. The location and amplitude of the response depends on both the location and strength of the stimulus. For spinal reflexes (e.g., flexor reflex), the sensory stimuli arise from receptors in muscles, joints, and skin, and the neural circuitry responsible for eliciting the motor response is contained entirely in the spinal cord. Homologous cranial-nerve reflexes are contained within the brain. Many reflexes are named according to the body part (not the nerve) stimulated during the test (e.g., "patellar reflex," "palpebral reflex"). Although the neuronal circuits that mediate reflexes are relatively simple, the brain frequently coordinates the action of several reflex circuits to generate more complex behaviors that clinical neurologists term reactions (e.g., placing reaction).

Postural reactions are complex responses that maintain an animal's normal, upright position under conditions of shifting loads. If an animal's weight is shifted from one side to the other, from front to rear or from rear to front, the increased load on the supporting limb or limbs requires increased tone in the extensor muscles to keep the limb from collapsing. Part of the alteration in tone is accomplished through spinal reflexes, but for the changes to be smooth and coordinated, the sensory and motor systems of the brain must be involved. Abnormalities of complex postural reactions (e.g., hopping) do not provide as anatomically precise information about neurological abnormalities as do reflex tests, which are more limited in scope. However, the intense demands on functional performance required by tests of postural reactions often reveal deficits in key neurological components that are not detected by observing gait (7). The basis(es) for the deficits may then be clarified by further testing of individual reflexes or by electrodiagnostic testing.

2.1.2.1. CRANIAL-NERVE REFLEXES

The somatosensory and somatomotor components of cranial nerve function are difficult to evaluate on more than a categorical (i.e., present/absent) scale. Nonetheless, the status of cranial-nerve reflexes is useful in describing the severity of effects of central nervous system (CNS) depressants, such as general anesthetics (9). The somatosensory component of the 5th cranial nerve and the somatomotor component of the 7th cranial nerve can be tested in rats by using either the palpebral or pinna reflexes. The palpebral reflex is tested by lightly touching the medial canthus (where the upper and lower eyelid meet by the nose) and observing closure of the palpebral fissure (6). The pinna reflex evaluates similar sensory and motor functions and can be performed by lightly touching the inner surface of the outer ear near the concha and observing the flattening of the pinna or shaking of the head that results (6). The pinna reflex can be standardized by using a single Semmes-Weinstein filament (Stoelting, Wood Dale, IL) to conduct the test. In the human neurology clinic, a series of filaments of ascending and descending size are typically used to estimate a threshold for light touch on glabrous (nonhairy) skin (10). However, in testing rats, a single nylon filament is used simply to standardize the procedure. The external ear of the rat has hairs, so that the procedure is not strictly analogous to the human test for cutaneous light touch.

Observations of general health provide indirect evidence for the integrity of certain cranial nerves. For example, normal chewing, eating, drinking, and/or swallowing are maintained by sensory and motor components of the 5th, 9th, 10th, and 12th cranial nerves. However, the small size of the rat makes it difficult to evaluate these functions by direct observation, and changes in food and water intake in toxicity studies are more likely to reflect malaise (see Subheading 2.1.4.2.) than neurological impairment. The somatomotor component of the 3rd, 4th, and 6th cranial nerves can also be evaluated by examining the position of the eye while pupil size is being evaluated (see below). The vestibular system coordinates the activity of the extraocular muscles and thus controls the position and movements of the eyes. Abnormalities in eye position and spontaneous eye movement (nystagmus) are frequently reported for animals with disease of the vestibular system *(7)*, but are rarely, if ever, reported for rats with toxicant-related damage to the vestibular system.

The autonomic component of cranial-nerve reflexes is evaluated by the pupillary size and pupillary reflex, which is typically tested by illuminating the retina with a hand-held light and observing the constriction of the pupil *(6)*. Pupil size and pupil reflex have been shown to be useful indicators of a variety of pharmacological changes that affect the autonomic nervous system *(11–14)*. Another group of endpoints (e.g., lacrimation, salivation) evaluate autonomic nervous-system function, although they are best suited for demonstrating excess lacrimation or salivation, which is useful for detecting chemicals with cholinergic or anticholinesterase activity *(15–17)*. Indeed, it is rare to see a report of insufficient lacrimation or insufficient salivation based on simple observations in a toxicity study.

2.1.2.2. Spinal Reflexes

The somatosensory and somatomotor components of spinal reflexes are tested by the flexor reflex, tail flick reflex, extensor thrust reflex, and grasp reflexes. To evaluate the flexor reflex, the tester supports the subject in the air by grasping the thorax from behind the rat. With the other hand, the tester grasps the toes on one hindlimb and pulls the leg into a position of partial extension. The toes are pinched, and the strength of the flexor response is evaluated. The reaction to the nociceptive stimulus (e.g., squirming or vocalization) may also be recorded. This test is probably more effective as an index of flexor muscle strength of the hind limbs than as a test of mechanical nociceptors, because the strength of the stimulus is uncontrolled, and it is difficult to resist the temptation to pinch "to effect" in order to elicit a response. However, absence of response to pinch may be informative as part of the overall evaluation of a CNS depressant or anesthetic *(9)*.

The tail-flick test is a commonly used test for nociceptive function. For this test, the subject is restrained manually and its tail is placed into a tray containing a heating element. The heating element is activated, and the latency to flick the tail away from the heat source is recorded, typically by a photocell-based system. In contrast to the flexor reflex, the tail-flick test is undoubtedly better as an indicator of nociceptive threshold and less effective as a test of motor function, because only a minimal response of the tail is necessary to trigger the photocell. The tail-flick test has been used primarily to demonstrate the reversible effects of analgesic drugs *(18–20)*, although it is effective in demonstrating persistent changes in nociceptive function that result from neurotoxicant-induced destruction of nociceptive afferents *(21,22)*. Tail temperature is an important variable for interpreting this test, because an initially low or high tail temperature changes the latency to excite thermal nociceptors *(23,24)*. Moreover, a wide variety of drugs and experimental conditions can alter the tail temperature *(25–27)*.

The extensor thrust reflex is used to evaluate the function of pressure receptors and stretch receptors in the foot pads as well as motor nerves to extensor muscles in the lower limb. To evaluate the extensor thrust reflex, the tester supports the subject in the air by grasping the thorax from behind. With the other hand, the tester gently but briskly presses the tips of the forefinger and middle finger into the middle of the plantar surface (i.e., footpads) of each hindlimb (one finger into each footpad). The rat will extend the hindlimbs, and the presence/strength of the extensor response is evaluated by digital palpation, or by using a strain gauge *(28)*. This test exemplifies the importance of considering both sensory and motor deficits in interpreting reductions in somatic reflexes, even though the strength of the response is the measured endpoint. Specifically, the extensor thrust response is reduced very early by low dose, subchronic dosing with acrylamide, and the effect appears to be related to a reduction in peripheral sensory function *(28)*.

The tactile palmar grasp reflex may be estimated by allowing the rat to grip a stable object (e.g., wire cage) with its forelimbs and exerting traction on the tail until the grip is broken. The strength of the palmar and plantar grasp reflexes can be quantified by attaching a T-bar or screen to a strain gauge by a procedure known as forelimb and hindlimb grip strength (FL-HLGS). Two types of gauges are available: an analogue type (e.g., Chatillon Model DPP–1 kg) and a digital type (Chatillon Model DFGS10). The analogue force gauge operates on the principle of Hooke's law. Specifically, a dial on a gauge indicates the degree of displacement of a spring under tension, which is assumed to be proportional to the applied force. The displacement of the spring introduces an error into measurement of the animal's strength forelimb grasp performance, since the animal may be able to "cheat" by capitalizing on the mechanical advantage afforded by pulling the T-bar close to its body at the very start of the test. In this position, the rat can use larger proximal limb muscles to assist in pulling the T-bar. The digital gauge produces a voltage signal that is proportional to applied force. The digital force gauge uses a resistive strain-gauge element whose displacement under applied force is negligible. Furthermore, the internal circuitry of the digital-force gauge compensates for strain-gauge temperature dependency, nonlinearity, and hysteresis.

It should be recognized that the FL-HLGS values may not reflect maximum muscular strength under certain testing conditions. This can be appreciated by noting the decrease in grip strength values that occur during repeated testing when tests are separated by only a few days. Under these conditions, grip strength values decrease by about 25% to plateau levels *(29)*. The decrease in grip performance probably reflects adaptation by the rats to the testing environment (i.e., decreased excitement). This issue is significant because motor units (i.e., an individual motor nerve and all of the muscle fibers that it innervates) are recruited in order of size. That is, a contraction of modest strength requires only small- to medium-sized motor units, and contractions of increased strength require the recruitment of successively larger motor units *(30,31)*. The size of the motor unit, in turn, is related to the size of the axon *(31)*. Thus, under some test conditions the grip strength test may not require the function of the largest motor-nerve fibers, which may be particularly vulnerable in certain toxic axonopathies *(32)*.

Even with its modest limitations, FL/HL-GS is one of the most practical and useful tests developed within the context of neurotoxicity testing *(33)* and has been used with great success to measure the effects of drugs and neurotoxicants *(14,16,28,29,33,34)* that affect somatomotor function. As might be expected, FL/HLGS is particularly useful for demonstrating the effects of neurotoxicants that damage the peripheral motor system *(29)*. For some neurotoxicants, hindlimb function is affected prior to forelimb function, and FLGS is then affected prior to, or to a greater extent, than HLGS *(35,36)*.

Nonetheless, it is important to recognize that motivational factors affect FL/HLGS performance, and FL/HLGS is not a specific measure for neuromuscular function, or for peripheral motor nerves. For example sedation can diminish FL/HLGS values *(37)*.

The function of the urinary and gastrointestinal systems provide clues to the status of both the autonomic and somatic component of spinal reflexes. Both urination and defecation are complex behaviors that require coordinated action of the somatic and autonomic nervous systems. Both activities require stimulation of smooth muscle by parasympathetic fibers, but sympathetic innervation is also required for optimal function. Both actions have a voluntary component, indicating significant control over the autonomic reflex by the brain. And both functions require the coordinated activity of sphincters, which include somatic muscle controlled by spinal reflexes *(38–41)*. Not surprising, micturition and defecation can be altered by an extremely wide variety of drugs and neurological interventions *(40,42)*.

It has been suggested or implied (e.g., ref. *43*) that counting the number of fecal boli and urine pools during the open-field test (*see* Subheading 2.1.4.3.) provides a measure of the autonomic component of defecation and micturition; and these measures are required by some guidelines for neurotoxicity testing (EPA OPPTS 870.6200). This approach is not consistent with the way in which autonomic nervous-system damage is expressed clinically as disorders of defecation and urination, and with the way that this dysfunction is evaluated clinically. Lesions that disrupt the innervation of the bowel are expressed as hyper—or hypomotility states and reflected by colic, abdominal distension, constipation, or diarrhea *(44)*. Body-weight loss is a frequent correlate. Thus, the appropriate endpoints are reflected in the subject's physical condition and quality (not number) of feces. Rodent fecal boli have been counted in novel open-field tests as a measure of emotional reactivity, which may indirectly stimulate defecation *(45)*. However, the counting of fecal boli is not particularly useful as a quantitative measure of autonomic function. Likewise, interruption of the bladder-reflex pathways by disease, drugs, or neurotoxicants is often expressed by observable signs including a change in void volume (increase or decrease) or urinary dribbling *(41,42,44,46–48)*. But the counting of urine pools, in the absence of void volume, provides little information. It should also be noted that obtaining accurate void volumes in groups of rats is a relatively trivial and noninvasive procedure that requires no food deprivation, aversive stimulation, or anesthesia. Each rat is given an oral water load by gavage, and the individual micturition events during the next hour are recorded by collecting the voids under the cage in a beaker attached to a load cell. A modest test system can determine void volumes accurately for 10–20 rats/h *(49)*.

The counting of fecal boli and urine pools in an open field as a measure of autonomic function is particularly problematic in repeat-dose toxicity studies, because defecation and urination decrease to very low levels after repeated experience with an initially novel environment. The limited value of these measures is confirmed by Catalano et al. *(50)*, who reported that counts of fecal boli and urine pools were among the least reliable endpoints in a functional observational battery (FOB).

A weak case can be made for recording the presence or absence of urine/feces in single-dose studies. Many rats will urinate or defecate during the first exposure to a novel chamber, and a failure of a group of rats to urinate or defecate could indicate a pharmacological effect *(41,42)*.

2.1.2.3. POSTURAL REACTIONS

Both the EPA and OECD guidelines for subchronic studies indicate the need to evaluate the reaction to proprioceptive stimulation *(3)*, and this is accomplished by various tests of postural reactions. The following discussion of these is intended to illustrate that tests of proprioception evaluate many and diverse nervous system structures, and help explain why they are such an important part of the evaluation of nervous-system function in safety studies.

Proprioception involves information about the position of the limbs (general proprioception) and head (special proprioception) in space during both static posture and movement. General proprioception is initiated by receptors in the muscles, tendons and joints that travel to the spinal cord in large myelinated fibers. Special proprioception is initiated by receptors (crista, macula) in the inner ear *(51)*.

Neurologists distinguish two types of general and special proprioception, which are mediated by separate projections of these peripheral afferent fibers from the limbs and head. Conscious proprioception is that function that enables an individual to be aware of the position of their limbs and head during static posture, and in the absence of visual information. For example, normal people can close their eyes and indicate verbally whether their right arm is by their side, at a 90° angle to their trunk, or straight up into the air. This proprioceptive sense depends on spinal projection fibers that travel in the dorsal columns of the spinal cord (fasciculi cuneatus and gracilis). Subsequently, information that travels in this pathway is relayed to somesthetic cortex via dorsal column nuclei in the medulla, internal arcuate fibers, medial lemniscus, and ventral posterior lateral thalamus. Unconscious proprioception enables the position of the limbs to be adjusted and coordinated smoothly during movement, even though the individual is unaware of the position of the limbs during the movement. This proprioceptive function depends on spinal projections of limb afferents that travel in the lateral columns (spinocerebellar pathways) to the cerebellum *(51)*.

Special proprioception involves the position of the head during static posture and movement. The afferents of this system comprise the peripheral vestibular system, which projects to the vestibular nuclei and cerebellum. The unconscious proprioception component depends on the direct projection of vestibular afferents to the cerebellum, and from projections from vestibular nuclei (vestibulospinal path) to motor systems in the spinal cord. The relative contribution of vestibular afferents for the conscious proprioception of the head is complicated because afferents from the muscles of the neck contribute significantly to the awareness of static head position *(51,52)*.

Conscious proprioceptive sense can be evaluated in rats by using the proprioceptive positioning reaction, which is commonly used by veterinary neurologists *(7)* but is relatively unknown to many neurotoxicologists. The test depends on the tendency of normal animals to keep their limbs in weight-bearing position directly under the body. The tester gently restrains the subject on a horizontal surface by grasping the thorax. The hind limb to be tested is flexed so that the dorsal surface of the paw is on the testing surface (usually a table top). The tester relaxes the restraint of the limb, but not the thorax. The rat will immediately return the paw to a weight-bearing position. Alternatively, the tester places a sheet of cardboard under a weight-bearing limb and moves the cardboard slowly in a lateral direction. As the limb reaches an abnormal position, the animal should return the limb to a normal position for bearing weight.

Unconscious proprioception is tested by a variety of postural reactions, including righting reactions, placing reactions, and the hopping reaction. Righting reactions have been evaluated by neuroscientists for many years, particularly to quantify the effects of CNS depressants. For example, onset and duration of the loss of the surface-righting reaction has been used to quantify "sleep time" of general anesthetic chemicals *(53,54)*, an effect that would be considered as evidence of neurotoxicity for a chemical not intended for surgical use. In its simplest form the surface righting reaction is trivial to conduct: the tester places the animal on its back on a horizontal surface. The subject is restrained briefly, then restraint is removed quickly. The normal rat quickly reassumes a normal standing position. For anesthetics, it may be sufficient to measure the onset and duration of loss of righting reaction. However, the righting reaction is complex, requiring the coordinated action of many different muscles in the neck, trunk, and limbs *(55)*. Considerably more information about neurological function may be derived with additional effort in recording and analyzing the righting reaction. For example, the latency and duration of the righting reaction may be measured *(56,57)*. Evaluation of qualitative effects may also be useful. For example, the position of the limbs should be evaluated immediately after the subject obtains a weight-bearing position, since proprioceptive deficits (e.g., bearing weight on the dorsal surface of a limb, especially a hindlimb) may be seen in animals that otherwise appear to right themselves normally. Finally, there may be value in examining the progression of the righting reaction. Generally, the reaction of proceeds rostrocaudally, with the head initiating the reaction, followed sequentially by the forelimbs and hind limbs. Some neurological deficits in rats are revealed by a change in the pattern or progression of the righting reaction in rats that right themselves successfully and quickly *(58)*. The surface righting reaction is of short duration (average duration is <0.40 s; *57,59*), so that analysis of video-taped responses is typically required to analyze the progression of the individual components of this reaction.

The aerial righting reaction is conducted by supporting the subject in the air with its back facing a horizontal surface. The tester's hands are removed rapidly and smoothly from the subject. The subject quickly rights itself in the air so that the weight-bearing surface of the paws is in an appropriate position when the subject reaches the horizontal surface. As for surface righting, the value of the test may be greatly improved by measuring the speed and progression of the reaction. The speed of the reaction can be measured in two ways. A simple approach is to begin the test about 5–10 cm from the surface and to raise the rat in 5-cm increments until righting has been accomplished successfully *(60)*. A ruler can be placed vertically adjacent to the surface to measure height accurately. This procedure has been used to quantify the effects of several CNS depressants that produce ataxia *(60)*. Alternatively, the speed of the response can be obtained by reviewing video tapes of the response. Review of video tapes can also reveal subtle changes in the character of the reaction, which may be the most significant indicators of variations in the response *(55,61)*. Unfortunately, many laboratories evaluate the response by holding the subject far from the landing surface (e.g., 30 cm) and recording the response categorically. This procedure extracts only a fraction of the information that may be available with only a little more effort.

The placing reaction is conducted in rats by suspending the subject in the air by holding it by the base of the tail, then moving it towards a horizontal surface (e.g., table top). When the vibrissae touch the edge of the table, the subject extends its neck, trunk, and forelimbs. As the table is reached, the subject will climb onto the surface. In many nonrodent animal species, vision plays an important part in this response. However, visual placing is not robust in rats *(62)*. Instead, the response is typically initiated by tactile information provided by the vibrissae. The mystacial vibrissae of the rat extend so far from the face that tactile placing initiated by cutaneous receptors is difficult to evaluate without shaving the vibrissae *(63)*.

The hopping reaction is conducted by holding the subject so that three limbs are tucked into the body surface, and much of the subject's body weight rests on the limb to be tested. The subject can be moved forward, medially or laterally (laterally is most effective; *57,62*). The subject will "hop" on the limb to maintain it in normal weight-bearing position. Hopping is generally considered by veterinary neurologists to be one of the most challenging tests for the subject to perform, and one of the most sensitive tests for detecting deficits *(7)*. Hopping requires the coordinated action of many muscles in the neck, trunk, and limbs. In particular, significant strength of limb extensor muscles is required. To illustrate, rats can hop on either forelimb or hindlimb at approx 7 hops/s while supporting approx 60% of their body weight on a single limb *(57)*. The reaction forces produced by the individual hops can be measured using a force plate, and the performance of hopping is impaired by acrylamide and haloperidol *(57)*.

Most laboratories do not evaluate hopping, partly because hopping requires considerable care on the part of the tester to ensure that the conditions of the test (e.g., speed of lateral movement, % body weight on the tested limb) are the same for each rat. As a result, there is very little known about the effects of neurotoxicants on this postural reaction.

The hindlimb landing foot-splay test is conducted by holding the rat horizontally a specified height (~20 cm) above a table top and dropping the rat. The distance between the hind feet upon landing is measured, generally by putting a drop of ink on the foot pads and dropping the rat onto a piece of paper. The hindlimb landing foot-splay test is popular because of its sensitivity to acrylamide neurotoxicity *(64,65)*. Considering the popularity of the splay test and its inclusion in the EPA neurotoxicity-testing guidelines (EPA OPPTS 870.6200), surprisingly little is known about this test. The anatomical basis for the test is unknown, and there is no obvious analogue used by veterinary or human neurologists. It is possible to hypothesize about the neurological basis for the test. The movement of the rat through space likely stimulates vestibular, tactile (vibrissae and other hairs), and visual receptors *(66)*. And extension of the limbs is an intuitively reasonable postural response in anticipation of landing *(52)*. However, the rationale for using the width of the response as in index of function is not at all clear. And while an increase in width has been reported for compounds producing a distal axonopathy with neurofilamentous accumulations, the interpretation of a decrease in width is not at all clear. This interpretation problem is curious, because reductions or loss of function is usually interpretable for tests of neurological function. Although the hindlimb landing foot-splay test is popular, the previously discussed tests of proprioception may be easier to interpret and relate to additional functional and morphological effects.

2.1.3. Special Sensory Evaluation

The function of general somatic afferents to skin, muscle, and joints is evaluated by observation of posture and gait (*see* Subheading 2.1.4.3.) and by the tests of reflexes and reactions described previously (*see* Subheading 2.1.2.2.). This section deals with the evaluation of tactile sensitivity and the function of the special senses: vision, audition, olfaction, and taste. To evaluate these functions requires the tester to present a variety of levels or types of stimuli and measure the reaction to each. Unfortunately, conducting this type of evaluation in laboratory animals generally requires sophisticated equipment and time-consuming procedures that are not currently available for use in laboratories conducting standard safety studies (e.g., *67*). Our discussion will be limited to those rapid tests that have reached some level of popularity.

The so-called touch response *(6,68)* is conducted by approaching the rat from the caudolateral aspect (from the side and behind) and touching the rump of the rat gently with a blunt object such as a pen or pencil. The tester records the reaction of the rat. There are many possible reactions, including flinching, jumping, slowly turning of the head or body, or walking away. As a measure of contact sensibility, this test has a plethora of problems in conduct and interpretation. First, it is difficult to stimulate the rat in a standard way, because a hand-held blunt object does not provide a standard pressure, and the rat can move before/during the presentation of the object. Second, tests of cutaneous sensibility are intended to evaluate cutaneous mechanoreceptors, not hairs, and are generally performed on glabrous (nonhairy) skin, such as a digit *(69)*. Third, many normal rats do not respond in a robust way to the stimulation. Thus, this test involves a stimulus that cannot be controlled and a response that cannot be predicted. Its utility as a test of tactile sensitivity is questionable.

The so-called visual approach response *(6,68)* is conducted by approaching the rat at nose level with the end of a blunt object and holding it approx 3 cm from the face for a few seconds, to give the rat time to respond. Possible reactions include whisking of the vibrissae, flinching, orientation (e.g., approaching or turning away from the object), biting, or defensive reaction (e.g., rearing into a "boxing" position). This test suffers from all of the deficiencies of the touch response (*see* above), and is not a robust test of vision.

The auditory startle test is conducted by measuring the flinch that occurs shortly after presentation of a brief, broad-band, high-amplitude auditory stimulus (e.g., metal clicker, snap of a metal clip on a clipboard, snap of fingers). In first-tier safety studies, the response is typically observed and recorded on a subjective ordinal scale (e.g., none, low, moderate, high). The response may also be evaluated quantitatively by presenting more precisely controlled auditory stimuli and recording the flinch with various electromechanical transducers *(70,71)*. The flinch represents the rapid, sequential contraction of muscles in the head and neck, forelimbs, axial region, and hindlimbs *(70)*. The core neuroanatomical elements underlying this response in the rat include receptors in the cochlea, auditory nerve, cochlear nuclei (ventral cochlear nuclei, cochlear root neurons), ventrolateral tegmental nucleus, nucleus reticularis pontis caudalis, reticulospinal tract, and spinal motor units *(70,71)*. The qualitative version of the test is not a robust test of auditory sensitivity, but is at least sufficient to detect rats with profound cochlear damage *(72)*, which show a reduced or absent response.

It should be obvious that the common tests of sensation do not measure *sensitivity*, but rather *reactivity* to stimulation. Reactivity to stimulation is also evaluated as the reaction to handling when the rat is removed from its home cage for hand-held observations. Taken together, these tests are probably better at providing a measure of CNS stimulants, CNS depressants, or general anesthetics than they are at detecting changes in sensation per se. An increased response to handling or external stimuli is a useful indicator of a variety of pharmacological effects *(68,73,74)* or brain lesions induced by physical or chemical agents *(75,76)*. A decreased reactivity to auditory or tactile stimulation is also a useful indicator of transient behavioral depression produced resulting from pharmacological effects (*68; see* Subheading 2.1.2.1.). However, in toxicity studies, decreased reactivity should be interpreted in the context of indicators of malaise such as decreased body weight, decreased grooming, and hypothermia (*see* Subheading 2.1.4.2.).

The chemical senses of olfaction and taste are not generally tested in neurotoxicity studies. Although the rat has a relatively large olfactory system, even complete removal of the olfactory bulbs produces few, if any, obvious changes in spontaneous behavior. A relatively simple olfactory-cued food-retrieval task has been developed and is quite effective in demonstrating olfactory deficits produced by toxicants *(77)*. The task involves locating a food pellet buried under a layer of bedding *(78)*. Unfortunately, even this relatively simple task is too complex to be utilized in standard safety studies, as the rats must be food deprived, and several acquisition sessions must be conducted before exposure to test chemicals can be evaluated. The primary taste modalities of salty, sweet, and bitter can be evaluated by a variety of procedures, all of which are too complex to be utilized in standard safety tests.

2.1.4. Observation of Spontaneous Behavior

Observation of spontaneous neurological abnormalities occurs during three parts of the clinical observations: in the home cage, while the rat is being held in the tester's hand, and during open-field testing.

2.1.4.1. HOME-CAGE OBSERVATIONS

In theory, home-cage observations provide an opportunity to record observations of behavior before the subject has been disturbed by the tester. In reality, it is very difficult to obtain meaningful information from observing rats at rest, especially if they are housed in typical wire cages. The vast majority of rats will be either sleeping or sitting still, and a feed container may also obscure the view. The cage can be opened to improve the view of the rat, but of course this disturbs the animal and eliminates the potential value of observing the animal in an undisturbed state.

2.1.4.2. HAND-HELD OBSERVATIONS

Some of the hand-held observations (e.g., respiratory sounds, skin lesions, and stains) are typical of classic clinical observations for general health that have been conducted for many years as part of regulated safety studies. Although these observations generally do not provide direct evidence of nervous system dysfunction, these measures of general health provide an extremely important context for interpreting many of the other observations. Among the hand-held observations, malaise is indicated by signs including hypothermia (cold to touch) and decreased grooming *(79)*.

The latter is evidenced by a rough hair coat and staining of the fur, particularly around the eyes, mouth, and distal extremities. It is important to recognize that malaise is not generally indicative of nervous-system dysfunction. Quite the contrary, malaise is an organized behavioral state that is coordinated by the nervous system, and which may have adaptive value in the face of disease *(79–83)*. Additional signs of malaise include reduced palpebral closure (*see* below), decreased strength, decreased reaction to handling, and decreased locomotor activity *(79–83)*.

Palbebral closure is a particularly important hand-held observation. Like any other somatic muscle, the muscle of the eyelids are innervated by somatic motor neurons. Thus, it would not be surprising to observe lid closure (i.e., ptosis) resulting from neurotoxicants that affect the activity of lower motor neurons. Indeed, in humans, ptosis is an early indicator of myasthenia gravis, a disease of the neuromuscular junction *(84)*. However, the importance of ptosis in toxicity studies relates primarily to Muller's superior tarsal muscle, a sympathetically innervated muscle that contributes to upper-eyelid retraction *(85,86)*. Thus, ptosis can be produced by a variety of chemicals with central or peripheral sympatholytic activity *(87–90)*. The degree of sympatholytic effect can be assessed *(91)* by recording the severity of ptosis using a semi-quantitative scale (e.g., wide open, quarter-closed, half-closed, etc.). However, ptosis is also a very common indicator of pain or malaise in rodents *(92)*, so that observations of ptosis need to be interpreted carefully in the context of signs of malaise discussed previously.

Although the vast majority of spontaneous movement abnormalities are best observed as part of the open-field observation (*see* below), a few of these observations are facilitated by a close examination of the hand-held rat. For example, fasciculation is a spontaneous, involuntary twitching of muscle fibers that may be observed as rippling of the skin if it involves subcutaneous muscles. Fasciculation is often confused with the term fibrillation, which is an abnormal electric potential characteristically emitted by denervated muscles *(93)*. Fasciculation has been reported as a consistent effect produced by chemicals that inhibit acetylcholinesterase *(94–96)*. Small amplitude resting tremors (a.k.a. fine tremors) of the distal extremities may be best observed as hand held observations, because the rat may be held for close examination, and because weight bearing may obscure the effect while the animal is in the open field. It is important to recognize that the amplitude of the tremor is related to the type, not severity, of a neurological change. That is, fine tremors are not necessarily a minor effect, nor a lesser affect than large amplitude tremors. Tremors have been reported in rats as a effect of the insect repellent diethyltoluamide (a.k.a. DEET) and various pyrethroids, chlorinated hydrocarbons, and acetylcholinesterase inhibitors. *(73,95–99)*. Tremors are also part of a behavioral/neurological syndrome associated with acute central serotonin excess *(100)*. It should be noted, however, that shivering and/or tremors are often observed as a thermogenic response of hypothermic mammals (e.g., after anesthesia; *101*). Thus, tremors observed in animals with signs of severe malaise need to be interpreted carefully.

2.1.4.3. Open-Field Observations

The requirement to observe rats in an open field is one of the most significant changes in the conduct of clinical observations mandated by the newer test guidelines. This effort is appropriate, because the open-field evaluations are sufficient to detect the

Table 1
Effects of Neurotoxicants Dosed at the MTD

Chemical class	Effect
Axonopathic, myelinopathic neuronopathic chemicals	Weakness, paralysis, obvious gait disorder *(109,229,230)*
Chlorinated hydrocarbon	Tremor, myoclonus *(98)*
CNS depressants	Ataxia, impaired righting reaction *(53–54,124,129–130)*
CNS stimulants	Stereotypy *(137)*
Excitotoxicants	Convulsion *(231)*
Organophosphate pesticides	Convulsion *(232)*
Pyrethroid insecticide	Tremor *(73)*

vast majority of known neurotoxicants. The sufficiency of the open field observations is based on the fact that regulatory guidelines typically require testing of materials at the maximum tolerated dose (MTD). At the MTD, neurotoxicants produce spontaneous neurological effects that are quite obvious (Table 1). However, open-field observations place a considerable burden on the expertise of the tester, because the scope of the possible observations is broad, and the use of appropriate terminology is essential. And unlike the endpoints in anatomical and clinical pathology, there are no duplicate samples to rerun, nor slides to send for peer review. In spite of this unique responsibility, personnel observing for neurological dysfunction in standard safety studies have far less training, proficiency evaluation, continuing education, and professional support than for their colleagues in anatomical or clinical pathology *(3)*.

The observations are conducted as the rat walks in a small arena that is called an open field. The duration of the test is typically 2–3 min., and the spontaneous movements typically evaluated in this test include the level of activity (ambulatory activity and rearing), posture, gait, and spontaneous movement abnormalities. The qualitative evaluation of auditory startle and excretions usually occurs in the open field, but these were discussed in Subheadings 2.1.2. and 2.1.3.

The level of activity is an overall assessment of ambulatory and nonambulatory movements in the open field, including walking, standing, rearing, sniffing, and head movements. In many cases, these behaviors do not occur uniformly during the entire period. Instead, there is an initial period of immobility, followed by a transition to the full locomotion pattern required for exploration. This transition evolves in a predictable sequence termed "warm up" *(102,103)*, to reflect the fact that behavior initially consists of small movements of individual body parts (head, trunk, limbs), then expands to include coordinated movement required for locomotion. However, the typical qualitative assessment of level of activity does not take warm up into account.

Rearing refers to the lifting of both forepaws from the floor. Adoption of this bipedal posture is almost certainly a challenge to the rat's postural control system. Not surprising, a wide variety of neurotoxicants decease rearing frequency *(68,104,105)*. It is tempting to interpret decreases in rearing as an animal model to the human "sway" test for postural instability *(106,107)* that may be conducted as part of a neurological examination. However, there are significant differences between rodent rearing and the human sway test. In humans, upright posture is the norm, and the conditions for maximizing human postural sway are relatively easily developed by asking the patient to close their eyes. In rats, rearing is a voluntary action and varies widely among normal animals, so that failure to rear cannot be equated with inability to rear. Furthermore, different labs may have different criteria for what constitutes a rear *(6)*, and rats can often rear both with and without the aid of the side wall in the open field. Thus, the count of spontaneous rearing is not analogous to the human sway test, because a human who was unable to maintain an upright posture without the aid of a wall would be considered to have significant dysfunction.

Another limitation of rearing as an indicator of neurotoxicity is that the stimulus factors underlying the initiation of rearing are unknown. For example, we have observed rats who rear in an apparent attempt at scanning the testing room for distal visual stimuli. Scanning for distal visual cures is an important part of rodent orientation/navigation *(108)*. However, we have observed no difference in rearing frequency in rats tested in both illuminated rooms and rooms lacking illumination (unpublished observations using infrared cameras and reflective markers) so that visual cues, distant or proximal, are not necessary for initiating the response.

In an open field the rat typically adopts a posture suitable for locomotion, with the trunk held off the ground, the head in line with the trunk, and the feet positioned to support body weight. The spinal column is slightly curved dorsally. Some spontaneous postural abnormalities (e.g., hunched posture, low carriage, writhing, head tilt) are most often associated with general toxicity, malaise, or infectious disease and are frequently observed in toxicity studies. Other postural abnormalities (e.g., knuckling, wide-based stance, catalepsy) are most often associated with neurological dysfunction and are infrequently observed in toxicity studies. Increased spinal curvature (hunched posture) is frequently associated with malaise, especially secondary to gastrointestinal irritation *(92)*. Low carriage is often caused by malaise, but may be caused by a variety of drugs and toxicants that render the rat too weak or uncoordinated to maintain the trunk and pelvis off the ground *(109)*. Weakness or proprioceptive deficit may also be associated with a posture sometimes called "knuckling," in which the dorsal surface of the paw(s) is held in contact with the ground *(109)*. Unilateral vestibular disease is associated with a characteristic postural abnormality: head tilt. Unilateral vestibular disease in rats is most often associated with infectious disease of the internal ear produced by *Mycoplasma pulmonis*, *Pasteurella pneumotropica*, or *Streptococcus pneumoniae (110)*. These diseases are rare in laboratory rat colonies meeting contemporary health standards. In contrast, vestibular toxicants such as iminodiproprionitrile generally produce a bilateral vestibular abnormality *(111)* that is associated with a syndrome including a postural change (wide-based stance), a gait abnormality (ataxia), and a spontaneous movement disorder (stereotypical, side-to-side head movements; *112*). The syndrome has been termed "waltzing disorder" *(113)*.

Catalepsy is a disorder associated most frequently with dopamine antagonist drugs (e.g., haloperidol) and includes akinesia (i.e., a marked reduction or absence of movement) and a postural abnormality characterized by exaggerated contact-related postural reactions. Specifically, the haloperidol-treated rat will remain in contact with any surface (e.g., floor, rods) that its paws contact. As a result, the paws of haloperidol-treated rats will remain in contact with surfaces (e.g., floor, rod, wire screen) even if their limbs are placed on the surfaces by the tester and the remainder of the body is required to maintain an unusual or awkward posture *(114–116)*. This tendency to maintain unusual postures may create an impression that that cataleptic rats are incapable of initiating movement. This impression is incorrect. For example, cataleptic rats perform air-righting reactions normally *(114)*. Muscle tone is not impaired. In fact muscle tone is increased when the rat's paws are in contact with surface. That is, the rats actively resist passive movement of its body when its limbs are in contact with a surface. This active resistance results from simultaneous contraction of normally antagonistic muscles. The state of the muscles is like that of a person who has climbed a high tree, then becomes "paralyzed" with fear as the ground is visualized. The current posture on the limb is defended by clinging and resisting displacement in any direction. This defense requires simultaneous activation of agonist and antagonist muscles around many joints. In the open field, haloperidol-treated rats have prolonged latencies to initiate movement and resist attempts to be pushed horizontally off their current location or to be prodded into movement *(114–116)*. Haloperidol-treated rats differ from rats dosed with other psychoactive substances (e.g., morphine) that may also be akinetic, but which do not resist passive displacement from their initial location on the floor of the open field *(116)*.

Gait abnormalities include ataxia and retropulsion. Retropulsion is an uncommon observation that indicates either persistent backward locomotion, or forceful, sudden backward movements. Sometimes the movement appears to be from extension of the forelimbs, which push the body backward *(6)*. Retropulsion has been reported occasionally as a sign of drug withdrawal *(117,118)* and for several neurotoxicants that affect vestibular function or supraspinal motor systems *(112,119–120)*.

The term "ataxia" is derived from the Greek:-a (= negative article) + taxi (= order). The literal translation is: "movement which is out of order." Most commonly the term ataxia is used to describe movements that are uncoordinated and clumsy. In quadripeds such as rodents, the term ataxia is most appropriately applied to a staggering, reeling, or lurching gait *(6)*. Such a gait is often accompanied by a wide-based stance, although a wide-based stance *per se* is not ataxia, but rather is a separate postural abnormality. Many years ago the term ataxia was used as a "catch all" term to describe impaired movement of any sort. The availability of training tools *(6)* for laboratory personnel may have improved this problem. Ataxia has been reported as a sign of neurotoxicity for many chemicals, and families of chemicals causing ataxia include insecticides *(121–122)*, anesthetics *(123)*, organic solvents *(124,125)*, heavy metals *(126)*, and many psychoactive drugs *(127–129)*.

In addition to ataxia and retropulsion, a wide variety of different gait abnormalities have been reported in the experimental literature. Many of these reports use specialized names (e.g., "waltzing," "duck-walking") whose definitions are not universally understood in the medical and toxicological community *(113,130)*. These types of terms are less meaningful than medically precise terms.

Spontaneous movement disorders include dyskinesias, convulsions, and stereotypical behavior *(7,131,132)*, and are part of the signs of neurological dysfunction associated with many neurotoxicants *(68,73,75 96–99,104,121,126,133–136)*. The term dyskinesia originates from the Greek "dyskinesia" (= difficulty of movement) and is a general term for a movement disorder. Common dysknesias include myoclonus, dystonia (myotonia), chorea, tics, and tremors. The term clonus is derived from the Greek "klonos" (= turmoil) and the term myoclonus refers to sudden, brief involuntary movements caused by muscular contractions (positive myoclonus) or inhibitions (negative myoclonus). These are brief, paroxysmal muscle jerks which often move an affected limb chaotically. The brief contractions of myoclonus should be distinguished from myotonia or dystonia, in which the contractions are sustained. Both myoclonic and myotonic contractions can be included in the term spasm. The term "tic" describes dyskinesia with a volitional component, and the term tic is best reserved for human conditions.

The movements of chorea resemble some types of myoclonic jerks in that the movements are brief and irregular (chaotic). The key feature of chorea is that the movements continue in a constant flow, randomly distributed over the body, with each involved muscle jerking randomly in time. The movements of chorea are neither repetitive nor rhythmical, and it is therefore impossible to know where or when to expect the next twitch. In contrast, myoclonus is characterized by distinctive and repetitive patterns of muscle jerking in which the same muscle groups contract time and time again, sometimes even rhythmically *(132)*. The muscle contractions of dystonia are more prolonged than those of myoclonus and distort the body into characteristic dystonic postures. Myoclonus and dystonia may occur in the same subject. The term spasm is a general term used to describe either a brief (i.e., myoclonic) or sustained (i.e., myotonic) muscle contraction. The term spasm is often used when the muscle contraction is associated with pain (e.g., occurs with vocalization).

Rhythmic myoclonus differs from tremor. The movements in tremor are rhythmic and oscillatory (sinusoidal). Rhythmic myoclonus is more like a "square wave" with an interval between each movement. Tremors are frequently classified as resting tremors (a.k.a. static tremors) or action tremors (a.k.a. kinetic tremors, intention tremors). Action tremors are markedly worsened by use of the affected body part(s), whereas the severity of resting tremors is independent of use of the affected limb. Many families of chemicals, especially insecticides and heavy metals, produce myoclonus or tremors at some dosing regimen *(75,96–99,104,124,126,133)*.

The terms seizure, convulsion, epilepsy and fit are synonyms for a brain disorder characterized by a paroxysmal cerebral dysrhythmia (i.e., an abrupt change in the electrical activity of the brain). The dysrhythmia has a sudden onset, frequently ceases spontaneously, and often recurs. The terms "seizure" and "convulsion" are used most frequently. The term "epilepsy" is often reserved for recurrent seizures of unknown cause (idiopathic). The term "fit" is used infrequently in the contemporary scientific literature.

Seizures often have three successive phases of independent duration and severity: (1) the aura (behavior during the pre-ictal period), (2) the ictus (the "attack" or "fit"), and (3) the recovery. Seizures can be described as partial (localizing signs) or generalized (no localizing signs). Partial seizures may evolve into generalized seizures. Seizures often occur immediately preceding death (agonal seizures). During the aura the subject exhibits behavioral changes (e.g., may become restless, exhibit frenzied activity, freeze, or stare into space). The ictus is characterized by involuntary muscle activity, which can be autonomic (e.g., pupillary dilation, vomiting, salivation, defecation, urination), somatic (e.g., chewing, paddling), or both. Many of the terms used to characterize dyskinesias are used as modifiers to describe abnormalities of somatic muscle activity expressed during a seizure (e.g., myoclonic convulsion, tonic/clonic convulsion). The recovery phase of the convulsion may last from minutes to days. Behavioral abnormalities may include long periods of sleeping, wandering, circling and/or bumping into objects *(7)*. Many families of chemicals, including insecticides, heavy metals, and excitatory amino acids, produce convulsions as a result of some dosing regimen *(68,97,121,126,136)*.

Stereotypy is the performance of an invariant sequence or repetition of specific gestures or movements that appear to be excessive or purposeless *(6)*. Behavior of a stereotypic rat will often occur out of context and with abnormally high frequency, to the exclusion of other behaviors. Examples of stereotypy include, but are not limited to, circling in tight circles, grooming whose duration continues well beyond the normal grooming action, persistent pacing (especially in one particular direction or around the perimeter of the open field), repetitive sniffing at one area, and head weaving. The behaviors themselves are normal; many rats occasionally groom or walk around in a circle. It is rather the frequency and persistence of these behaviors that distinguish them as stereotypic. Stereotypy is associated with chemicals that directly or indirectly affect activity at dopaminergic or cholinergic synapses in the brain *(137–139)*.

2.2. Measurement of Locomotor Activity

2.2.1. Introduction

This quantification of locomotor activity is distinct from the qualitative assessment of motor activity performed during the observation of open-field behavior. In theory, measurement of locomotor activity should quantify and improve the precision of what has already been learned from the qualitative observation of movement during the observation of behavior in the open field. In this capacity, it would be analogous to the measurement of grip strength, which provides a quantified estimate of strength to provide perspective for the qualitative estimate of strength recorded as a hand-held observation (e.g., palmar grasp). However, the term "locomotor activity" can be applied to a wide variety of test systems that measure quite different aspects of the behavior (e.g., exploration, navigation, emotional reactions) that occur while a rat ambulates in an enclosure. Unfortunately, none of the currently available systems is complete enough to provide a quantitative version of the qualitative endpoints that are examined in the open field through observation.

The measurement of locomotor activity of rats as part of a neurotoxicity battery is controversial. Some neurotoxicologists favor the use of locomotor activity measurements *(140)*, and locomotor activity is measured as a part of several test guidelines (EPA OPPTS Guidelines 870.3100, 870.6200; OECD guideline 407, 408). Other neurotoxicologists argue that locomotor activity data are both too variable and too difficult to interpret to be used as a primary measure of neurotoxicity *(141)*. Some psychopharmacologists have made similar arguments *(142,143)*. Some testing guidelines for neurotoxicity (e.g., draft Food and Drug Administration [FDA] guidelines for food additives; *144*) do not include measurement of locomotor activity.

The following section includes descriptions of some of the many test systems that have been used to measure locomotor activity, and will provide sufficient historical and contemporary data to clarify the strengths and limitations in interpretation associated with the locomotor activity testing most commonly performed as part of toxicity studies.

2.2.2. Technical Considerations

There are at least three technical aspects that must be considered to appreciate the similarities and differences among test-systems for measuring locomotor activity: (1) the test environment (2) the transducer(s) or detector device(s), and (3) the quantitative analysis applied to the raw data.

2.2.2.1. TEST ENVIRONMENT

The testing environment is an important factor, and consists of the floor, walls, and enclosure. The are three common shapes for the floor of locomotor activity test devices: (1) square/rectangular, (2) round, and (3) figure-eight. Square or rectangular devices are the most common, probably due to the ease of construction *(145)*. Round enclosures have the advantage of a similarity to circular open fields that were particularly popular among experimental psychologists several decades ago *(146)*. Figure-eight "mazes" are configured to resemble tunnels that may be more like rodents' natural environment than the other two types of devices. The walls/ceiling of the square or circular devices are typically high enough to permit or even to encourage the rat to rear to examine the vertical surface of the test chamber. The walls/ceiling of the figure-eight maze are generally short, increasing the resemblance of the maze to a tunnel.

The type of enclosure and level of illumination are particularly important factors to consider when evaluating locomotor activity data. In general, relatively high levels of illumination tend to increase the duration of the warm-up period and reduce the level of activity, ostensibly by increasing emotional reactions (e.g., fear, anxiety), which reduces exploration and/or elicit "freezing" behavior *(147,148)*. Access to distal visual cues is another important factor. Rodents navigate in their environment by using a variety of ideothetic and allothetic cues. Ideothetic cues arise from the animal's own movement and are provided by vestibular receptors and muscle/joint receptors (i.e., proprioceptors; *see* Subheading 2.1.2.3.). Ideothetic cues are likely to play a greater role in navigation in large environments with many turns (e.g., figure-eight maze) than in small symmetric enclosures. Allothetic cues include stable external visual, olfactory, and auditory stimuli *(149,150)*. The availability of distal visual cues is particularly important when the rats are tested in an enclosure with low walls. Obviously, if the walls and ceiling of the enclosure are high and opaque, then the contribution of the distal visual cues to the behavior of the animals is essentially eliminated.

2.2.2.2. ACTIVITY DETECTOR

There are two common types of detector systems used to quantify the behavior of rats in a test chamber: photocell-based systems and video-based systems. In photocell-based systems, lines of photocells are placed at regular intervals along the perimeter of the test chamber. Typically, the photocells are placed about 1 inch apart. In some photocell-based systems there are two levels of photocells. A lower row of photocells is placed approx 3–6 cm from the floor, and this row detects horizontal activity (i.e., ambulation). A second row of photocells is placed 10–15 cm from the floor, and this row of photocells detects rearing. In video-based systems, one or more cameras are used to record the behavior of the rat. These two types of systems vary considerably in terms of cost, speed of data acquisition, resolution of behavior, and interpretability of the data. In general, video-based systems cost more and are slower to operate, but provide much higher resolution, and better identification of individual behaviors (see below). Video-based systems are slower to operate because the raw data are often analyzed off-line with either visual review *(151)* or image processing software *(152,153)*, which are used to identify individual behaviors (e.g, standing, turning, grooming). Either of these approaches can be very time-consuming. In contrast, photocell counts can be returned almost immediately to the experimenter. The resolution of behavior is particularly important for endpoints such as walking speed, consistency of walking path, and turning. The relatively large distance between photocells in most commercially available locomotor activity devices results in inherent and important limitations in resolution. However, photocell-based systems are the norm for standard toxicity studies.

2.2.2.3. ANALYSIS

There are roughly two types of analyses of locomotor activity data, which we will arbitrarily term macroanalysis and microanalysis. The term macroanalysis implies gross characteristics of the behavior including path length (i.e., total horizontal activity), spatial distribution of locomotion (e.g., in center or periphery of enclosure), temporal distribution of locomotion (e.g., in a 40-min session, the level of activity is generally decreases across successive 10-min intervals), and speed of ambulation. The term microanalysis includes smaller components of the rats' behavior. The smaller components may be either small segments of the locomotion path *(154,155)*, or individual behaviors such as sitting, standing, sniffing, grooming, or turning, *(152,153)*.

2.2.3. *Approaches to Measurement and Evaluation of Locomotor Activity*

Measurement of locomotor activity and/or exploration in a novel environment has been a very popular test in experimental psychology, psychopharmacology, and neuroscience. Variations of this test have been used for many years to provide an index of sensory function *(153)*, motor function *(153)*, emotionality *(148)*, and cognition *(156)*. This test has also been used to evaluate the effects of a variety of psychoactive compounds *(157)*.

There are two general approaches. The first is to place the rat in a relatively sterile, symmetric enclosure and to measure as many aspects of the ambulation and/or movements as possible. The second approach is to focus on a specific aspect of the ambulation and/or movements (e.g., turning, thigmotaxis). For the latter approach the investigator may make a subtle variation in the environment (e.g., place an object[s] for investigation, alter the lighting conditions). The following illustrates some of the wide variety of pharmacological and neurotoxicological phenomena that can be detected and characterized using locomotor activity systems.

Schwarting and colleagues *(153)* used a video-based locomotor activity system to study changes in sensory and motor systems in the brain. Specifically, they investigated brain systems involved in the motor actions needed to attend to sensory phenomena. In rats, these brain systems include sensory afferents from the mystacial vibrissae and dopaminergic components of the nigroneostriatal system. In brief, this group reported that either unilateral vibissaectomy or unilateral nigrostriatal lesions resulted in asymmetric locomotion. Specifically, unilateral vibrissaectomy produced contralateral thigmotaxis or peritaxis (i.e., the rat moved in a circular direction that kept its intact vibrissae in contact with the wall or periphery of the open field). Unilateral nigrostriatal lesions produced by injections of the neurotoxicant 6-hydroxydopamine resulted in ipsilateral turning or rotation, (i.e., the rat moved in a circular direction, which maintained its intact vibrissae-nigrostriatal system towards the wall [thigmotaxis] or periphery [peritaxis] of the open field). This application of the locomotor activity test requires proprietary software that enables the researchers to identify turning behavior in either clockwise or counterclockwise directions in increments as small as quarter-turn (i.e., 90°).

The temporal and spatial pattern of locomotion in an open field have also been used as an index of emotionality, particularly as an index of anxiety or fear. This interpretation of open-field behavior is an extension of the earliest application of the open field test, in which the level of activity and number of fecal boli emitted during the test were used primarily as indices of emotionality *(146,148)*. The most common paradigm for using locomotor activity as a measure of anxiety begins by placing the subject in the center of the open field. The relevant endpoint may be the duration of "freezing" (cowering), which is measured as the latency to leave the center of the open field and begin ambulation. Or the endpoint may be the percentage of time spent adjacent to the walls of the enclosure (i.e., thigmotaxis). Typically the open field will be illuminated fairly brightly to encourage freezing. Changes in freezing and thigmotaxis have been used to document changes in anxiety produced by genetic variations or by anxiogenic or anxiolytic drugs *(158,159)*. However, the open field model of anxiety has been superceded recently by more specific models of anxiety, such as the elevated plus maze *(160)*.

Some groups of drugs (e.g., psychomotor stimulants, N-methyl-D-aspartate [NMDA] receptor antagonists) disorder movement, and measurement of locomotion has been a popular approach for characterizing these effects *(161,162)*. For example, lower effective doses of dopaminergic agonists (e.g., amphetamine, quinpirole, apomorphine) produce hyperactivity reflected by an increase in photocell counts or path length *(163,164)*. Higher doses often result in stereotypic behavior, in which a single behavior is repeated, to the exclusion of other normal behaviors *(137)*. Stereotypy is of two types: (1) response stereotypy, in which the same behavior (e.g., sniffing, grooming) is repeated *(6)* and (2) locomotor stereotypy, in which the same path is traversed repeatedly or the same area of the open field is investigated to exclusion of other areas *(139,161)*. To characterize these and other effects of various psychoactive drugs with a photocell-based system, Paulus and Geyer published several versions of a quantitative analysis that focused on the temporal and spatial features of activity *(154,155,163–165)*. Specifically, they analyzed locomotion in terms a dynamical entropy exponent (h) and a spatial scaling exponent (d). The exponent h quantified the extent of the predictability of the next movement based on the current position and current direction. A high h was generated by a wide variety of different, unpredictable motor movements. In contrast, repeated movements (e.g., stereotypical behavior) yielded a low h. The exponent d quantified the relationship between the contribution of local circumscribed motor behavior and the contribution of long distance-covering or straight motor movements to the overall observed motor behavior. The d values ranged from 1.0 for perfectly straight line movements to 2.0 for highly local movements with consecutive small movements in close proximity. Paulus and Geyer *(154)* developed an additional term, $f(d)$, which described the contribution of micro-event subsequences with different local spatial exponents. This function quantified how sequences of behavioral events form macroscopic behavior patterns. These exponents were used successfully to quantify the effects of various dopamine agonists and hallucinogens, but the approach has not been used widely outside of this laboratory (e.g., *166*).

Kernan and Mullenix developed a statistical approach for analyzing movements in an open field that resembled that of Paulus and Geyer in that it included elaborate statistical analysis of sequences of movements over time. It differed in that they used a video-based system and pattern recognition software to identify individual postures (e.g., standing, sitting, lying down) and behavioral acts (e.g., walking, sniffing, grooming) that occurred in a relatively small enclosure. Their system reported the number of times that a specific behavior was initiated, the total time spent in specific behaviors, and most importantly, the K function, a measure of the distribution of behavioral acts with respect to time *(167)*. This system was used to report effects (e.g., sodium flouride, triethyltin, childhood leukemia medications) or lack of effects (e.g., for aspartame, phenylalanine) for several chemicals *(168–171)*.

Neither the Paulus/Geyer nor the Kernan/Mullinex approach has been used extensively in toxicology outside of their laboratories. One obvious technical impediment to widespread use was the dependence on custom software that was not commercially available. An additional conceptual impediment was the presentation of their results in derived statistical measures (e.g., $f(d)$, K-function), which were difficult to compare with the results of other investigators who described the effects of drugs and neurotoxicants on the motor behavior using more traditional neurological and psychological terminology.

Several investigators have argued that a specific reference point or points must be identified to appreciate the orderliness of rat behavior in an open field. For example, Golani and colleagues examined the rat exploration of a large open field and reported that locomotion could be understood only after identifying the rat's home base(s). The home base was identified as the place in the open field where the rat stopped most often and for the longest time, and where the incidence of grooming and rearing was high *(151)*. Locomotor activity was analyzed in terms of "trips," defined as excursions to and from the home base. They observed that trips consisted of low velocity and intermittent locomotion away from the home base followed by high velocity, continuous locomotion during the return to the home base *(172)*. Eilam and Golani used this model to describe the locomotor stereotypy in amphetamine-treated rats *(173)*. Eilam et al. described changes in exploration in rats treated with anti-cholinergic neuron antibodies *(174)*. Although total path length was not affected, the treatment resulted in a reduction in the explored space and a decrease in the number of round trips to the home base(s).

In addition to quantifying some macroscopic aspects of rat behavior in a novel environment, Golani and colleagues also published an elegant description of the microscopic aspects of behavior in normal and brain-damaged rats. Eilam and Golani used a video-based system followed by visual review to analyze behavior shortly after a rat is placed in a large novel environment *(102)*. During this time there is a transition ("warm up") from the initial "freezing" to full locomotion required for exploration. Warm up proceeds along three dimensions: anatomical, spatial, and amplitude. The progression of events in warm-up can be appreciated by considering the following sequence of movements:

AAAAABABAABABBCBABABABCACB

For the anatomical dimension, A, B, and C represent the head, torso, and pelvis, respectively. For the spatial dimension they represent lateral, forward, and vertical movement, respectively. For the amplitude dimension they represent increasing amplitudes of movement. Warm-up proceeds lawfully along all of the dimensions simultaneously. Thus, a body part cannot move along a spatial dimension unless the part anterior to it has already moved along the same dimension. And every part of the trunk must first move laterally, then forward, then up. Once a new type of movement has been performed, the rat repeats it and reverts to it unpredictably later in the test period. And there is a gradual, but interrupted increase in the amplitude of movements along all of the spatial dimensions. Also, the parts of the trunk switch repeatedly between clockwise or counterclockwise movement.

The approach taken by Eilam and Golani provides detailed information about both macroscopic and microscopic aspects of motor function and exploratory behavior. However, their test system employs an unusually large open field, so that it is difficult to test the large number of animals required for safety studies. And the analysis requires painstaking review of videotaped behavior, which also limits its utility for safety testing purposes.

2.2.4. Locomotor Activity Testing in Standard Toxicity Studies

The typical locomotor activity measurement system and testing paradigm used in regulated toxicity studies is plain. Specifically, most laboratories place the subjects into small, sterile enclosures with high walls for 30–60 min and measure the activity with photocells. Indeed, many locomotor activity devices are simply small clear Plexiglas cubes housed in a sound-attenuating chamber. The statistical analysis generally includes only a measure of total activity (e.g., number of movements, path length) and the temporal distribution of activity in 3–4 time bins of 10–15 min. When normal animals are studied, the latter analysis generally reveals a decrease in activity as a function of duration in the enclosure.

The small size of the enclosure limits the duration and importance of warm-up phenomena, and the unavailability of distal cues minimizes the influence of allothetic cues. Some commercially available photocell-based devices claim (175) to provide microanalysis of behavior (e.g., turning, stereotypy). But at best, the microanalysis is almost certainly much lower than that provided by video-based systems. We recommend that users of commercially available photocell-based systems check with the supplier to determine the statistical algorithms used to obtain derived measures. There are commercially available video systems, but these are primarily tracking devices, and do not provide much by way of microanalysis of individual behaviors.

The routine use of small, sterile enclosures and photocell-based detection means that the standard assessment of behavior in a novel environment assesses only a fraction of the behaviors typically emitted during normal rat exploration or navigation. Moreover, the typical system does not provide even a fraction of the data provided by the human observer in the open-field tests. For example, changes in posture, gait, and spontaneous movement abnormalities are not measured. Proponents of locomotor activity as a tool in neurotoxicity testing generally justify its inclusion on the basis that it is a quantitative test, and that the decrease in activity over time reflects a learning phenomenon known as habituation *(176)*. Both arguments are weak. First, the mere ability to quantify an endpoint does not just justify its inclusion (e.g., we don't measure the length of the tail). The second issue, the temporal changes in locomotor activity and their relationship to habituation, is more complicated. Habituation is a hypothetical learning mechanism used to explain a progressive decrease in responsiveness during repeated presentations of a stimulus. For example, presentation of a novel auditory stimulus will generally elicit an orienting response that includes somatic (movement of eyes, head, neck, and other body parts) and autonomic components (changes in respiration and cardiovascular endpoints). With repeated presentations of the stimulus, there is a progressive decrease in the amplitude of these responses *(143)*. The interpretation of locomotor activity as habituation rests on the assumption that locomotion reflects exploration of a novel environment, and that the reduction in locomotion over time reflects acquisition of the stimulus features of the environment, which become progressively less novel. This interpretation has been challenged *(143)*. First, the definition of habituation implies that habituation is best measured when the stimulus is discrete, limited to one sensory system, can be controlled and the response(s) measured. Current tests of locomotor activity provide none of these. Instead, the rat may attend to any aspect of the environment, and the relationship of exploration to ambulation is confounded with the sensory system used for investigating. Specifically, sniffing or palpation (i.e., with the vibrissae) of the floor often occurs while the rat is moving in the chamber with its head down. In contrast, visual scanning or palpation of the walls and corners with the vibrissae often occur while the rat is stopped. Thus, ambulation cannot be used as an unambiguous measure of exploration. Second, there is evidence to suggest that locomotion in novel environments may indicate attempts to escape the environment as much as it may indicate exploration *(143)*. Thus, escape and exploration are confounded, and changes in the rate of locomotion over time cannot be interpreted unambiguously using a cognitive model *(143)*.

Several reviews have indicated that studies of chemicals on behavior in the open field are largely uninterpretable *(142,143)*, especially when ambulation is the only endpoint taken. File has even suggested that: "The popularity of this technique must depend on its economy and ease of execution rather than on any desire to analyse the meaning of any observed drug effects" *(143)*. File has also suggested that an independent measure of exploration (e.g., head poking into a hole board) might be a useful addition to a locomotor-activity test system *(143)*. Hole-poking is now measured by some investigators *(177–181)*, but questions still remain about the utility and interpretation of this endpoint *(182)*.

Guidelines for standard toxicity studies require locomotor activity only for repeat-dosing studies (EPA OPPTS 870.3100; OECD #408). This restriction is particularly curious, because the most frequent use of locomotor activity in research is to evaluate the effects of single doses of drugs. Despite the difficulties involved in interpreting locomotor activity data, the neurotoxicity literature suggests that dose-related hyperactivity raises suspicion about a possible neurotoxic effect. For example, a variety of psychoactive drugs *(157,161–164)* and chemicals that injure the hippocampus *(75)* or vestibular system *(183)* have been shown to produce hyperactivity that is measurable in standard locomotor-activity devices. Likewise, hypoactivity has been a useful indicator of pharmacological and injurious effects of neurotoxicants *(184,185)*. However, the interpretation of hypoactivity as a neurotoxic effect is especially problematic because it is not unusual for one or more levels of any test material to produce some malaise *(186)*.

3. CRITICAL EVALUATION OF THE CURRENTLY AVAILABLE TESTS

Protection of the nervous system is an important public-health concern, and an enormous amount of intellectual energy has been expended in the pursuit of an acceptable approach for testing chemicals. The simple, crucial question is: "How well do the currently available tests work?" There are both historical and contemporary data to help address this question. The clinical observations are linked historically to the neurological examination used for many years in human and veterinary medicine. The locomotor activity test is linked with decades of experimental studies in psychopharmacology and neuroscience. For both categories of tests, there is also significant contemporary information about their operating characteristics as functional indicators of neurotoxicants. However, before embarking on this analysis, it is important to discuss the general principles for this critique.

3.1. General Criteria for Evaluating an Individual Test or Test Battery

It is absolutely essential to understand that an individual test, groups of similar tests and the entire test battery must be evaluated in the context in which it is used. A number of factors contribute to this context:

1. *What question(s) is the experiment designed to address?* A diverse battery of qualitative observations may be most appropriate for a Tier 1 (screening) study of a chemical with unknown effects. However, if the study intended to provide a precise evaluation of a well-characterized effect of a chemical, then a smaller number of quantitative tests is probably more appropriate. A systematic checklist of observations may be appropriate for a subchronic or chronic test design conducted with low doses of a chemical, because signs of toxicity evolve relatively slowly. However, multiple signs of neurotoxicity can occur within seconds during a single-dose toxicity study using high doses. Under these test conditions, observing with a checklist may be too cumbersome, and some neurological changes could be missed as a result. In this case, it may be more appropriate to record "by exception" (i.e., only abnormalities are recorded).
2. *What quality of technology is commercially available for conducting the test?* For regulated toxicology studies, the value of a functional endpoint varies with the quality of the technology available for recording it. For example, the popularity of FLGS and HLGS is partly a function of the availability of analogue and digital strain gauges for measuring this endpoint. In contrast, many potentially useful tests and test systems are not commercially available *(28,57)*, and are not used in regulated safety studies.
3. *What is the level of expertise of people conducting the test?* The value of an endpoint or test battery varies with the individual responsible for conducting the test. For example, most test batteries include an evaluation of the subjects for spontaneous movement abnormalities. But if the tester cannot distinguish among ataxia, tremor, and myoclonus, the value of these observations is reduced.

    A related issue is the relationship between the relative level of expertise required to conduct the test and the availability of adequate numbers of professionals trained in the technology. For example, the attractive features of neurophysiological endpoints are well-documented *(187)*, but there are relatively few people trained to conduct this type of testing. As a result, neurophysiological endpoints are rarely collected during safety studies.

4. *What is the level of expertise of people who interpret the results?* As summarized earlier, the typical safety study presents the reviewer with data in the domains of anatomical pathology, clinical pathology, and clinical observations. The functional tests for neurotoxicity are part of the latter domain. The value of the functional data depend on the ability of the reviewer to combine these data in a way that is consistent with generally accepted scientific and/or medical practice *(3)*.

5. *What additional endpoints will be collected concurrently during the test?* Changes in any functional test are interpreted by using the context provided by other functional endpoints, and by changes in endpoints included in the other major test categories of results, namely anatomical and clinical pathology. For a simple example, failure to flex the leg in response to a toe pinch could reflect loss of consciousness, reduced nociceptive capacity, or inability to move the leg. Furthermore, any of these could be related to malaise, which is often caused by the high doses of test substances used in safety studies. To differentiate among these possibilities requires additional information about neurological status (e.g., speed of righting reaction, grip strength, the presence of neuropathological lesions and their location), general health status, and an algorithm for combining the results. The process for combining the results is superficially similar to differential diagnosis as it is practiced in a neurology clinic. The results of a good test or test battery are capable of being evaluated in this way *(3)*.

A related issue is the ability of a test in one area of technology (e.g., neuropathology) to compensate for areas of function which are particularly difficult to assess in animals. For example, a test battery that lacks an effective test of vision could still be considered appropriate if the structures underlying vision (i.e., retina and central projections) were assessed adequately by the neuropathological endpoints. Likewise, a cumbersome or marginally effective functional test could still be considered a necessary and valuable part of the testing battery if it evaluated a part of the nervous system (e.g., cochlea) that was even more difficult to evaluate routinely using neuropathological procedures.

The initial critique of clinical observations will be organized into major groups of functions: somatic sensory and motor, special sensory/nociceptive, and autonomic functions. After these are discussed separately, the utility of the entire battery (clinical observations, locomotor activity, and neuropathology) will be analyzed.

3.2. Evaluation of Specific Functional Endpoints

3.2.1. Somatic Sensory and Motor Endpoints

The observations include some spinal reflexes, postural reactions, and the observations of gait, posture, and spontaneous movement abnormalities in the open field. The veterinary neurology literature indicates that, taken together, these tests help to evaluate possible dysfunction to a large number of nervous system components *(7,8)*. It is difficult to imagine that any neurotoxicant that produced a significant alteration in somatic sensory or motor function could fail to be detected by this collection of tests when dosed at the MTD. This impression is supported by a large literature that documents these endpoints as indicators of neurotoxicant-related damage in peripheral somatosensory and somatomotor nerves *(35,43)*, vestibular system *(112)*, cerebellum *(188)*, and basal ganglia *(184)*. These endpoints also detect a variety of pharmacological effects, including those produced by general anesthesia *(123,189)*, opiates *(90,116)*, ethanol *(189)*, and other psychoactive compounds *(118,137)*. These endpoints also demonstrate the transient neurotoxic effects of many varieties of pesticides, including organophosphates *(122)*, carbamates *(122)*, chlorinated hydrocarbons *(133)*, and pyrethroids *(121)*. They also demonstrate the effects of heavy metals *(75,126)* and excitotoxicants *(136)*.

It can be argued that current test batteries lack a test of light-touch awareness. In humans, this sensation is initiated by low-threshold cutaneous mechanoreceptors which are innervated by large, myelinated sensory fibers. Conscious perception of light touch requires transmission of the information to the dorsal columns of the spinal cord, dorsal column nuclei in the medulla, medial lemniscus, ventral posterior thalamic nuclei, and somesthetic cortex. The involvement of large myelinated sensory fibers is significant, because these fibers are particularly sensitive in some neurotoxic axonopathies, like that produced by acrylamide *(190)*. Moreover, changes in cutaneous sensitivity are sensitive indicators of acrylamide neurotoxicity in humans and animals *(191,192)*.

In humans, screening for tactile sensitivity on glabrous skin is accomplished by using a series of tests that require a verbal report from the patient *(10; see* Chapter 20 by Albers). Rats do not give verbal reports, so an analogous test cannot be conducted. The reflex arc (not conscious awareness) stimulated by light touching can be tested with either the canthal reflex or pinna reflex, but both sites contain abundant hairs. Rat paws contain glabrous skin, and the presence or absence of the contact placing response initiated by the paws can be tested in rats. The forelimb-placing response has been shown to be an effective tool for demonstrating lesions in somesthetic cortex *(63)*. Although this test can be performed without using sophisticated equipment, extraordinary measures must be taken to eliminate the contribution of visual stimuli and afferents from the mystacial vibrissae. Even then, contact sensitivity is not assessed, since it is impossible to vary the level of stimulation systematically.

Although the rat has little glabrous skin for testing contact sensitivity, the mystacial vibrissae perform a similar function to human fingers (e.g., palpation of the environment), which requires many of the same neurological structures (e.g., ventral posterior lateral thalamus, somesthetic cortex; *193–195)*. Rats and hamsters with reduced visual information and light-touch cues (i.e., either blindfolded or vibrissaectomized and tested in the dark) show characteristic changes in exploration of a novel open field. Specifically, they walk slowly and with a hunched posture, with their nose to the floor. They also make few head scans, which enable the vibrissae to touch various objects *(196,197)*. Thus, it might be possible to test for large deficits in light touch function in rats by careful observation or measurement of spontaneous locomotor activity in environments that are either dark or illuminated by infrared light.

3.2.2. Special Sensory and Nociception Endpoints

Of the special senses, the only modality with even a crude functional test is audition, which is assessed as part of the auditory startle test. Auditory startle is probably better positioned as a test of deafness than as a test of hearing, as rats with profound cochlear damage do demonstrate a decreased auditory startle reaction *(72)*. Testing for deficits in olfaction, vision, and taste is poor or nonexistent. Current guidelines do not require a quantitative test of nociception, and the common qualitative tests (e.g., flexor reflex) do not really evaluate pain sensitivity.

3.2.3. Autonomic and Thermoregulatory Endpoints

The current test batteries contain several endpoints relevant for assessing autonomic nervous-system function. Specifically, the evaluation of pupil size, pupillary reflex, and lacrimation/salivation is sufficient to detect changes in parasympathetic activity (12–17). Decreases in the sympathetic tone should be reflected by ptosis (87–90). Detecting sympathomimetic effects on cranial-nerve autonomic reflexes may be problematic, but most sympathomimetics produce hyperactivity and stereotypy at some dose (198). Although it is clear that these autonomic endpoints are adequate to detect pharmacological effects, their ability to detect damage to autonomic nerve fibers is unclear. Part of the difficulty is that there are few model compounds for studying autonomic neuropathy in rats. Vacor and vincristine produce convincing autonomic neuropathy in humans (199,200), but as yet there are no parallel studies in rats. Perinatal dosing with capsaicin reduces the number of unmyelinated sensory nerve fibers, some of which are involved in autonomic reflexes. Although enlarged bladders have been reported in rats dosed perinatally with capsaicin, in general, capsaicin-treated rats show very few spontaneous signs of autonomic nervous system dysfunction in urinary, cardiovascular, digestive, or respiratory function. Instead, the functional changes observed after systemic capsaicin dosing are revealed only through quantitative measures of selected autonomic reflexes (5,21,22). It should be noted that several agents (e.g., capsaicin, guanethidine, clonidine) that diminish autonomic function also have deleterious effects based on sexual behavior, reproductive performance, and/or histopathology of primary and secondary sex organs in rats (201–208). Thus, standard reproductive toxicity studies may provide additional information about autonomic nervous-system status.

Obvious changes in the temperature of distal body parts (e.g., "warm to touch," "cold to touch") may be observed and reported as part of hand-held clinical observations. While these types of observations may reflect thermoregulatory responses to dosing of test chemicals, they do not constitute an evaluation of thermoregulatory function, which is not generally addressed in standard safety studies.

3.3. Evaluation of the Test Battery

3.3.1. Introduction

Standard toxicity studies are typically conducted using at least three dose groups and a control group, and the highest dose is usually the MTD. The purpose of the neurological assessment is to detect effects that signify possible neurological dysfunction. Additional anatomical and clinical pathology endpoints are used to characterize any neurotoxicity (e.g., by identifying neuropathological effects) or to help differentiate neurotoxic effects from effects due to malaise or toxicity to another organ system. In standard studies, all tissues for histopathology are fixed by immersion, embedded in paraffin, and examined after sectioning and staining with hematoxylin and eosin (H&E). Clinical pathology endpoints include serum chemistry and hematological endpoints.

The current guidelines for repeated dose studies call for more effort than do the guidelines for single-dose studies. Specifically, guidelines for repeat-dose studies specify that the rat be removed from its home cage, and specify a need for evaluation of grip strength and locomotor activity. For both single-dose and repeat-dose studies, functional effects may be transient or persistent. Since the guidelines for repeat-dose studies are more complete than those for single-dose studies, the discussion proceeds better if the multiple-dose studies are discussed first.

3.3.2. Repeated Dose Studies

Although there are exceptions, in repeated-dose studies the functional effects generally evolve relatively slowly, over days or weeks. In this context, a systematic recording of all observations—normal behavior and abnormalities—is appropriate. The need to record as many endpoints as possible, and as quantitatively as possible, is justified by the fact that iterative (i.e., tiered) testing with subchronic studies is expensive and time-consuming. This situation is quite different for clinical neurological testing, in which several levels of technology of ever-increasing sophistication can be employed quickly, and the number of tiers of tests does not, per se, increase cost. Thus, in repeat-dose toxicity studies it makes sense to try to both screen for effects and, if effects are observed, to include sufficient observations to establish a no-adverse-effect level (NOAEL) for neurotoxicological effects. This NOAEL may reflect the limitations of the endpoint, which may not be the most scientifically robust way of measuring the neurotoxic effect when only a single study is conducted. The situation in toxicity testing might be improved if it were possible to incorporate special end-of-study testing based on interim observations. For example, it has been suggested that electrophysiological endpoints could be incorporated this way *(187)*. However, current test guidelines and Good Laboratory Practices make it very cumbersome to engage in this practice on an occasional basis.

Since functional effects generally evolve over days to weeks, there is adequate time for functional signs of malaise (e.g., decreased food intake and body weight; rough hair coat; staining around eyes, nose, mouth, and paws) to develop. Moreover, there is time for organ-system toxicity to be reflected by changes in clinical pathological and anatomical pathological endpoints. Thus, the conditions provided by repeated-dose studies are reasonable for estimating the contribution of malaise or organ-system toxicity to any neurological signs.

Our review clearly suggests that the current test batteries are not equally strong in all three areas of function (i.e., somatic sensory, and motor, special sensory and autonomic). The battery contains many endpoints capable of detecting effects on somatic sensory and motor systems. While the tests available for measuring somatic reflexes and postural reactions in the rat are nowhere near as extensive as those available for evaluating humans and domestic animals, neurotoxicants tend to affect categories of nerves (e.g., somatic motor nerves, large sensory nerves). Thus, complete anatomical coverage is probably not as important as assuring that important categories of nerves are evaluated. Also, most neurotoxicants that affect somatic sensory and motor function affect more than one endpoint when dosed at the MTD. For example, although subchronic dosing with acrylamide affects large sensory fibers early in the course of the toxicity, continued dosing at the MTD for 91-d produces obvious changes in grip strength. Thus, although the test battery lacks a test of tactile sensitivity, the absence of such a test is not an impediment to detecting the neurotoxicity of acrylamide. Likewise, repeated dosing of the striatal neurotoxicant 3-nitropropionic acid produces stiffness, ataxia, slowness of movement, and a wide-based stance *(209)*. In the context of clear neurological signs such as these, histopathological effects are useful to characterize the neurotoxicity, but are not needed for detection.

In contrast to the number of endpoints for documenting changes in somatic sensory and motor function, the evaluation of special senses (i.e., vision, hearing, olfaction, taste) and nociception is relatively meager. Behavioral and electrophysiological tests are available for measuring special senses in rats *(67,187)*, but regulatory agencies have been reluctant to require them in standard acute and subchronic test guidelines. The absence of such tests from the guidelines almost certainly reflects the fact that these tests are generally very consumptive of time, money, and expertise. For vision and olfaction, the absence of an adequate functional test is probably compensated by the availability of histopathological sections of the retina (including optic nerve) and olfactory epithelium from both of these senses. The sense of taste is not covered directly at all, but there is little indication from the literature suggesting that the absence of a test for taste should be cause for concern. However, the absence of a functional test of audition may be a significant omission. Unlike the visual and olfactory receptors, the auditory receptors are not routinely afforded a histopathological examination. Histological processing of the cochlea is extremely difficult, because the cochlea is housed in the temporal bone. Currently, the auditory startle test is the only endpoint that involves an auditory stimulus. The auditory startle reaction may be reduced or absent after dosing of chemicals (e.g., IDPN) that produce total or near-total cochlear damage *(72)*, but may not be sensitive to the effects of chemicals (e.g., styrene), which produce more localized cochlear damage *(210)*. Concern for ototoxicity is amplified by the endemic low grade hearing loss in the human population, especially during aging. The high endemic level makes it difficult to detect insidious ototoxic effects in the human population. Concern for ototoxicity is further heightened by data suggesting that chemical ototoxicity may be additive to effects of other conditions (e.g., loud noise, aging) that predispose the cochlea to damage *(211)*. Again, these types of effects of exposure would be very difficult to detect in the human population. In view of the relatively large number of ototoxic chemicals, it has been suggested that testing for ototoxicity in routine safety studies should be improved *(210)*.

Only a few endpoints contribute to the functional examination of the autonomic nervous system, and these endpoints are is probably best suited to detect transient (i.e., pharmacological) effects (*see* Subheading 3.3.3.) resulting from single doses of chemicals. Like audition, the functional evaluation on the autonomic nervous system is especially important, because effects on this system are not covered well by traditional histopathology. In this case, the problem for histopathology lies in nerves that subserve autonomic function. Many of these nerves are small and unmyelinated, and are not readily evaluated by traditional histopathological techniques. In particular, there is special concern for evaluating unmyelinated afferents that contribute the sensory part of many autonomic reflexes. In part, the concern arises from the literature dealing with capsaicin. When dosed repeatedly at the MTD to adult rats, capsaicin damages the central and peripheral terminals of these afferents *(212–215)*. This damage would not be detected by histopathological approaches currently used in standard acute or subchronic dosing studies. Indeed, this damage would not likely be detected by histopathology according to current EPA Neurotoxicity guidelines (EPA OPPTS 870.6200). Despite the widespread damage to afferent terminals, rats treated with capscaicin appear grossly normal, and show no changes in gait, posture, or somatic reflexes and reactions. In general, the damage to unmyelinated afferents is revealed only by behavioral or physiological procedures in which protective behavioral or autonomic reflexes are elicited by potentially damaging or irritating stimulation *(5)*. Perhaps the simplest assay for unmyelinated sensory afferents is the blepharospasm or "eye-wipe" test, in which a dilute solution of a mild irritant (e.g., 1% zingerone) is placed into the eye, and the number of wipes with the forepaw is counted *(216)*. This test generally takes less than a minute to conduct, which is an indication of the mild level of irritation produced by the procedure. As an alternative, the tail-flick test is also sensitive to damage to unmyelinated afferents *(217)*.

The contribution of locomotor activity data to the neurological assessment is minimal, and it is difficult to fathom why it is required for repeat dose studies. Clearly, the quantification of locomotor activity does not have the same relationship to observation of open field behavior that grip strength has to hand-held estimations of strength. On the contrary, human observation of behavior in the open field is far more informative than photocell counts of locomotor activity. Clearly, measurement of locomotor activity has no impact on the assessment of autonomic function. As was described in Subheading 2.2., enhanced measurement of movements in a novel environment have been used appropriately by neuroscientists to assess a variety of sensory and motor functions. Unfortunately, the typical unenhanced test systems used in standard toxicity studies does not provide this type of information.

3.3.3. Single-Dose Studies

Guidelines for single-dose studies (e.g., EPA OPPTS 870.1100; OECD 401) differ from guidelines for repeat-dose studies in that the single-dose guidelines lack language that explicitly require that the animal be removed from its home cage and observed in an arena. It should be obvious that hand-held observations and observations in the open field are essential parts of any neurological evaluation, and it is difficult to understand why the requirements differ for the two guidelines. A reasonable compromise is to place the animals into large, clear, plastic shoe-box cages for observation after dosing. There is sufficient room to encourage walking, and the observer can examine multiple animals concurrently for spontaneous movement abnormalities. Animals can be removed easily for hand-held observations based on predetermined timing in the protocol and/or observations of spontaneous abnormalities that require closer attention. All of these observations can be recorded "by exception" (*see* below).

Single doses of neurotoxicants can produce transient or persistent neurological effects, and these effects can be associated with pharmacological mechanisms as well as neuropathological changes. Although there are exceptions, transient functional effects usually reflect pharmacological rather than neuropathological mechanisms. For many chemicals that cause transient effects, signs of neurotoxicity begin within minutes after dosing, and multiple functional effects can be observed to begin, change in severity, and recede with different time courses over a few minutes to hours. As was the case for subchronic dosing, the commonly used endpoints are capable of detecting a tremendous variety of pharmacological effects of chemicals dosed at the MTD *(11,13,14,16,53,54,60,68,73,87,90,91,96–101,104,105,121,122,125,130,134,135, 137,138,185).*

In the context of single-dose studies and the typical rapid time course of effects, it is probably better to record observations "by exception" (i.e., only abnormalities are recorded), rather than record every endpoint, even ones that are not affected. To be certain, the qualitative observations and procedures are performed systematically, but time is preserved for recording abnormalities. Functions not recorded as abnormal are presumed to be normal. Saving time is necessary to provide for iterations of observations that are required to document the detailed temporal progression of functional changes. The need for iterative observations is particularly important because of the desirability of discriminating neurotoxicity from other forms of toxicity, especially malaise.

To appreciate the need for iterative observations in acute toxicity studies, it is useful to compare the situation with that provided by a repeat dose study (Subheading 3.3.2.). In repeat dose studies, the typically slow evolution of neurological changes allow time for comparison of a variety of endpoints that help determine the presence and degree of malaise or effects on other organ systems. In single-dose toxicity studies, it is often the case that either no clinical pathological or anatomical pathological endpoints are recorded, or there is insufficient time for changes in these endpoints to occur. Thus, in acute toxicity studies, this discrimination between malaise and neurotoxicity depends on the dose-response and the temporal evolution of changes in various endpoints. That is, effects observed only at near-lethal doses and temporally close to death are more likely to be related to malaise. While this discrimination may be straightforward in some cases, other types of toxicity may require very detailed observations. For example, detailed observations of individual animals may be required to discriminate agonal convulsions from a convulsant that produces death after status epilepticus. The issue is further complicated by the fact that many neurotoxicants produce physical and behavioral signs of malaise. This fact is evidenced by the number of neurotoxicants that have been used as unconditioned stimuli in conditioned taste aversion studies *(218–222)*. Thus, it needs to be remembered that not only can malaise produce signs of neurotoxicity, but neurotoxicants can produce signs of malaise. Discriminating the malaise component from any neurotoxicity component requires detailed information. And in acute toxicity studies, that level of detailed information requires sufficient iterations of observations—up to and including continuous observations in severely affected animals. Conducting these iterations is hindered by the time required to record observations of normal behaviors.

Some have attempted to resolve the uncertainty in discriminating neurotoxicity from other changes by introducing the concept of "level of concern" *(4)*. This term implies that chemicals that produce unequivocal signs of neurotoxicity (e.g., paralysis, brain lesions) engender a high level of concern, whereas a lower level of concern is afforded chemicals in which the evidence of neurotoxicity is less, or even equivocal. Unfortunately, it is not yet clear how the level of concern should be translated into risk management by a regulatory body. Thus, a very real possibility exists that a chemical could be regulated or a "neurotoxicant" label applied to a chemical based on equivocal effects.

It is not possible to depend solely on observational endpoints to distinguish between neurotoxicants that have solely a pharmacological action and those that produce neuropathological effects. Numerous examples exist of chemicals which produce only transient signs of toxicity, but that also produce significant neuropathology. For example, the metabotropic glutamate-receptor antagonist MK801 produces transient neurological signs including stereotypy, ataxia, and loss of righting reaction. Standard neuropathological processing (e.g., H & E staining) is sufficient to demonstrate the lesions in the cingulate cortex *(223)*, but cupric-silver staining for degenerating neurons reveals damage to neuronal-cell bodies and process at more sites, including the hipppocampus and entorhinal cortex *(224)*. Transient signs of motor dysfunction are also produced by the neurotoxicant 3-acetylpyridine, for which neuropathologic lesions are most obvious in the inferior olivary nucleus and several cranial nerve nuclei *(225)*. However, cupric-silver staining reveals much more widespread damage including the diagonal-band nucleus, substantia nigra (SN), and hippocampus *(226)*. The functional and morphological effects of capsaicin are especially problematic. High systemic doses of capsaicin produce transient functional signs that include hypothermia, ptosis, and a flattened posture (*see* ref. *227* for a summary). There is widespread damage to unmyelinated sensory terminals in many organ systems including urinary, cardiovascular, and respiratory *(212,213)*. There is also damage in brain regions including the inferior olive, interpeduncular nucleus, suprachiasmatic nucleus, septum, and posterior hypothalamus *(214,215)*, which is revealed only by cupric-silver staining. Taken together, the results of these studies indicate the need to use the best possible technology to detect and characterize morphological effects of neurotoxicants. The data also suggest that, in general, biomarkers of damage (e.g., silver-degeneration stains) are superior to traditional staining procedures (e.g., Nissl stains or H & E) for demonstrating damage. Now that efficient and reliable techniques are available for performing silver-degeneration stains *(228)*, regulatory agencies should begin to encourage their use in regulated studies.

4. SUMMARY

The current testing strategy for detection of potential neurotoxicants includes observations of rats given a range of doses, which includes the MTD. The literature suggests that this strategy is effective, because the vast majority of neurotoxicants will produce clear signs of neurotoxicity at these high doses. Locomotor activity is measured under some subchronic testing guidelines, but commercially available technology provides only modest information, it is not clear that this test adds significant value to the observational tests under current testing conditions.

REFERENCES

1. U. S. Congress, Office of Technology Assessment. (1990) *Neurotoxicity: Identifying and Controlling Poisons of the Nervous System.* Document OAT-BA-436. U. S. Government Printing Office, Washington, D.C.
2. Hutchings, D. E., Callaway, C. W., and Sobotka, T. J. (1987) Symposium introduction. Predicting neurotoxicity and behavioral dysfunction from preclinical toxicologic data. *Neurotoxicol. Teratol.* **9(6),** 397–401.
3. Ross, J. F., Mattsson, J. L., and Fix, A. S. (1998) Expanded clinical observations in toxicity studies: historical perspectives and contemporary issues. *Regul. Toxicol. Pharmacol.* **28,** 17–26.
4. U. S. Environmental Protection Agency (1998) Guidelines for Neurotoxicity Risk Assessment. *Fed. Reg.* **63(93),** 26,925–26,954.

5. Buck, S. H. and Burks, T. F. (1986) The neuropharmacology of capsaicin: review of some recent observations. *Pharmacol. Rev.* **38,** 179–226.

6. Moser, V. C. and Ross, J. F. (eds.) (1996) Training Video and Reference Manual for a Functional Observational Battery. American Industrial Health Council. Washington, DC.

7. Oliver, J. E. and Lorenz, M. D. (1983) *Handbook of Veterinary Neurologic Diagnosis.* W.B. Saunders, Philadelphia.

8. Redding, R. W. and Braund, K. G. (1978) Neurological examination, in *Canine Neurology: Diagnosis and Treatment* (Hoerlein, B. F., ed.), W.B. Saunders, Philadelphia, PA, pp. 53–70.

9. Mason, D. E. and Brown, M. J. (1997) Monitoring of Anesthesia, in *Anesthesia and Analgesia in Laboratory Animals* (Kohn, D. F, Wixxson, S. K., White, W. J., and Benson, G. J., eds.), Academic Press, New York, NY, pp. 73–81.

10. Lindblom, U. and Tegner, R. (1989) Quantification of sensibility in mononeuropathy, polyneuropathy, and central lesions, in *Quantification of Neurologic Deficit* (Munsat, T. L., ed.), Butterworth, Boston, MA, pp. 171–185.

11. Hsu, W. H. and Kakuk, T. J. (1984) Effect of amitraz and chlordimeform on heart rate and pupil diameter in rats: mediated by alpha 2-adrenoreceptors. *Toxicol. Appl. Pharmacol.* **73,** 411–415.

12. Soli, N. E., Karlsen, R. L., Opsahl, M., and Fonnum, F. (1980) Correlations between acetylcholinesterase activity in guinea-pig iris and pupillary function: a biochemical and pupillographic study. *J. Neurochem.* **35,** 723–728.

13. Daniotti, S. and Del Soldato, P. (1984) Comparative studies of the effects of some antimuscarinic agents on gastric damage and pupillary reflex in the rat. *Br. J. Pharmacol.* **82,** 305–307.

14. Moser, V. C. (1991) Investigations of amitraz neurotoxicity in rats. IV. Assessment of toxicity syndrome using a functional observational battery. *Fundam. Appl. Toxicol.* **17,** 7–16

15. Kennedy, G. L. (1986) Acute toxicity studies with oxamyl. *Fundam. Appl. Toxicol.* **6,** 423–429.

16. Moser, V. C. (1995) Comparisons of the acute effects of cholinesterase inhibitors using a neurobehavioral screening battery in rats. *Neurotoxicol. Teratol.* **7,** 617–625.

17. Bartolomeo A. C., Morris, H., Buccafusco, J. J., Kille, N., Rosenzweig-Lipson, S., Husbands, M. G., et al. (2000) The preclinical pharmacological profile of WAY–132983, a potent M1 preferring agonist. *J. Pharmacol. Exp. Ther.* **292,** 584–596.

18. Janss, A. J., Jones, S. L., and Gebhart, G. F. (1987) Effect of spinal norepinephrine depletion on descending inhibition of the tail flick reflex from the locus coeruleus and lateral reticular nucleus in the rat. *Brain Res.* **400,** 40–52.

19. Hough, L. B., Nalwalk, J. W., Li, B. Y., Leurs, R., Menge, W. M., Timmerman, H., et al. (1997) Novel qualitative structure-activity relationships for the antinociceptive actions of H2 antagonists, H3 antagonists and derivatives. *J. Pharmacol. Exp. Ther.* **83,** 1534–1543.

20. McCormack, K., Prather, P., and Chapleo, C. (1998) Some new insights into the effects of opioids in phasic and tonic nociceptive tests. *Pain* **78,** 79–98.

21. Holzer, P., Jurna, I., Gamse, R., and Lembeck, F. (1979) Nociceptive threshold after neonatal capsaicin treatment. *Eur. J. Pharmacol.* **58,** 511–514.

22. Nagy, J. I. and van der Kooy, D. (1983) Effects of neonatal capsaicin treatment on nociceptive thresholds in the rat. *J. Neurosci.* **13,** 1145–1150.

23. Roane D. S., Bounds J. K., Ang C. Y., and Adloo A. A. (1998) Quinpirole-induced alterations of tail temperature appear as hyperalgesia in the radiant heat tail-flick test. *Pharmacol. Biochem. Behav.* **59,** 77–82.

24. Hole, K. and Tjolsen, A. (1993) The tail-flick and formalin tests in rodents: changes in skin temperature as a confounding factor. *Pain* **53,** 247–254.

25. Gordon, C. J. (1991) Toxic-induced hypothermia and hypometabolism: do they increase uncertainty in the extrapolation of toxicological data from experimental animals to humans? *Neurosci. Biobehav. Rev.* **15,** 95–98.

26. Gordon, C. J. and Rowsey, P. J. (1998) Poisons and fever. *Clin. Exp. Pharmacol. Physiol.* **25,** 145–149.

27. Gordon, C. J. (1990) Thermal biology of the laboratory rat. *Physiol. Behav.* **47,** 963–991.

28. Ross, J. F., Handley, D. E, Fix, A. S., Lawhorn, G. T., and Carr, G. J. (1997) Quantification of the hindlimb extensor thrust response in rats. *Neurotoxicol. Teratol.* **19,** 405–411.

29. Ross, J. F. and Lawhorn, G. T. (1990) ZPT-related distal axonopathy: behavioral and electrophysiologic correlates in rats. *Neurotoxicol. Teratol.* **12,** 153–159.

30. Kimura, J. (1996) Electrodiagnosis of neuromuscular disorders, in *Neurology in Clinical Practice* (Bradley, W. G., Daroff, R. B., Fenichel, G. M., and Marsden, C. D., eds.), Butterworth-Heinemann, Boston, MA, pp. 477–498.

31. De Luca, C. J. (1978) Towards understanding the EMG signal, in *Muscles Alive* (Basmajian, J. V., ed.), Williams and Wilkins, Baltimore, MD, pp. 53–78.

32. Spencer, P. S. and Schaumburg, H. H. (1977) Ultrastructural studies of the dying-back process. IV. Differential vulnerability of PNS and CNS fibers in experimental central-peripheral distal axonopathies. *J. Neuropathol. Exp. Neurol.* **36,** 300–320.

33. Meyer, O. A., Tilson, H. A., Byrd, W. C., and Riley, M. T. (1979) A method for the routine assessment of fore—and hindlimb grip strength of rats and mice. *Neurobehav. Toxicol.* **1,** 233–236.

34. Nevins, M. E., Nash, S. A., and Beardsley, P. M. (1993) Quantitative grip strength assessment as a means of evaluating muscle relaxation in mice. *Psychopharmacology (Berl.)* **110,** 92–96.

35. Shell, L., Rozum, M., Jortner, B. S., and Ehrich, M. (1992) Neurotoxicity of acrylamide and 2,5-hexanedione in rats evaluated using a functional observational battery and pathological examination. *Neurotoxicol. Teratol.* **14,** 273–283.

36. Pryor, G. T. and Rebert, C. S. (1992) Interactive effects of toluene and hexane on behavior and neurophysiologic responses in Fischer-344 rats. *Neurotoxicology* **13,** 225–234.

37. Roks, G., Deckers, C. L., Meinardi, H., Dirksen, R., van Egmond, J., and van Rijn, C. M. (1999) Effects of polytherapy compared with monotherapy in antiepileptic drugs: an animal study. *J. Pharmacol. Exp. Ther.* **288,** 472–477.

38. Wein, A. J. and Raezer, D. M. (1979) Physiology of micturition, in *Clinical Neuro-Urology* (Krane, R. J. and Siroky, M. B., eds.), Little, Brown and Co., Boston, MA, pp. 1–33.

39. Rushton, D. N. (1996) Sexual and sphincter dysfunction, in *Neurology in Clinical Practice* (Bradley, W. G., Daroff, R. B., Fenichel, G. M., and Marsden, C. D., eds.), Butterworth-Heinemann, Boston, MA, pp. 407–420.

40. Mathias, C. J. (1996) Disorders of the autonomic nervous system, in *Neurology in Clinical Practice* (Bradley, W. G., Daroff, R. B., Fenichel, G. M., and Marsden, C. D., eds.), Butterworth-Heinemann, Boston, MA, pp. 1953–1981.

41. Bird, T. D. (1984) Autonomic nervous system dysfunction, in *Signs and Symptoms in Neurology* (Swanson, P. D., ed.), J. B. Lippincott, New York, NY, pp. 303–328.

42. Brust, J. C. M. (1996) *Neurotoxic Side Effects of Prescription Drugs.* Butterworth-Heinemann, Boston, MA.

43. Moser, V. C., Anthony, D. C., Sette, W. F., and MacPhail, R. C. (1992) Comparison of subchronic neurotoxicity of 2-hydroxyethyl acrylate and acrylamide in rats. *Fundam. Appl. Toxicol.* **18,** 343–352.

44. Oribe, E. and Appenzeller, O. (1995) Autonomic nervous system, *in Guide to Clinical Neurology* (Mohr, J. P. and Gautier, J. C., eds.), Churchill Livingstone, New York, NY, pp. 521–540.

45. Pletnikov, M. V., Rubin, S. A., Schwartz, G. J., Moran, T. H., Sobotka, T. J., and Carbone, K. M. (1999) Persistent neonatal Borna disease virus (BDV) infection of the brain causes chronic emotional abnormalities in adult rats. *Physiol. Behav.* **66,** 823–831.
46. Sharkey, K.A. , Williams, R. G., Schultzberg, M., and Dockray, G. J. (1983) Sensory substance P-innervation of the urinary bladder: possible site of action of capsaicin in causing urine retention in rats. *Neuroscience* **10,** 861–868.
47. Durant, P. A. and Yaksh, T. L. (1988) Micturition in the unanesthetized rat: effects of intrathecal capsaicin, N-vanillylnonanamide, 6-hydroxydopamine and 5,6-dihydroxytryptamine. *Brain Res.* **451,** 301–308.
48. Horvath, G., Morvay, Z., Kovacs, M., Szikszay, M., and Benedek, G. (1994) An ultrasonographic method for the evaluation of dexmedetomidine on micturition in intact rats. *J. Pharmacol. Toxicol. Methods.* **32,** 215–218.
49. Carpenter, F. G. (1981) Atropine and micturition responses by rats with intact and partially innervated bladder. *Br. J. Pharmacol.* **73,** 837–842.
50. Catalano, P. J., McDaniel, K. L., and Moser, V. C. (1997) The IPCS Collaborative Study on Neurobehavioral Screening Methods: VI. Agreement and reliability of the data. *Neurotoxicology* **18,** 1057–1064.
51. De Lahunta, A. (1977) *Veterinary Neuroanatomy and Clinical Neurology.* W. B. Saunders, Philadelphia, PA.
52. Ghez, C. (1991) Posture, in *Principles of Neural Science* (Kandel, E. R., Schwartz, J. H., and Jessell, T. M., eds.) Appleton and Lange, Norwalk, CT, pp. 596–607.
53. Bol, C. J., Vogelaar, J. P., and Mandema, J. W. (1999) Anesthetic profile of dexmedetomidine identified by stimulus-response and continuous measurements in rats. *J. Pharmacol. Exp. Ther.* **291,** 153–160.
54. Gustafsson, L. L., Ebling, W. F., Osaki, E., and Stanski D. R. (1996) Quantitation of depth of thiopental anesthesia in the rat. *Anesthesiology* **84,** 415–427.
55. Pellis, S. M. (1996) Righting and the modular organization of motor programs, in *Measuring Movement and Locomotion: From Invertebrates to Humans* (Ossenkopp, K.-P., Kavaliers, M., and Sanberg, P. R., eds.), Chapman and Hall, New York, NY, pp. 115–132.
56. Dingwall, B., Reeve, B., Hutchinson, M., Smith, P. F., and Darlington, C. L. (1993) The tolerometer: a fast, automated method for the measurement of righting reflex latency in chronic drug studies. *J. Neurosci. Methods* **48,** 111–114.
57. Handley, D. E., Ross, J. F., and Carr, G. J. (1998) A force plate system for measuring low-magnitude reaction forces in small laboratory animals. *Physiol. Behav.* **64,** 661–669.
58. Pellis, S. M., Pellis, V. C., Chen, Y-C., Barzci, S., and Teitelbaum, P. (1989) Recovery from axial apraxia in the lateral hypothalamic labyrinthectomized rat reveals three elements of contact righting: cephalocaudal dominance, axial rotation and distal limb action. *Behav. Brain Res.* **35,** 241–251.
59. De Ryck, M., Schallert, T., and Teitelbaum, P. (1980) Morphine versus haloperidol catalepsy in the rat: a behavioral analysis of postural support mechanisms. *Brain Res.* **201,** 143–172.
60. Frye, G. D. and Breese, G. R. (1982) GABAergic modulation of ethanol-induced motor impairment. *J. Pharmacol. Exp. Ther.* **223,** 750–756.
61. Pellis, S. M., Pellis, V. C., and Teitelbaum, P. (1991) Air righting without the cervical righting reflex in adult rats. *Behav. Brain Res.* **45,** 185–108.
62. Brooks, C. M. (1933) Studies on the cerebral cortex. II. Localized representation of hopping and placing reactions in the rat. *Am. J. Physiol.* **105,** 162–171.
63. Glassman, R. B. (1994) Behavioral effects of SI versus SII cortex ablations on tactile orientation-localization and postural reflexes of rats. *Exp. Neurol.* **125,** 125–133.
64. Fullerton, P. M. and Barnes, J. M. (1966) Peripheral neuropathy in rats produced by acrylamide. *Br. J. Ind. Med.* **23,** 210–221.
65. Edwards P. M. and Parker, V. H. (1977) A simple, sensitive, and objective method for early assessment of acrylamide neuropathy in rats. *Toxicol. Appl. Pharmacol.* **40,** 589–591.

66. Pellis, S. M., Pellis, V. C., and Whishaw, I. Q. (1996) Visual modulation of air righting by rats involves calculation of time-to-impact, but does not require the detection of the looming stimulus of the approaching ground. *Behav. Brain Res.* **74,** 207–211.

67. Crofton, K. M. (1990) Reflex modification and the detection of toxicant-induced auditory dysfunction. *Neurotoxicol. Teratol.* **12,** 461–468.

68. Moser, V. C., McCormick, J. P., Creason, J. P., and MacPhail, R. C. (1988) Comparison of chlordimeform and carbaryl using a functional observational battery. *Fundam. Appl. Toxicol.* **11,** 189–206.

69. Dyck, P. J. and O'Brien, P. C. (1989) Approaches to quantitative cutaneous sensory assessment, in *Quantification of Neurologic Deficit* (Munsat, T. L., ed.), Butterworth, Boston, MA, 187–195.

70. Yeomans, J. S. and Frankland, P. W. (1995) The acoustic startle reflex: neurons and connections. *Brain Res. Brain Res. Rev.* **21,** 301–314.

71. Lee, Y., Lopez, D. E., Meloni, E. G., and Davis M. (1996) A primary acoustic startle pathway: obligatory role of cochlear root neurons and the nucleus reticularis pontis caudalis. *J. Neurosci.* **16,** 3775–3789.

72. Llorens, J. and Crofton, K. M. (1991) Enhanced neurotoxicity of 3,3'-iminodipropionitrile following carbon tetrachloride pretreatment in the rat. *Neurotoxicology* **12,** 583–594.

73. McDaniel, K. L. and Moser, V. C. (1993) Utility of a neurobehavioral screening battery for differentiating the effects of two pyrethroids, permethrin and cypermethrin. *Neurotoxicol. Teratol.* **15,** 71–83.

74. Freund, G. (1975) Induction of physical dependence on alcohol in rodents. *Adv. Exp. Med. Biol.* **56,** 311–325.

75. Moser, V. C. (1996) Rat strain- and gender-related differences in neurobehavioral screening: acute trimethyltin neurotoxicity. *J. Toxicol. Environ. Health* **47,** 567–586.

76. Harrell, L. E. and Balagura, S. (1975) Septal rage: mitigation by pre-surgical treatment with p-chlorophenylalanine. *Pharmacol. Biochem. Behav.* **3,** 157–159.

77. Genter, M. B., Owens, D. M., Carlone, H. B., and Crofton, K. M. (1996) Characterization of olfactory deficits in the rat following administration of 2,6-dichlorobenzonitrile (dichlobenil), 3,3'-iminodipropionitrile, or methimazole. *Fundam. Appl. Toxicol.* **29,** 71–77.

78. Alberts, J. R. and Galef, B. G., Jr. (1971) Acute anosmia in the rat: a behavioral test of a peripherally-induced olfactory deficit. *Physiol. Behav.* **6,** 619–621.

79. Hart, B. L. (1988) Biological basis of the behavior of sick animals. *Neurosci. Biobehav. Rev.* **12,** 123–137.

80. Kent, S., Bret-Dibat, J. L., Kelley, K. W., and Dantzer, R. (1996) Mechanisms of sickness-induced decreases in food-motivated behavior. *Neurosci. Biobehav. Rev.* **20,** 171–175.

81. Kent, S., Bluthe, R. M., Kelley, K. W., and Dantzer, R. (1992) Sickness behavior as a new target for drug development. *Trends Pharmacol. Sci.* **13,** 24–28.

82. Profet, M. (1992) Pregnancy sickness as adaptation: a deterrent to maternal ingestion of teratogens, in *The Adapted Mind: Evolutionary Psychology and the Generation of Culture* (Barkow, J. H., Cosmides, L., and Tooby, J., eds.), Oxford University Press, New York, NY, pp. 327–365.

83. Linthorst, A. C. and Reul, J. M. (1998) Brain neurotransmission during peripheral inflammation. *Ann. NY Acad. Sci.* **840,** 139–152.

84. Sanders, D. B. and Howard, J. F., Jr. (1996) Disorders of neuromuscular transmission, in *Neurology in Clinical Practice* (Bradley, W. G., Daroff, R. B., Fenichel, G. M., and Marsden, C. D., eds.), Butterworth-Heinemann, Boston, MA, pp. 1983–2001.

85. Bang, Y. H., Park, S. H., Kim, J. H., Cho, J. H., Lee, C.J., and Roh, T. S. (1998) The role of Muller's muscle reconsidered. *Plast. Reconstr. Surg.* **101,** 1200–1204.

86. Beard, C. (1985) Muller's superior tarsal muscle: anatomy, physiology, and clinical significance. *Ann. Plast. Surg.* **14,** 324–333.

87. Zochodne, D. W., Ward, K. K., and Low, P. A. (1988) Guanethidine adrenergic neuropathy: an animal model of selective autonomic neuropathy. *Brain Res.* **461,** 10–16.

88. Brimijoin, S. and Lennon, V. A. (1990) Autoimmune preganglionic sympathectomy induced by acetylcholinesterase antibodies. *Proc. Natl. Acad. Sci. USA* **87,** 9630–9634.

89. Campbell, A. and Baldessarini R. J. (1981) Effects of maturation and aging on behavioral responses to haloperidol in the rat. *Psychopharmacology (Berl.)* **73,** 219–222.

90. Benvenga, M. J., Del Vecchio, R. A., Capacchione, J. F., and Jerussi, T. P. (1992) An in vivo alpha–2 assay reversal of opioid-induced muscular rigidity and neuroleptic-induced ptosis. *J. Pharmacol. Toxicol. Methods* **27,** 45–50.

91. Aceto, M. D. and Harris, L. S. (1965) Effect of various agents on reserpine-induced blepharoptosis. *Toxicol. Appl. Pharmacol.* **7,** 329–336.

92. Danneman, P. J. (1997) Monitoring of analgesia, in *Anesthesia and Analgesia in Laboratory Animals* (Kohn, D.F, Wixxson, S. K., White, W. J., and Benson, G. J., eds.), Academic Press, New York, NY, pp. 83–103.

93. Goodgold, J. and Eberstein, A. (1977) *Electrodiagnosis of Neuromuscular Diseases.* Williams and Wilkins, Baltimore, MD, pp. 91–96.

94. Okamoto, M, Walewski, J. L., Artusio, J. F., Jr., and Riker, W. F., Jr. (1992) Neuromuscular pharmacology in rat neonates: development of responsiveness to prototypic blocking and reversal drugs. *Anesth. Analg.* **75,** 361–371.

95. Bois, R. T., Hummel, R. G., Dettbarn, W. D. and Laskowski, M. B. (1980) Presynaptic and postsynaptic neuromuscular effects of a specific inhibitor of acetylcholinesterase. *J. Pharmacol. Exp. Ther.* **215,** 53–59.

96. Gupta, R. C. and Dettbarn, W. D. (1992) Potential of memantine, D-tubocurarine, and atropine in preventing acute toxic myopathy induced by organophosphate nerve agents: soman, sarin, tabun and VX. *Neurotoxicology* **13,** 649–661.

97. Hoskins, B., Fernando, J. C., Dulaney, M. D., Lim, D. K., Liu, D. D., Watanabe, H. K., and Ho, I. K. (1986) Relationship between the neurotoxicities of Soman, Sarin and Tabun, and acetylcholinesterase inhibition. *Toxicol. Lett.* **30,** 121–129.

98. Williams, J., Montanez, S., and Uphouse, L. (1992) Effects of chlordecone on food intake and body weight in the male rat. *Neurotoxicology* **13,** 453–462.

99. Ambrose, A. M., Huffman, D. K., and Salamone, R. T. (1959) Pharmacologic and Toxicologic studies on *N,N*-Diethyltoluamide. I. *N,N*-Diethyl-*m*-Toluamide. *Toxicol. Appl. Pharmacol.* **1,** 97–115.

100. Sternbach, H. (1991) The serotonin syndrome. *Am. J. Psychiatry* **148,** 705–713.

101. Grahn, D. A., Heller, M. C., Larkin, J. E., and Heller, H. C. (1996) Appropriate thermal manipulations eliminate tremors in rats recovering from halothane anesthesia. *J. Appl. Physiol.* **81,** 2547–54.

102. Eilam, D. and Golani, I. (1988) The ontogeny of exploratory behavior in the house rat (Rattus rattus): the mobility gradient. *Dev. Psychobiol.* **21,** 679–710.

103. Whishaw, I. Q. and Gorny, B. P. (1991). Postprandial scanning by the rat (Rattus norvegicus): the importance of eating time and an application of "warm-up" movements. *J. Comp. Psychol.* **105,** 39–44.

104. Plummer, J. L., Gourlay, G. K., Cmielewski, P. L., Odontiadis, J., and Harvey, I. (1995) Behavioural effects of norpethidine, a metabolite of pethidine, in rats. *Toxicology* **95,** 37–44.

105. Moser, V. C. (1991) Investigations of amitraz neurotoxicity in rats. IV. Assessment of toxicity syndrome using a functional observational battery. *Fundam. Appl. Toxicol.* **17,** 7–16.

106. Yokoyama, K., Araki, S., Murata, K., Nishikitani, M., Nakaaki, K., Yokota, J., et al. (1997) Postural sway frequency analysis in workers exposed to n-hexane, xylene, and toluene: assessment of subclinical cerebellar dysfunction. *Environ. Res.* **74,** 110–115.

107. Nieschalk, M., Ortmann, C., West, A., Schmal, F., Stoll, W., and Fechner G. (1999) Effects of alcohol on body-sway patterns in human subjects. *Int. J. Legal Med.* **112,** 253–260.

108. Arbib, M. A. (1997) From visual affordances in monkey parietal cortex to hippocampo-parietal interactions underlying rat navigation. *Philos. Trans. R. Soc. Lond. B Biol. Sci.* **352,** 1429–1436.

109. Spencer, P. S., Couri, D., and Schaumburg, H. H. (1980) N-hexane and Methyl-n-butyl ketone, in *Experimental and Clinical Neurotoxicology* (Spencer, P. S. and Schaumburg, H. H., eds.), Williams and Wilkins, Baltimore, MD, pp. 456–475.

110. Sharp, P. E. and La Regina, M. C. (1998). Veterinary care, in *The Laboratory Rat* (Sharp, P. E. and La Regina, M. C., eds.) CRC Press, Boca Raton, FL, pp. 65–127.

111. Llorens, J., Dememes, D., and Sans, A. (1993) The behavioral syndrome caused by 3,3'-iminodipropionitrile and related nitriles in the rat is associated with degeneration of the vestibular sensory hair cells. *Toxicol. Appl. Pharmacol.* **123,** 199–210.

112. Moser, V. C. and Boyes, W. K. (1993) Prolonged neurobehavioral and visual effects of short-term exposure to 3,3'-iminodipropionitrile (IDPN) in rats. *Fundam. Appl. Toxicol.* **21,** 277–290.

113. Rudberg, T. (1957) Occurrence of the "waltzing syndrome" in mice after administration of aminodiproprionitrile. *Acta. Pharmacol. Toxicol.* **13,** 233–239.

114. Cordover, A. J, Pellis, S. M., and Teitelbaum, P. (1993) Haloperidol exaggerates proprioceptive-tactile support reflexes and diminishes vestibular dominance over them. *Behav. Brain Res.* **56,** 197–201.

115. Pellis, S. M., Chen, Y. C., and Teitelbaum, P. (1985) Fractionation of the cataleptic bracing response in rats. *Physiol. Behav.* **34,** 815–823.

116. De Ryck, M. and Teitelbaum, P. (1983) Morphine versus haloperidol catalepsy in the rat: an electromyographic analysis of postural support mechanisms. *Exp. Neurol.* **79,** 54–76.

117. Aceto, M. D., Scates, S. M., Lowe, J. A., and Martin, B. R. (1996) Dependence on delta 9-tetrahydrocannabinol: studies on precipitated and abrupt withdrawal. *J. Pharmacol. Exp. Ther.* **278,** 1290–1295.

118. Martin, W. R, Sloan, J. W., and Wala, E. P. (1993) Precipitated abstinence in the diazepam-dependent rat. *Pharmacol. Biochem. Behav.* **46,** 683–688.

119. Chiueh, C. C., Markey, S. P., Burns, R. S., Johannessen, J. N., Pert, A., and Kopin, I. J. (1984) Neurochemical and behavioral effects of systemic and intranigral administration of N-methyl-4-phenyl-1,2,3,6-tetrahydropyridine in the rat. *Eur. J. Pharmacol.* **100,** 189–194.

120. Zang, X. P., Tanii, H., Kobayashi, K., Higashi, T., Oka, R., Koshino, Y., and Saijoh, K. (1999) Behavioral abnormalities and apoptotic changes in neurons in mice brain following a single administration of allylnitrile. *Arch. Toxicol.* **73,** 22–32.

121. Pham, H. C., Navarro-Delmasure, C., Pham, H. C., Clavel, P., van Haverbeke, G., and Cheav, S. L. (1984) Toxicological studies of deltamethrin. *Int. J. Tissue React.* **6,** 127–133.

122. Moser, V. C. (1999) Comparison of aldicarb and methamidophos neurotoxicity at different ages in the rat: behavioral and biochemical parameters. *Toxicol. Appl. Pharmacol.* **157,** 94–106.

123. Shimoyama, M., Shimoyama, N., Inturrisi, C. E., and Elliott, K. (1997) Oral ketamine produces a dose-dependent CNS depression in the rat. *Life Sci.* **60,** PL9–PL14.

124. Himnan, D. J. (1984) Tolerance and reverse tolerance to toluene inhalation: effects on open-field behavior. *Pharmacol. Biochem. Behav.* **21,** 625–631.

125. Hougaard, K., Ingvar, M., Wieloch, T., and Siesjo, B. K. (1984) Cerebral metabolic and circulatory effects of 1,1,1-trichloroethane, a neurotoxic industrial solvent. 1. Effects on local cerebral glucose consumption and blood flow during acute exposure. *Neurochem Pathol.* **2,** 39–53.

126. Ross, J. F, Sahenk, Z., Hyser, C., Mendell, J. R., and Alden, C. L. (1988) Characterization of a murine model for human bismuth encephalopathy. *Neurotoxicology* **9**, 581–586.

127. Danysz, W., Essmann, U., Bresink, I., and Wilke, R. (1994) Glutamate antagonists have different effects on spontaneous locomotor activity in rats. *Pharmacol. Biochem. Behav.* **48**, 111–118.

128. Larson, S. J. and Siegel, S. (1998) Learning and tolerance to the ataxic effect of ethanol. *Pharmacol. Biochem. Behav.* **61**, 131–142.

129. Colpaert, F. C., Desmedt, L. K., and Janssen, P. A. (1976) Discriminative stimulus properties of benzodiazepines, barbiturates and pharmacologically related drugs; relation to some intrinsic and anticonvulsant effects. *Eur. J. Pharmacol.* **37**, 113–123.

130. Daughtrey, W. C., Gill, M. W., Pritts, I. M., Douglas, J. F., Kneiss, J. J., and Andrews, L. S. (1997) Neurotoxicological evaluation of methyl tertiary-butyl ether in rats. *J. Appl. Toxicol.* **17(Suppl. 1)**, S57–S64.

131. Lange, A. E. (1996) Movement disorder symptomatology, in *Neurology in Clinical Practice* (Bradley, W. G., Daroff, R. B., Fenichel, G. M., and Marsden, C. D., eds.), Butterworth-Heinemann, Boston, MA, pp. 299–320.

132. Marsden, C. D., Hallett, M., and Fahn, S. (1982) The nosology and pathophysiology of myoclonus, in *Movement Disorders* (Marsden, C. D., and Fahn, S., eds.), Butterworth Scientific, London, pp. 299–320.

133. Hwang, E. C. and Van Woert, M. H. (1978) p,p'-DDT-induced neurotoxic syndrome: experimental myoclonus. *Neurology* **28**, 1020–1025.

134. Moser, V. C. and MacPhail, R. C. (1989) Neurobehavioral effect of triadimefon, a triazole fungicide, in male and female rats. *Neurotoxicol. Teratol.* **11**, 285–293.

135. Haggerty, G. C. and Brown, G. (1996) Neurobehavioral profile of subcutaneously administered MK–801 in the rat. *Neurotoxicology* **17**, 913–921.

136. Appel, N. M, Rapoport, S. I., O'Callaghan, J. P., Bell, J. M., and Freed, L. M. (1997) Sequelae of parenteral domoic acid administration in rats: comparison of effects on different metabolic markers in brain. *Brain Res.* **754**, 55–64.

137. Canales, J. J. and Graybiel, A. M. (2000) A measure of striatal function predicts motor stereotypy. *Nat. Neurosci.* **3**, 377–383.

138. Mathur, A., Shandarin, A., LaViolette, S. R., Parker, J., and Yeomans, J. S. (1997) Locomotion and stereotypy induced by scopolamine: contributions of muscarinic receptors near the pedunculopontine tegmental nucleus. *Brain Res.* **775**, 144–155.

139. Fritts, M. E., Mueller, K., and Morris, L. (1998) Locomotor stereotypy produced by dexbenzetimide and scopolamine is reduced by SKF 83566, not sulpiride. *Pharmacol. Biochem. Behav.* **60**, 639–644.

140. MacPhail, R. C., Peele, D. B., and Crofton, K. M. (1989) Motor activity and screening for neurotoxicity. *J. Am. Coll. Toxicol.* **8**, 117–125.

141. Maurissen, J. P. and Mattsson, J. L. (1989) Critical assessment of motor activity as a screen for neurotoxicity. *Toxicol. Ind. Health.* **5**, 195–202.

142. Kumar, R., Stolerman, I. P., and Steinberg, H. (1970) Psychopharmacology, in *Annual Review of Psychology* (Mussen, P. H. and Rosenzweig, M. R., eds.), Annual Reviews, Inc. Palo Alto, CA, pp. 595–628.

143. File, S. (1981) Pharmacological manipulations of responses to novelty and their habituation, in *Theory in Psychopharmacology* (Cooper, S. J., ed.), Academic Press, New York, NY, pp. 197–232.

144. Sobotka, T. J., Ekelman, K. B., Slikker, W., Jr, Raffaele, K., and Hattan, D. G. (1996) Food and Drug Administration proposed guidelines for neurotoxicological testing of food chemicals. *Neurotoxicology* **17**, 825–836.

145. Kulig, B. V. and Lammers, J. H. C. M. (1992) Assessment of neurotoxicant-induced effects on motor function, in *Neurotoxicology* (Tilson, H. A. and Mitchell, C. L., eds.), Raven Press, New York, NY, pp. 147–179.

146. Walsh, R. N. and Cummins, R. A. (1976) The open-field test: a critical review. *Psych. Bull.* **83**, 482–504.
147. Robbins, T. W. (1977) A critique of the methods available for the measurement of spontaneous motor activity, in *Principles of Behavioral Pharmacology* (Iversen, L. L., Iversen, S. D., and Snyder, S. H., eds.), Plenum Press, New York, NY, pp. 37–80.
148. Archer, J. (1973) Tests for emotionality in rats and mice: a review. *Anim. Behav.* **21**, 205–235.
149. Etienne, A. S., Maurer, R., and Seguinot, V. (1996) Path integration in mammals and its interaction with visual landmarks. *J. Exp. Biol.* **199**, 201–209.
150. Whishaw, I. Q and Brooks, B. L. (1999) Calibrating space: exploration is important for allothetic and idiothetic navigation. *Hippocampus* **9**, 659–667.
151. Eilam, D. and Golani, I. (1989) Home base behavior of rats (Rattus norvegicus) exploring a novel environment. *Behav. Brain Res.* **34**, 199–211.
152. Kernan, W. J., Jr., Mullenix, P. J., and Hopper, D. L. (1989) Time structure analysis of behavioral acts using a computer pattern recognition system. *Pharmacol. Biochem. Behav.* **34**, 863–869.
153. Schwarting, R. K. W., Fornaguera, J., and Huston, J. P. (1996) Automated video-image analysis of behavioral asymmetries, in *Motor Activity and Movement Disorders: Research Issues and Applications* (Sanberg, P. R., Ossenkopp, K.-P., and Kavaliers, M., eds.), Humana Press, Totowa, NJ, pp. 141–174.
154. Paulus, M. P. and Geyer, M. A. (1993) Quantitative assessment of the microstructure of rat behavior: I, f(d), the extension of the scaling hypothesis. *Psychopharmacology (Berl.)* **113**, 177–186.
155. Paulus, M. P., Callaway, C. W., and Geyer, M. A. (1993) Quantitative assessment of the microstructure of rat behavior: II. Distinctive effects of dopamine releasers and uptake inhibitors. *Psychopharmacology (Berl.)* **113**, 187–198.
156. Gallistel, C. R. (1989) Animal cognition: The representation of space, time and number. *Ann. Rev. Psychol.* **40**, 155–189.
157. Ericson, E., Samuelsson, J., and Ahlenius, S. (1991) Photocell measurements of rat motor activity. A contribution to sensitivity and variation in behavioral observations. *J. Pharmacol. Methods* **25**, 111–122.
158. Hine, B. (1995) Differential open field reactivity in HAS and LAS rats. *Physiol. Behav.* **57**, 301–306.
159. Treit, D. and Fundytus, M. (1988) Thigmotaxis as a test for anxiolytic activity in rats. *Pharmacol. Biochem. Behav.* **31**, 959–962.
160. Hogg, S. (1996) A review of the validity and variability of the elevated plus-maze as an animal model of anxiety. *Pharmacol. Biochem. Behav.* **54**, 21–30.
161. Mueller, K., Hollingsworth, E. M., and Cross, D. R. (1989) Another look at amphetamine-induced stereotyped locomotor activity in rats using a new statistic to measure locomotor stereotypy. *Psychopharmacology (Berl.)* **97**, 74–79.
162. Krebs-Thomson, K., Lehmann-Masten, V., Naiem, S., Paulus, M. P., and Geyer, M. A. (1998) Modulation of phencyclidine-induced changes in locomotor activity and patterns in rats by serotonin. *Eur. J. Pharmacol.* **343**, 135–143.
163. Paulus, M. P. and Geyer, M. A. (1991) A scaling approach to find order parameters quantifying the effects of dopaminergic agents on unconditioned motor activity in rats. *Prog. Neuropsychopharmacol. Biol. Psychiatry* **15**, 903–919.
164. Paulus, M. P. and Geyer, M. A. (1991) A temporal and spatial scaling hypothesis for the behavioral effects of psychostimulants. *Psychopharmacology (Berl.)* **104**, 6–16.
165. Paulus, M. P., Geyer, M. A., Gold, L. H., and Mandell, A. J. (1990) Application of entropy measures derived from the ergodic theory of dynamical systems to rat locomotor behavior. *Proc. Natl. Acad. Sci. USA* **87**, 723–727.

166. Teicher, M. H, Klein, D. A., Andersen, S. L., and Wallace, P. (1995) Development of an animal model of fluoxetine akathisia. *Prog. Neuropsychopharmacol. Biol. Psychiatry* **19,** 1305–1319.

167. Mullenix, P. J. (1996) The computer pattern recognition system for study of spontaneous behavior of rats, in *Motor Activity and Movement Disorders: Research Issues and Applications* (Sanberg, P. R., Ossenkopp, K.-P., and Kavaliers, M., eds.), Humana Press, Totowa, NJ, pp. 141–174.

168. Mullenix, P. J., Denbesten, P. K., Schunior, A., and Kernan, W. J. (1995) Neurotoxicity of sodium fluoride in rats. *Neurotoxicol. Teratol.* **17,** 169–177.

169. Mullenix, P. J., Kernan, W. J., Schunior, A., Howes, A., Waber, D. P., Sallan, S. E., and Tarbell, N. J. (1994) Interactions of steroid, methotrexate, and radiation determine neurotoxicity in an animal model to study therapy for childhood leukemia. *Pediatr. Res.* **35,** 171–178.

170. Mullenix, P. J., Tassinari, M. S., Schunior, A., and Kernan, W. J. (1991) No change in spontaneous behavior of rats after acute oral doses of aspartame, phenylalanine, and tyrosine. *Fundam. Appl. Toxicol.* **16,** 495–505.

171. Kernan, W. J., Hopper, D. L., and Bowes, M. P. (1991) Computer pattern recognition: spontaneous motor activity studies of rats following acute exposures to triethyltin. *J. Am. Coll. Toxicol.* **10,** 705–718.

172. Tchernichovski, O. and Golani, I. (1995) A phase plane representation of rat exploratory behavior. *J. Neurosci. Methods* **62,** 21–27.

173. Eilam, D. and Golani, I. (1990) Home base behavior in amphetamine-treated tame wild rats (Rattus norvegicus). *Behav. Brain Res.* **36,** 161–170.

174. Eilam, D., Szechtman, H., Faigon, M., Dubovik, V., Feldon, J., and Michaelson, D. M. (1993) Disintegration of the spatial organization of behavior in experimental autoimmune dementia. *Neuroscience* **56,** 83–91.

175. Sanberg, P. R., Zoloty, S. A., Willis, R., Ticarich, C. D., Rhoads, K., Nagy, R. P., et al. (1987) Digiscan activity: automated measurement of thigmotactic and stereotypic behavior in rats. *Pharmacol. Biochem. Behav.* **27,** 569–572.

176. MacPhail, R. C. and Tilson, H. A. (1995) Behavioral screening tests: past, present and future, in *Neurotoxicology, Approaches and Methods* (Chang, L. W. and Slikker, W., Jr., eds.), Academic Press, New York, NY, pp. 231–238.

177. Geyer, M. A., Russo, P. V., and Masten, V. L. (1986) Multivariate assessment of locomotor behavior: pharmacological and behavioral analyses. *Pharmacol. Biochem. Behav.* **25,** 277–288.

178. Krebs-Thomson, K. and Geyer, M. A. (1998) Evidence for a functional interaction between 5-HT1A and 5-HT2 receptors in rats. *Psychopharmacology (Berl.)* **140,** 69–74.

179. Koek, W. and Slangen, J. L. (1984) Acute effects of naloxone and naltrexone, but lack of delayed effects, on exploratory behavior in the rat. *Psychopharmacology (Berl.)* **84,** 383–387.

180. Morita, T., Sonoda, R., Nakato, K., Koshiya, K., Wanibuchi, F., and Yamaguchi, T. (2000) Phencyclidine-induced abnormal behaviors in rats as measured by the hole board apparatus. *Psychopharmacology (Berl.)* **148,** 281–288.

181. Kronthaler, U. O. and Schmidt, W. J. (1996) 1S,3R-ACPD has cataleptogenic effects and reverses MK–801-, and less pronounced, D,L-amphetamine-induced locomotion. *Eur. J. Pharmacol.* **316,** 129–136.

182. Bilkei-Gorzo, A. and Gyertyan, I. (1996) Some doubts about the basic concept of hole-board test. *Neurobiology (Bp)* **4,** 405–415.

183. Crofton, K. M. and Knight, T. (1991) Auditory deficits and motor dysfunction following iminodipropionitrile administration in the rat. *Neurotoxicol. Teratol.* **13,** 575–581.

184. Borlongan, C. V., Koutouzis, T. K., Freeman, T. B., Hauser, R. A., Cahill, D. W., and Sanberg, P. R. (1997) Hyperactivity and hypoactivity in a rat model of Huntington's

disease: the systemic 3-nitropropionic acid model. *Brain Res. Brain Res. Protoc.* **1,** 253–257.

185. Emerich, D. F., Zanol, M. D, Norman, A. B., McConville, B. J., and Sanberg, P. R. (1991) Nicotine potentiates haloperidol-induced catalepsy and locomotor hypoactivity. *Pharmacol. Biochem. Behav.* **38,** 875–880.

186. Gerber, G. J. and O'Shaughnessy, D. (1986) Comparison of the behavioral effects of neurotoxic and systemically toxic agents: how discriminatory are behavioral tests of neurotoxicity? *Neurobehav. Toxicol. Teratol.* **8,** 703–710.

187. Mattsson, J. L., Boyes, W. K., and Ross, J. F. (1992) Incorporating evoked potentials into neurotoxicity test schemes, in *Neurotoxicology* (Tilson, H. A., ed.), Raven Press, Ltd., New York, NY, pp. 125–145.

188. Widdowson, P. S, Wyatt, I., Gyte, A., Simpson, M. G., and Lock, E. A. (1996) L-2-chloropropionic acid-induced neurotoxicity is prevented by MK–801: possible role of NMDA receptors in the neuropathology. *Toxicol. Appl. Pharmacol.* **136,** 138–145.

189. Gougos, A., Khanna, J. M., Le, A. D., and Kalant, H. (1986) Tolerance to ethanol and cross-tolerance to pentobarbital and barbital. *Pharmacol. Biochem. Behav.* **24,** 801–807.

190. Le Quesne, P. M. (1980) Acrylamide, in *Experimental and Clinical Neurotoxicology* (Spencer, P. S. and Schaumburg, H. H., eds.), Williams and Wilkins, Baltimore, MD, pp. 309–325.

191. Maurissen, J. P., Weiss, B., and Davis, H. T. (1983) Somatosensory thresholds in monkeys exposed to acrylamide. *Toxicol. Appl. Pharmacol.* **71,** 266–279.

192. Deng, H., He, F., Zhang, S., Calleman, C. J., and Costa, L G. (1993) Quantitative measurements of vibration threshold in healthy adults and acrylamide workers. *Int. Arch. Occup. Environ. Health* **65,** 53–6.

193. Carvell, G. E. and Simons, D. J. (1990) Biometric analyses of vibrissal tactile discrimination in the rat. *J. Neurosci.* **10,** 2638–2648.

194. Simons, D. J. (1985) Temporal and spatial integration in the rat SI vibrissa cortex *J. Neurophysiol.* **54,** 615–635.

195. Waite, P. M. E. (1973) Somatotopic organization of vibrissal responses in the ventrobasal complex of the rat thalamus. *J. Physiol. London* **228,** 527–540.

196. Whishaw, I. Q. and Maaswinkel, H. (1998) Rats with fimbria-fornix lesions are impaired in path integration: a role for the hippocampus in "sense of direction." *J. Neurosci.* **18,** 3050–3058.

197. Wineski, L. E. (1983) Movements of the cranial vibrissae in the Golden hamster (Mesocircetus auratus). *J. Zool. Lond.* **200,** 261–280.

198. Antoniou, K., Kafetzopoulos, E., Papadopoulou-Daifoti, Z., Hyphantis, T., and Marselos, M. (1998) D-amphetamine, cocaine and caffeine: a comparative study of acute effects on locomotor activity and behavioural patterns in rats. *Neurosci. Biobehav. Rev.* **23,** 189–196.

199. Ludolph, A. C. and Spencer, P. S. (2000) Pyriminil, in *Experimental and Clinical Neurotoxicology*, 2nd ed. (Spencer, P. S. and Schaumburg, H. H., eds.), Oxford University Press, New York, NY, pp. 1048–1049.

200. Schaumburg, H. H. (2000) Vinca alkaloids, in *Experimental and Clinical Neurotoxicology*, 2nd ed. (Spencer, P. S. and Schaumburg, H. H., eds.), Oxford University Press, New York, NY, pp. 1232–1236.

201. Meston, C. M., Moe, I. V., and Gorzalka, B. B. (1996) Effects of sympathetic inhibition on receptive, proceptive, and rejection behaviors in the female rat. *Physiol. Behav.* **59,** 537–542.

202. Rosa e Silva, A. A., Prajiante, T. M., Almeida, F. H., Guimaraes, M. A., and Lunardi, L. O. (1997) Ovarian granulosa and theca interstitial cells: a morphological and physiological analysis in guanethidine denervated rats at pre-puberty. *Cell. Mol. Biol. (Noisy-le-grand)* **43,** 409–416.

203. Carvalho, T. L., Guimaraes, M. A., Kempinas, W. G., Petenusci, S. O., and Rosa e Silva, A. A. (1996) Effects of guanethidine-induced sympathectomy on the spermatogenic and steroidogenic testicular functions of prepubertal to mature rats. *Andrologia* **28**, 117–122.

204. Kempinas, W. G., Petenusci, S. O., Rosa e Silva, A. A., Favaretto, A. L., and Carvalho, T. L. (1995) The hypophyseal-testicular axis and sex accessory glands following chemical sympathectomy with guanethidine of pre-pubertal to mature rats. *Andrologia* **27**, 121–125.

205. Carvalho, T. L., Kempinas, W. G., and Favaretto, A. L. (1993) Morphometric evaluation of the rat testis, epididymis and vas deferens following chemical sympathectomy with guanethidine. *Anat. Anz.* **175**, 453–457.

206. Lamano-Carvalho, T. L., Favaretto, A. L., Petenusci, S. O., and Kempinas, W. G. (1993) Prepubertal development of rat prostate and seminal vesicle following chemical sympathectomy with guanethidine. *Braz. J. Med. Biol. Res.* **26**, 639–646.

207. Stefanick, M. L., Smith, E. R., Szumowski, D. A., and Davidson, J. M. (1985) Reproductive physiology and behavior in the male rat following acute and chronic peripheral adrenergic depletion by guanethidine. *Pharmacol. Biochem. Behav.* **23**, 55–63.

208. Traurig, H. H., Papka, R. E., and Rush, M. E. (1988) Effects of capsaicin on reproductive function in the female rat: role of peptide-containing primary afferent nerves innervating the uterine cervix in the neuroendocrine copulatory response. *Cell Tissue Res.* **253**, 573–581.

209. Koutouzis, T. K., Borlongan, C. V., Scorcia, T., Creese, I., Cahill, D. W., Freeman, T. B., and Sanberg P. R. (1994) Systemic 3-nitropropionic acid: long-term effects on locomotor behavior. *Brain Res.* **646**, 242–246.

210. Mattsson, J. L. (2000) Ototoxicity: an argument for evaluation of the cochlea in safety testing in animals. *Toxicol. Pathol.* **28**, 137–141.

211. Cary, R., Clarke, S., and Delic, J. (1997) Effects of combined exposure to noise and toxic substances—critical review of the literature. *Ann. Occup. Hyg.* **41**, 455–465.

212. Ritter, S. and Dinh, T. T. (1992) Age-related changes in capsaicin-induced degeneration in rat brain. *J. Comp. Neurol.* **318**, 103–116.

213. Ritter, S. and Dinh, T. T. (1988) Capsaicin-induced neuronal degeneration: silver impregnation of cell bodies, axons, and terminals in the central nervous system of the adult rat. *J. Comp. Neurol.* **271**, 79–90.

214. Chung, K, Klein, C. M., and Coggeshall, R. E. (1990) The receptive part of the primary afferent axon is most vulnerable to systemic capsaicin in adult rats. *Brain Res.* **511**, 222–226.

215. Chung, K., Schwen, R. J., and Coggeshall, R. E. (1985) Ureteral axon damage following subcutaneous administration of capsaicin in adult rats. *Neurosci. Lett.* **53**, 221–226.

216. Szolcsanyi, J., Jancso-Gabor, A., and Joo, F. (1975) Functional and fine structural characteristics of the sensory neuron blocking effect of capsaicin. *Naunyn. Schmiedebergs Arch. Pharmacol.* **287**, 157–169.

217. Perkins, M. N. and Campbell, E. A. (1992) Capsazepine reversal of the antinociceptive action of capsaicin in vivo. *Br. J. Pharmacol.* **107**, 329–333.

218. Nishida, N., Farmer, J. D., Kodavanti, P. R., Tilson, H. A., and MacPhail, R. C. (1997) Effects of acute and repeated exposures to Aroclor 1254 in adult rats: motor activity and flavor aversion conditioning. *Fundam. Appl. Toxicol.* **40**, 68–74.

219. Peele, D. B., Farmer, J. D., and MacPhail, R. C. (1987) Conditioned flavor aversions: applications in assessing the efficacy of chelators in the treatment of heavy-metal intoxication. *Toxicol. Appl. Pharmacol.* **88**, 397–410.

220. MacPhail, R. C. (1982) Studies on the flavor aversions induced by trialkyltin compounds. *Neurobehav. Toxicol. Teratol.* **4**, 225–230.

221. Parker, L. A., Hutchison, S., and Riley, A. L. Conditioned flavor aversions: a toxicity test of the anticholinesterase agent, physostigmine. *Neurobehav. Toxicol. Teratol.* **4**, 93–98.

222. Wayner, E. A., Singer, G., Wayner, M. J., and Barone, F. C. (1980) The taste aversion induction properties of two long duration barbiturates. *Pharmacol. Biochem. Behav.* **12,** 807–810.

223. Fix, A. S, Horn, J. W., Wightman, K. A., Johnson, C. A., Long, G. G., Storts, R. W., et al. (1993) Neuronal vacuolization and necrosis induced by the noncompetitive N-methyl-D-aspartate (NMDA) antagonist MK(+)801 (dizocilpine maleate): a light and electron microscopic evaluation of the rat retrosplenial cortex. *Exp. Neurol.* **123,** 204–215.

224. Horvath, Z. C., Czopf, J., and Buzsaki, G. (1997) MK-801-induced neuronal damage in rats. *Brain Res.* **753,** 181–195.

225. Anderson, W. A. and Flumerfelt, B. A. (1980) A light and electron microscopic study of the effects of 3-acetylpyridine intoxication on the inferior olivary complex and cerebellar cortex. *J. Comp. Neurol.* **190,** 157–174.

226. Balaban, C. D. (1985) Central neurotoxic effects of intraperitoneally administered 3-acetylpyridine, harmaline and niacinamide in Sprague-Dawley and Long-Evans rats: a critical review of central 3-acetylpyridine neurotoxicity. *Brain Res.* **356,** 21–42.

227. Nagy, J. I. Capsaicin: a chemical probe for sensory neuron mechanisms, in *Handbook of Pscychopharmacology*, vol. 15 (Iversen, L. L., Iversen, S. D., and Snyder, S. H., eds.), Plenum Press, New York, NY, pp. 185–235.

228. Switzer, R. C. 3rd. (2000) Application of silver degeneration stains for neurotoxicity testing. *Toxicol. Pathol.* **28,** 70–83.

229. LeQuesne, P. M. (1980) Acrylamide, in *Experimental and Clinical Neurotoxicology* (Spencer, P. S. and Schaumburg, H. H., eds.), Williams and Wilkins, Baltimore, MD, pp. 309–325.

230. Watanabe, I. (1980) Organotin (Triethyltin) in *Experimental and Clinical Neurotoxicology* (Spencer, P. S. and Schaumburg, H. H., eds.), Williams and Wilkins, Baltimore, MD, pp. 545–557.

231. Olney, J. W. (1980) Excitotoxic mechanisms of neurotoxicity, in *Experimental and Clinical Neurotoxicology* (Spencer, P. S. and Schaumburg, H. H., eds.), Williams and Wilkins, Baltimore, MD, pp. 272–294.

232. Davis, C. S. and Richardson, R. J. (1980) Organophosphorus compounds in *Experimental and Clinical Neurotoxicology* (Spencer, P. S. and Schaumburg, H. H., eds.), Williams and Wilkins, Baltimore, MD, pp. 527–544.

20

Neurological Assessment

The Role of the Clinician in Clinical Neurotoxicology

James W. Albers

1. INTRODUCTION

Neurology is a branch of the medical sciences that deals with the human nervous system, under normal circumstances and in disease. The principles of clinical neurology are analogous to those used in animal neurotoxicology. Both fields utilize the scientific method to formulate and test hypotheses, albeit under different testing conditions. The animal neurotoxicologist evaluates behavior and neuropathologic changes in groups of animals in response to controlled manipulation of the environment that includes detailed knowledge about the exposure to a given test substance. The primary questions to the neurotoxicologist are what neurologic problems are caused by exposure to the substance in question and what mechanisms produce the problem. In contrast, the neurologist utilizes results from the clinical evaluation of a single patient to formulate a differential diagnosis, the initial step in identifying the underlying pathophysiology and developing a treatment plan. The primary questions to the neurologist are what explanations exist to explain the patient's problem and what can be done to correct or modify it. The neurologist frequently faces the problem of detecting and treating nervous-system dysfunction independent of any initial information related to an underlying cause or etiology. Nevertheless, identifying the cause of a problem represents an important goal. Commonly, a neurologic evaluation is requested because of symptoms experienced by an individual patient, presented in the form of complaints, that suggest nervous system dysfunction. In theory, symptoms referable to the nervous system are important in localizing and characterizing the underlying problem. In practice, numerous physiological and psychological responses to a variety of stimuli produce symptoms that, in spite of suggesting neurologic dysfunction, are benign and not indicative of neuropathology.

The clinical neurologic examination is a highly structured portion of the medical evaluation. The examination was developed and refined during the early to mid–1900s *(1)*. It derives from an understanding of the cellular and anatomic components of the nervous system, as well as from an understanding of the nervous system's response to injury. Like other areas of medicine and the biologic sciences in general, the most

From: Handbook of Neurotoxicology, Vol. 2
Edited by: E. J. Massaro © Humana Press Inc., Totowa, NJ

difficult determination is distinguishing normal from abnormal function. The spectrum of differences in human performance, and the effects of education, motivation, learning, and training accentuate the difficulty. Portions of the neurologic examination are subjective and susceptible to patient effort and cooperation *(2)*. Experienced clinicians recognize the importance of motivation on test results, and they utilize an arsenal of clinical tests to enhance effort or identify poor cooperation. Even the objective portions of the examination are open to examiner interpretation *(3)*. Fortunately, all signs are not of equal importance. A hierarchy of findings exists relative to pathologic importance, with certain clinical findings having greater clinical importance relative to others. When symptoms or signs suggest a neurologic abnormality, numerous tests are available to the neurologist to further evaluate for potential anatomic, chemical, electrophysiologic, immunologic, and even genetic abnormalities. Proper utilization and interpretation of these tests requires understanding of the sensitivity and specificity of individual examinations in the context of the overall evaluation. The art of medicine reflects the neurologist's ability to interpret the results of the history, clinical evaluation, and laboratory tests; to recognize the difference between physiologic, psychologic, and pathologic abnormalities; to formulate a treatment plan; and to satisfactorily convey the combined information to the patient.

The neurologist plays an additional role of recognizing and studying neurotoxic disorders *(4,5)*, usually at the level of clinical observation as opposed to laboratory investigation. Such observations are limited to natural or accidental experiments as opposed to controlled manipulation of the environment. The obvious exception is the use of the neurologic evaluation in clinical pharmacological investigations. Many neurotoxic disorders were first recognized or suspected by clinicians. Examples include 1-methyl-4-phenyl-1,2,3,6-tetrahydropyridine (MPTP)-induced parkinsonism *(6)*, l-tryptophan-induced neurotoxicity *(7)*; pyridoxine-induced sensory neuronopathy *(8)*, and numerous other neurologic disorders related to adverse medication effects. Eventually, some presumed neurodegenerative disorders may prove to have a toxic etiology *(9)*. Once a definite neurologic impairment has been identified in the individual patient, the clinician's ability to establish a neurotoxic cause is limited by several factors. The most common limitation faced by the clinician is the absence of a measure of exposure *(10)*. Even when estimates of exposure exist, most initial impressions rely on the temporal association between exposure to a potential neurotoxin and a subsequent neurologic event. While important, temporal association is only one of several important considerations in establishing causation. More commonly, the neurologist as a neurotoxicologist plays the role of generating hypotheses that can be tested under more controlled circumstances. The following sections describe the components of the neurologic evaluation and address the strengths and weaknesses of this methodology relative to clinical neurotoxicology.

2. THE NEUROLOGIC EVALUATION

The neurologic examination is one portion of the overall medical examination, and at least some portion of a general medical examination is performed as part of every neurologic examination. For all practical purposes, the evaluation of a patient with potential neurotoxic exposure is identical to the neurologic evaluation performed on any patient with complaints of any etiology referable to the nervous system. The evalu-

Table 1
The Medical History: Information Typically Obtained by the Physician

Chief complaint(s)
    Primary symptoms important to the patient
History of present illness
    Including onset, temporal profile, provoking or relieving factors
Past medical and surgical histories
    Specific illnesses (medical and psychological), operations, and serious injuries
    Known allergies, medication sensitivities
    Travel history
    Medications (current and past use), including blood transfusions
    Prior neurologic procedures and results
        (EMG, EEG, evoked potential studies, CCT, MRI, PET, SPECT, angiogram)
Family history
    Describe particular disease or cause of death for blood relatives
Social history
    Marital status
    Children
    Education (years completed and grades)
    Tobacco and alcohol use (current and past)
    Use of drugs other than prescribed medications
    Hobbies
Occupational history
    Employment status
    Types of previous jobs (chronological list)
    Special training or skills
    Occupational exposure to chemicals
    Job or hobbies involving repetitive or forceful hand exertions
Review of systems
    General inquiry about additional symptoms not elicited above

ation depends in part on the patient's complaints and the subsequent findings, but it is relatively independent of the underlying cause of the symptoms or signs.

2.1. Clinical History

Almost all medical examinations begin with a history obtained from the patient (Table 1). Notable exceptions include evaluation of patients who are unable to provide information. The history is used to determine what chief complaints (symptoms) are troubling the patient. For most neurologic problems, the history is useful in localizing the problem to one of several broad anatomic categories. The description, distribution, and temporal profile of individual complaints is important. Patients must describe in detail their presenting complaints because initial descriptions often represent the patient's interpretation of their problem. For example, a complaint of "dizziness" may represent several different symptoms including syncope, postural unsteadiness, true vertigo, or even unsteady gait. The complaint of "numbness" may represent tingling or paresthesias, loss of sensation, or even weakness. Once the chief complaints are iden-

Table 2
Components of the General Medical Examination

Vital signs (resting and orthostatic blood pressure, pulse rate)
Head and neck (masses, bruits)
Pulmonary (auscultation of breath sounds)
Cardiac (heart sounds or murmur)
Abdomen (tenderness, masses, sounds)
Extremities (bulk, range of motion, masses)
Vascular (pulses)
Musculoskeletal (range of motion, straight leg raising)
Lymphatic (nodes)
Skin

tified, the history of present illness further examines the symptoms described by the patient. The temporal profile of each complaint is established in terms of onset, progression, severity, and frequency if intermittent. Associated relieving or provocative factors are identified. The review of systems is a direct inquiry about other potential symptoms that the patient may have forgotten or felt unimportant. Information related to any other past or current medical problems, as well as inquiry about family, social, and occupation histories, is obtained. This includes information related to potential toxic exposures, including those associated with use of prescription and over-the-counter medications.

2.2. Clinical Examination

The clinical examination represents the most fundamental level of testing in the evaluation of a suspected neurologic disorder. The neurologic examination constitutes an important component of the physical examination, performed in combination with a general physical examination. Most, but not all, of the information necessary to localize a neurologic lesion can be obtained from a careful history. The examination serves as an independent source of information for patients who are poor observers, have trouble communicating, or provide incomplete or misleading information. The primary purpose of the examination is to document evidence of clinically evident abnormalities or impairments (signs). The initial goal of the neurologist is to determine whether or not there is clinical evidence of a neurologic impairment, and, if signs are present, to localize the abnormalities to broad regions of the nervous system. The examination includes substantial redundancy that can be used to verify internal consistency, increasing the certainty of any suspected impairment. While the history is almost entirely subjective, the neurologic examination consists of objective and subjective portions. For example, reflexes are relatively independent of patient effort and are considered objective, whereas components of the sensory examination depend on the patient's cooperation and interpretation of events. In other words, a patient cannot "cause" his or her reflexes to disappear, but a patient can deny feeling the vibration from a tuning fork.

Individual components of the general physical examination and the neurologic examination are listed in Tables 2 and 3. The neurologic examination includes evaluation of mental status, cranial nerves, motor and sensory systems, reflexes, and several addi-

Table 3
Components of the Neurologic Examination

Mental status
    General appearance (e.g., tense, hostile, agitated, uncooperative, inappropriate, tangential, hallucination, depressed)
    Level of alertness (lethargic, obtunded, coma)
    Cognition, including orientation, attentiveness, language (receptive and expressive), judgment, memory (immediate recall, intermediate, long-term), abstract reasoning (similarities, proverbs), arithmetic calculations, follow multiple step command
    Knowledge of current events
    Mini-mental status examination (MMSE)
Cranial nerves
    Olfaction, vision, pupillary size and response to light, ophthalmoscopy, visual fields, eye movements, ptosis, nystagmus (physiologic and optokinetic), facial sensation, facial symmetry, hearing, speech, and examination of jaw, palate, pharynx, neck, and tongue muscles.
Motor
    Station (eyes open and closed [Romberg])
    Gait (casual, tandem, arm swing, walk on toes and heels)
    Adventitious (involuntary) movements
        Tremor (resting, postural)
        Myoclonus
        Chorea
        Asterixis
        Tic
        Fasciculations
        Myokymia
    Coordination (finger-to nose and heel-to knee)
    Alternate motion rate
    Strength, bulk, and
    Tone (resistance to passive limb movement)
Sensory
    Vibration, pin-pain, joint position, light touch, and cold sensations
    Dual simultaneous stimulation
    Stereognosis
    Quantitative touch-pressure
Reflexes
    Muscle stretch (jaw, biceps brachii, triceps, brachioradialis, quadriceps, hamstring, gastrocnemius)
    Pathologic (Glabellar, snout, grasp, palmomental, Hoffmann, Chaddock, Babinski)
Additional provocative tests as indicated
    Volitional hyperventilation, Tinel and Phalen signs, Adson maneuver

tional miscellaneous tests that are performed in response to particular complaints or findings. The mental status examination includes evaluation of cognition, orientation, attentiveness, language, judgment, memory (immediate recall, intermediate, long-term), abstract reasoning (similarities, proverbs), and arithmetic calculations. Evaluation of the cranial nerves includes examination of olfaction, vision and pupillary size and response to light, ophthalmoscopy, visual fields, eye movements including documentation of abnormal nystagmus, facial sensation, facial symmetry, hearing, speech, and examination of the palate, neck muscles, and tongue. The motor evaluation includes examination of station and gait (casual gait, tandem, and standing with eyes closed [Romberg]); observation for involuntary movements; tests of coordination (finger-to nose and heel-to knee) and alternate motion rate; and measures of strength, bulk, and tone or resistance to passive movement of the limbs. Sensory evaluation includes tests of vibration, pin-pain, joint position, light touch, and cold sensations, as well as evaluation of dual simultaneous stimulation. Muscle stretch reflexes are examined in the upper and lower extremities, and the presence or absence of pathologic reflexes is documented. Additional provocative tests include observation during volitional hyperventilation or following positional maneuvers. Cervical and lumbosacral range of motion, straight leg raising, and limb range of motion are examined as part of the general musculoskeletal evaluation.

The neurologic examination is efficient, reliable, and reproducible, with demonstrated clinical validity and sensitivity *(11–14)*. The full clinical examination allows recognition of patterns of abnormalities potentially related to toxic exposure or other causes. Yet, the neurologist's most difficult task is identifying normal function. In addition to age, gender and body size are important considerations in defining abnormality *(15,16)*. In the context of establishing clinical evidence of neurotoxicity, the sensitivity of the clinical neurologic examination is important. Issues related to sensitivity in general are beyond the scope of this chapter, but clinical abnormalities are frequently present in asymptomatic individuals. Sensitivity has been addressed extensively for many peripheral disorders *(15,17)*. For example, the ability to detect neuropathy in patients with diabetes mellitus is well-established for a variety of different measures. In general, there is substantial concordance between the different measures used to detect neuropathy *(15)*. Electrodiagnostic measures are considered by most to represent the "gold standard" for identifying neuropathy, and nerve conduction studies are capable of detecting subclinical diabetic neuropathy in asymptomatic, clinically intact diabetic patients. Importantly, the clinical detection threshold for neuropathy coincides with or is close to the point at which symptomatic neuropathy develops *(15,18)*. Although the magnitude of clinical neurologic impairments typically are registered in broad terms of mild, moderate, or severe abnormality, many components of the examination are amenable to quantification *(19–21)*.

2.3. Neurologic Impression

The mechanism by which the neurologic impression is derived likely differs among neurologists, and it ultimately depends on the judgment of adequately trained and experienced physicians, not on the results of single clinical or laboratory tests *(22)*. Results obtained from the history (symptoms) and physical examination (signs) are the basis of the initial overall neurologic impression and eventually the differential diagnosis (Table 4). The differential diagnosis is the fundamental component of any clinicopathologic exercise *(23)*. In essence, it is simply a list of possible explanations for the patient's problem that are compatible with the presenting symptoms and signs, although incidental or unrelated signs or laboratory findings complicate the task

Table 4
Questions Addressed by the Neurologist in Formulating the Differential Diagnosis

Is there evidence of any neurologic problem?
What is the general level of the suspected disorder?
    Supratentorial
    Posterior fossa
    Spinal cord
    Peripheral
    Multiple levels or diffuse
What is the location of the suspected disorder within the level selected?
    Left side, right side, midline, nonfocal and diffusely located
What is the temporal profile of the onset and progression of the suspected disorder?
    Acute (seconds to minutes), subacute (days to weeks), chronic (months to years)
What general diagnostic category is suggested by the temporal profile?
    Vascular, traumatic, infections or inflammatory, degenerative, neoplastic ("new growth");
        toxic, or metabolic
What possible explanations exist (differential diagnosis) to explain the suspected problem?
What tests would help confirm, refute, or refine individual hypotheses in the differential
    diagnosis?
    Tests of blood and urine
    Electrophysiologic evaluations
    Imaging studies
    Functional imaging studies
    Therapeutic (e.g., pharmacological) trial
What is the most likely final explanation (diagnosis) for the patient's problem?

(24,25). The differential diagnosis may or may not include information related to the etiology (cause) of the patient's problem.

2.3.1. Localization

The neurologic impression is developed by first localizing the problem in the nervous system. This is accomplished as the result of several steps, each reflecting the answer to a specific question *(26–28)*.

2.3.1.1. LEVEL OF ABNORMALITY

The first question relates to localization of any suspected disorder to one or more of several broad levels of the nervous system. These include the supratentorial (e.g., the cerebrum and related structures located above the cerebellar tentorium), posterior fossa, spinal, and peripheral neuromuscular levels. Supratentorial disorders typically produce abnormality among tests of cognition, memory, mood, language, vision, motor function, and sensation. Unilateral disorders produce contralateral symptoms and impairments including hemiparesis, hemisensory loss, and hemianopsia with involvement of the face, trunk, and extremities. The sensory impairment associated with supratentorial lesions typically involves discrimination functions such as localization, two-point discrimination, and dual simultaneous stimulation.

The posterior fossa encompasses the brain stem, cerebellum, and 10 of the 12 cranial nerves (the olfactory and optic nerves are part of the supratentorial level). Unilateral posterior fossa lesions produce a combination of unique symptoms and signs that reflect involvement of exiting cranial nerves and transversing sensory and motor pathways before they cross in the medulla. Lesions in this localization produce ipsilateral abnormalities of the head and contralateral abnormalities of the trunk and extremities. Symptoms suggestive of posterior fossa involvement include diplopia, dysarthria, dysphagia, dysphonia, dysequilibrium, incoordination, and crossed motor and sensory impairments producing weakness or sensory loss of one side of the face and the opposite side of the body.

Spinal-cord lesions are the only nervous-system disorders capable of producing a level of abnormality, with intact function above and impaired function below that level. Unilateral spinal-cord lesions produce a characteristic syndrome below the lesion of ipsilateral weakness, hyperreflexia, pathologic reflexes such as Babinski and Chaddock responses, and impaired vibration, touch, and joint position sensations in association with contralateral impairment of pain and temperature sensations.

Symptoms and signs of peripheral nervous system (PNS) involvement depend on the components involved. The components include the peripheral sensory and motor nerves, the muscles, and the neuromuscular junction. Recognition of peripheral-nerve disorders requires knowledge of the distribution of sensory and motor innervation of individual nerves. Generalized or diffuse dysfunction of peripheral nerves (polyneuropathy) produces a characteristic stocking-glove distribution sensory loss, distal weakness, and distal decrease or loss of muscle stretch reflexes. Generalized dysfunction of muscles (myopathy) produces proximal greater than distal weakness with preservation of sensation and reflexes. Neuromuscular junction abnormalities produce fluctuating weakness with abnormal fatigability, with a predilection of extraocular, bulbar, and proximal limb muscle involvement.

2.3.1.2. LOCATION WITHIN LEVEL

The second question is relatively simple and straightforward. It addresses the location of the responsible lesion within the level selected. Possible responses include lesions that are focal on the right or left side of the nervous system, focal but involving midline structures, or nonfocal and diffusely located. Correct localization depends on an understanding of neuroanatomic principles. In the context of this chapter, neurotoxic effects are typically bilateral and symmetrical.

2.4. Diagnostic Categories

The answers to the first two localization questions derive from information obtained from the neurologic examination. The next question involves identification of possible diagnostic categories using results from the first two questions plus information about the temporal profile of symptoms *(26,28,29)*. For example, symptoms having a temporal profile of acute (minutes), subacute (hours to days), or chronic (weeks to months) translate into vascular (including acute trauma), inflammatory, and neoplastic or degenerative categories, respectively. Similarly, the distribution of signs into focal or diffuse locations as described earlier allows further subdivision into additional categories. An acute focal lesion is characteristic of an infarction or stroke, whereas a subacute diffuse disorder characterizes an inflammatory meningitis or encephalitis. It is unlikely that all neurologists approach impairment identification as described earlier, but this model of problem solving emphasizes description of the logic involved.

Based on these considerations, the neurologist might summarize an initial impression as a progressive focal, right-sided supratentorial lesion, likely representing a neoplasm or new growth. A patient with a "stroke" might be described as having an acute onset, unilateral, focal posterior fossa impairment, consistent with a vascular etiology. A peripheral disorder associated with a neurotoxic exposure might be summarized as a subacute onset, symmetrical, distal greater than proximal sensorimotor polyneuropathy. The neurologist's description at this point usually does not include information about specific causes for the problem. For example, vascular disorders could be related to embolic, thrombotic, or inflammatory (vasculitis) problems related to several different causes. As mentioned earlier, almost all neurotoxic disorders produce bilateral neurologic impairments. This is important, because if the results of the neurologic examination identify a focal impairment, a neurotoxic explanation is extremely unlikely and other explanations should be explored. The temporal profile of most neurotoxic disorders is chronic, similar to the majority of metabolic disorders. Like metabolic disorders, however, there are exceptions, and neurotoxic syndromes also may have acute or subacute presentations.

After localizing the neurologic impairment to broad areas of the nervous system and establishing a general diagnostic category, the neurologist next develops a preliminary differential diagnosis or list of possible explanations for the symptoms and signs. Commonly, additional diagnostic or laboratory testing is obtained to further refine the differential diagnosis in an attempt to formulate a final impression. Ironically, there are many neurologic disorders that can be identified with confidence and treated successfully without knowledge about the actual cause of the problem. For many disorders, the cause remains uncertain even when the underlying pathophysiology is at least partially understood. This process of developing the differential diagnosis is addressed next, followed by review of the different forms of neurodiagnostic testing and the accepted process of establishing the specific cause for an identified problem.

3. ESTABLISHING A CLINICAL DIAGNOSIS

The most important role played by the neurologist is establishing the diagnosis for the patient's problem. This process is supplementary to the process of establishing the presence of a neurologic impairment. In fact, some neurologic diagnoses can be established with virtual certainly in the absence of an identifiable impairment. For example, diagnoses such as complex partial epilepsy, sleep apnea, or migraine headache are not associated with abnormal findings on the clinical neurologic examination, yet they can be identified with confidence.

3.1. Use of Neurologic Symptoms

The process of developing a differential diagnosis begins as the patient presents a description of chief complaints. The list of possibilities is refined based on the results of the neurologic examination. Only occasionally are symptoms sufficiently characteristic to be considered "cardinal" or diagnostic of one specific diagnosis. The recurrent abrupt onset of a unilateral pulsatile headache with nausea and vomiting, preceded by a visual aura without evidence of residual neurologic signs is characteristic of migraine, but other disorders including structural lesions may produce similar symptoms and signs *(30)*.

3.1.1. Nonspecific Symptoms

Unfortunately, transient, nonspecific neurologic symptoms are quite prevalent in the general population and rarely of clinical importance or utility in establishing a diagnosis. Many transient symptoms are related to normal physiologic variation. These normal physiologic events produce symptoms that are for the most part ignored unless attention is drawn to them or concern develops that they indicate a problem. For example, momentary lightheadedness or dizziness after standing may reflect postural hypotension due to dysautonomia, but most frequently this symptom is a normal physiologic response to assuming an upright posture. A similar sensation in response to rapid head movement is another normal physiologic response of no pathologic importance. Fleeting or momentary extremity numbness and tingling related to limb position, such as when awaking from sleep or after sitting in a crossed-leg position, simply reflects local limb ischemia or physiologic nerve compression. As a general rule, fleeting or intermittent symptoms are unlikely to reflect neurologic impairment, the obvious exceptions being seizure and fatigue-related impairments of neuromuscular transmission.

3.1.2. Influence of Anxiety and Depression

Emotions are the source of innumerable physiologic symptoms that are frequently interpreted as indication of an underlying physical illness. Unfortunately, there is a general tendency to deny psychological explanations for apparent physical symptoms. Because of the nature of these symptoms, the neurologist is frequently consulted to establish the neurologic explanation for the problem. Most neurologists are well-acquainted with the frequency of such symptoms in the population of referred patients, and some neurologists estimate that up to 50% of their referral practice relates to psychologically related symptoms. One of the greatest challenges is distinguishing neurologic symptoms having a psychological basis from those having an organic explanation.

The influence of anxiety and depression in any neurologic practice is substantial. The tendency by most patients is to assume that any symptom attributed to a psychological explanation must be imagined and is therefore discounted by the physician. Actually, the opposite is true. The autonomic nervous system probably has not evolved substantially over the past several thousand years, although our environment has changed greatly. Several thousand years ago our nervous system reflected an ability to rapidly respond to physical threat. This response is often described in terms of the classic "fight or flight" response, but it also influenced other activities including sleep. Our ancestors who slept soundly probably were at great disadvantage compared to those who were more anxious and easily aroused from sleep in response to any potential danger. In the face of immediate danger, such as the appearance of a predatory animal, an involuntary response is mediated by the central, peripheral, and autonomic nervous systems. The resultant autonomic nervous system response produces sympathetic stimulation and parasympathetic suppression. Information is communicated as encoded data in the nervous system by electrical impulses along axons or transmitted chemically at junctions (synapses) with dendrites on nerve, muscle, or gland cells. The chemicals involved in such transmission are known as neurotransmitters. Certain specialized neurons in the brain communicate with body organs by releasing chemical substances (hormones) into the blood. The resultant response to danger or threat produces several physiologic results, including increased respiratory and cardiac rates, diversion of blood from our gastrointestinal system to our muscles, increased perspiration in anticipation of increased body temperature from muscular activity, and dilation of pupils to let in maximal light. All of these responses are appropriate for physical activity associated with fight or flight.

In modern society, the attack of a predator animal usually takes place over the telephone or in response to an overwhelming family or work schedule. The "attack" is at a cognitive level, in association with anticipated events. The sympathetic response in these situations is no different than the response associated with attack by a predator. Unfortunately, in the absence of physical activity, most of the physiologic responses are misdirected. For example, diversion of blood to muscle that are inactive reduces the contribution of venous return associated with contracting muscle, producing decreased venous blood flow and symptoms of lightheadedness and dizziness characteristic of pre-syncope. Physiologic hyperventilation in the absence of physical activity produces hypocapnia and secondary cerebral vasoconstriction. The resultant dizziness or lightheadedness is disconcerting but also of no pathologic significance. An increased arousal state interferes with restful sleep, resulting in the consequent chronic fatigue.

Depression in response to life events also produces a variety of neurologic symptoms that are not obviously related to the depression, *per se*. Depression of any cause is associated with frequent sleep arousal and a terminal sleep disturbance with early morning awakening. Poor sleep produces fatigue and exhaustion. For reasons unclear, depression interferes with concentration and memory. The prevalence of depression-related cognitive impairment is common, and the term "pseudo-dementia" is used to identify patients whose apparent dementia is in fact related to an abnormal mood and reversible with treatment of the underlying depression. Other physical symptoms, including headache and some diffuse pain syndromes, are directly related to impaired mood, without other organic explanation for the pain syndrome and resolution with reversal of the mood disorder.

3.2. Use of Signs

Identification of neurologic signs is important in defining the neurologic impairment and in establishing a differential diagnosis.

3.2.1. Objective and Subjective "Signs"

Signs identified during the neurologic examination are generally considered "objective" compare to subjective symptoms described by the patient. Unfortunately, objectivity in this context is a relative concept and few components of the neurologic examination are not influenced by the patient's effort and cooperation.

Few would argue that the reflex examination is not objective. Muscle stretch reflexes vary slightly in response to anxiety, but they are independent of patient motivation or effort. The most important finding, that of absent reflexes in distal extremities, depends only on the skill of the examining neurologist. Even documentation of absent reflexes may be misleading unless further qualified, because absent reflexes may re-appear with facilitation as during the Jendrastic maneuver, a finding of less clinical importance than true areflexia. Because reflex variability is a minor consideration, documentation of normal ankle reflexes by one examiner and absent ankle reflexes by another likely reflects failure by the second examiner to properly obtain the reflexes.

Some signs are far more open to examiner interpretation than are other signs. For example, measurement of strength depends on a cooperative, motivated patient. However, like the reflex examination, demonstration of full strength even for a moment suggests intact function in most situations. The experienced examiner does not simply attempt to overcome the patient in examining strength, but rather asks the patient to overcome the examiner as increasingly greater force is applied. For example, in testing the triceps muscle, the physician secures the forearm at 45° to the arm and instructs the patient to "push" the examiner away. In this context, the examiner must provide increasing resistance using his mechanical advantage to resist the patient's efforts. Examination of patients with true peripheral weakness demonstrates smooth release, as opposed to the sudden collapse of the patient with decreased effort. "Clasp-knife" weakness suggestive of upper motor neuron abnormality should not occur in isolation. Instead, the presence of pronator drift, increased resistance to passive manipulation, impaired alternate motor rate, increased muscle-stretch reflexes, and pathologic reflexes all support an upper motor-neuron impairment. The alternate motion rate depends on maximal subject effort, and a nonspecific reduced rate in the absence of other evidence of basal ganglia dysfunction would be of limited importance. Similarly, examination of coordination and gait require good patient effort, and slow deliberate responses do not always indicate neurologic dysfunction.

The sensory examination is almost entirely subjective and dependent on patient cooperation and effort. Report of "dull" following application of a sharp pin to the skin is a subjective response, whereas jumping in response to application of the pin would be an objective indication the pin was painful. The clinical sensory examination has substantial redundancy, and isolated or poorly reproducible findings are of limited importance. The reported inability to perceive light touch yet correctly performing dual simultaneous stimulation would be internally inconsistent, because the more difficult task demonstrates normal performance whereas the simpler task is performed incorrectly. Inability to identify objects placed in the hands with the eyes closed (astereognosis), yet intact ability to manipulate the objects could not be explained by a PNS disorder.

Redundancy also exists across tests seeming to evaluate different function because portions of the nervous system are common to both evaluations. Internal consistency or concordance of clinical findings is an important concept because of substantial overlap in the neurologic examination. For example, impaired joint position sensation in the toes and ankles could not be reconciled with normal stance with eyes closed, because the latter requires precise information about joint position and both tests evaluate in part function of large myelinated nerve fibers. Peripheral loss of vibration, fine touch, and joint position sensations with a positive Romberg sign could not be attribute to a peripheral neuropathy in the presence of normal ankle reflexes. Inability to feel light touch, yet correctly moving the touched finger with the eyes closed during examination of coordination would represent an inconsistency.

3.2.2. Specificity

Few signs are pathognomonic of a given disorder, although exceptions exist. Waxing and waning neurologic signs over weeks to months in association with persistent double vision and eye movement abnormalities indicating an internuclear ophthalmoplegia strongly suggests the diagnosis of multiple sclerosis (MS) *(31)*. Subacute onset of a generalized movement disorder in a young adult noted to have Kaiser Fletcher rings on ophthalmologic examination strongly suggests a diagnosis of Wilson's disease *(32)*. The presence of Mees' lines in the nails of a patient with a severe distal neuropathy suggests arsenic intoxication *(33,34)*. More frequently, however, individual signs useful in localizing the neurologic lesion are not useful in establishing a specific diagnosis or cause of the neurologic problem. For example, evidence of impaired cognition with disorientation, abnormal postural tremor, slowed coordination, akathesia, and prominent primitive reflexes would suggest a clinical diagnosis of encephalopathy but not a specific etiology. But if these signs appeared in combination with evidence of midline cerebellar degeneration and a distal sensorimotor polyneuropathy, the possibility of hepatic-related neurologic dysfunction would become a prime consideration *(35)*.

Abnormal signs do not always indicate underlying pathology. Isolated abnormalities frequently are found in the clinically normal, asymptomatic population, independent of any identifiable disease but often in association with advancing age. For example, some primitive or atavistic reflexes such as palmomental, snout, or suck reflexes exist in a substantial proportion of normal subjects with advancing age *(36)*. A neurologist identifying such reflexes cannot therefore conclude that a specific disease exists. Ankle reflexes, whose absence is considered among the most sensitive indicators of neuropathy, are decreased or absent in 5% in healthy subjects older than 50 yr, limiting their value as a sign of polyneuropathy and necessitating a grading change with age *(18)*. Even diffusely absent reflexes may not suggest underlying pathology, because some individuals, particular athletic males, have diffuse hypo- or areflexia with no other abnormal findings and no evidence of any underlying pathology. Healthy subjects retain their ability to walk on toes and heels regardless of age, excessive weight, or lack of physical fitness, but the ability to arise from a kneeled position is lost in more than 5% of persons 60 yr and older *(18)*. Certain tests, including the sensory examination, are subjective and abnormalities limited to tests requiring the patient's interpretation must be assessed cautiously. In addition, decreased touch sensation in a person with highly callused hands or decreased distal touch and vibration sensations in an overweight individual occur commonly, in the absence of an underlying peripheral nerve disorder *(16,37)*.

3.3. The Differential Diagnosis Process

The differential diagnosis is a list of explanations capable of accounting for the patient's symptoms and signs. Invariably, the list includes some items that are more likely than others to account for the patient's symptoms and signs. The process of formulating a differential diagnosis requires careful characterization of any neurologic impairment with a logical step-by-step inclusion or exclusion of diagnostic possibilities *(22)*. This process has as its goal identification of the correct diagnosis. Logical algorithms can be derived that mimic or model the diagnostic process, but the process also depends on clinical judgment based on extensive neurobiological and clinical knowledge and training *(22)*. Additional diagnostic methodologies exist, including the "shotgun" and "gestalt" approaches *(22)*. The "shotgun" approach refers to reliance on a battery of clinical, laboratory, and imaging tests to identify abnormalities presumably important to the clinical problem, without detailed characterization of the neurologic impairment or determination of how likely any identified abnormalities are to explain the patient's symptoms. The "gestalt" approach refers to the pattern recognition technique in which the diagnosis is identified by recognition of a clinical pattern of symptoms, course, or disease associations. The two approaches differ substantially in the required amount of examiner experience and both have limitations.

The more conventional differential diagnosis approach begins by localizing and characterizing the neurologic impairment using results of the history and neurologic examination as described previously *(22)*. Based on the initial diagnostic impression, imaging, electrophysiologic, laboratory, and other tests are used to confirm the correctness of the anatomic and pathologic impressions. The diagnostic process begins as a list of possible explanations for information derived from the patient, findings obtained from the neurologic examination (signs), and results of diagnostic testing. The differential diagnosis process is based on the scientific method as an iterative hypothesis-generating/hypothesis-testing procedure. This process proceeds over time, frequently using additional information from neurodiagnostic or laboratory testing, repeat neurologic examinations to evaluate for improvement or progression, or even response to treatment. These additional evaluations or observations result in an increasingly shorter list of possible explanations for the patient's problem until only one likely diagnosis remains or the disorder remains undiagnosed *(22)*.

The differential diagnosis process sometimes but not always includes knowledge of the cause of the underlying problem. For example, a diagnosis of meningiococcal meningitis infers that the meningiococcal bacteria is the cause of the patient's problem. For other disorders, the diagnosis and successful treatment of the patient's problem reflects an understanding of the underlying pathophysiology independent of understanding the actual cause of the problem. Examples include identification of disorders such as migraine headache, Parkinson's disease (PD), inflammatory polyneuropathy, polymyositis, or myasthenia gravis.

4. NERVOUS-SYSTEM RESPONSE TO TOXIC EXPOSURE

There are innumerable substances that, when present in sufficient quantities and over sufficient periods of time, can interfere with or injure the nervous system. There is no single, defined neurologic response to chemical agents. The net effect produced by any substance to which an individual is exposed depends on many factors, including portal of body entry, distribution in tissues, ability to enter the nervous system, site of attack, concentration at the target site, duration of exposure, rate of breakdown, toxicity of metabolic products, and efficiency of excretion. Dose (concentration of the substance) is an important concept because certain doses may be harmless or even have nutrient value, whereas higher doses elicit profound, long-lasting, or irreversible changes. Duration of exposure is a key consideration in determining whether a particular concentration of a substance will be neurotoxic. The idea of a delayed-response following exposure to a neurotoxic substance is a consideration. Important examples of delayed neurotoxicity exist, but they are relative few in number *(38)*. Nevertheless, the idea of irreversible damage to a population of neurons, insufficient to produced clinical dysfunction but sufficient to later emerge following normal age-related attrition of the same cell population, is of interest and may be important in some neurodegenerative disorders.

Although there is no single, defined response to chemical agents, there are several well-recognized general patterns of response. Many neurotoxic substances affect the nervous system as part of a wider systemic response, with abnormalities presenting in distinctive patterns involving the nervous system as well as other systems. For example, arsenic intoxication produces a sensorimotor peripheral neuropathy, but also causes multiorgan involvement with anemia, gastritis, hepatitis, dermatitis, and other well-defined abnormalities such a Mees' lines in the nails *(33)*. Some neurotoxins are highly selective in damaging specific portions of the nervous system without causing other abnormalities. For example, the essential vitamin pyridoxine (vitamin B_6), when given in sufficient doses, causes selective injury to sensory cells in the dorsal-root ganglion, producing a sensory neuropathy or neuronopathy without producing other neurologic or systemic findings *(39,40)*. Similarly, MPTP, a designer meperidine-analog inadvertently developed and distributed as a synthetic heroin, causes a form of parkinsonism by producing selective injury to neurons in the zona compacta of the substantia nigra (SN) *(6)*.

The nervous system is divided into central and peripheral components. This division is somewhat contrived because there is substantial overlap in structure and function between the two components. Nevertheless, the division is useful in considering neurotoxic disorders and describing their evaluation. The central nervous system (CNS) consists primarily of those parts of the nervous system contained within the skull and the vertebral column. The CNS is responsible for initiating, receiving, and integrating signals needed to maintain internal homeostasis, cognition, awareness, memory, language, personality, behavior, sleep and wakefulness, locomotion, sensation, vision, balance, and many other bodily functions. The PNS consists of nerve cells and their processes that convey sensory, motor, and autonomic information to and from the CNS. Included are receptors and free nerve endings located in the skin, mucous membranes, and deep tissues that initiate information for touch, joint position, muscle motion, pressure, vibration, temperature, and pain sensations. Sensory nerves transmit signals from these receptors to the CNS where they are processed, integrated, and stored. Motor nerves transmit information originating in the CNS to muscles. In addition to volitional activation, much of the information transmitted by motor nerves results in reflex movements, such as maintaining posture. Autonomic nerves also convey information from the CNS to the periphery. This information concerns activities that usually are not under volitional control, including activation of smooth muscle within blood vessels and the viscera, the heart, and endocrine glands.

4.1. Central Nervous System

The CNS can be influenced by exposure to neurotoxins in several ways. The most common neurotoxic syndromes involving the CNS produce an acute or chronic encephalopathy. For the most part, the resultant neurologic symptoms and signs are independent of the underlying cause. For this reason, similar CNS syndromes result from numerous causes including prolonged hypoxia, hepatic dysfunction, uremia, hyperglycemia, or neurotoxins directly injuring neurons in the cortex. Patients with acute, mild "encephalopathy" associated with acute exposure to a variety of substances complain of headache and lightheadedness but demonstrate few neurologic signs. Symptoms rapidly resolve after removal from exposure.

A common model for CNS neurotoxicity producing acute and chronic encephalopathy is that which results from exposure to ethyl alcohol (common alcohol) *(35,41)*. Acute exposure has a dramatic impact on the CNS causing intoxication or drunkenness, resulting in impaired cognition, judgment, and coordination. In this form of acute intoxication, confusion, increased irritability, and altered levels of consciousness develop. Examination demonstrates altered judgment and disorientation, nystagmus, and ataxia prior to more severe alteration of consciousness. With increasing dose, the acute sedative properties of ethyl alcohol progress from increasing somnolence, to coma, or even death. The acute effects of sublethal exposures resolve in hours after removal from additional exposure without evidence of residual impairment.

Chronic or repeated acute exposures to ethyl alcohol, typically in association with nutritional deficiency, may produce neurochemical and structural changes in the CNS. Sudden withdrawal from alcohol after prolonged exposure results in effects opposite to those associated with acute exposure, producing agitation, tremulousness, hallucinosis, and generalized major motor seizures. This withdrawal state is an indirect neurotoxic effect, as chronic exposure produces temporary, reversible neuropharmacological effects on the CNS that are not related to permanent injury.

Chronic alcohol exposure in some individuals is associated with variable degrees of permanent encephalopathy characterized by dementia, cerebral atrophy, and slowing of the background electroencephalogram. The concept of a chronic, irreversible encephalopathy from alcohol is controversial. This is because the effects of chronic exposure are difficult to distinguish from the effects of malnutrition that almost always accompanies chronic alcoholism. These anatomical and physiological abnormalities have limited diagnostic importance other than to indicate the magnitude of abnormality. A progressive encephalopathy is associated with alcohol-related hepatic failure. This encephalopathy eventually terminates in a chronic vegetative state, requiring assistance in activities of daily living, including feeding and personal hygiene. These abnormalities do not occur in isolation, however, and symptomatic patients demonstrate many findings. Abnormalities include evidence of cerebellar degeneration with unsteady gait and incoordination; peripheral neuropathy with distal sensory loss, weakness, and areflexia; myopathy with proximal weakness; and additional neurologic findings such as asterixis (an involuntary flap of the outstretch hands), a finding associated with chronic hepatitis and cirrhosis.

In chronic, progressive toxic encephalopathy such as associated with chronic liver failure, the early nonspecific behavioral abnormalities (irritability, confusion, and anxiety) are followed by personality change, inappropriate behavior, impaired cognition, and disorientation. At this level of impairment, the neurologic examination demonstrates postural tremor, slowed coordination, and restlessness, typically in association with asterixis, dysarthria, akathesia, gross ataxia, and the appearance of primitive reflexes (palmomental, snout, suck, and grasp). As delirium develops, reflexes become hyperactive, and pathologic Babinski and Chaddock reflexes become evident, sometimes in association with myoclonus. Progression is associated with deterioration of consciousness and decerebrate posturing develops.

An additional syndrome associated with alcoholism and malnutrition is the Wernicke-Korsakoff syndrome *(42)*. Wernicke's syndrome refers to the subacute onset of encephalopathy with impaired extra-ocular eye movements and peripheral neuropathy that is potentially reversible with administration of thiamine *(42,43)*. Korsakoff's syndrome refers to a chronic residual amnestic state in which there is a relative inability to record new memories *(42,44)*.

A nonspecific psycho-organic syndrome has been attributed by some to chronic low-level or repeated high-level occupational exposure to organic solvents used as paint thinners or degreasers *(45)*. Substantial controversy exists as to whether exposure to these substances, in the absence of hypoxia, produces permanent neurologic damage in the form of a chronic toxic encephalopathy. Of note, the psycho-organic syndrome typically does not progress to the level of impairment where neurologic or electrophysiologic signs are evident. At this mild or equivocal level of abnormality, conventional neuropsychological testing is important *(46)*. Despite the initial enthusiasm linking solvents and chronic encephalopathy, the bulk of scientific evidence suggests that factors other than occupational exposure to solvents explain the purported symptoms *(47–53)*.

4.2. Peripheral Nervous System

The PNS is generally a sensitive indicator of nervous system involvement from neurotoxic chemicals.*(54)* Many neurotoxins produce recognizable effects on the PNS as part of their overall effect when given in sufficient dose and over a sufficient period of time. This is important because the most objective and quantifiable evaluation techniques available to the neurologist evaluate the PNS. The characteristic PNS abnormality following neurotoxic exposure is peripheral neuropathy. "Neuropathy" is a general term that literally means "sick nerve" that is used to denote damage to the PNS. The term "mononeuropathy" indicates involvement of a single peripheral nerve. "Polyneuropathy" is used to indicate diffuse involvement of multiple nerves, and the terms "neuropathy," "peripheral neuropathy," and "polyneuropathy" are used interchangeably in reference to such involvement of the PNS. Different forms of peripheral neuropathy exist, including those classified as sensory, motor, sensorimotor, and/or autonomic, depending upon the predominant class of nerve fibers involved.

A clinical diagnosis of peripheral neuropathy is based on a characteristic set of neurologic symptoms and signs. A diagnosis of confirmed peripheral neuropathy requires evidence of appropriate electrodiagnostic or neuropathologic abnormalities *(55,56)*. The clinical findings consist of symmetric abnormalities of sensation and/or strength that are most prominent distally, in the feet and hands. This is because most toxic or metabolic neuropathies are length dependent and characterized by a distal "axonal, dying-back neuropathy," demonstrating abnormalities involving the longest nerve segments *(57–59)*. Muscle-stretch reflexes are diminished and almost always absent at the ankles in any peripheral neuropathy of clinical significance involving large myelinated fibers (the most common type of involvement). Electrodiagnostic findings provide supportive, objective evidence of peripheral neuropathy, and also provide information regarding the underlying pathophysiology *(56)*. These findings usually can determine whether the neuropathy involves the cell body (neuronopathy), nerve roots (polyradiculopathy), or the axon, in addition to indicating whether there is evidence of

Table 5
Electrophysiologic and Imaging Tests Useful in Evaluating the Central Nervous System (CNS)

Electrophysiology
    Electroencephalogram (EEG)
    Quantitative EEG (QEEG) and EEG Brain Mapping
    Evoked potential studies
        Visual evoked responses (VER)
        Brain stem auditory evoked responses (BAER)
        Somatosensory evoked potentials (SSEP)
    Event-related potentials (e.g., P–300)
    Blink reflexes
Imaging
    Computerized tomography (CT)
    Magnetic resonance imaging (MRI)
    Single photon emission computed tomography (SPECT)
    Positron emission tomography (PET)

Adapted with permission from ref. *(121)*.

primary demyelination. When electrodiagnostic studies are normal, the likelihood of detecting a clinically significant peripheral neuropathy is virtually excluded.

5. USE OF DIAGNOSTIC TESTS

After a differential diagnosis has been developed, specific tests are available to refine the differential diagnosis by examining relevant aspects of neurologic function or structure *(60,61)*. Some tests are used to assure the organic nature of a suspected disorder. Depending on test results, items are eliminated from consideration or new items added to the differential diagnosis. This iterative process of formulating a clinical hypothesis and performing diagnostic studies to refine the diagnosis forms the basis of clinical medicine. Available tests include measures of cognition and affect, imaging studies of anatomy and structure, metabolic studies of neuroanatomic function, electrophysiologic studies of the CNS and PNS, and a variety of ancillary laboratory studies that evaluate other organ systems or measure the body burden of a specific substance. The latter include laboratory evaluations of blood, urine, hair, nails, and cerebrospinal fluid (CSF). Test results are interpreted in the context of the complete examination, and minor deviations from normal may be clinical irrelevant. Histologic examination of nerve, muscle, and other tissues may contribute to a diagnosis.

Specific diagnostic tests are of limited value until the tests themselves have been evaluated. At a minimum, the sensitivity and specificity of any measure must be known before it can be effectively used diagnostically. All tests have limitations, and indiscriminate use in suspected occupational or environmental disorders is inconsistent with their intended application. Most neurodiagnostic tests have limited use in establishing the cause of neurologic problem. This is because few neurotoxic problems have cardinal electrophysiological features sufficiently characteristic as to be considered diagnostic. Measures purporting to identify subclinical group differences in cross-sectional

Table 6
Physiologic, Electrophysiologic, and Neuropathology Tests Useful in Evaluating the Autonomic (ANS) and Peripheral (PNS) Nervous Systems

ANS
  Q-SART
  Sympathetic skin response (SSR)
  R-R interval
PNS
  Quantitative measures
    Quantitative sensory testing (QST)
    Posturography
  Electrophysiology
    Electromyography
      Nerve conduction studies (sensory and motor)
      Repetitive motor nerve stimulation
    Needle electromyography
      Conventional
      Single fiber
    Blink reflexes
  Neuropathology
    Nerve and muscle biopsy

Adapted with permission from ref. *(121)*.

studies of suspected neurotoxic disorders must be interpreted cautiously because of numerous confounders that influence such data.

Tests frequently used to evaluate different levels of the nervous system are listed in Tables 5 and 6. Many of these tests are sensitive to neurologic dysfunction. Others, such as EMG studies, localize abnormality to a degree not clinically possible. When used appropriately, many of these tests can be considered extensions of the clinical neurologic examination. The material that follows reviews diagnostic tests frequently used in studies of potential neurotoxic disorders. Neurobehavioral evaluations are discussed in a separate chapter, and specific laboratory tests that may be useful in establishing an elevated body burden of a specific potential neurotoxin also are not addressed.

5.1. Imaging

Imaging studies are important in the evaluation of patients with CNS disorders potentially related to neurotoxic exposure. In the context of suspected neurotoxicity, the most important contributions are to provide objective evidence of neuronal loss and to identify disorders other than neurotoxic exposure to account for the neurologic findings. Computerized tomography (CT) and magnetic resonance imaging (MRI) are capable of identifying structural abnormalities. Both are sensitive to disorders that produce cerebral atrophy, and any neurotoxin producing neuronal death has the potential to produce symmetrical atrophy identifiable by imaging studies, depending on the location and extent of involvement. Unilateral abnormalities cannot be attributed to toxic exposure. Imaging studies of patients with acute encephalopathy are unremarkable unless there is a pre-existing abnormality. In chronic encephalopathy of sufficient magnitude, imaging abnormalities reflect the magnitude of neuronal loss. Study of imaging results associated with hypoxic encephalopathy is useful in predicting the types and sensitivity of potential imaging abnormalities that occur in response to neurotoxic exposure. Depending on the magnitude and duration of hypoxia or anoxia, a spectrum of imaging abnormalities exist *(62–68)*. Like any disorder producing neuronal death, the abnormalities are not immediately apparent, but develop sequentially after the initial injury. CT and MRI imaging studies are obtained in response to a clinical suspicion that a structural abnormality exists, and indiscriminate use as screening evaluations is never justified.

Additional neuroimaging studies including single photon emission computed tomography (SPECT) and positron emission tomography (PET) are considered "functional imaging studies" because they provide information on some factor such as regional cerebral blood flow (rCBF) in addition to anatomic structure. At present, these are specialized tests of uncertain sensitivity or specificity that have little general application or acceptance for establishing specific diagnoses. SPECT measures regional blood flow and, in general, the resultant images reflect regional cerebral metabolism *(69)*. PET utilizes positron emitting radiopharmaceuticals to provide images of the distribution of these biological compounds that reflects the metabolic, biochemical, or pharmacological processes *(70)*. Both SPECT and PET studies may demonstrate abnormality in response to neurotoxic injury, and even those neurotoxins highly selective for only one specific cell type (e.g., MPTP and neuronal damage in the zona compacta of the SN) produce identifiable PET abnormalities *(9,71)*. PET is complimentary to structural imaging studies, with proven clinical efficacy in the evaluation of dementia, movement disorders, and in localization of brain tumors and seizure foci *(70)*. At present, few controlled experimental studies of SPECT or PET exist and sensitivity and specificity rates are unavailable *(72)*. Most current information is derived from nonreplicated, unpublished or anecdotal observations. This makes the application of such information, particularly in forensic situations, inappropriate. The Society of Nuclear Brain Imaging Council recently cautioned that use of these studies to provide "objective evidence" of impairment potentially leads to insupportable conclusions when used to link a neurophysiological parameter (such as blood flow or metabolism) to clinical dysfunction *(72)*. It is equally inappropriate to interpret SPECT or PET information to infer evidence that any neurologic condition is caused by a specific substance-induced illness or injury.

5.2. Electrophysiology

5.2.1. Electroencephalogram (EEG)

The EEG consists of electrical signals recorded from the scalp that are generated by neural tissue within the brain. The resultant waveforms are inspected visually and interpreted subjectively. Interpretation includes evaluation of the waveform amplitude, frequency, coherence, symmetry, and responsiveness. Criteria used to define abnormality are somewhat arbitrary, and minor inter-observer differences exist in the determination of normal and abnormal. In addition, the EEG is influenced by numerous factors that may be difficult to control, including the level of arousal.

The EEG plays an important role in the evaluation of encephalopathy by providing an objective measure of severity. There is a relatively good relationship between the EEG abnormality and the level of encephalopathy in acute encephalopathy *(73,74)*. Sensitivity for detecting encephalopathy is modest, but most patients with clinically evident encephalopathy have an abnormal EEG. The earliest characteristic EEG finding in encephalopathy is diffuse intermittent or continuous slowing of the background rhythm into the low alpha or high theta frequency range. With progressive deterioration, a dominant theta frequency becomes widespread and the EEG demonstrates poor reactivity, especially to visual stimuli. As the level of encephalopathy deteriorates, intermittent delta frequency appears, maximal over anterior regions. In patients with severe encephalopathy, large amplitude irregular delta activity predominates, followed by progressive loss of amplitude and reactivity. Burst-suppression patterns precede loss of all electrical activity, coinciding to loss of cerebral function.

A major limitation of the EEG is the poor specificity associated with slowing of the background rhythm. Slowing is a nonspecific finding that does not distinguish between the many forms of encephalopathy *(73,74)*. Triphasic waves are recorded in hepatic encephalopathy, but also occur with other forms of encephalopathy, including those associated with water intoxication, hypercalcemia, thyroid disease, renal failure, and hypoxia. The presence of triphasic waves best correlates with the level of consciousness, and they are most are prominent in obtunded patients *(73)*. The EEG is more likely to be abnormal in acute encephalopathy than in chronic encephalopathy. In chronic encephalopathy, any objective evidence of cerebral dysfunction is an important finding supportive of an organic etiology. For example, in chronic renal failure, the EEG typically becomes abnormal only when deterioration of mental status is clinically evident. The best examples of toxic encephalopathy occur with barbiturate intoxication. EEG abnormalities are as described earlier, and the degree of abnormality correlates well with the degree of mental alteration and level of intoxication. In addition, symmetrical beta activity appears in frontal head regions, representing a common medication effect. Degenerative disorders producing encephalopathy also demonstrate reduced frequency and abnormal background rhythm regulation. Disorders producing cortical gray matter dysfunction produce primarily irregular slowing and reduced amplitude. Those associated with subcortical gray matter involvement demonstrate bilateral synchronous, semi-rhythmic slow activity or spike-wave complexes *(73)*.

5.2.2. Quantitative EEG (QEEG) and EEG Brain Mapping

QEEG is the result of mathematical manipulation or processing of the conventional EEG signal in order to highlight particular components of interest such as epileptiform discharges or to transform the signal to emphasize some particular information such as slow-frequency activity. Excessive slow activity is a common finding in toxic encephalopathy, and one potential application might be a frequency domain analyses to quantify the power of the low-frequency signal. Quantification of this type permits statistical comparisons between individual patients and normative data, between groups of patients, and between successive measurements of the same individual. Brain mapping is the result of a topographic display of the QEEG data. This includes amplitude and frequency representations. QEEG and brain mapping have theoretical potential advantages over conventional EEG studies, but at present they are research tools and have had limited application in the evaluation of encephalopathy or dementia. As such, they have unknown sensitivity and specificity *(74)*.

QEEG has had limited application in attempts to identify differences between groups of subjects. This is because any identified differences may simply reflect different levels of arousal that are too subtle to be detected in the conventional EEG. Committees of the American Academy of Neurology (AAN) and the American Clinical Neurophysiology Society (ACNS) concluded that QEEG and brain mapping are predisposed to false-positive errors that limit their clinical potential *(75)*. QEEG techniques vary between laboratories, and clinical utility using one technique cannot be generalized to other techniques. EEG artifacts that are easily identified by an experienced electroencephalographer on conventional EEG sometimes appeared in unusual ways in QEEG analyses. In addition, data-processing algorithms generate new artifacts that are difficult to identify, and analyses sometimes include hundreds of comparisons that produce "abnormalities" by chance alone. In the evaluation of a patient with suspected dementia or encephalopathy, the finding of focal or generalized background slowing supports an organic disorder as opposed to an affective disorder such as depression. In making determinations about focal or generalized background slowing, QEEG likely parallels the role of conventional EEG *(74)*.

The American Psychiatric Association (APA) Task Force on Electrophysiological Assessment concluded that QEEG can assist in detecting excessive slow activity in organic disorders *(76)*. However, retrospective evaluations of QEEG techniques comparing disparate groups usually are uncontrolled and are neither random or masked, making it difficult to evaluate their clinical utility. Further, evaluations of individual techniques are often conducted by investigators involved in the commercialization of the instrument, making it difficult to assess bias *(75)*. There is little information on how EEG brain-mapping can impact the diagnosis of individual patients. The information on brain mapping sensitivity and specificity fail to substantiate a role for these tests in the clinical diagnosis of individual patients *(77)*. Abnormalities identified by these techniques are nonspecific for the cause and type of pathology and do not necessarily correspond to any symptoms *(74,77)*.

The AAN and the ACNS assessed medical-legal abuse in relationship to brain mapping and QEEG *(75)*. Difficulties identified were "false-positive" and "false-negative" results at odds with other clinical measures. Both reports expressed concern that results can be influenced dramatically during the relatively subjective process of selecting portions of the EEG signal for evaluation and quantitative analyses. Test-retest reproducibility was poor, and there are few objective safeguards to limit statistical or selection-bias errors *(75)*. The major concern in application of studies of unproved sensitivity, specificity, and reproducibility is the resultant confusion caused by their introduction. Prospective controlled studies have not as of yet satisfactorily evaluated test specificity or sensitivity of QEEG techniques. At present, QEEG and brain mapping should be used only by physicians highly skilled in conventional EEG, and then only as an adjunct to interpretation of the traditional EEG *(75)*. Use in any other context has been classified as Class III quality (evidence provided by expert opinion, nonrandomized historical controls, or case reports) *(75)*.

5.2.3. Evoked Potential Studies

Evoked potential (EP) studies record electrical signals generated within the nervous system in response to a specific peripheral stimulus (visual, auditory, tactile, or percutaneous electrical shock) *(74)*. These surface recordings are made of electrical activity generated from peripheral nerve, plexus, spine, or brain, reflecting the functional integrity of the afferent pathways.

Visual-evoked potentials (VEPs) are recorded from the scalp in response to visual stimuli, usually a shifting checkerboard pattern. They are sensitive to optic nerve and anterior chiasm disorders. Brain-stem auditory evoked potentials (BAEPs) evaluate the integrity of the auditory portion of cranial nerve VIII or the auditory pathways in the brain stem. Somatosensory evoked potentials (SSEPs) are analogous to sensory nerve-conduction studies. As such, they reflect activity in large myelinated peripheral axons and posterior and lateral afferent spinal-cord pathways. The SSEP amplitude is lower than sensory-nerve recordings and varies considerably in response to averaging technique, electrode montage, muscle activity, and stimulation paradigm, limiting the usefulness of SSEP amplitude measures. The most reliable EP abnormalities are those related to afferent pathway-conduction slowing. Most neurotoxins produce neuronal death and axonal loss. This results in loss of response but little in the way of conduction slowing, limiting the sensitivity of SSEP measures to detect neurotoxic injury. In addition, selective loss of small myelinated fibers typically does not produce SSEP abnormalities, although SSEPs recorded in response to thermal stimuli provide a possible mechanism to evaluate small fiber neuropathy.

EP studies are most commonly used to identify clinically silent lesions in demyelinating disease such as MS, and these studies have had limited application in neurotoxicology evaluations *(74,78)*. This is because more sensitive and specific tests exist for detection of demyelination. MRI imaging is particularly sensitive to myelin abnormalities, resulting in decreased clinical demand for EP studies because of their relative insensitivity and lack of specificity. Nevertheless, EP studies are occasionally abnormal when other clinical and laboratory studies are normal. BAEP abnormalities were reported in toluene abusers at a time when no other clinical or electrophysiological abnormalities were identified, suggesting a potential screening role for this test *(79)*. Nevertheless, at present, this proposed application has yet to be evaluated in a controlled environment.

5.2.4. Event-Related Potentials

Event-related potentials are specialized EEG techniques used to explore specific cortical processes, including those purportedly related to cognition and attention*(80)*. In these recordings, a specific event is time-locked to the EEG in order to explore temporally associated activity. One such event-related potential is the P-300, a potential generated in response to a random auditory signal that the patient is instructed to count, thereby encouraging attention to the stimuli. The P-300 is sometimes referred to as a cognitive evoked potential, attributing some cognitive significance to its presence. Nevertheless, the role of this signal in relation to cognition is controversial, and the P-300 may be an electrophysiological correlate of selected attention *(80–82)*. At present, application of this technique is limited, and the sensitivity and specificity of the test is undefined.

5.2.5. Blink Reflexes

Blink-reflex studies are evoked responses recorded from the orbicularis oculi muscles in response to percutaneous electrical stimulation of the supra-orbital nerve. They reflect neural activity along peripheral and central pathways, including a polysynaptic-pathway component that crosses the midline *(83)*. The afferent limb of the blink reflex is mediated by the trigeminal nerve, and the efferent component is mediated by the facial nerve. Blink reflex measures include ipsilateral and contralateral response latencies. Like other evoked response measures, their utility has not been established in neurotoxic disorders. This complex polysynaptic reflex is sensitive to cueing, indicating that attention influences test results *(84)*. It is likely that numerous other intervening factors influencing results, as well. The sensitivity and specificity of the blink-reflex measures are unknown.

5.2.6. Electromyography

"Electromyography" is the term used to describe nerve conduction studies (NCSs) and the needle electromyography examination (NEE). These electrodiagnostic tests are the most important tests available to evaluate PNS function. They are sensitive and specific for disorders of the lower motor neuron, the dorsal root ganglion and its peripheral axon, the neuromuscular junction, and muscle fibers. In general, most electromyographers consider nerve NCSs and the NEE extensions of the neurologic examination. NCSs are noninvasive, and the NEE examination minimally invasive. Their most important role is to localize abnormality to specific levels of the PNS. A secondary role includes identification of the most likely pathophysiology, producing a more manageable differential diagnosis.

The electrodiagnostic evaluation of patients with suspected neuropathy includes sensory and motor NCSs, evaluation of late responses, the NEE, and occasionally other studies such as sympathetic skin responses (SSRs). The combined evaluation is used to confirm clinical findings and localize specific abnormalities to a degree not clinically possible. The electrodiagnostic evaluation is an extension of the clinical examination, with established reference values, reproducibility, limitations, and guidelines for appropriate utilization *(85–89)*. The results of the evaluation allow classification of the neuropathies into broad categories that suggest the underlying pathophysiology. This information helps focus the differential diagnosis and directs the subsequent evaluation. Electrodiagnostic results often suggest a specific diagnosis, either alone or when combined with other clinical and laboratory information. Factors such as age, limb temperature, and body size influence normal values, and awareness of these influences increases the sensitivity and accuracy of electrodiagnostic testing *(37,90–93)*. Electrodiagnostic studies also play an important role in evaluation of the efficacy and detection of subclinical neurotoxicity of therapeutic agents.

Sensory and motor NCSs and the NEE evaluate slightly different components of the nervous system *(56)*. NCSs are noninvasive and provide the most useful information in the evaluation of neuropathy. These tests technically are "evoked response" studies, and an electrical signal generated by peripheral nerve or muscle is recorded in response to a percutaneous stimulus. The NEE has a secondary role in the evaluation of neuropathy, being used primarily to document the distribution of axonal lesions and to identify

Table 7
Questions Addressed by the Electrodiagnostic Examination in Characterizing Peripheral Dysfunction

Is there evidence of:

Polyneuropathy, mononeuropathy multiplex, or polyradiculopathy?
Sensory, motor, or combined involvement?
Substantial conduction slowing (myelin or membrane) or amplitude loss (axon)?
Impaired neuromuscular transmission?
Isolated muscle fiber involvement?

Adapted with permission from ref. *(74)*.

disorders such as polyradiculopathy that may be clinically indistinguishable from neuropathy.

Information derived from the electrodiagnostic examination can identify different types of neuropathy but cannot diagnose toxic neuropathy in isolation *(74)*. Several questions addressed by the electrodiagnostic examination are listed in Table 7. The questions do not address whether a specific toxin produced abnormality, but instead begin by localizing any abnormality to a focal, multifocal, or diffuse distribution. In the case of a diffuse polyneuropathy, the presence of predominant sensory or motor involvement is established, followed by determination of whether the abnormalities are characterized by substantial conduction slowing or simply loss of amplitude. This classification separates peripheral disorders into broad categories based on electrodiagnostic evidence of sensory or motor involvement combined with the presence or absence of substantial nerve conduction slowing (uniform or multifocal) *(55)*. The answers to these questions do not produce a diagnosis of toxic neuropathy in isolation, nor are the findings restricted to toxic neuropathies. This classification represents one method of identifying peripheral disorders using electrodiagnostic test results. The classification is easy to apply, but it does have limitations. The categories are not exclusive, and several neurotoxic disorders present with very different electrophysiologic features, depending on the severity and timing of testing in terms of the clinical course. The importance of this classification system is that it reduces to an extent not clinically possible the number of disorders that must be considered in the differential diagnosis.

Table 8 classifies several types of toxic neuropathy using electrophysiological test results. This classification reduces the number of disorders that must be considered in the differential diagnosis of any possible neuropathy. The definition of decreased motor nerve-conduction velocity is important in this classification. Criteria exist to identify nerve conduction slowing consistent with segmental demyelination, but other disorders including axonal degeneration, axonal stenosis, channelopathies, and selective loss of large myelinated fibers also produce similar findings. Conduction slowing as used in this classification includes any slowing that cannot be attributed to axonal loss lesions alone. In general, conduction velocities less than 80% of the lower limit of normal or distal latencies and F wave latencies exceeding 125% of the upper limit of normal fulfill this requirement *(94,95)*. The results of the electrodiagnostic examination also distinguish acquired neuropathies, including those associated with neurotoxic disor-

Table 8
Toxic Neuropathy Classified by Electrodiagnostic Findings

Motor or motor > sensory, conduction slowing
    Arsenic (shortly after acute exposure)
    Amiodarone
    Carbon disulfide
    Cytosine arabinoside (ara-C)
    Methyl n-butyl ketone
    n-Hexane
    Saxitoxin (sodium channel blocker)
    Suramin
    Swine flu vaccine
Motor or motor > sensory, no conduction slowing
    Cimetidine
    Dapsone
    Disulfiram (carbon disulfide?)
    Doxorubicin
    Hyperinsulin/hypoglycemia
    Nitrofurantoin
    Organophosphorus esters (OPIDN)
    Vincristine
Sensory only (neuropathy or neuronopathy)
    Cisplatin
    Ethyl alcohol
    Metronidazole
    Pyridoxine
    Thalidomide
    Thallium (small fiber)
Sensorimotor, no conduction slowing
    Acrylamide
    Amitriptyline
    Arsenic (chronic)
    Carbon monoxide
    Colchicine (neuromyopathy)
    Ethambutol
    Ethyl alcohol
    Ethylene oxide
    Elemental mercury
    Gold
    Hydralazine
    Isoniazid
    Lithium
    Metronidazole
    Nitrofurantoin
    Nitrous oxide (myeloneuropathy)
    Paclitaxel
    Perhexiline
    Phenytoin
    Thallium
    Vincristine

Adapted with permission from ref. *(121)*.

ders, from hereditary disorders associated with conduction slowing *(96)*. Partial conduction block along motor axons and increased temporal dispersion are important features associated with some acquired neuropathies. Absence of these features suggests uniform involvement of all fibers and supports a hereditary rather than acquired etiology.

The NEE is a sensitive indicator of partial denervation of any cause, and even mild axonal loss of motor fibers produces easily identified abnormalities such as fibrillation potentials. The NEE is an important component of the electrodiagnostic examination, but it has a secondary role in the evaluation of neurotoxic disorders compared to NCSs. A prominent exception is in the evaluation of toxic myopathy, although the abnormalities are nonspecific. Separation of a muscle fiber from the nerve innervating it, regardless of cause, results within weeks in the appearance of abnormal insertional activity characterized by positive waves and fibrillation potentials. These spontaneous discharges represent involuntary muscle fiber potentials associated with denervation acetylcholine (ACh) hypersensitivity due to proliferation of ACh receptors on the muscle-fiber surface. They are easily recognized, not easily confused with other NEE signals, and not present in normal muscle. The NEE is a sensitive indicator of partial denervation or muscle-fiber necrosis.

5.2.7. Repetitive Motor-Nerve Stimulation

Repetitive motor-nerve stimulation is the most frequently used technique available to evaluate neuromuscular transmission *(97)*. Impaired neuromuscular transmission is identified as a decline (decrement) in the motor response recorded with repeated depolarization of the nerve at low rates (e.g., 3 Hz) of stimulation *(98,99)*. Ordinarily, ACh released from the nerve terminal in response to depolarization produces an endplate potential larger than necessary to generate a muscle action potential. The normal neuromuscular junction shows no variation in amplitude or configuration with repetitive stimulation. A normal response depends on the availability of ACh, inactivation of ACh in the synaptic cleft, and functioning ACh receptors. Abnormality of any of these may result in impairment of neuromuscular transmission. Application of this technique in neurotoxic disease associated with chemical exposure is limited. Examples include demonstration of abnormal neuromuscular transmission in acute organophosphorus intoxication or after therapeutic use of penicillamine *(100–102)*. There are, however, several biologic neurotoxins that interfere with neuromuscular transmission, including botulinum toxin, alpha-bungarotoxin, and curare *(103–106)*.

5.2.8. Single Fiber Electromyography (SFEMG)

Single fiber electromyography (SFEMG) was first described by Elkstedt and Stalberg *(107,108)*. It is a method for extracellular recording of single muscle fiber action potentials (MFAPs) using an electrode with a small recording surface (25 μm) located on the shaft of the SFEMG electrode. When MFAPs are recorded from the same motor unit during minimal activation, there are small variations in the timing of the action potentials. This variation is called jitter. Jitter reflects the small difference in the time required for an endplate potential to reach threshold prior to development of the MFAP. When the amplitude of the endplate potential is well above threshold, there is little variability in the timing of MFAP discharge and jitter values are small. When the endplate potential is just above threshold, there is great variability in the timing of

MFAP discharge and jitter values are large. With substantial neuromuscular transmission impairment, the endplate potential fails to reach threshold and a MFAP is not generated. The decremental response recorded in patients with defective neuromuscular transmission during repetitive motor stimulation is related to blocking of individual MFAPs. The measure used to describe jitter is the mean consecutive interpotential difference (MCD). Because there is substantial variability in the MCD among normal MFAP pairs, at least 15–20 potential pairs are studied for any muscle and the results expressed as an average MCD, the percentage of pairs having an abnormal MCD, and the percentage of pairs demonstrating intermittent blocking. Normal values vary slightly from laboratory to laboratory, being dependent on technique, patient age, and the muscle tested. SFEMG also can be used to determine muscle-fiber density. The number of individual MFAPs from a single motor unit is counted during a single electrode placement, and the average number of MFAPs calculated from multiple electrode insertions in different locations within the muscle. In association with axonal sprouting and reinnervation, muscle fiber density increases, making SFEMG a sensitive method of identifying previous denervation.

SFEMG is commonly used to evaluate neuromuscular transmission in patients with suspected myasthenia gravis, but it also has been utilized in a variety of physiologic and pathologic conditions of neuromuscular transmission and muscle-fiber density, including those related to neurotoxicity (e.g., penicillamine-induced myasthenia gravis). SFEMG is an objective and extremely sensitive measurement of neuromuscular transmission. However, an abnormal SFEMG is not specific for any particular disorder of neuromuscular transmission, and false-positive studies occur in a variety of disorders associated with partial denervation and reinnervation (e.g., motor-neuron disease, polymyositis, chronic neuropathy).

5.2.9. Tests of Autonomic Nervous System Function

The sympathetic skin response (SSR) is a readily available measure of autonomic function *(109)*. Whereas standard conduction studies primarily evaluate large myelinated nerve fibers, SSRs evaluate small nerve-fiber function. The SSR is differentially recorded from skin between areas of high and low sweat-gland density. SSRs normally appear spontaneously or in response to a variety of stimuli such as electrical stimulation, loud noise, or an emotionally charged question. The purpose of the stimulus is to illicit an autonomic response to startle, not to directly depolarize the nerve. SSRs are used to document autonomic impairment in disorders such as inflammatory or diabetic neuropathy, but they have limited application in neurotoxic disorders. In general, neither their sensitivity nor specificity is known. Other tests of autonomic nervous function exist (e.g., R-R interval, Q-SART, skin biopsy to assess small unmyelinated nerve fibers or sweat glands), but are beyond the scope of this chapter. At present, none of these has had extensive application or evaluation in the neurotoxic disorders.

5.3. Other Laboratory Testing

The role of traditional laboratory measures in the evaluation of suspected neurotoxic disorders relates primarily to identifying systemic disorders associated with neurologic dysfunction. For example, arsenic-induced toxic neuropathy is associated with anemia, pancytopenia, and abnormal liver function tests; and l-tryptophan intoxication is associated with an increased total eosinophil count and evidence of vasculitis *(33,110–112)*. In addition, the excretion of some substances like arsenic and certain heavy metals can be measured in the urine and other tissues such as hair *(113,114)*. Unfortunately, the metabolism of most other chemicals is sufficiently rapid to make detection in body tissues difficult. In select situations, surrogates of exposure exist. For example, after acute organophosphate exposure, plasma butyryl (pseudo) cholinesterase (BuChE) and red blood cell acetylcholinesterase (AChE) levels are reduced when measured soon after poisoning, although neither is directly related to neurotoxicity *(115,116)*.

The evaluation of individual laboratory tests of blood and urine is beyond the scope of this chapter. It is important to recognize, however, that the role of random screening is limited and finding an abnormal value does not insure that the cause has been established as competing explanations commonly exist. Consider, for example, the increased excretion of urinary arsenic or mercury associated with ingestion of some seafood. The numerous commercially available tests purporting to associate abnormal antibodies or borderline-elevations of trace substances in response to some chemical exposure are, for the most part, of unknown reproducibility, sensitivity, or specificity. Frequently, control population information is unavailable or undefined. Until further evaluated, application of such measures has unknown utility. None of these measures is useful for screening purposes, other than in those industrial hygiene applications that monitor exposure to a specific chemical in an occupational setting.

Tissue biopsy occasionally is utilized in neurotoxicology evaluations. In patients with solvent-induced neuropathy associated with n-hexane intoxication, peripheral nerve biopsy shows characteristic focal axonal swellings consisting of neurofilament aggregates. Biopsy of skin, fascia, muscle, and nerve from patients with eosinophilia-myalgia syndrome associated with l-tryptophan intoxication typically demonstrates perivascular inflammation with lymphocytes and rare eosinophils in connective tissue. In other neurotoxic disorders, tissue biopsy is rarely indicated, other than to document the presence of problems unrelated to toxic exposure.

5.4. *Quantitative Measures of Neurologic Function*

5.4.1. *Quantitative Sensory Tests (QSTs)*

QSTs have been used to assess toxic neuropathy, and these psychomotor tests have application in clinical, pharmacological, and neurotoxicology studies *(117,118)*. These psychophysical measures derive from the well-established quantitative hearing tests (audiometry) used in the evaluation of hearing loss, including that related to ototoxicity. Further, experience with audiometry formed the basis for the numerous paradigms used to evaluate cutaneous sensation. The validity of QSTs is established, and inter-examiner comparisons are favorable, including comparison of paramedical personnel. Different sensory modalities such as vibration and thermal sensations can be evaluated, corresponding to different nerve-fiber populations. The testing is noninvasive and well-tolerated, and the quantitative results allow parametric statistical analyses and detection of subtle group differences in controlled clinical trials. QSTs also are used in monitoring longitudinal change in sensation over time. In some comparisons, such as the prospective study of pyridoxine neurotoxicity, thermal changes detected by QSTs occurred earlier and were more severe than changes in vibration sensation or changes in sural nerve action-potential amplitude *(119)*. In contrast, other comparisons of QST and NCS results, as in the evaluation of diabetic polyneuropathy, found QSTs complimentary but ancillary to NCSs, with the sural nerve recording being the best single predictor of mild neuropathy *(120)*. Disadvantages of QSTs include the time required to perform such studies; the need for patient cooperation; sensitivity to subtle motivational factors, learning and age-effects; and the inability to distinguish central from peripheral disorders *(121,122)*.

5.4.2. Posturography

Static posturography records minute swaying of the body during quiet stance, providing a quantitative measure of postural movement. The static platform senses vertical and shear forces exerted by the feet. The measures allow calculation of the amplitude and rate of sway. Dynamic posturography uses the same technique to record sway in response to perturbation of the platform, often combined with visual stimuli. The most common application is in the evaluation of patients with suspected vestibular disorders. The AAN Therapeutics and Technology Assessment Subcommittee evaluated the clinical utility of posturography *(123)*. In their review, specificity was found to be poor and information regarding test sensitivity or the importance of patterns of abnormality reported was limited. In addition, results are dependent on subject cooperation in maintaining a stable posture. Small volitional shifts in posture dramatically influence the test results, reducing test objectivity. In a cooperative, motivated subject, test results are repeatable. However, posturography is not useful in localizing lesions in the nervous system, nor does it establish a specific diagnosis *(123)*.The subcommittee expressed doubt that posturography will become an efficacious diagnostic test.

6. ESTABLISHING CAUSATION

Establishing the cause of many clinical problems is difficult, and many common neurologic disorders are idiopathic and of unknown etiology. For the most part, it is difficult to establish the etiology of a neurotoxic disorder because there is no one specific presentation. There are, however, several characteristic presentations that suggest the possibility of a toxic cause for the neurologic presentation. Like any clinical diagnosis, the initial clue in suspecting a toxic etiology may be recognition of a cardinal systemic feature suggesting exposure to a specific toxin. This recognition usually stems from a high level of suspicion after eliminating other competing causes. Suffice it to say that one of the fundamental principles of pharmacology and toxicology is that exposure to any neurotoxic substance produces a characteristic syndrome or pattern of neurologic effects, not a random collection of disparate signs. Only rarely, however, are clinical findings so characteristic as to suggest a specific disorder. Occasionally the results of a laboratory test will suggest the cause of a neurotoxic problem. Occasionally a toxic etiology is proposed because no immediate etiology is apparent (as in probable "toxic-metabolic" neuropathy). Unfortunately, there is no guarantee that the only cause that can be thought of is the explanation for the patient's problem. The patient with a neurologic disorder of uncertain cause understandably searches for any possible explanation for their problem. Exposure to potential neurotoxins occurs frequently, and a neurotoxic explanation for a given problem sometimes becomes self evident. Nevertheless, association is only one of several criteria used to identify a cause-effect relationship between a potential toxin and a neurologic disorder.

Table 9
Questions Useful in Establishing a Toxic Etiology

Appropriate timing of exposure and signs?
High relative risk based on epidemiology studies or case reports?
Biologically plausible?
Dose-response relationship?
Removal from exposure modifies effect?
Existence of animal model?
Consistency among studies conducted at different times and in different settings?
Relative specificity of cause-effect?
Evidence of analogous problems caused by similar agents?
Other causes eliminated?

Clinical medicine is based on the scientific method of hypothesis generation and testing, and most clinicians apply general scientific principles in the formulation of any differential diagnosis without giving thought to the process. Although it is difficult to establish the etiology of some neurotoxic disorders, there are criteria useful in establishing etiology. The cause or etiology of a problem is commonly inferred by addressing a series of questions sometimes referred to as the Bradford Hill criteria *(124)*. This process probably has its most direct application to infectious diseases, but it is an exercise that clinicians use daily in identifying any number of vascular, metabolic, infectious, neoplastic, or toxic etiologies. Table 9 lists several of the questions important in determining whether a specific toxin is capable of causing toxic neuropathy, as modified from those first outlined by Sir Austin Bradford Hill *(124)*. These questions are used to distinguish causation from association. In the appropriate clinical setting, specific laboratory tests may be useful in establishing an increased body burden of a potential neurotoxin or identifying characteristic pathologic features of toxic exposure.

The most directly relevant of the Bradford Hill criteria used to establish a neurotoxic etiology are the presence of an appropriate exposure, biologic plausibility, and elimination of competing causes. Although a difficult diagnostic step is recognizing the potential relationship of a toxic exposure and the neurologic disorder, a common diagnostic error is failure to adequately address competing causes. The term "consistent with" is frequently used to link a particular finding to a toxic etiology, without recognizing or acknowledging that the neurologic findings are "consistent with" numerous other etiologies. For example, a patient with excessive alcohol exposure who develops a pure sensory neuropathy with stocking-glove sensory loss, areflexia, and absent sensory nerve-action potentials may have an alcohol-associated sensory neuropathy. But a clinically indistinguishable neuropathy occurs in association with Sjogren's syndrome; neoplasm (paraneoplastic syndrome); hereditary sensory neuropathy; Friedreich's ataxia; human immunodeficiency virus; idiopathic sensory ganglionitis; nutritional disorders (e.g., vitamin E deficiency); the Fisher variant of Guillain-Barre syndrome; and numerous PNS toxins including Vacor, cisplatin, metronidazole, pyridoxine, thalidomide, and thallium *(55,56)*.

Errors of exclusion or reliance on isolated abnormalities as indicative of a disease process are diagnostic errors frequently observed in trainees or inexperienced clinicians. The presence of these errors seems particularly true with respect to the evaluation of suspected neurotoxic disorders. This may be because the cause is thought to be established before the clinical syndrome is evaluated, for example when the patient is evaluated after reporting potential neurotoxic exposure. These errors are more frequent when clinicians are asked to address clinical problems outside of their specialty. For example, a neurologist who incidentally identifies a cardiac dysrhythmia in a patient with toxic exposure is more likely to associate a toxic cause to the problem than an experienced cardiologist who might recognize a normal physiologic variant. In the presence of nonspecific complaints or unexplained findings and a known exposure, the diagnostic reasoning sometimes seems based on incomplete knowledge and can be summarized as follows: "Since I cannot think of any other explanation, the one possible explanation I can think of must explain the neurologic findings." Obviously, failure to recognize the numerous items typically included in the differential diagnosis of progressive cerebellar ataxia does not exclude them from consideration. A physician who is not familiar with familial spinocerebellar degeneration is not going to make the diagnosis. For relatively rare disorders, diagnostic uncertainty is common, and such uncertainty is the accepted reason for referral to a specialist.

The dose of any substance to which a patient is exposed is an important concept. It is well-established that certain doses to virtually any substance (e.g., oxygen, water, aspirin, vitamin B_6, etc.) may be harmless, whereas increased doses may elicit profound, long-lasting, and even irreversible changes. Duration of exposure is another key consideration in determining whether a particular concentration of a substance will be neurotoxic. Clinical evaluations frequently fail to address dose, assuming that exposure to any amount of a neurotoxin is sufficient to fulfill the criterion related to exposure.

The first step in establishing causation is to demonstrate that there is evidence of a clinically significant neurologic impairment. As described, this requires documentation of appropriate neurologic signs, usually with imaging or electrophysiologic confirmation. The pattern of neurologic abnormality must be considered, and the mere presence of an isolated sign cannot be used as an indication of neurologic damage caused by neurotoxic exposure. This includes reliance on vague abnormalities on conventional neurologic testing such as increased sway on standing with the eyes closed without breaking stance, difficulty hopping, patchy sensory loss, or demonstration of isolated atavistic reflexes. As described previously, the inherent redundancy in the neurologic examination provides substantial opportunity to corroborate any individual findings. Maintaining balance with the eyes closed is one measure of large nerve fiber-sensory function and abnormal results are corroborated by tests of sensation (touch, vibration, and joint-position sensation) and evaluation of muscle-stretch reflexes. Solitary "abnormalities" on neurologic examination are rarely of clinical importance as isolated findings.

The temporal profile of the neurologic problem and the type and rate of progression are important concepts not addressed in the Bradford Hill criteria. The most obvious exposure criterion is addressed in the criteria, namely, the problem can not precede exposure. For most neurotoxic syndromes, late progression following an isolated acute exposure in the absence of an acute response is unusual. In general, even delayed responses are measured in terms of days or weeks, not months or years. While isolated exceptions exist, progressive neurologic disorders are the exception, not the rule. Most neurotoxic disorders resolve or improve after removal from exposure, unless the exposure is exceptionally large and the initial neurologic impairment is particularly severe. This is particularly true of the PNS, but even severe CNS injuries such as those associated with cerebral hypoxia demonstrate change and improvement over time. Very severe forms of metabolic encephalopathy such as those associated with hepatic failure, reverse after the metabolic abnormality is corrected. Therefore, progression of any neurologic syndrome following removal from exposure should stimulate search for an alternate explanation to toxic exposure. On rare occasions, inadvertent re-exposure to a purported neurotoxin after resolution of a neurologic disorder provides information important is associating the substance with or excluding it from consideration as the possible cause of the neurologic disorder.

7. NEUROLOGIC TESTING IN GROUP COMPARISONS

The neurologic examination has its primary application in individual patient evaluations, and most of the tests described are used conventionally in the evaluation of patients with suspected neurologic disorders. Unfortunately, few neurologic signs or test abnormalities are specific for a neurotoxic impairment, and therefore the evaluation cannot directly identify a neurotoxic disorder. Neurologic tests occasionally are applied to groups of individuals. This application may be less familiar to the clinical neurologist, and, in this setting, understanding the numerous forms of unintentional bias becomes important in interpreting any identified group differences.

Quantitative neurologic tests such as NCSs play an important role in clinical pharmacological studies *(19,60)*. Electrophysiologic measures frequently are used to fulfill entry criteria and identify appropriate candidates for inclusion in the study. In addition, the quantitative nature of many neurologic tests makes them appropriate end-point measures. In their most common application, electrophysiologic measures are used to evaluate the efficacy of a specific treatment in prospective, randomized cohort studies. For example, the Diabetic Care and Complication Trial (DCCT) compared intensive diabetic therapy to conventional diabetic care *(125)*. Significant nerve conduction differences were observed between the treatment groups, all favoring better performance (e.g., faster conduction) in the intensive therapy group. Nonparametric multivariate tests of the NCS measures demonstrated a strong effect in favor of intensive treatment and established that the electrophysiological abnormalities associated with diabetic neuropathy are delayed or prevented by intensive treatment. NCSs were among the most sensitive measures of efficacy relative to other measures, but the results from clinical examinations supported the positive NCS findings. Prospective cohort studies have the advantage of using the patient as his or her own control, thereby minimizing extraneous effects, including inadvertent selection bias. Cohort and case-control studies are the only studies able to establish a direct cause-effect relation, and cohort studies are the foundation for evaluation therapeutic agents.

In another use, electrophysiologic measures are occasionally monitored in pharmaceutical trials to identify suspected or unsuspected neurotoxicity of the study medication. For example, sensory nerve-conduction studies are used to monitor patients receiving cisplatin, a chemotherapeutic medication known to be neurotoxic *(126,127)*. Repetitive motor nerve-stimulation studies and occasionally SFEMG are used to detect impaired neuromuscular transmission among patients receiving penicillamine because of the myasthenia gravis-like syndrome associated with this medication *(102)*. In both examples, the neurotoxicity of each agent is well-established. In contrast, nerve-conduction studies are used in some pharmaceutical studies to identify potential peripheral neurotoxicity even when suspicion of such toxicity is low *(128)*.

Electrophysiologic measures also have been used to evaluated subjects exposed to occupational or environmental neurotoxins. Unlike the pharmaceutical cohort studies, most environmental or occupational studies make cross-sectional comparisons between the group of interest and an unexposed or historical control group. The major limitation of cross-sectional studies is inherent selection bias that is difficult to identify or control, and many unsuspected factors potentially influence the test results. For this reason, cross-sectional studies are considered hypothesis generating, incapable of establishing the cause of any identified group differences. This contrasts to the hypothesis testing capability of cohort or case-control studies. Cross-sectional studies, while not directly able to establish cause-effect relationships, often are used to demonstrate dose-response relationships, an important part of any evaluation. In addition, a negative cross-sectional study is useful in establishing that the group of interest has not experienced adverse exposure-related effects.

As described, selection bias is an important problem in cross-sectional studies. An example of possible, inadvertent selection bias follows. An evaluation of 138 chloralkali workers with occupational exposure to elemental mercury was conducted in the 1980s using electrodiagnostic and clinical evaluations to document neurologic impairment *(129)*. This cross-sectional study was designed so that examiners were masked to mercury exposure levels and workers were not told of the specific study question. Workers were randomly selected from those eligible to participate in an effort to minimize selection bias. The evaluation identified abnormalities suggestive of a mild, asymptomatic neuropathy among exposed workers, including electrodiagnostic evidence of a mild sensorimotor polyneuropathy. Of the 138 workers, 18 were found to have mild clinically evident neuropathy. When the 18 were compared to the remaining 120 workers, the workers with mild yet clinically evident neuropathy demonstrated significantly elevated urine mercury indices, prolonged distal latencies, and reduced sensory amplitudes. Further comparison of NCS results for all workers to historical control data matched by sex and age demonstrated many significant differences, all favoring poorer performance in the mercury-exposed workers. Important findings included lower median and ulnar sensory amplitudes and prolonged distal latencies in the worker population compared to the historical control group. Sural amplitudes were only lower for those workers with clinically evident neuropathy. This finding was surprising because sural NCSs are generally considered a more sensitive indicator of sensory neuropathy than upper extremity sensory NCSs.

Multiple linear regression analysis of the clinical and electrodiagnostic measures vs urine mercury indexes demonstrated several significant correlations of the clinical grading of sensory loss and the ulnar and median sensory latencies with mercury indexes. These differences persisted even with age, height, weight accounted for in the analyses. The findings were interpreted to identify a toxic neuropathy associated with mercury exposure. An alternative explanation was that the reduced sensory amplitudes could have been explained by hand size, because the manual laborers studied were heavier and probably had larger hands than unexposed workers (hand size was not measured). This argument did not appear to explain the longer latencies, however. Although the relationship between mercury exposure and weight was not explained, it was hypothesized that larger individuals were more likely to work as manual laborers in the exposed areas, and that larger workers might conceivably accumulate greater amounts of mercury, producing increased toxicity.

It now is established that many anthropometric factors, including height, weight, body mass index (BMI), and finger circumference account for substantial variability in clinical and electrodiagnostic measures *(37,37,93,130)*. The relationship with finger size is clear, with large fingers dispersing the fixed number of receptors and with increasing finger diameter producing a decreased sensory amplitude because the recording electrode is separated farther from the digital nerves compared to smaller finger size *(37,131)*. The relationships between other variables such as BMI and sensory latencies are not as intuitively obvious. Nevertheless, given this new information, at least some of the clinical and electrodiagnostic results obtained for the chlor-alkali workers may have reflected differences in BMI, not mercury exposure. In retrospect, "normal" values for unexposed workers matched for age and BMI are comparable to those reported for exposed workers in the original manuscript, indicating that mercury exposure probably did not explain all of the electrodiagnostic findings *(92,132)*. The relationship between mercury exposure and BMI that was identified was unsuspected and unappreciated as important. Unfortunately, it produced an unexpected selection bias that no statistical manipulation is capable of correcting.

8. CONCLUSION

The neurologic examination is one of the most fundamental forms of standardized clinical testing capable of detecting subtle but clinically important abnormalities potentially associated with neurotoxic exposure. The neurologist routinely interprets symptoms and signs in establishing the extent and clinical significance of neurologic dysfunction. Whenever possible, the neurologist also is responsible for defining the etiology of a specific problem prior to recommending treatment. The iterative process of establishing a neurologic diagnosis includes interpreting results obtained from clinical, laboratory, electrodiagnostic, and imaging studies. During the neurologic evaluation, systemic illnesses producing neurologic abnormalities are often detected, as are normal patterns of physiological or psychological variation that mimic neurologic disease.

When cognitive dysfunction is suspected, the neurologist uses the results of standardized clinical neuropsychological evaluations, performed in consultation with a clinical neuropsychologist. The formal neuropsychological test measures are important in quantifying cognitive impairments and in evaluating nonspecific complaints such as decreased memory or concentration. The neuropsychologic evaluation also may identify altered mood, abnormal anxiety states, motivational factors, and psychopathology. Occasionally, selected psychomotor or psychosensory tests supplement the neurologic and neuropsychologic examinations. These measures are most often used to identify subtle differences between exposed and unexposed populations, particularly when a specific abnormality such as diminished sensation, impaired coordination, or abnormal tremor is suspected. In this context, results obtained in cross-sectional evaluations are subject to selection bias. Few of these specialized measures have had widespread application in standardized form, and their sensitivity and specificity have limited evaluation.

Many of the electrophysiologic tests used to investigate neurologic function are standardized, with widespread application as part of the clinical neurologic evaluation. The PNS is a common target of neurotoxic substances, and the conventional EMG examination is used to evaluate patients with suspected peripheral neuropathy. The sensitivity and specificity of NCSs are established, and these objective measures are independent of patient cooperation or motivation. Other electrodiagnostic studies such as EEG and evoked responses have extensive clinical application, but their application in potential neurotoxic evaluations is less well established.

Standard neuroimaging techniques are most useful in identifying anatomic or structural CNS problems. In clinical neurotoxicology evaluations, imaging studies typically are used to exclude other disorders; they are not screening examinations and their use usually is not justified unless there is a demonstrable neurologic impairment or strong suspicion of a structural defect. SPECT and PET are specialized functional imaging techniques of research interest with uncertain sensitivity or specificity. They have little general application or acceptance for establishing specific diagnoses at present, and no direct role in identifying neurotoxicity.

Identifying individual patient abnormalities differs from identifying exposed vs control group differences. The individual patient evaluation uses standard neurologic test results to develop a differential diagnosis. This preliminary list of possible explanations for the patient's problem is used to determine what additional testing will be helpful in establishing a final diagnosis. The conventional examination also is important in establishing the clinical significance of a specific effect. Group evaluations often include additional quantitative measures important in determining whether any effect can be demonstrated between groups. Group comparisons may be important in establishing dose-response relationships, but cross-sectional studies are sensitive to selection bias and are considered hypothesis generating rather than hypothesis-testing studies. The neurologist's experience in evaluating adverse neurologic effects from pharmaceutical agents is directly applicable to the evaluation of symptomatic or asymptomatic individuals with occupational or environmental exposures to potential neurotoxins. Clinical neurotoxicology is a multidisciplinary effort; the standardized neurologic and neuropsychologic evaluations are the most important tests in defining clinical abnormalities and establishing cause-effect relationships.

ACKNOWLEDGMENT

Supported in part by a DOW Chemical Company Foundation SPHERE (Supporting Public Health and Environmental Research Efforts) Award.

REFERENCES

1. Dejong, R. N. (1979) *The Neurologic Examination*, 4th ed., Harper and Row, New York.
2. Potvin, A. R., Tourtellotte, W. W., Pew, R. W., and Albers, J. W. (1973) Motivation and learning in the quantitative examination of neurological function. *Arch. Phys. Med. Rehabil.* **54,** 432–440.
3. Tourtellotte, W. W. and Syndulko, K. (1989) Quantifying the neurologic examination:

principles, constraints, and opportunities, in *Quantification of Neurologic Deficit* (Munsat, T. L., ed.), Butterworths, Boston, pp. 7–16.

4. Rosenberg, N.L. (1991) *Occupational and Environmental Neurology*. Butterworth-Heinemann, Boston.

5. Feldman, R. G. (1999) Recognizing the chemically exposed person, in *Occupational and Environmental Neurotoxicology*, Lippincott Raven, Philadelphia, pp. 7–12.

6. Langston, J. W., Ballard, P. A., Tetrud, J. W., and Irwin, I. (1984) Chronic parkinsonism in humans due to a product of meperidine-analog synthesis. *Science* **11**, 160–165.

7. Kaufman, L. D., Seidman, R. J., and Gruber, B. L. (1990) L-tryptophan-associated eosinophilic perimyositis, neuritis, and fasciitis. A clinicopathologic and laboratory study of 25 patients. *Medicine* **69**, 187–199.

8. Schaumburg, H., Kaplan, J., Windebank, A., Vick, N., Rasmus, S., Pleasure, D., and Brown, M. J. (1983) Sensory neuropathy from pyridoxine abuse. *N. Engl. J. Med.* **309**, 445–448.

9. Calne, D. B., Eisen, A., and McGeer, E. (1986) Alzheimer's disease, Parkinson's disease, and motoneuron disease: abiotrophic interaction between aging and environment? *Lancet* **2**, 1067–1070.

10. Taubes, G. (1995) Epidemiology faces its limits. *Science* **269**, 164–169.

11. Vogel, H.-P. (1992) Influence of additional information on interrater reliability in the neurologic examination. *Neurology* **42**, 2076–2081.

12. McCombe, P. F., Fairbank, J. C. T., Cockersole, B. C., and Pynsent, P. B. (1989) Reproducibity of physical signs in low-back pain. *Spine* **14**, 908–918.

13. Dyck, P.J., Kratz, K.M., Lehman, K.A., Karnes, J.L., Melton, L.J., O'Brien, P.C., et al. (1991) The Rochester Diabetic Neuropathy Study: design, criteria for types of neuropathy, selection bias, and reproducibility of neuropathic tests. *Neurology* **41**, 799–807.

14. Cornblath, D. R., Chaudhry, V., Carter, K., Lee, D., Seysedadr, M., Miernicki, M., and Joh, T. (1999) Total neuropathy score. Validation and reliability study. *Neurology* **53**, 1660–1664.

15. Albers, J. W., Brown, M. B., Sima, A. A. F., and Greene, D. A. for the Tolrestat Study Group for the Early Diabetic Intervention Trial (1996) Nerve conduction measures in mild diabetic neuropathy: the effects of age, sex, type of diabetes, disease duration, and anthropometric factors. *Neurology* **46**, 85–91.

16. Dyck, P. J., Litchy, W. J., Lehman, K. A., Hokanson, J. L., Low, P. A., and O'Brien, P. C. (1995) Variables influencing neuropathic endpoints: the Rochester Diabetic Neuropathy Study of Healthy Subjects. *Neurology* **45**, 1115–1121.

17. Dyck, P. J., Karnes, J. L., O'Brien, P. C., Litchy, W. J., Low, P. A., and Melton, L. J. (1992) The Rochester Diabetic Neuropathy Study: reassessment of tests and criteria for diagnosis and staged severity. *Neurology* **42**, 1164–1170.

18. Abou-Donia, M. B. and Lapadula, D. M. (1990) Mechanisms of organophosphorus esterinduced delayed neurotoxicity: Type I and type II. *Pharmacol. Toxicol.* **30**, 405–440.

19. Potvin, A. R., Tourtellotte, W. W., and Potvin, J. H. (1985) *Quantitative Examination of Neurologic Functions. Vol. I: Scientific Basis and Design of Instrumented Tests; Vol. II: Methodology for Test and Patient Assessments and Design of a Computer-Automated System.* CRC Press, Boca Raton, FL.

20. Albers, J. W. (1988) Standardized neurological testing in neurotoxicology studies, in *Proceedings of the Third International Symposium on Neurobehavioral Methods in Occupational and Environmental Health* (Anger, W. K., Durao, A., Johnson, B. L., and Xintaras, C., eds.), Pan American Health Organization, Washington, DC, pp. 1–18.

21. Munsat, T. L. (1989) *Quantification of Neurologic Deficit*. Butterworths, Boston.

22. Miller, A. S., Willard, V., Kline, K., Tarpley, S., Guillotte, J., Lawler, F. H., and Pendell, G. M. (1998) Absence of longitudinal changes in rheumatologic parameters after silicone breast implantation: a prospective 13-year study. *Plastic Recon. Surg.* **102**, 2299–2303.

23. Eddy, D. M. and Clanton, C. H. (1982) The art of diagnosis. Solving the clinicopathological exercise. *N. Engl. J. Med.* **306**, 1263–1268.

24. Kassirer, J. P. (1992) Clinical problem-solving: a new feature in the Journal. *N. Engl. J. Med.* **326**, 60–61.

25. Pauker, S. G. and Kopelman, R. I. (1992) Clinical problem-solving. Trapped by an incidental finding. *N. Engl. J. Med.* **326**, 40–43.

26. Mayo Clinic and Mayo Foundation (1981) *Clinical Examinations in Neurology*, 5th ed. W.B. Saunders, Philadelphia.

27. Gelb, D. J. (1995) *Introduction to Clinical Neurology*. Butterworth-Heinemann, Boston.

28. Gilman, S. (1999) *Clinical Examination of the Nervous System*, McGraw-Hill, New York.

29. Daube, J. R., Westmorland, B., Sandok, B. A., and Reagan, T. (1986) *Medical Neurosciences. An Appropach to Anatomy, Pathology, and Physiology by Systems and Levels*, 2nd ed. Little, Brown and Co., Boston.

30. Stang, P. E., Yanagihara, T., Swanson, J. W., and Beard, C. M. (1992) Incidence of migraine headache: a population-based study in Olmsted County, Minnesota. *Neurology* **42**, 1657–1662.

31. McFarland, H. F. and Dhib Jalbut, S. (1989) Multiple sclerosis: possible immunological mechanisms. *Clin. Immunol. Immunopathol.* **50**, S96–S105.

32. Scully, R. E. (1984) Case records of MGH. *N. Engl. J. Med.* **311**, 1170–1177.

33. Donofrio, P. D., Wilbourn, A. J., Albers, J. W., Rogers, L., Salanga, V., and Greenberg, H. S. (1987) Acute arsenic intoxication presenting as Guillain-Barre-like syndrome. *Muscle Nerve* **10**, 114–120.

34. Lerman, B. B., Ali, N., and Green, D. (1980) Megaloblastic, dyserythropoietic anemia following arsenic ingestion. *Ann. Clin. Lab. Sci.* **10**, 515–517.

35. Victor, M. (1989) Neurologic disorders due to alcoholism and malnutrition, in *Clinical Neurology* (Joynt, R. J., ed.), J.B. Lippincott, Philadelphia, pp. 1–94.

36. Jacobs, L. and Gossman, D. (1980) Three primitive reflexes in normal adults. *Neurology* **30**, 184–188.

37. Stetson, D. S., Albers, J. W., Silverstein, B. A., and Wolfe, R. A. (1992) Effects of age, sex, and anthropometric factors on nerve conduction measures. *Muscle Nerve* **15**, 1095–1104.

38. Albers, J. W., Kallenbach, L. R., Fine, L. J., Langolf, G. D., Wolfe, R. A., Donofrio, P. D., et al. (1988) Neurological abnormalities associated with remote occupational elemental mercury exposure. *Ann. Neurol.* **24**, 651–659.

39. Schaumburg, H. H., Kaplan, J., Windebank, A. J., Vick, N., Rasmus, S., Pleasure, D., and Brown, M. J. (1983) Sensory neuropathy from pyridoxine abuse: a new megavitamin syndrome. *N. Engl. J. Med.* **309**, 445–448.

40. Albin, R. L., Albers, J. W., Greenberg, H. S., Townsend, J. B., Lynn, R. B., Burke, J. M. J., and Alessi, A. G. (1987) Acute sensory neuropathy-neuronopathy from pyridoxine overdose. *Neurology* **37**, 1729–1732.

41. Fraser, C. L. and Arieff, A. I. (1985) Hepatic encephalopathy. *N. Engl. J. Med.* **313**, 865–873.

42. Victor, M., Adams, R. D., and Collins, G. H. (1989) *The Wernicke-Korsakoff Syndrome and Related Neurologic Disorders Due to Alcholism and Malnutrition*. Contemporary Neurology Series, vol. 3, F.A. Davis, Philadelphia.

43. Reuler, J. B., Girard, D. E., and Cooney, T. G. (1985) Wernicke's encephalopathy. *N. Engl. J. Med.* **312**, 1035–1039.

44. Scully, R. E., Mark, E. J., and McNeely, B. U. (1986) Case records of the Massachusetts General Hospital. Case 33–1986. *N. Engl. J. Med.* **315**, 503–508.

45. Arlien-Soborg, P., Bruhn, P., Gyldensted, C., and Melgaard, B. (1979) Chronic painters' syndrome. Chronic toxic encephalopathy in house painters. *Acta Neurol, Scand.* **60**, 149–156.

46. Report of the Therapeutics and Technology Subcommittee of the American Academy of Neurology, (1996) Assessment: neuropsychological testing in adults. Considerations for neurologists. *Neurology* **47,** 592–599.

47. Albers, J. W., Wald, J. J., Werner, R. A., Franzblau, A., and Berent, S. (1999) Absence of polyneuropathy among workers previously diagnosed with solvent-induced toxic encephalopathy. *J. Occup. Environ. Med.* **41,** 500–509.

48. Albers, J. W., Wald, J. J., Garabrant, D. H., Trask, C. L., and Berent, S. (2000) Neurologic evaluation of workers previously diagnosed with solvent-induced toxic encephalopathy. *J. Occup. Environ. Med.* **42,** 410–422.

49. Gade, A., Mortensen, L., and Bruhn, P. (1988) "Chronic painter's syndrome." A reanalysis of psychological test data in a group of diagnosed cases, based on comparisons with matched controls. *Acta Neurol. Scand.* **77,** 293–306.

50. Errebo-Knudsen, E. O. and Olsen, F. (1987) Solvents and the brain: explanation of the discrepancy between the number of toxic encephalopathy reported (and compensated) in Denmark and other countries [letter]. *Br. J. Indust. Med.* **44,** 71–72.

51. Errebo-Knudsen, E. O. and Olsen, F. (1986) Organic solvents and presenile dementia (the painters' syndrome). A review of the Danish literature. *Sci. Total Environ.* **48,** 45–67.

52. Maizlish, N. A., Langolf, G. D., Whitehead, L. W., Fine, L. J., Albers, J. W., Goldberg, J., and Smith, P. (1985) Behavioural evaluation of workers exposed to mixtures of organic solvents. *Br. J. Indust. Med.* **42,** 579–590.

53. Bolla, K. I., Schwartz, B. S., Agnew, J., Ford, P. D., and Bleecker, M. L. (1990) Subclinical neuropsychiatric effects of chronic low-level solvent exposure in US paint manufacturers. *J. Occup. Med.* **32(8),** 671–677.

54. Albers, J. W. and Bromberg, M. B. (1995) Chemically induced toxic neuropathy, in *Occupational and Environmental Neurology*, (Rosenberg, N. L., ed.), Butterworth-Heinemann, Boston, pp. 175–233.

55. Donofrio, P. D. and Albers, J. W. (1990) Polyneuropathy: classification by nerve conduction studies and electromyography. *Muscle Nerve* **13,** 889–903.

56. Albers, J. W. (1993) Clinical neurophysiology of generalized polyneuropathy. *J. Clin. Neurophysiol.* **10,** 149–166.

57. Spencer, P. S. and Schaumburg, H. H. (1976) Central peripheral distal axonopathy: the pathology of dying-back polyneuropathies, in *Progress in Neuropathology*, vol. III (Zimmerman, H., ed.), Grune and Grune-Stratton, New York, pp. 253–250.

58. Dyck, P. J. (1982) Current concepts in neurology. The causes, classification, and treatment of peripheral neuropathy. *N. Engl. J. Med.* **307,** 283–286.

59. Sterman, A. B. (1985) Toxic neuropathy (editorial). *Mayo Clin. Proc.* **60,** 59–61.

60. Albers, J. W. (1990) Standardized neurological testing in neurotoxicology studies, in *Advances in Neurobehavioral Toxicology: Applications in Environmental and Occupational Health* (Johnson, B. L., ed.), Lewis Publishers, Chelsea, pp. 151–164.

61. Junck, L., Albers, J. W., and Drury, I. J. (2000) Laboratory evaluation, in *Clinical Examination of the Nervous System* (Gilman, S., ed.), McGraw-Hill, New York, pp. 269–303.

62. Eisenberg, H. M., Gary, H. E., Jr., Aldrich, E. F., Saydjari, C., Turner, B., Foulkes, M. A., et al. (1990) Initial CT findings in 753 patients with severe head injury. A report from the NIH Traumatic Coma Data Bank. *J. Neurosurg.* **73,** 688–698.

63. Varnell, R. M., Stimac, G. K., and Fligner, C. L. (1987) CT diagnosis of toxic brain injury in cyanide poisoning: considerations for forensic medicine. *Am. J. Neuroradiol.* **8,** 1063–1066.

64. Tippin, J., Adams, H. P., Jr., and Smoker, W. R. (1984) Early computed tomographic abnormalities following profound cerebral hypoxia. *Arch. Neurol.* **41,** 1098–1100.

65. Kinkel, W. R., Jacobs, L.. and Kinkel, P. R. (1980) Gray matter enhancement: a computerized tomographic sign of cerebral hypoxia. *Neurology* **30,** 810–819.

66. D'Arceuil, H. E., de Crespigny, A. J., Rother, J., Seri, S., Moseley, M. E., Stevenson, D. K., and Rhine, W. (1998) Diffusion and perfusion magnetic resonance imaging of the evolution of hypoxic ischemic encephalopathy in the neonatal rabbit. *J. Mag. Res. Imag.* **8,** 820–828.

67. van der Knaap, M. S., Jakobs, C., and Valk, J. (1996) Magnetic resonance imaging in lactic acidosis. *J. Inher. Metab Dis.* **19,** 535–547.

68. Latchaw, R. E. and Truwit, C. E. (1995) Imaging of perinatal hypoxic-ischemic brain injury. *Sem. Ped Neurol.* **2,** 72–89.

69. American Academy of Neurology (1991) SPECT and neurosonology qualifications approved. *Neurology* **41,** 13A.

70. American Academy of Neurology (1991) Assessment: positron emission tomography. *Neurology* **41,** 163–167.

71. Calne, D. B. and Snow, B. J. (1993) PET imaging in Parkinsonism. *Adv. Neurol.* **60,** 484–487.

72. Society of Nuclear Brain Imaging Council (1996) Ethical clinical practice of functional brain imaging. *J. Nucl. Med.* **37,** 1256–1259.

73. Markand, O. N. (1984) Electroencephalography in diffuse encephalopathies. *J. Clin. Neurophysiol.* **1,** 357–407.

74. Aminoff, M. J. and Albers, J. W. (1999) Electrophysiologic techniques in the evaluation of patients with suspected neurotoxic disorders, in *Electrodiagnosis in Clinical Neurology* (Aminoff, M. J., ed.), Churchill Livingstone, New York, pp. 721–734.

75. Nuwer, M. (1997) Assessment of digital EEG, quantitative EEG, and EEG brain mapping: report of the American Academy of Neurology and the American Clinical Neurophysiology Society. *Neurology* **49,** 277–292.

76. American Psychiatry Association (1991) Quantitative electroencephalography: a report on the present state of computerized EEG technology. American Psychiatry Association Task Force on Quantitative Electrophysiological Assessment. *Am. J. Psychiatry* **148,** 961–964.

77. Assessment: EEG brain mapping. (1989) Report of the American Academy of Neurology Therapeutics and Technology Assessment Committee. *Neurology* **39,** 1100–1101.

78. Arezzo, J. C., Simson, R., and Brennan, N. E. (1985) Evoked potentials in the assessment of neurotoxicity in humans. *Neurobehav. Toxicol. Teratol.* **7,** 299–304.

79. Rosenberg, N. L., Spitz, M. C., Filley, C. M., Davis, K. A., and Schaumburg, H. H. (1988) Central nervous system effects of chronic toluene abuse—clinical, brainstem evoked response and magnetic resonance imaging studies. *Neurotoxicol. Teratol.* **10,** 489–495.

80. Matsumoto, J. Y. (1996) Movement-related potentials and event-related potentials, in *Clinical Neurophysiology* (Daube, J. R., ed.), FA Davis, Philadelphia, pp. 141–144.

81. Polich, J., Moore, A. P., and Wiederhold, M. D. (1995) P300 assessment of chronic fatigue syndrome. *J. Clin. Neurophysiol.* **12,** 186–191.

82. Geisler, M. W. and Polich, J. (1992) P300 and individual differences: morning/evening activity preference, food, and time-of-day. *Psychophysiology* **29,** 86–94.

83. Small, G. W. and Borus, J. F. (1983) Outbreak of illness in a school chorus. Toxic poisoning or mass hysteria? *N. Engl. J. Med.* **308,** 632–635.

84. Sanin, L. C., Kronenberg, M. F., and Stetkarova, I. (1993) Potentiation of the R Component of blink reflex by anticipation (abstr). *Neurology* **43,** A289–A290.

85. American Association of Electrodiagnostic Medicine (1992) Guidelines in electrodiagnostic medicine. *Muscle Nerve* **15,** 229–253.

86. Dyck, P. J. (1990) Invited review: limitations in predicting pathologic abnormality of nerves from the EMG examination. *Muscle Nerve* **13,** 371–375.

87. American Association of Electrodiagnostic Medicine (1997) Proposed policy for electrodiagnostic medicine. AAEM, Rochester, MN.

88. Chaudhry, V., Cornblath, D. R., and Mellits, E. D. (1991) Inter- and intra-examiner reliability of nerve conduction measurements in normal subjects. *Ann. Neurol.* **30,** 841–843.

89. Campbell, W. W. and Robinson, L. R. (1993) Deriving reference values in electrodiagnostic medicine. *Muscle Nerve* **16**, 424–428.

90. Denys, E. H. (1991) The influence of temperature in clinical electrophysiology. *Muscle Nerve* **14**, 795–811.

91. Swift, T. R., Ward, L. C., and Soudmand, R. (1981) Height determines nerve conduction velocity in the legs. *Neurology* **31(Part II)**, 66.

92. Stetson, D. S., Silverstein, B. A., Keyserling, W. M., Wolfe, R. A., and Albers, J. W. (1993) Median sensory distal amplitude and latency: comparisons between nonexposed managerial/professional employees and industrial workers. *Am. J. Ind. Med.* **24**, 175–189.

93. Robinson, L. R., Rubner, D. E., Wahl, P. W., Fujimoto, W. Y., and Stolov, W. C. (1993) Influences of height and gender on normal nerve conduction studies. *Arch. Phys. Med. Rehabil.* **74**, 1134–1138.

94. Bromberg, M. B. (1991) Comparison of electrodignostic criteria for primary demyelination in chronic polyneuropathy. *Muscle Nerve* **14**, 968–976.

95. Report from an Ad Hoc Subcommittee of the American Academy of Neurology AIDS Task Force (1991) Research criteria for diagnosis of chronic inflammatory demyelinating polyneuropathy (CIDP). *Neurology* **41**, 617–618.

96. Lewis, R. A. and Sumner, A. J. (1982) Electrodiagnostic distinctions between chronic familial and acquired demyelinative neuropathies. *Neurology* **32**, 592–596.

97. Ozdemir, C. and Young, R. R. (1976) The results to be expected from electrical testing in the diagnosis of myasthenia gravis. *Ann. NY Acad. Sci.* **274**, 203–225.

98. Albers, J. W. and Leonard, J. A.,Jr. (1992) Nerve conduction studies and electromyography, in *Neurosurgery: The Scientific Basis of Clinical Practice* (Crockard, A., Hayward, R., and Hoff, J. T., eds.), Blackwell Scientific Publications Ltd., Oxford, UK, pp. 735–757.

99. Massey, J. M. (1990) Electromyography in disorders of neuromuscular transmission. *Semin. Neurol.* **10**, 6–11.

100. Namba, T., Nolte, C. T., Jackrel, J., and Grob, D. (1971) Poisoning due to organophosphate insecticides. Acute and chronic manifestations. *Am. J. Med.* **50**, 475–492.

101. Kinnby, B., Konsberg, R., and Larsson, A. (1988) Immunogenic potential of some mercury compounds in experimental contact allergy of the rat oral mucosa. *Scand. J. Dent. Res.* **96**, 60–68.

102. Albers, J. W., Hodach, R. J., Kimmel, D. W., and Treacy, W. L. (1980) Penicillamine-associated myasthenia gravis. *Neurology* **30**, 1246–1250.

103. Cherington, M. (1998) Clinical spectrum of botulism. *Muscle Nerve* **21**, 701–710.

104. Albers, J. W. and Wald, J. J. (1997) Neuroanesthesia and neuromuscular diseases, in *Textbook of Neuroanesthesia with Neurosurgical and Neuroscience Perspectives* (Albin, M. S., ed.), McGraw-Hill, New York, pp. 453–499.

105. Lingle, C. J. and Steinbach, J. H. (1988) Neuromuscular blocking agents. *Int. Anesthesiol. Clin.* 26, 288–301.

106. Goetz, C. G. and Cohen, M. M. (1990) Neurotoxic agents, in *Clinical Neurology*, vol. 2 (Baker, A. B. and Baker, L. H., eds.), J.B. Lippincott Co., Philadelphia, p. 9.

107. Stalberg, E., Ekstedt, J., and Broman, A. (1974) Neuromuscular transmission in myasthenia gravis studied with single fibre electromyography. *J. Neurol. Neurosurg. Psychiatry* **37**, 540–547.

108. Sanders, D. B. and Stalberg, E. V. (1996) AAEM Minimongraph #25: single-fiber electromyography. *Muscle Nerve* **19**, 1069–1083.

109. Shahani, B. T., Halperin, J. J., Bolu, P., and Cohen, J. (1984) Sympathetic skin responses—a method of assessing unmyelinated axon dysfunction in peripheral neuropathies. *J. Neurol. Neurosurg. Psychiatry* **47**, 536–542.

110. Troy, J. L. (1991) Eosinophilia-myalgia syndrome. *Mayo Clin. Proc.* **66**, 535–538.

111. Kamb, M. L., Murphy, J. J., Jones, J. L., Caston, J. C., Nederlof, K., Horney, L. F., et al. (1992) Eosinophilia-myalgia syndrome in L-tryptophan-exposed patients. *JAMA* **267**, 77–82.

112. Winkelmann, R. K., Connolly, S. M., Quimby, S. R., Griffing, W. L., and Lie, J. T. (1991) Histopathologic features of the L-tryptophan-related eosinophilia-myalgia (fasciitis) syndrome. *Mayo Clin. Proc.* **66**, 457–463.

113. Poklis, A. and Saady, J. J. (1990) Arsenic poisoning: acute or chronic? Suicide or murder? *Am. J. Forensic Med. Pathol.* **11**, 226–232.

114. Windebank, A. J. (1993) Metal neuropathy, in *Peripheral Neuropathy* (Dyck, P. J., Thomas, P. K., Griffin, J. W., Low, P. A., and Poduslo, J. F., eds.), W.B. Saunders, Philadelphia, pp. 1549–1570.

115. Lotti, M. (1991) The pathogenesis of organophosphate polyneuropathy. *Crit. Rev. Toxicol.* **21**, 465–487.

116. Richardson, R. J. (1995) Assessment of the neurotoxic potential of chlorpyrifos relative to other organophosphorus compounds: a critical review of the literature. *J. Toxicol. Environ. Health* **44**, 135–165.

117. Bleecker, M. L. (1986) Vibration perception thresholds in entrapment and toxic neuropathies. *J. Occup. Med.* **28**, 991–994.

118. Bleecker, M. L. (1985) Quantifying sensory loss in peripheral neuropathies. *Neurobehav. Toxicol. Teratol.* **7**, 305–308.

119. Berger, A. R., Schaumburg, H. H., Schroeder, C., Apfel, S., and Reynolds, R. (1992) Dose response, coasting, and differential fiber vulnerability in human toxic neuropathy: a prospective study of pyridoxine neurotoxicity. *Neurology* **42**, 1367–1370.

120. Redmond, J. M. T., McKenna, M. J., Feingold, M., and Ahmad, B. K. (1992) Sensory testing versus nerve conduction velocity in diabetes polyneuropathy. *Muscle Nerve* **15**, 1334–1339.

121. Albers, J. W. and Berent, S. (1999) Neurotoxicology, in *Diagnostic Testing in Neurology* (Evans, R. W., ed.), W.B. Saunders, Philadelphia, pp. 257–271.

122. Albers, J. W. (1999) Toxic neuropathies, in *Continuum: Lifelong Learning in Neurology: Neurotoxicology* (Bleecker, M. L., ed.), Lippincott Williams & Wilkins, Baltimore, MD, pp. 27–50.

123. American Academy of Neurology (1992) Assessment: posturography. Report of the Therapeutics and Technology Assessment Subcommittee, American Academy of Neurology, Minneapolis, MN.

124. Hill, A. B. (1965) The environment and disease: association or causation? *Proc. R. Soc. Med.* **58**, 295–300.

125. Diabetes Control and Complications Trial (DCCT) Research Group (1995) Effect of intensive diabetes treatment on nerve conduction in the Diabetes Control and Complications Trial. *Ann. Neurol.* **38**, 869–880.

126. Daugaard, G. K., Petrera, J., and Trojaborg, W. (1987) Electrophysiological study of the peripheral and central neurotoxic effect of cis-platin. *Acta Neurol. Scand.* **76**, 86–93.

127. Van Der Hoop, R. G., Vecht, C. J., Van Der Burg, M. E. Elderson, A., Boogerd, W., Heimanns, J. J., et al. (1990) Prevention of cisplatinum neurotoxicity with an ACTH(4–9) analogue in patients with ovarian cancer. *N. Engl. J. Med.* **322**, 89–94.

128. Protocol #27, 201-27. ER Squibb and Sons (1988) Efficacy and safety of SQ 31,000 in the treatment of hypercholesterolemia relative to the degree of dietary intervention: neurotoxicity study for Squibb 31,000.

129. Albers, J. W., Cavender, G. F., Levine, S. P., and Langolf, G. D. (1982) Asymptomatic sensorimotor polyneuropathy in workers exposed to elemental mercury. *Neurology* **32**, 1168–1174.

130. Stetson, D. S. (1991) Median and Ulnar Conduction Measures in Control and Industrial Populations: Associations with Ergonomic Risk Factors. PhD Thesis, University of Michigan, Ann Arbor, MI.
131. Bolton, C. F. and Carter, K. M. (1980) Human sensory nerve compound action potential amplitudes: variation with sex and finger circumference. *JNNP* **43,** 925–928.
132. Rivner, M. H., Swift, T. R., Crout, B. O., and Rhodes, K. P. (1990) Toward more rational nerve conduction interpretations: the effect of height. *Muscle Nerve* **13,** 232–239.

21

Human Neuropsychological Testing
and Evaluation

Stanley Berent and Christine L. Trask

1. INTRODUCTION

1.1. Historical Context

Psychology reflects the scientific study of behavior, in human as well as in animal models. From a very early time, people have noticed and have been interested in the concept of individual differences. Aristotle directly commented on this with reference to the idea that intelligence is not equally distributed in all organisms *(1)*. Individual differences more accurately characterize behavior than does commonality. Yet, the availability of this "fact" of behavior to scientific study was debated for hundreds of years. It was not until the nineteenth century that any meaningful scientific method of inquiry was applied to variable behaviors.

Dozens of names can be associated with the history of psychology, names from antiquity as well as more modern times. While it is beyond the scope of this manuscript to review this history in detail, some of these names include individuals known for their work in anatomy, biology, astronomy, medicine, physics, physiology, and other fields as well, or even more so, than in psychology. Some notable names include such eminent scholars as Darwin, Titchner, James, Ebbinghaus, Mill, Herbart, Galton, and others. However, it was Cattell as much as any one, who, building upon the evolutionary viewpoint of Francis Galton, defined the quantitative approach to the systematic study of individual differences *(1)*. In fact, Lewis Terman in his presidential address to the American Psychological Association in 1923 credited Cattell with the first use of the term, "mental test" *(2)*. Besides Cattell, other scholars sought to explain the purpose of testing. For example, Binet and Henri in 1896 first defined "the method of mental tests as the selection of a number of tasks designed to give detailed information on individual differences" *(2)*.

To a large extent, modern psychology can be described as the scientific study of individual differences. The early workers were able to successfully develop approaches to the study of behavior in a manner that met with acceptance by others in the scientific community, furthering our understanding of behavior, allowing for applications to practical problems, and making contributions to science beyond psychology itself. Since

From: Handbook of Neurotoxicology, Vol. 2
Edited by: E. J. Massaro © Humana Press Inc., Totowa, NJ

the mid- to latter-nineteenth century and the early part of the twentieth century continuing to the present, psychologists have built upon these methods and procedures.

From an early period, the method of psychological testing won a place of central importance in the study of individual differences. Together with the methods of experimental science and other endeavors such as medicine, it has become clear that such testing, when applied in prescribed and appropriate ways, can provide an effective tool for the study of behavior and for addressing the many challenges in so doing. This chapter focuses on this approach and the specialized application of these methods called "neuropsychology."

2. THE NEUROPSYCHOLOGICAL APPROACH TO DETECTING CENTRAL NERVOUS SYSTEM DYSFUNCTION

The central nervous system (CNS), and more specifically the brain, regulates most human thoughts, feelings, and actions. It is no surprise, therefore, that stimulation of or damage to the CNS is often reflected in behavioral symptoms. In addition, damage to particular regions of the brain in some instances become associated with particular behavioral sequelae. For example, injury to Broca's area has been shown to result in an expressive aphasia *(3)*. The predictability of these phenomena has allowed science and medicine to approach the problem of studying the brain by "tracing back" from behavior. Because the brain is not easily accessible to direct observation, this approach at times may be the only way to study the functioning CNS.

Aside from allowing for direct inquiry aimed at enhancing our knowledge of brain-behavior relationships, the methods of psychology also provide tools for understanding the meaning of information that comes from other methods used to study the CNS. For example, positron emission tomography (PET), magnetic resonance imaging (MRI), and electroencephalography (EEG) have allowed us to image chemical, metabolic, and other functional and structural aspects of the CNS. However, we do not always understand the relationships between the data derived from these images and underlying brain function. A systematic and objective measurement of behavior can be used to compliment other approaches and to provide practical meaning to these images.

There are challenges to being able to effectively use behavioral information to study the CNS as well. Problems associated with the behavioral approach include decisions about how to objectively and quantitatively measure behavior. One must consider how to use the techniques within a scientific context, to ask scientifically meaningful questions within an acceptable scientific paradigm. Consideration must be given as to the meaningfulness of data derived, drawing on knowledge regarding psychometric theory but also on a wider scientific knowledge base, which includes behavioral and medical theories of disease, normal and abnormal behavior, nosology, and others.

3. THE NEUROPSYCHOLOGICAL EVALUATION

In general, the process of neuropsychological evaluation consists of documenting the existence and nature of an impairment, defining the problem in terms of the nervous system, discovering the etiology if possible, and recommending further evaluation or treatment. There are questions that can be answered through the neuropsychological process and others that can not. In general, the neuropsychologist can deal only with observable events, or those with objective behavioral analogs. A battery of neuropsychological tests typically sample multiple domains of functioning, including: intelligence, academic skills (e.g., reading, spelling, arithmetic), attention, learning and memory, language, visuospatial processing, executive skills, sensory-motor, and emotional.

The first question to be formally asked in this process is usually about the presence or absence of abnormality. To answer this question requires a knowledge of normal and abnormal behavior, as well as the psychometric characteristics of the measure. In order to appropriately select tests and formulate hypotheses, a neuropsychologist often initially collects the patient's subjective report of symptoms from clinical interview or questionnaire. These symptoms, together with results from neuropsychological tests, are examined in relationship to a reference group. In evaluating performance, the problem of individual differences must also be considered. That is, people vary one from another, sometimes substantially, along a continuum for any given behavior. A number of moderator variables have been identified that are important to consider in interpreting neuropsychological test performance, including age, gender, handedness, motivation, education, pre-existing psychological or cognitive disorders, language or cultural differences, and certain medical conditions *(4)*. As will be discussed more fully later in this chapter, the factors leading to individual differences are many and complex. The neuropsychologist must consider these in interpreting his results.

In addition to determining the presence or absence of an impairment, the neuropsychologist is often asked to assess if there has been a decline in functioning in some areas. It helps when effective indices of pre-morbid functioning exist. This can often be obtained from patients' academic records or other past documentation of performance or ability. The overall level of educational attainment may also offer some information, as grade level often yields correlations of about 0.70 with Wechsler Full Scale IQ score *(5)*, although qualitative information, such as the failure of a grade or placement in special education, can significantly alter interpretations *(6)*. At other times some acceptable degree of estimation of base-line functioning can be made on the basis of current examination results. Particular skills, such as reading, have been theorized to be less vulnerable to cognitive disruptions and have been used to estimate premorbid functioning (e.g., Nelson and O'Connell *[7]*), although others have suggested that these tasks may still underestimate intellectual functioning for patients with language-based deficits *(8)*. There have also been attempts to predict premorbid intellectual levels via regression equations on the basis of several demographic characteristics, such as age, sex, race *(9,10)*.

From a practical clinical viewpoint, the suspicion of abnormal behavior is raised whenever there has been some trauma, or even possible trauma, to the CNS. A patient is referred, for example, because they have been exposed to a toxic substance such as a solvent or heavy metal. The referral asks if the patient evidences any behavioral consequence as a result of the exposure. Have they been damaged from a neuropsychological perspective? While in this case the question begins with a possible cause, exposure to a substance, at other times the referral is generated from a change in behavior. To give a clinical example, a person with previously diagnosed mental retardation shows a dramatic change in behavior, becoming aggressive and destructive, whereas before he had been more docile. Does this change in behavior reflect underlying neurologic dysfunction? Both instances reflect common and reasonable questions. In clinical practice, the process in both instances begins with an inquiry into complaints, or symptoms, the patient may be evidencing. Such symptoms are usually bothersome or painful to the individual, or someone close to the person, either because of their nature or because of the stress that results from the concern itself. The patient's symptoms are seen by the neuropsychologist as a problem that deserves professional attention. From a clinical diagnostic viewpoint, however, the patient's complaints alone do not provide the entire story. To understand the individual's clinical picture, it is necessary to determine objective signs that substantiate and more fully elucidate the nature of these symptoms in terms of CNS dysfunction. In approaching this goal, the neuropsychological method employs a careful history and interview of the patient and, at times, others close to the patient, a review of past records that includes the results of others' evaluations and laboratory test results, and, most often, psychometric examination. The use of psychometric testing is almost unique to psychologists and allows the neuropsychologist to systematically obtain a scientifically based, objective and quantitative appraisal of the patient's functioning and to establish signs that may elucidate the patient's clinical status and lead to a definitive diagnosis.

Sometimes, the neuropsychological evaluation begins and ends with only this question about presence of abnormality. If there is a finding of abnormality, a series of further clinical questions are usually addressed. These questions must be asked in ways that are answerable by behavioral measurement. The measurements to be made, and, hence, the specific tests to be employed, are determined by the data needed to answer the question(s). Following the objective documentation of abnormality, some of the most often asked questions include the following:

- What is the specific nature or pattern of the abnormality?
- What behavioral domains are affected?
- What is(are) the level(s) of severity?
- Is the pattern suggestive of acute, subacute, or chronic disorder?
- Is the observed picture progressively worsening, static, or resolving?
- Does the pattern of deficit suggest focal or general neurological involvement?
- To what extent are motivation, depression, and other non-neurological factors involved in the behavior observed?
- What is its functional significance for other aspects of the individual's life?
- What are the implications for diagnosis, treatment, prognosis, etiology?

To summarize the steps in the clinical neuropsychological approach, the response to a referral of a patient with questions about CNS dysfunction, regardless of the suspected cause, begins with an interview and a description of the patient's chief complaints. There will be a review of the patient's medical, psychosocial, occupational, school, and other histories. The psychometric examination will usually follow. Information from the history and interview (symptoms) and the examination (signs) are used to identify and document any abnormality and to formulate diagnostic impressions. Factual historical information (e.g., school performance, employment records, results of past objective testing) should be obtained whenever possible. After all information is reviewed, the neuropsychologist will prepare a written report outlining any recommendations for treatment or additional consultations that might be suggested.

4. BASIC PSYCHOMETRIC CONSIDERATIONS

In the neuropsychological approach to behavioral measurement, the word "test" has special meaning. Although in conversation, many will use this term in too casual a manner, it is actually a technical term that denotes that the instrument referred to has met certain psychometric requirements. The psychometrics of an instrument chiefly refer to its reliability and validity.

4.1. Reliability

The degree to which test scores are free from errors of measurement reflecting imprecision is termed, "reliability" *(11)*. Put another way, reliability is the index of a test's consistency, e.g., consistent results between items in a given administration or between two or more administrations of the same test. Interestingly, the reliability of a test determines the upper limit for the test's validity. In other words, a test that is not reliable can not be valid, although tests that are reliable may not be valid. While the user of a test is not generally required to independently establish a test's reliability, the user should be aware of the extent to which differences between forms or administrations of a given test reflect variations in the measuring device vs changes in the person being measured, e.g., changes in behavior that result from exposure to a chemical, progression of a disease or disorder, or other event affecting the individual's behavior.

It is important to acknowledge that every measurement includes some error. The results of psychological tests are no exception to this rule. This is neither bad nor good but is a fact of measurement that must be recognized, specified, and considered in making conclusions based on the measurement obtained. This error is expressed as the error of measurement and should be specified by the test publisher in the published manual or related material. To give an example, the published error of measurement on a commonly used intelligence test is ± 5 points. Thus, the observed score (k) on any given occasion would actually be $k \pm 5$ (depending on the confidence interval chosen, e.g., ± 3 points at a 68% confidence level). If $k = 100$, then the actual score lies between 95 and 105. This has important implications for the interpretation of test scores. Should a test be administered, for instance, to the same person on two separate occasions, yielding scores of 95 and 100, respectively, in practice the two scores would be considered to be the same. As in any scientific enterprise, conclusions that are based on psychological test findings are probability statements, and this includes the error of measurement. This error score will vary depending on the exactness required in a given instance. Professional convention leads to the use of ± 5 points as in the example given. In order to be 99% accurate, a larger confidence interval (± 13 points) would be required. While less than perfect, these 10–26 point variations compare favorably to other tests used to measure medical and physical aspects of human functioning, such as MRI or PET.

There are a number of subtypes of reliability, and the reliability of a psychological test may be reported as test-retest, alternate form, split-half, and other measures of internal consistency. The reliability of a given test is determined through formal scientific inquiry and is usually represented by correlation analysis. Test-retest reliability is used to establish the stability of a particular test score over time. The time interval between administration of the test may be particularly important in this process. When close together in time, successive administration of a test may lead to artificial inflation

of the test-retest correlation because "practice effects," that is, the effects of test familiarity on subsequent test performance. A practice effect is another variable that must be
considered in interpretation of test results in individual cases as well as in the initial
determination of the test's reliability.

The relationship between performances on alternate forms of a test is also used to
assess the stability of the test's measurement. Interestingly, practice effects can be seen
between alternate forms of a test similarly to that seen in subsequent administrations of
the same test *(12)*. While re-administering too close in time can affect the test score, so
can waiting too long before a subsequent administration of the test. The longer the
interval between test measurements, the more likely there will be intervening variables
to consider in interpreting the test results, e.g., changes in normal development, other
changes in the individual's experience history, and so on. These, of course, can confound the relationship between the two measurements and potentially explain differences in test scores between the two administrations.

Methods for assessing internal consistency include Cronbach's coefficient alpha *(13)*
for tests with items with multiple choice responses (e.g., "always," "sometimes," or
"never") or the Kuder-Richardson formula 20 *(14)* for dichotomously scored items
(e.g., "true/false," "yes/no"). Split-half reliability, which examines the intercorrelations
among all test items and estimates the potential effect of shortening or lengthening the
instrument, is often measured with the Spearman-Brown formula, described by Charles
Spearman and William Brown in 1910 *(15)*. Internal consistency can not be determined for all types of tests. Measures of internal consistency are not meaningful, for
example, on tasks that primarily assess "speed" as opposed to accuracy of response.

Raters are used in the construction of some items to be used in tests and for setting
the standards for test scores. The variability between individual scorers will change as
a function of the complexity of the items being rated. Deciding how to score a complex
drawing on a test such as the Rey-Osterrieth complex figure, for instance, will likely
lead to more variability between raters than will assessing "right" or "wrong" on a task
such as the Halstead Category Test. While the raters may be individuals with a high
degree of sophistication regarding the content areas of the items to be employed, it is
important to establish inter-rater reliability for all subjectively rated criteria.

The reliability of a test is an important but complex issue. Aside from the considerations already mentioned, the reliability of a test instrument can be influenced by other,
extraneous factors. As the length of a test increases, for example, the reliability of the
measurement often increases as well. Reliability can also be influenced by the nature
of the scores obtained, such as the variability in a given type of score being used. It will
also be influenced by any restriction in the possible range of scores. For instance, if the
distribution of scores is restricted in range, the reliability coefficient will be lower than
if the score range is more expansive. Of course, individual factors, such as attempts at
"guessing," "malingering," or variations in the test situation, may also act as confounds
in assessing the reliability of a test.

Anastasi *(12)*, a relatively early and extremely influential worker in this area, suggested using different reliability measurements to parcel out "true" variance in the construct of interest from error of the measuring device by interpreting test-retest
differences as variance due to time, alternate form immediate administration as variance due to content, and alternate form delayed administration as variance due to both

time and content. She also suggested that split-half measurements reflect variance due to content sampling, that KR–20 and Cronbach's coefficient alpha reflect variance due to content sampling and heterogeneity, and that inter-scorer reliability reflects variance due to examiner and style of individual administration. These considerations should be attended to and resolved in the process of test development. The results of such analyses should be published and the adequacy of these analyses considered by the test user when selecting a particular test.

4.2. Validity

Simply stated, validity refers to the extent to which scores from a given test relate to the theoretical construct it is designed to measure. Whereas reliability reflects the consistency or precision of a measure, validity refers to the accuracy of the measure. How well, for example, does a test of anxiety actually measure anxiety? Validity is empirically established during test construction using formal mathematical methods, and information regarding the test's validity should be presented in the manual accompanying the test as well as in published scientific literature. There also are general reference materials that review the technical aspects of commercially available tests, e.g., The *Mental Measurements Yearbook (16)* and *Tests in Print (17)*. Published standards also exist for developing formal tests *(11)*, and these standards reflect the paramount importance placed by the field of psychology on the criterion of validity. Validity, these standards state, determines the "…appropriateness, meaningfulness, and usefulness of the specific inferences made from test scores" *(11)*. The term "validity" is actually complex and can be expressed in several ways.

The simplest form of validity is face validity. This concept refers to the apparent meaningfulness of a test item, or collection of such items. To give an example, the question, "Do you tend to forget things easily?" would reflect good face validity for a test item designed to measure a construct such as "memory." While common-sensical, simple, straightforward, and often a good place to start in test item construction, face validity alone is not sufficient to qualify an item for final inclusion in a formal psychological test.

A face-valid item is a good place to start in selecting test items, but formal statistically based research will be brought into play. Correlation methods are most often used to formally establish a test's actual validity. Through this formal step in the process of test construction, items that informally appear to reflect some underlying construct, e.g., memory, may be found to have minimal statistical relationship to the behavior of interest. Through this statistical process, interestingly, other items that at first appear to be unrelated may prove to be strongly related to the construct.

As an aside, some items with good face validity might be dropped from the final collection of test items even when they are shown to meet more formal validity criteria. As will be discussed several times in this chapter, issues such as response set, bias, motivation, and other aspects of behavior present special challenges in the testing of all living organisms, and this is especially pertinent in human behavioral testing. Items, or tasks to be performed, which carry high face validity, for example, could lead a person to inflate their positive responses to such items, whereas such symptom or deficit inflation might be less likely on tasks with low face validity. These and other extra-test considerations will need to be considered in test construction as well as in the selection of tests for application in a given research or clinical situation.

Another aspect of validity is content validity. Content validity refers to the comprehensiveness and representativeness of the test's content in relation to its intended aspect of behavioral measurement. The test will need to sample behavior, e.g., knowledge, performance, and so on, that is relevant to and representative of its stated purpose. In assessing memory, for example, relevant and representative content might include measures of verbal and visual learning and recall, recognition memory, short- and long-term memory, and the like. What to include is determined by the knowledge bases of relevant fields of study, and during test construction experts from these fields might be asked to generate the specific content areas that should be included. The draft test might be reviewed later to insure that its content is consistent with the experts' understanding of the construct being measured. In contrast to the mathematical requirements for criterion and construct validity to be discussed next, content validity is typically established based on expert judgment.

A test's criterion validity is defined by the strength of the relationship, measured mathematically, between the test and some other, independent criterion. A test's criterion validity may be further differentiated to address the concurrent or predictive aspects of a test. Concurrent validity for a test of reading comprehension, for example, can be determined by mathematically correlating performance on the test with scores on another, perhaps already established and standardly used reading measure that is administered concurrently. This method is widely employed and represents using a comprehensively studied and well established measure as a "gold standard" to establish and document the validity of the new test. This practice is acceptable, and one used commonly by fields other than psychology, but it does necessitate unequivocal scientific proof that the criterion instrument is itself valid. At best, however, a new test which is developed using concurrent validity will remain an approximation of the old, criterion test *(12)*. For this and other reasons, the test developer, as well as the person choosing to use such a test, should ask why the original measure is not sufficient to use. Is there a compelling reason to develop or use the new test? The answer to this question may be "yes," the new test may be shorter, more modern in context, more economical, simpler, or more easy to use, to give a few examples.

Predictive validity is determined by formally correlating the current test score to some future outcome criterion. For instance, measures of intellectual performance may be correlated with future school grades, successful completion of a course of study, or some other observable criterion used to define the construct of intelligence. The measure of a test's criterion validity can never be stronger than the criterion against which it is compared. Given the many nonintellectual factors that affect a person's grades in school, for example, one would not expect to find a perfect relationship between school grades and earlier performance on a test of intellectual ability. A perfect correspondence may not be required in every instance, however, and the test user will need to consider the test's technical aspects such as its predictive validity in making a decision about its use in a given situation.

Typically, a test is designed to measure some specified theoretical construct or aspect of behavior. Consistent with the science underlying the psychometric approach, the construct to be measured must be definable in terms of observables. A few examples of constructs are anxiety, depression, intelligence, and memory. Since these and other behavioral constructs of interest are seldomly observable directly, analogs must be identified that are known to reflect aspects of the target behavior. In this respect, the psychometric approach is similar to many other fields that employ measurement in the service of scientific inquiry. Nuclear medicine, for example, might employ a chemical ligand with characteristics similar to some other chemical of interest but that is not directly accessible for observation. In similar fashion, an emotional state such as "anxiety" may not be observable directly, but aspects of anxiety might be identified that can be observed and that mirror what we think of as "anxiety," e.g., increases in heart rate, changes in skin conductance, and so on. The extent to which a given test is shown to relate to such constructs is termed its "construct validity."

Even though the construct, e.g., anxiety, may be theoretical from a scientific viewpoint, it or its analogue must have clear boundaries and definitions to be used in a psychological test. The extent to which a given test corresponds or fails to correspond to the target construct is assessed by measures of convergent and discriminant validity. That is, the test scores should be shown to be strongly associated with other measures of similar abilities (convergence) and shown to have minimal relationship with extraneous concepts (discrimination). Campbell and Fiske *(18)* introduced the multi-trait/multi-method, designed to examine these patterns of relationships in test construction. Without going into great detail, this method involves examining two or more traits or behaviors with two or more methods (e.g., self-report inventory, observation ratings, test performance). The method results in a matrix containing four types of correlation coefficients: monotrait-monomethod, monotrait-heteromethod, heterotrait-monomethod, and heterotrait-heteromethod. Convergent validity is established through this procedure when measurements of the same trait have a high correlation (e.g., high monotrait-heteromethod coefficients), regardless of the type of method used. Divergent validity is established when a low correlation (e.g., low heterotrait-monomethod and low heterotrait-heteromethod coefficients) is found between different traits, even when employing the same method of measurement.

Discriminant and convergent validity may also be discussed in terms of a test's sensitivity and specificity, usually discussed with regard to a particular question the behavioral measure is used to answer. Concepts of sensitivity and specificity have been used commonly in medicine to characterize clinical diagnostic tests (e.g., Kraemer *[19]*), and these concepts are applicable to psychological tests as well. Sensitivity refers to capacity of a test to detect signs of behavioral dysfunction or variations in behavior when they occur. General intellectual measures, for instance, may not be sensitive to early signs of dementia even though they may be accurate, and valid, indicators of the intellectual construct they are designed to measure. The field of psychology usually defines sensitivity mathematically as a ratio of the true positives of a given test to the sum of its true positives and false-negatives *(19)*. Specificity, on the other hand, refers to the "uniqueness" of a given test's scores, meaning that the test does not report an effect when it is absent. Specificity can be represented mathematically as the ratio of true negatives to the sum of true negatives plus false-positives *(19)*. To give two examples, an error score on a test of complex problem solving, called the Halstead Category Test (HCT), has been shown to be "sensitive" to neurological dysfunction in frontal regions of the human brain *(20)*. Despite this sensitivity, are the scores on this test specific to only frontal dysfunction or can neurologic dysfunction in other brain regions, or even extra-neurologic factors, lead to similar error scores? Since the answer to this question is yes, we can say that the HCT is sensitive to neurologic dysfunction of the frontal lobes of the brain but is not specific to such dysfunction. Additional techniques would need to be employed in order to diagnose accurately the dysfunction that leads to the poor score on the HCT. The spelling subtest of the *Wide Range Achievement Test-Third Edition (21)* to give a second example, is sensitive to a person's spelling accuracy, but the scores on this test are not specific to underlying disorder. A low score could reflect neurological dysfunction of one or more types, but it might also result from past educational shortcomings, failure to understand the test directions, inattention, or even lack of motivation.

A weakness of many psychological tests is that resultant scores might result from one of a number of possible causes or even be multiply determined. Of course, no matter how sensitive a test might be to a given disorder, or construct, its specificity will be limited by the nature of the disorder or construct itself. Some diseases, for instance, may overlap in their manifestations with other illnesses. A sensitive test might be expected to faithfully measure this condition while failing to specify any of the underlying conditions specifically. For reasons such as this, issues of specificity are not unique to psychological tests, but that does not excuse the need to address these issues further than they may have been addressed to date.

It should be kept in mind that there are aspects to validity that transcend the strictly mathematical. Cronbach *(22)* identified an additional perspective of validity, which he termed, "functional validity." Others have used other terms to describe similar ideas, e.g., "ecological validity" *(23)*. For Cronbach, the worth of a test (its functional validity) should be evaluated against its truth (statistical validity) in making decisions about its usefulness. That is, even if a test can validly measure memory functioning, how do scores on that measure relate to practical behaviors of interest such as remembering to take medications or remembering a particular work-related task? From this perspective, the ultimate relevance of test scores to real-world events might carry greater weight in clinical practice than the relationship of test scores to theoretical constructs with only hypothetical relationship to practical outcomes.

4.3. Other Issues in Test Construction and Selection

In addition to the basic psychometric properties of a test, it is also important to consider the standardization and normative samples that are available for a measure (*see* Table 1).

4.3.1. Standardization

Before a behavioral measure can be formally termed a "test," the device must be "standardized." That is, a standard procedure for administering the test should be specified. For the results of such a device to be meaningful, of course, the person administering the test must follow the standardized procedure exactly. In some cases (e.g., a paper and pencil inventory such as the Minnesota Multiphasic Personality Inventory [MMPI]) this is fairly easily accomplished by becoming familiar with a few basic and general rules of test administration and by carefully following the instructions in the manual. Basic considerations in test administration can be found in such publications

Table 1
Qualities of a "Good" Test

Reliable (reliability coefficients > .70)
    Demonstrated by:
        Alternate forms
        Test-retest
        Internal consistency
        Inter-rater reliability
Valid
    Assessed in terms of:
        Face validity
        Content validity
        Criterion validity (predictive and concurrent)
        Construct validity (discriminant and convergent)
        Functional validity
Sensitive and specific
Standardized
Appropriate normative groups

as Anastasi's *(12)* or Cronbach's *(24)* textbooks on psychological testing. In other instances (e.g., the Wechsler Intelligence Scales or the Halstead-Reitan Neuropsychological Test Battery), considerable training may be required for proper test administration or interpretation. In addition to textbooks as those listed previously, there are published guidelines and texts that address a variety of clinical practice issues (e.g., *The TCN Guide to Professional Practice in Clinical Neuropsychology [25]* and Division 40's guidelines *[26]*).

As in science more generally, the concept of standardization is important in psychology. Its importance in the measurement of behavior can not be overestimated. Standardization applies to every aspect of the test, and this includes such seemingly extra-test considerations as the instructions and examples given to the subject before the actual test is administered. It also applies to the timing of stimulus presentations, the nature of responses given to a subject's questions, the physical environment of the test situation, and other details of the test situation. Standardization extends to test scoring as well. Should the standardized procedure of test administration be altered, the reliability and validity of the instrument is compromised. This is as true in psychological testing as in any other measurement enterprise, e.g., deciding whether to measure a person's weight or height with shoes on or off.

4.3.2. Normative Data

Psychological tests can be used to measure aspects of behavior, and these data can be used in controlled experiments where the meaningfulness of the results is determined by statistical comparison to one or more "control" groups. To be meaningful in the context of measurement of an individual, however, a test must be "normed." That is, there will be some prescribed method for relating the observed test score(s) to a representative population sample. Normative data, or "norms," aid in understanding what a particular score on a test means. A relatively low score on a verbal learning task might be expected of someone with a life-long record of low intellect and academic

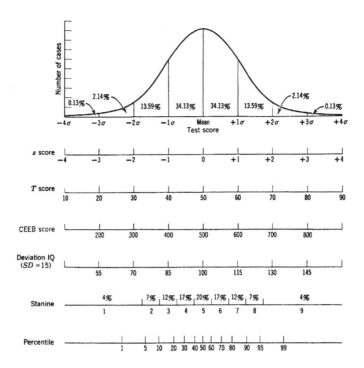

Fig. 1. The normal curve, depicting standard deviations, corresponding percentiles, and standard scores. Reprinted with permission of Pearson Education, Inc., Upper Saddle River, NJ 07458 *(12)*.

achievement, for instance, whereas in another person it might reflect a cognitive impairment. Normative data for verbal learning that takes into account level of intellect and education will aid in making proper distinctions in a such an instance. Norms do not remove the paramount importance placed on validity and reliability issues mentioned earlier. It is also worth mentioning that in the experimental setting, when a statistically significant difference in a test measure is found between two or more groups, norms aid in determining whether or not that difference holds clinical relevance in addition to strictly statistical significance.

Normative data are usually developed through formal research by administering the test to a large and representative group of subjects. Important factors to consider in evaluating the adequacy of a particular normative sample include representativeness, size, and relevance to the population of interest. Psychological tests often generate scores that are standardized or presented in terms of percentile rank and based on the normative sample. Such scores allow comparison of an individual's performance across different tests. The standardized scores and percentile ranks are usually based on either the assumption, the knowledge from previous study, or both that the population's performance on this measure reflects a characteristic numeric distribution. For most human behaviors, the scores approximate a normal distribution or bell-shaped curve (*see* Fig. 1).

The "normative" group determines the average performance expected for a given individual in terms of the specified test score and provides an indication of "normally" expected variability in performance. It is through such normative based testing that a "raw" test score will come to have clinically relevant meaning. By scaling the raw score, we are able to compare the individual performance to a meaningful referent group and determine the score's significance. For example, commonly used tests of intelligence have been normed against a sample that reflects an average index score of 100, with a standard deviation of ±15. An observed index score of 85 in this instance, then, falls one standard deviation below the average and is at the 15th percentile in comparison to the referent population (i.e., better than only 15% of the referent population). The adequacy of the test, therefore, is intimately related to the adequacy of the sample against which the test has been normed. Some measurements may also generate age-equivalent or grade-equivalent scores, and not all measured variables are normally distributed (e.g., relative handedness is not normally distributed in the general population). The reference group(s) will determine the shape of the distribution, as well as its average performance level and variability.

4.4. When is Behavior Abnormal?

Concerns about the distinction between normal vs abnormal are more relevant in the clinical setting than in the research arena. As reflected in writings from the early part of this century (e.g., Whipple *[27]*), the distinction between the two settings, clinical and research, may largely be a matter of aims. In both settings, there is interest in alterations in behavior. In research endeavors, the aim is to study the effect of some independent (experimental) variable in terms of its altering another dependent variable(s) while holding other potentially intervening (nuisance) variables constant. For example, neuroepidemiological studies focusing on differences between "cases" and "controls," or studies focusing on "dose-response" relationships may be useful in establishing clinically relevant variables that differentiate between groups or are sensitive to the experimental variable. This information may help further our understanding of a clinically important topic area but are usually of unknown significance in evaluating an individual case. In these research endeavors, there may be a need to define the dependent response as normal or abnormal only during the conclusion stage of the method when the researcher is attempting to generalize the findings to a larger population and when the researcher is attempting to comment on the meaningfulness of the findings. In contrast, the problem of knowing that a given behavior is, in fact, abnormal is perhaps more immediately relevant in the clinical context where clinical diagnosis is often a primary motivation for conducting the study. Regardless of the setting, there are essentially two primary models for determining abnormality *(28)*. These are limited to statistical and qualitative approaches to defining normality or its exception.

The statistical approach rests on a definition of normality on the basis of what most people do in a specified population sample. The sample determines the nature of the distribution, often normally distributed in the case of most behavioral variables (*see* Fig. 1). Abnormality in the statistical model is usually defined by exclusion, i.e., departure from the mean of the distribution by some specified variance. While the statistical approach is attractive, perhaps especially to scientists, because of its inherent objectivity and quantitative nature, it carries with it serious drawbacks as well. For instance, normality is basically defined as what most people do in a given population. What happens when the majority in that population is considered to be deviant according to the consensual judgment of others? An example might be a society prone to intolerance, one in which its members often attack others who are not recognized as conforming to their standards. In such a case, the statistical model would describe as "normal" a great many behaviors that by other standards would be considered deviant.

Qualitative approaches can be divided into those which specify specific, positive criteria of normality and those which list specific pathognomonic behaviors considered to represent abnormality. The qualitative models have many weaknesses as well. The criteria are often vague, failing to lend well to attempts at standardization or operationalism. There is usually considerable subjectivity in the original determination of the criteria, and current values with time limited relevance are often employed in their construction. These models are perhaps most effective when their criteria are derived from empirical research, but, even then, considerable subjectivity remains.

An approach to defining normality that combines statistical and qualitative models may be the most effective. The statistical allows for quantitative and objective definition of behavioral variables, especially in terms of understanding the magnitude of a specified variable. Employing such variables to study specified conditions and developing a knowledge base from ongoing, systematic study can allow for an effective definition of normal or abnormal, at least in the defined context. Knowing the expected course of progression in a disease such as Alzheimer's, for instance, and discovering an objective and quantitative behavioral corollary to the disease endpoint would allow for a psychometric definition of abnormality within that context.

Clinicians must also be aware of the context of their diagnoses. For example, the positive or negative predictive power of a specific test score rests, in part, on the presumed base rate for that disorder in the population. If clinicians assume that there is an equal likelihood of every disorder, diagnostic accuracy may be compromised *(29)*.

4.5. The Concept of Bias in Neuropsychology

The validity of a test is usually established in the environment of scientific research, with the luxury of an acceptable level of control over potential nuisance variables. The environment of everyday life is never ideal and an individual's performance on a test can reflect multiple factors that may compromise the accuracy or meaningfulness of a particular set of test scores even when the test has well-established validity. Such factors include test-based variables, examiner peculiarities, and unique aspects of the individual. Some more specific examples of such variables include the individual's comprehension of the given directions for completing the tasks, individual variations in degree of novelty of the test items, and even cultural bias of test items.

The measurement of behavior through psychological testing has found success and applicability in science, and its quantitative and objective nature has lead to widespread use of these methods in society at large. With the recognition of its strengths has come increased awareness of weaknesses as well. Legislative action, as in the case of Larry P. vs Riles *(30)*, for instance, was based on the realization that the established validity of a test in a subculture may not generalize to another and led to laws restricting the use of standardized achievement tests when determining mental retardation. While psychologists have long known about and struggled with such challenges to the effective measurement of behavior, it will be an ongoing effort to discover relevant issues and make appropriate adjustments to our procedures.

Variables, such as age, socio-economic status, or cultural background, may affect a given individual's motivation for testing, response set, or test-taking approach. Other issues that must be considered in properly understanding the results of testing include the appropriateness of standardization samples, potential biases in the language used by the examiner, and the possible adverse consequences of the test results to the person taking the tests to job or social role. Further, members from minority cultures could experience the same task demands in testing situations differently from the majority on which validity studies were based, leading to differential motivation in performing a task and confounding the results of their performance *(31,32)*. Even the base rate of the "usual" speed with which a person approaches a given task can vary between individuals from different cultures, a factor Hinkle *(33)* has termed the "tempo of life."

While we are interested in individual differences, these differences may reflect factors that interact with and potentially confound the aspect of behavior being measured in a specific test instance. In addition to issues associated with cultural groups, some relevant factors of this type include skill level, anxiety, motivation, physical limitations, deficiencies in educational opportunities, or unfamiliarity with testing situations *(34)*. Variations in individual motivation may be particularly important to consider when interpreting the results of psychological measurements. Persons involved in litigation, for example, may reflect an approach to the test situation that differs from others in the general population, among other consequences producing unique base-rates of reported symptoms *(35,36)*.

The specific nature of motivational intrusion may vary based on the extent that the symptoms are under conscious control and what type of gain is sought by the patient *(37)*. For example, there are psychiatric conditions, such as Somatization Disorder and Conversion Disorder, which present with physical symptoms that stem from psychological processes not under a person's conscious control. In contrast, some people present with physical or psychological symptoms that are under conscious control, but have no obvious gain for the patient. This condition is typically referred to as Factitious disorder. Malingering refers to symptoms that are consciously produced or exaggerated and is directed towards obtaining some benefit, such as a settlement. Estimates of the base rate of malingering in groups of people involved in litigation or "other benefit-seeking" situations have been reported from 7.5–15% *(38)* to 18–33% *(39)*. Research has also shown that people involved in litigation typically report higher levels of neurotoxic and neuropsychologic symptoms in comparison to people not in litigation *(35,40)*. In order to be able to evaluate the potential for such psychiatric phenomena, it is essential that neuropsychological test results be interpreted by appropriately trained individuals who are knowledgeable, not only about physical based pathology, but who are also familiar with symptoms and signs associated with psychopathology.

Specific measurement techniques have been studied with regard to their usefulness in identifying motivational intrusion. A common technique has been the use of a simplistic task to assess faking or exaggeration. For example, the Rey's 15-Item recall test presents the patient with a simple array of 15 objects to recall. Research has suggested that recall of less than seven items is suggestive of faking or exaggeration of impairment *(41)*. Other potential signs of malingering include suggestion of performance below chance level on common measures or suggestion of excessive inconsistency both within and across tests *(42)*. Malingering has also been associated with an "atypical" response style on neuropsychological tests, in combination with vague and unusual somatic complaints *(43)*. In addition, research has suggested that attempting to "warn" patients about the presence of symptom validity assessment techniques tends to result in a more sophisticated and subtle pattern that is more difficult to detect *(44)*.

Within research protocols, it may be worthwhile to ask a group of "simulators" to participate in the study along with actual patients *(45)*. In this paradigm, simulators are told to act as if they were a real subject and to attempt to deceive a blind experimenter. If the simulators' test performance can pass as a real subject's, it suggests that demand characteristics of the tests or experimental conditions may be accounting for, at least, some of the results.

Any or all of the issues just mentioned might impact on the validity of a test instrument for a given person *(46)*. It is the job of psychology, then, to do more than simply develop technically sound instruments for the measurement of behavior. Variables that may result in different validity coefficients for various individuals and subgroups must be identified and accounted for in validation studies. The training of individuals who will administer and interpret the tests must include not only the development of sensitivity to these issues but methods for dealing with them effectively as well.

5. THE NEUROPSYCHOLOGICAL APPROACH IN RESEARCH

5.1. *The Scientific Method*

Neuropsychology considers itself to be a field that is based on science. In general, this manifests in several ways: it employs objective and quantitative methods to the extent possible; the work of neuropsychology is aimed at contributing to an expanding knowledge base that is archived through publication and related professional communications; it attempts to deal with observable and operational variables; and it employs the scientific method whenever feasible. In the simplest terms, the scientific method consists of defining a problem (question) or problems (questions) and proposing an answer to the problem or problems (the hypothesis[es]). The question must be testable, that is, stated in terms of observables and stated as a proposition that is falsifiable. A research design is created that will allow for observations of variables relevant to testing the hypothesis while controlling for extraneous factors that could confound the results obtained. These results are analyzed mathematically, leading to probability statement about the likelihood that the test proposition is true. Conclusions are drawn from this test, recognizing the limits to which the observations can be generalized beyond the immediate test situation and other constraints that limit what can be said from a cause and effect viewpoint. Most often, this method employs a controlled experiment to test the proposed hypothesis, but neuropsychology also strives to approximate the scientific approach in all of its activities. In practice, the approximation is never perfect, and careful attention must be given to the limitations of the knowledge obtained from either arena.

5.2. Differences Between the Research and Clinical Approach in Neuropsychology

As already discussed, the clinical approach in neuropsychology is to use psychometric tests, together with other sources of information, in order to quantify and describe an individual's current level of functioning. The aims of clinical and research endeavors vary. In 1914, Whipple explicitly differentiated the two approaches, stating that the primary difference was in the objective *(27)*. While psychological tests could be used in experiments, the aim of testing was primarily diagnostic, to analyze, measure, and rank aspects of behavior in an individual. The aim of the psychological experiment is theoretical, to discover new facts, principles, or laws for the science of psychology (or science in general). In other words, the goal of research is to increase our scientific knowledge base. Others, such as Stern *(47)* and Dunlap *(48)*, carried on these definitions and distinctions, providing the basic understandings that have carried to this day.

In research, the objective is to evaluate potential relationships between variables, searching for cause-and-effect relationships. The scientific method often attempts to simplify nature in order to better understand the components. In order to isolate changes, researchers need to follow a systematic, scientific approach regardless of challenges. As with clinical endeavors, not all questions will lend to this approach. In order to measure constructs, we must work with observables and be able to apply principles of measurement to the variables of interest. Instead of working from a clinical referral, research is initiated by the specification of a question(s) that is derived from and accounts for prior work on the topic. In addition to careful and systematic review of literature on the topic of interest, one must examine critically the areas of inconsistency and unknowns in the current literature. This is used as the impetus to formulating a question that is amenable to scientific method and answerable by obtainable, observational, psychometric data.

5.3. Research Design

Within many of the biological sciences, the "gold standard" of research has been the use of the experimental model. In order to be able to draw causal conclusions, a high degree of experimental control, including the ability to randomize, or to randomly assign subjects into different treatment conditions, is essential. The use of randomization, in combination with double blinding, is believed to control for potential experimenter and participant biases *(49)*. However, in the area of human neurotoxicology, a true experimental model is sometimes not possible. In addition, the high variability associated with most behavioral variables leaves it unlikely that the precision of the controlled laboratory will ever be obtained in this area of inquiry. Acknowledging such challenges, a scientific approach to human behavioral topics can still be accomplished.

Neurotoxicology research has often relied on the use of animals models, which can conform to experimental conditions of random assignment to exposure conditions (i.e., dose, frequency, duration, and timing) and provide support of a causal link *(50)*. However, as in any analog study, the results are more meaningful with increased similarity between the "analog" and the desired population. As a result, reliance on animal models alone is insufficient, as there can be significant differences in susceptibility of the species. For example, there has been some suggestion that nonhuman primates are more vulnerable when exposed to polychlorinated biphenyls (PCBs) than humans *(51)* More-over, some of the behaviors that one would like to model (e.g., internal emotional disruption) may not lend itself to observable behaviors in animal studies. And lastly, the increased control utilized in experimental design that allows for cause-effect analyses, is often at the expense of external validity. As noted by Kazdin *(45)*, "design features that make an experiment more sensitive as a test of the independent and dependent variables tend to limit the generality of the findings." Conversely, features of an experiment that enhance generality of the results tend to increase variability and to decrease the sensitivity of the experimental test. For example, procedures that can regulate and quantify dose or exposure, such as the use of gavage or intravenous administration, can result in different outcomes than studies with inhalation or dermal absorption (e.g., Baelum *[52]*). In order to establish a causal relationship between exposure to a neurotoxic agent and specific neurobehavioral outcomes in exposed persons requires evidence from both animal and human research.

In human studies, true experimental models may not be a viable method for assessing neurotoxic effects given ethical and moral guidelines. For instance, the APA ethical principles state "Research procedures likely to cause serious or lasting harm to a participant are not used unless the failure to use these procedures might expose the participant to risk of greater harm or unless the research has great potential benefit and fully informed and voluntary consent is obtained from each participant" *(53)*. As a result of these considerations, human neurotoxicology research tends to utilize what have been called "quasi-experimental models," where randomization is not possible *(45)*. There are two major types of quasi-experimental models, a cross-sectional design and a cohort (longitudinal) design. Cross-sectional designs can have important implications for causal hypotheses. For example, case-control studies can be particularly well suited to studying conditions that are relatively infrequent where it would not be possible to obtain a sufficient sample size using random sampling. Typically, case-control studies are more efficient in terms of their costs while still providing an opportunity to study the magnitude and type of relationship between the independent and dependent variables. Case-control studies are also useful in generating hypotheses related to causal relationships. Longitudinal or developmental cohort designs can strengthen the evidence by providing temporal relationship between antecedent events and outcomes *(45)*.

Although a single quasi-experimental study may not be able to establish cause-and-effect relationships, the pattern of research outcomes can be examined and evaluated. In particular, the use of quantitative review techniques, such as meta-analysis, that permits comparison of research outcomes and effect sizes, is preferred over simple tallying of positive and negative findings *(61)*. However, the accuracy or validity of the findings of a meta-analysis is dependent on the quality of the original research. Further, a consistent error that occurs across studies may be incorrectly reported as a treatment-related effect in a meta-analysis.

Within epidemiological research, several theorists have proposed a variety of criteria for establishing causation. In 1965, Sir Bradford Hill formulated a set of criteria for assessing causation in regards to chemical hazards *(62)*. The evidence of causation is determined by the strength, consistency, and specificity of the association between the agent and symptoms/signs. In addition, there must be evidence of a temporal relationship and a dose-response relationship. The hypothesized mechanism must be biologically plausible and must be coherent within accepted scientific theory. This relationship should also be supported by evidence from experimental and analog studies. For example, a repeated positive response to a specific treatment can be documented experimentally and similar effects may be seen in other species or with other similar chemicals.

5.4. Issues Related to Sample Selection

5.4.1. Comparison Groups

The strength of a quasi-experiment often rests on its ability to control for potential group differences, as random assignment in true experimental models is believed to result in equivalent groups *(45)*. However, the likelihood of equivalent groups is related to the sample size, and inequality in groups may be particularly problematic when working with small samples *(54)*. Moreover, the use of randomization of human subjects has sometimes been argued to be in opposition to a physician's duty to act in the patient's best interest *(55,56)*. Some have argued that randomization is only appropriate where true "equipoise" exists and the null hypothesis is truly supported *(57)*.

Many studies in human neurotoxicology rely on "convenient" or serendipitous samples obtained from patients seeking care at a particular clinic. Research in treatment-seeking for psychiatric patients has found support of Berkson's bias, which suggests that those persons with comorbid disorders are more likely to seek treatment *(58)*. Convenient samples from clinics may be overrepresentative of more severe cases with more comorbid and complicating factors and may not be representative of the larger population. Samples can also introduce bias on the basis of difference in several moderating variables, such as age, general health status, or body mass. For example, because of solvents' affinity for lipids or fats, they are believed to have a longer biological half life in persons who are obese as compared to thin persons *(59)*. If potential confounding variables are identified, researchers can attempt to control for potential moderating effects by either matching the groups on the characteristics or attempting to use statistical controls, such as analysis of covariance. Early research in human neurotoxicology has been characterized by weaknesses in the quantification of individual exposure and dose levels, as well as failure to control for relevant confounding factors *(60)*.

In addition to normal control groups, where the objective is to identify differences between a healthy and potentially impaired group, the use of pathology comparison groups is important in determining the specificity of the findings. For example, in order to determine the significance of neuropsychological abnormalities in a potentially exposed group, it may be most useful to compare their performances to both a normal control group, as well as to a group of patients with anxiety or depression (pathology comparison group). This may allow researchers to assess the potential specificity of the findings.

5.4.2. Volunteerism

A general principle in ethics is respecting the rights of people to make their own decisions. As a result, the Ethical Principles of Psychologists and Code of Conduct *(63)* states that informed consent for research can only be set aside in situations involving anonymous questionnaires, naturalistic observations, or some kinds of archival research. As a result, much of the research involving human participants must rely on volunteers. Those persons who volunteer for experiments have been found to often be better educated, have a higher occupational status, be more self-disclosing, have a higher need for social approval, and be more sociable *(64,65)*. In order to minimize potential effects from volunteerism, it is important for researchers to actively recruit subject participation and increase the range of potential subjects instead of merely using ready volunteers.

5.4.3. Power

The power of a research study is determined by the size of the effect, as well as the sample size. Often, issues of power are discussed only in relationship to the sample size. Within research, the phrase "bigger is better" is often echoed. As a study's sample size increases, the power of the study to find significant results increases. If power is too low, it is possible to miss important relationships. However, in extremely large samples, the high level of power may permit detection of minuscule differences that have no clinical significance. In reporting research results, information related to the measured effect size is important in helping to determine the potential clinical significance of the research findings *(66)*.

In neurotoxicology, researchers are often looking for subtle effects within a noisy background of individual variance. When faced with relatively subtle effects, the traditional solution has been to increase power by increasing the study's sample size. In neurotoxicology, this may not be possible. Actually confirmed events of neurotoxic exposure to some agents may be quite rare. In those situations, a detailed case study, which can often resemble a clinical examination, may be the most appropriate way to provide rich descriptive data on an infrequent and rare condition. However, researchers need to make clear the limitations of case studies. When examining a single person, the possibility for alternate explanations is great. Rather than confirming or attempting to provide support of a hypothesis, case studies often yield the most useful research information when they "provide a counterinstance" to a previously assumed relationship *(45)*.

5.5. Issues Related to Design and Procedures

5.5.1. Reactivity

As previously mentioned, ethical considerations for people's autonomy and personal rights demands the use of informed consent for participation in experimental research. Therefore, participants are often aware of the nature and the purpose of a planned study. If participants' behavior is changed as a result of having participated in a study, the study would be said to be "reactive." Concern has been raised that in-depth questioning of people's symptoms may lead to an iatrogenic effect *(67,68)*. In particular, during informed consent, participants might be told that the purpose of the study is to identify possible negative effects from neurotoxic exposures. Having been informed that symptoms are expected following an exposure may make participants increasingly aware of nonspecific symptoms and attribute those symptoms to the presumed exposure. For example, in a multicenter clinical trial on the benefits of aspirin in the treatment of unstable angina, researchers found that inclusion of potential gastrointestinal side effects in the consent form was associated with a significantly higher rate of subjects withdrawing from the study, attributing subjective and minor gastrointestinal symptoms to the drug therapy *(69)*.

Previous research has noted that studies of different occupational and environmental exposures report similar increases in nonspecific symptoms, such as headache, fatigue, and memory problems, suggesting that common psychological factors are responsible, as compared with unique factors from specific toxins *(69)*. During early, exploratory studies it might be useful to examine the relationship of symptom reports with potential confounding variables, such as participants' knowledge or expectation of effects from a toxin. In subsequent studies, one strategy to deal with participants' potential reactivity to symptoms may be to include "filler" items, symptoms that are not expected to be associated with the particular neurotoxin. By being able to examine both the specificity, as well as the sensitivity, of their symptom report, research can better measure and assess the reactivity. Advances in computer-administered testing can also be used to help streamline measurement and reduce reactivity. For example, based on hierarchical arrangement of items, computers can "tailor" the questions asked of participants, selecting appropriate follow-up questions and omitting irrelevant items.

5.5.2. Measurement

In addition to the neuropsychological tests that have been traditionally used in clinical settings, attempts have been made in human neurotoxicology research to develop standardized test batteries to facilitate comparison of results across studies. These batteries are often designed to specifically select measures that have been shown to be sensitive to neurotoxin exposures. However, they often do not include measurement of potential moderating variables or functions that would be expected to be resistant to effects of exposure, such as reading ability or general intellectual functioning. The approach of only selecting measures that may be sensitive to effects of toxins often neglects the importance of sensitivity or discriminant validity.

The World Health Organization (WHO) Neurobehavioral Core Test Battery provides measurement of affect, attention/response speed, auditory memory, manual dexterity, perceptual motor speed, and visual perception/memory, and motor steadiness *(71)*. This group of "core" tests was developed as a way to measure specific functions that are often disrupted by exposure to neurotoxins and to provide a battery of tests with limited verbal demands that could be employed in a variety of cultural settings *(71)*. However, researchers have also found that the sensitivity of individual tasks appeared to vary across studies *(72)*.

The advent of the computer has also influenced the process of testing in human neurotoxicology. The use of computer-administered tests have several advantages for research applications. Computer based testing is often more cost-efficient as it decreases the need for highly training personnel for data collection and testing can be repeated without "fatigue" factors. Moreover, computerization allows for consistency in the standardization of the administration of tests and recording of small changes in response time can be calculated. However, there are also significant weaknesses to the use of computer-administered testing. As noted by Letz, computer-based tests often utilized a restricted modality of stimuli and responses *(73)*. Test stimuli are typically visually presented and responses are frequently based on manual responding with measurement of the speed of the response. There has been some suggestion that computer-administered tests may have an increased level of "method" variance than traditional examiner-administered tests, which may obscure detection of the actual "trait" or "construct" variance *(74)*. In addition, computer-administered testing often neglects the importance of qualitative behavioral observations with regard to motivational effort and emotional factors. Moreover, although computer-aided testing may allow for increased precision in response time measurement, it can be difficult to ascertain the clinical and functional significance of these differences. A trained neuropsychologist is required to synthesize historical and observational information with collected test data.

As noted in the section on basic psychometrics, the reliability and validity of a measurement determine its meaningfulness. However, other sources of bias and error can occur in data collection. The perceived emotional valence and cognitive expectations that often accompany environmental exposures (perceived or real) can exert a strong effect on subjects' report of symptoms and interpretation of bodily sensations. For example, in a study examining the relationship between anesthesia exposure and miscarriage, Axelsson and Rylander compared women's self-reports of a history of miscarriage to medical records *(75)*. They found that women were more likely to report having had a miscarriage if they also were exposed to anesthesia than women who miscarried in the absence of any exposure. Kihlstrom noted that participants' perceptions about a study and their expectations can influence how they perform *(76)*.

Even early in the history of psychology, it was found that it is possible to induce the majority of a sample to report the presence of an odor by suggesting its presence and using a visual analogue, such as pouring distilled water onto a cotton pad *(77)*. Odor has been suggested to be a possible mediating factor in the expression of physical symptoms for environmental exposures. For example, Baelum found that the report of symptoms associated with solvent exposure using an alternate route of exposure and in the absence of odor was particularly low and did not reflect a dose-response relationship *(52)*.

Research has also suggested that there may be significant interactions between people's responses to chemicals and a host of psychological factors, including cognitive expectations and perceived odor. For example, Dalton and colleagues examined 90 naive control subjects' responses to acetone *(78)*. Subjects were either given a positive, negative, or neutral bias towards acetone and were then asked to rate the intensity of odor and irritation. They found that subjects with a negative cognitive bias towards acetone reported significantly higher levels of odor and irritation and reported significantly more health symptoms than the other groups. The impact of odor may also be moderated by demographic variables, such as gender. Women have been reported to have lower odor-detection thresholds than men *(79)* and have also been reported to be more sensitive to suggestion *(80)*. Women have also been found to be more likely to report symptoms of sick-building syndrome *(81–84)* and multiple chemical sensitivies *(85)*. In an experimental paradigm, Gilbert, Sabini, and Knasko demonstrated that women, in comparison to men, were more likely to demonstrate improvement on a information processing task (e.g., digit deletion task) with the suggestion of a pleasant odor or in the context of no odor *(86)*. Men, however, were more likely to perform better when there was no suggestion of the valence of the odor.

Expectation bias needs to be specifically evaluated in order to interpret research results. In studying group differences from chemical exposures, it is important to assess participants perceived evaluations of their exposure, in addition to their reported symptoms. The perceived short- or long-term risks associated with an environmental exposure can be a significant confounding factor *(67)*. For example, in a study of the level of symptom report for residents living near a hazardous waste-disposal site, researchers found that the level of symptom report was related to hypochondriacal traits in both the experimental and control groups. Moreover, for residents living close to the site, their opinion about the potential environmental effects of waste sites was also a significant moderating variable associated with the level of reported symptoms *(87)*.

In addition, the presence of other sources of psychological stress may be a potential indirect or moderating variable. For example, Citterio and colleagues found complaints of headaches to be one of the most common symptoms of sick-building syndrome *(81)*. Within their sample, they also found a significant and negative correlation between headaches and their reported "comfort" in the workplace. Similarly, Ooi and Goh found a trend for increasing prevalence of sick-building syndrome among workers with reported high levels of physical and mental stress and perceived low "climate of cooperation" in their workplace *(88)*.

5.5.3. Blinding and Placebo Controls

One of the traditional forms of research to establish the effectiveness of a medication is to conduct a double-blind, placebo-control study. A placebo typically refers to an inert agent that is not expected to alter behavior. In a placebo-control, one group would receive the active pharmacological agent, whereas the other group would receive the "placebo." Double-blinding refers to the condition when neither the participant nor the researcher is aware of which persons are receiving the active medication or the inert placebo. Theoretically, this type of design is supposed to control for possible psychological or "anticipatory" factors, outside of the actual biochemical effects, that may occur with medications. Without blinding, it has been asserted that experimenter expectancies may exert an effect on the outcome. For example, in conducting a meta analysis of studies on the effects of carbon monoxide, Benignus noted that 75% of the single-blind (participant-blinded only) studies found significant results as compared with only 26% of double-blind studies *(89)*. However, studies have also found that attempts to blind researchers are often ineffective, demonstrating that researchers can often correctly guess a participant's group status *(90,91)*.

One method for routinely measuring the efficacy of blinding in a study is by asking observers to guess the status of selected participants *(92)*. In some studies, it may also be relevant to ask participants to guess their treatment group or exposure status in order to further evaluate the quality of the "blinding" of the study. Ney, Collins, and Spencer also suggested that researchers should measure the participants' and observer's assessment of a possible attributional factor, namely, whether the change is believed to result from the intended independent variable or from other intervening confound variables *(93)*. Although the use of double-blind techniques are well-known, it is rare for researchers to systematically evaluate the effectiveness of blinding techniques in a study *(93,94)*. It may be difficult to fully evaluate the integrity of blinding procedures, however, it is important to understand the potential source of bias this might introduce.

Double-blind techniques have not been extensively used in studies of environmental exposure. In particular, it often problematic to blind the subjects in exposure studies. For example, in case-control studies of environmental exposure, participants are often self-identified as "exposed" or not. In addition, informed consent procedures or the nature of some measures (such as, "Questionnaire for environmental-induced illness") may provide subjects with information about the presumed hypothesis under study. Although it may not be possible to blind subjects in environmental-exposure studies, researchers should attempt to assess the potential effect the knowledge of the exposure might have. For example, this would likely including measurement of the participants expectations about the potential results of exposure, as well as assessment of other potential moderating variables, such as perception of risk or work satisfaction.

In neuropsychological studies, blinding of the experimenter is often easier to accomplish. The use of technicians to actually administer tests is one way to attempt to keep "data collectors" blind. Technicians do not need to be informed about the exposure status of participants, nor do they need to be informed about the specific hypothesis under examination. Poststudy techniques, such as polling technicians to determine how readily they were able to determine the status of participants, can help determine some of the limitations in the effectiveness of this blinding. These field studies can also be supplemented and supported by analogue, experimental research where double blind conditions may be better implemented.

6. CONCLUSION

Neuropsychology has a history of specialization in the area of testing and measurement, examining the relationship between brain disruption and observable behavioral changes. In particular, neuropsychological approaches to assessment of environmental exposure can be used fruitfully in either the clinical or the research setting. Within the clinical arena, it is particularly important to evaluate a patient's complaints within the larger context of the psychometric test data. In particular, comprehensive evaluation requires analysis of patterns of results, such as consistency between historical records and current performance, the relationship to normative data, and consideration of differential diagnosis, including examination of base-rates of competing disorders. Selection of specific test batteries reflects coverage of the major domains of behavior, as well as knowledge of individual instruments' psychometric properties.

Within research, the scientific method is applied to assess the merit of specific hypotheses. The selection of the research design and statistical tools for analysis create particular strengths and limitations for each study. Although ethical and practical concerns often preclude the use of true experimental models, a body of research from quasi-experimental and analogue studies can be used to evaluate the strength of presumed causal relationships between environmental agents and neuropsychological symptoms in humans. Attempts to measure and control for potentially biasing factors, such as experimenter expectancies, demand characteristics, and other moderating variables, can strengthen the quality of research results (*see* Table 2).

Whether in the role of researcher, clinician, or consumer of knowledge generated by neuropsychological methods, the many principles and cautions discussed in this chapter should be considered. The following table provides a checklist which may be consulted when planning or reviewing such work.

Table 2
Some Important Issues to Consider When Planning or Evaluating
Behavioral Studies

1. Hypothesis
   * Is the problem area appropriately defined?
   * Is the type of study apparent (e.g., hypothesis generating vs hypothesis testing)?
   * Are the hypotheses clearly stated?
   * How well do the hypotheses relate to the stated problem?
2. Research design
   * What type of design is proposed?
       "True" experimental design vs quasi-experimental design vs case study
       Cross-sectional (case-control) vs longitudinal (cohort) design
   * Are the hypotheses truly testable by the proposed methods?
   * Are the proposed methods and procedures appropriate, safe, and ethical?
3. Sample selection
   * Who are the subjects and how are they selected?
       Convenient sample vs random selection
   * What type of comparison or control group is being used?
       Matched controls
       Normal and/or pathology controls
4. Exposure assessment
   * How was the intensity or level of exposure determined?
   * How was the duration of exposure determined?
5. Selection of tests or measurement
   * Is formal psychometric testing to be used?
       * Are the proposed measures reliable and valid?
       * Are they administered in an acceptably standardized manner by qualified personnel?
       * Are scores based on an appropriate normative sample?
6. Procedures
   * What are potential sources of bias or reactivity and how will they be controlled?
       * What is the nature of the informed consent process?
         (For example, might the informed consent process itself be a source of bias?)
       * Are subject(s) blinded?
       * Is the researcher blinded?
       * What are the limitations of blinding?
           Was the effectiveness of the blind measured?
           Were the potential consequences of a lack of blinding explicitly evaluated?
           How was expectation bias from knowledge or belief of exposure evaluated?
       * What are the consequences of the limitations of blinding on the conclusions drawn?
   * How will extraneous variables, including issues of motivation, be controlled?
7. Analyses
   * Are the statistical methods appropriate and sufficient to test the stated hypotheses?
   * Did the study have adequate power to detect true effects?
   * Is there a potential risk of elevated Type I errors?
       * How many dependent variables were assessed?
       * How many comparisons were conducted?
       * Was there any attempt to manage Type I error rates (e.g., Bonferroni technique, more conservative *p*-value, etc.)?

Table 2 (*continued*)

8. Discussion
    *   Are all the hypotheses addressed?
    *   Are the study conclusions supported by the data?
    *   What is the strength of the current finding?
            Was dose-response relationship discussed?
            Was there a clear pattern or syndrome of effects that was consistent with a toxicity-mediated effect?
            Are these findings specific to the exposure or associated with other possible etiologies?
            Are potential confounds, such as subjects' expectations of exposure-related effects, measured and incorporated into the interpretation of the results?
            Is there a clear temporal relationship between the exposure and onset of symptoms?
    *   How consistent is this finding with previous research?
            Was this syndrome consistent with existing animal and human studies?
            Are the resulting symptoms consistent with the level of exposure?
    *   To what extent do the study's findings contribute to our understanding of the problem addressed?
    *   Are limitations of the study and its findings appropriately discussed?
            How were "true" effects distinguished from Type I errors?
            How were randomization, blinding, and expectation bias addressed?

ACKNOWLEDGMENTS

Supported in part by a DOW Chemical Company Foundation SPHERE (Supporting Public Health and Environmental Research Efforts) Award, and funding from CSX Transportation, Inc. and the National Institutes of Health (NS 15655, AG 08671 and AG 07378). The authors wish to thank Joel Mattsson for his helpful editorial and conceptual suggestions.

REFERENCES

1. Murphy, G. (1949) *Historical Introduction to Modern Psychology*. Harcourt, Brace & World, New York.
2. Hilgard, E. R. (ed.) (1978) *American Psychology in Historical Perspective: Addresses of the Presidents of the American Psychological Association*. American Psychological Association, Washington, DC.
3. Mohr, J. P. (1976) Broca's area and Broca's aphasia, in *Studies in Neurolinguistics* (Whitaker, H. and Whitaker, H. A., eds.), Academic Press, New York, pp. 201–235.
4. Rozensky, R. H., Sweet, J. J., and Tovian, S. M. (1997) *Psychological Assessment in Medical Settings*. Plenum, New York.
5. Matarazzo, J. D. (1972) *Wechsler's Measurement and Appraisal of Adult Intelligence*, 5th ed. Williams & Wilkins, Baltimore, MD.
6. Wilson, R. S. and Stebbins, G. T. (1991) Estimating premorbid and preexisting neuropsychological deficits, in *Forensic Neuropsychology: Legal and Scientific Bases* (Doer, H. O. and Carlin, A. S., eds.), Guilford Press, New York, pp. 89–98.
7. Nelson, N. E. and O'Connell, A. (1978) Dementia: the estimation of premorbid intelligence levels using the New Adult Reading Test. *Cortex* **14**, 234–244.

8. Stebbins, G. T., Gilley, D. W., Wilson, R. S., Bernard, B. A., and Fox, J. H. (1990) Effects of language disturbances on premorbid estiamtes of IQ in mild dementia. *Clin. Neuropsychol.* **4**, 64–68.

9. Barona, A., Reynolds, C. R., and Chastain, R. (1984) A demographically based index of premorbid intelligence for the WAIS-R. *J. Consult. Clin. Psychol.* **52**, 885–887.

10. Eppinger, M. G., Craig, P. L., Adams, R. L., and Parsons, O. A. (1987) The WAIS-R index for estimating premorbid intelligence: Cross-validation and clinical utility. *J. Consult. Clin. Psychol.* **55**, 86–90.

11. American Psychological Association (1985) *Standards for Educational and Psychological Testing*. APA, Washington, DC.

12. Anastasi, A. (1976) *Psychological Testing*, 4th ed. Macmillan Publishing Company, New York.

13. Cronbach, L. J. (1951) Coefficient alpha and the internal consistency of tests. *Psychometrika* **16**, 297–334.

14. Kuder, G. F. and Richardson, M. W. (1937) The theory of the estimation of test reliability. *Psychometrika* **2**, 151–160.

15. Walker, H. M., and Lev, J. (1953) *Statistical Inference*. Holt, New York.

16. Mitchell, J. V., Jr. (ed.) (1998) *The Mental Measurements Yearbook*. Buros Institute of Mental Measurements, University of Nebraska, Lincoln, NE.

17. Buros Institute of Mental Measurements (1999) *Tests in Print*. Buros Institute of Mental Measurements, University of Nebraska-Lincoln, Lincoln, NE.

18. Campbell, D. T., and Fiske, D. W. (1959) Convergent and discriminant validation by the multitrait-multimethod matrix. *Psychol. Bull.* **56**, 81–105.

19. Kraemer, H. C. (1982) Estimating false alarms and missed events from interobserver agreement: comment on Kaye. *Psychol. Bull.* **92**, 749–754.

20. Reitan, R. M. (1955) Investigation of the validity of Halstead's measures of biological intelligence. *Arch. Neurol. Psychiatry* **73**, 28–35.

21. Wilkinson, G. S. (1993) *Administration Manual for the Wide Range Achievement Test*. Wide Range, Wilmington, DE.

22. Cronbach, L. J. (1988) Five perspectives on validity argument, in *Test Validity* (Wainer, H., and Braun, H. I., eds.), Lawrence Erlbaum Associates, Hillsdale, NJ, pp. 3–17.

23. Wilson, B. A. (1993) Ecological validity of neuropsychological assessment: do neuropsychological indexes predict performance in everyday activities? *Appl. Prevent. Psychol.* **2**, 209–215.

24. Cronbach, L. J. (1984) *Essentials of Psychological Testing*. Harper and Row, New York.

25. Adams, K. M. and Rourke, B. P. (1992) *The TCN Guide to Professional Practice in Clinical Neuropsychology*. Swets & Zeitlinger, Berwyn, PA.

26. Division 40 Task Force on Education, Accreditation, and Credentialing (1989) Guidelines regarding the use of nondoctoral personnel in clinical neuropsychological assessment. *Clin. Neuropsychol.* **3**, 23–24.

27. Whipple, G. M. (1914) *Manual of Mental and Physical Tests*. Warwick and York, Baltimore.

28. Berent, S. (1986) Modern approaches to neuropsychological testing, in *Advances in Neurology* (Smith, D., Treiman, D., and Trimble, M., eds.), Raven Press, New York, pp. 423–434.

29. Gouvier, W. D. (1999) Base rates and clinical decision making in neuropsychology, in *Forensic Neuropsychology: Fundamentals and Practice* (Sweet, J. J., ed.), Swets & Zeitlinger, Lisse, Netherlands, pp. 27–37.

30. Larry P v Riles, No. C–71–2270 RFP (1979), *aff'd*, No. 80-4027 DC No. CV 71-3370 (9th Cir. 1984)

31. Brescia, W. and Fortune, J. C. (1989) Standardized testing of American Indian students. *College Student J.* **23**, 98–104.

32. Loewenstein, D. A., Arguelles, T., Arguelles, S., and Linn-Fuentes, P. (1994) Potential cultural bias in the neuropsychological assessment of the older adult. *J. Clin. Exp. Neuropsychol.* **16,** 623–620.

33. Hinkle, J. S. (1994) Practitioners and cross-cultural assessment: a practical guide to information and training. *Measure. Eval. Counsel. Dev.* **27,** 103–115.

34. Deutsch, M., Fishman, J. A., Kogan, L., North, R., and Whiteman, M. (1964) Guidelines for testing minority group children. *J. Social Issues* **20,** 129–145.

35. Dunn, J. T., Lees-Haley, P. R., Brown, R. S., and Williams, C. W. (1995) Neurotoxic complaint base rates of personal injury claimants: implications for neuropsychological assessment. *J. Clin. Psychol.* **51,** 577–584.

36. Lees-Haley, P. R. (1992) Neuropsychological complaint base rates of personal injury claimants. *Forensic Rep.* **5,** 385–391.

37. Cullum, C. M., Heaton, R. K., and Grant, I. (1991) Psychogenic factors influencing neuropsychological performance: somatoform disorders, factitious disorders, and malingering, in *Forensic Neuropsychology: Legal and Scientific Bases* (Doeer, H. O. and Carlin, A. S., eds.), Guilford Press, New York, pp. 141–171.

38. Trueblood, W. and Schmidt, M. (1993) Malingering and other validity considers in the neuropsychological evaluation of mild head injury. *J. Clin. Exp. Neuropsychol.* **15,** 578–590.

39. Binder, L. (1993) Assessment of malignering after mild head trauma with the Portland Digit Recognition Test. *J. Clin. Exp. Neuropsychol.* **15,** 170–182.

40. Lees-Haley, P.R. and Brown, R.S. (1993) Neuropsychological complaint base rates of 170 personal injury claimants. *Arch. Clin. Neuropsychol.* **8,** 203–209.

41. Lee, G. P., Loring, D. W., and Martin, R. C. (1991) Rey's 15-item visual memory test for the detection of malingering: normative observations on patients with neurological disorders. Paper presented at the 19th annual meeting of the International Neuropsychological Society, San Antonio, TX.

42. Sweet, J. J. (1999) Malingering: differential diagnosis, in *Forensic Neuropsychology: Fundamentals and Oractice* (Sweet, J. J., ed.), Swets & Zeitlinger, Lisse, pp. 255–285.

43. Klonoff, P.S. and Lamb, D.G. (1998) Mild head injury, significant impairment on neuropsychological test scores, and psychiatric disability. *Clin. Neuropsychol.* **12,** 31–42.

44. Youngjohn, J. R., Lees-Haley, P. R., and Binder, L. M. (1999) Comment: Warning malingerers produces more sophisticated malingering. *Arch. Clin. Neuropsychol.* **14,** 511–515.

45. Kazdin, A. E. (1998) *Research Design in Clinical Psychology,* 3rd ed. Allyn and Bacon, Boston.

46. Reynolds, C. R. and Brown, R. T. (eds.) (1984) *Perspectives on Bias in Mental Testing.* Plenum, New York.

47. Stern, W. (1911) *Die Differentielle Psychologie in Ihren Methodischen Grundlagen.* J.A. Barth, Leipzig.

48. Dunlap, K. (1922) *The Elements of Scientific Psychology.* C.V. Mosby, St. Louis.

49. Byar, D. P., Simon, R. M., Friedewald, W. T., Schlesselman, J. J., DeMets, D. L., Elenberg, J.H., Gail, M. H., and Ware, J. H. (1976) Randomized clinical trials: Perspectives on some recent ideas. *N. Engl. J. Med.* **295,** 74–80.

50. Stanton, M. E. and Spear, L. P. (1990) Workshop on the qualitative and quantitative comparability of human and animal developmental neurotoxicity. Work Group I report: comparability of measures of developmental neurotoxicity in humans and laboratory animals. *Neurotoxicol. Teratol.* **12,** 261–267.

51. Kimbrough, R. D. (1995) Polychlorinated biphenyls (PCBs) and human health: an update. *Crit. Rev. Toxicol.* **25,** 133–163.

52. Baelum, J. (1999) Acute symptoms during non-inhalation exposure to combinations of toluene, trichloroethylene, and *n*-hexane. *Intl. Arch. Occup. Environ. Health* **72,** 408–410.

53. American Psychological Association (1987) *Ethical Principles in the Conduct of Research with Human Participants.* American Psychological Association, Washington, DC.

54. Hsu, L. M. (1989) Random sampling, randomization, and equivalence of contrasted groups in psychotherapy outcome research. *J. Consult. Clin. Psychol.* **57,** 131–137.

55. Schafer, A. (1985) The randomized clinical trial: for whose benefit. *IRB: Rev. Human Sub. Res.* **7,** 4–6.

56. Weinstein, M. C. (1974) Allocation of subjects in medical experiments. *N. Engl. J. Med.* **291,** 1278–1285.

57. Freedman, B. (1987) Equipoise and the ethics of clinical research. *N. Engl. J. Med.* 317, 141–145.

58. Glabaud de Fort, G. E., Newman, S. C., and Bland, R. C. (1993) Psychiatric comorbidity and treatment seeking: sources of selection bias in the study of clinical populations. *J. Nervous Mental Dis.* **181,** 467–474.

59. Cohr, K. H. (1985) Definition and practical limitation of the concept organic solvents, in *Chronic Effects of Organic Solvents on the Central Nervous System and Diagnostic Criteria (Document 5)* (Joint WHO/Nordic Council of Ministers Working Group, eds.), World Health Organization, Regional Office for Europe, Copenhagen.

60. Baker, E .L., Jr. (1985) Epidemiologic issues in neurotoxicity research. *Neurobehav. Toxicol. Teratol.* **7,** 293–297.

61. Hartman, D.E. (1991) Neuropsychology and the (neuro) toxic tort, in *Forensic Neuropsychology: Fundamentals and Practice* (Sweet, J. J., ed.), Swets & Zeitlinger, Lisse, pp. 255–285.

62. Hill, A. B. (1965) The environment and disease: association or causation? *Proc. R. Soc. Med.* **58,** 295–300.

63. American Psychological Association (1992) *Ethical Principles of Psychologists and Code of Conduct.* American Psychological Association, Washington, DC.

64. Rosenthal, R. and Rosnow, R. L. (1991) *Essentials of Behavioral Research: Methods and Data Analysis,* 2nd ed. McGraw-Hill, New York.

65. Rosenthal, R. and Rosnow, R. L. (1975) *The Volunteer Subject.* Wiley, New York.

66. Kraemer, H.C. (1992) Reporting the size of effects in research studies to facilitate assessment of practical or clinical significance. *Psychoneuroendocrinology* **17,** 527–536.

67. Lees-Haley, P. R. and Brown, R. S. (1992) Biases in perception and reporting following a perceived toxic exposure. *Percept. Motor Skills* **75,** 531–544.

68. Williams, C. W. and Lees-Haley, P. R. (1993) Perceived toxic exposure: a review of four cognitive influences on perception of illness. *J. Social Behav. Personality* **8,** 489–506.

69. Myers, M. G., Cairns, J. A., and Singer, J. (1987) The consent form as a possible cause of side effects. *Clin. Pharmacol. Therap.* **42,** 250–253.

70. Spurgeon, A., Gompertz, D., and Harrington, J. M. (1996) Modifiers of non-specific symptoms in occupational and environmental syndromes. *Occup. Environ. Med.* **53,** 361–366.

71. Johnson, B. L., Baker, E. L., Gilioli, R., Seppalainen, A. M., El Batawi, M., Hanninen, H., and Zintaras, C. (eds.) (1987) *Prevention of Neurotoxic Illness in Working Populations.* John Wiley & Sons, New York.

72. Liang, Y.-X., Chen, Z.-Q., Sun, R.-K., Fang, Y.-F., and Yu, J.-H. (1990) Application of the WHO Neurobehavioral Core Test Battery and other neurobehavioral screening methods, in *Advances in Neurobehavioral Toxicology: Applications in Environmental and Occupational Health* (Johnson, B. L., ed.), Lewis Publishers, Chelsea, MI, pp. 225–243.

73. Letz, R. (1990) The Neurobehavioral Evaluation System: an international effort, in *Advances in Neurobehavioral Toxicology: Applications in Environmental and Occupational Health* (Johnson, B. L., ed.), Lewis Publishers, Chelsea, MI, pp. 189–199.

74. Law, D., Lash, A. A., Bowler, R., Estrin, W., and Becker, C. E. (1990) Evaluation of the construct validity of examiner-administered and computer-administered neuropsychologi-

cal tests, in *Advances in Neurobehavioral Toxicology: Applications in Environmental and Occupational Health* (Johnson, B. L., ed.), Lewis Publishers, Chelsea, MI, pp. 263–271.

75. Axelsson, G. and Rylander, R. (1984) Use of questionnaires in occupational studies of pregnancy outcomes: validation of questionnaire reported miscarriage, malformation, and birth weight. *Intl. J. Epidemiol.* **13,** 94–98.

76. Kihlstrom, J. (1995) From the subject's point of view: the experiment as conversation and collarboration between investigator and subject. Keynote address presented at the meeting of the American Psychological Society, New York.

77. Slosson, E. E. (1899) A lecture experiment in hallucinations. *Psychol. Rev.* 6, 407–408.

78. Dalton, P., Wysocki, C. J., Brody, M. J., and Lawley, H. J. (1997) The influence of cognitive bias on the perceived odor, irritation, and health symptoms from chemical exposure. *Intl. Arch. Occup. Environ. Health* **69,** 407–417.

79. Koelega, H. S. and Koster, E. P. (1974) Some experiments on sex differences in odor perception. *Ann. NY Acad. Sci.* **237,** 234–236.

80. Eagly, A. H. (1983) Gender and social influence: A social psychological analysis. *Am. Psychol.* **38,** 971–981.

81. Citterio, A., Sinforiani, E., Verri, A., Cristina, S., Gerosa, E., and Nappi, G. (1998) Neurological symptoms of the sick building syndrome: analysis of a questionnaire. *Funct. Neurol.* **13,** 225–230.

82. Stenberg, B. and Wall, S. (1995) Why do women report 'sick building symptoms' more often than men? *Social Sci. Med.* **40,** 491–502.

83. Burge, S., Hedge, A., Wilson, S., Bass, J. J., and Robertson, A. (1987) Sick building syndrome: a study of 4343 office workers. *Ann. Occup. Hygiene* **31,** 493–504.

84. Skov, P., Valbjorn, O., and Pedersen, B. V. (1989) The Danish Indoor Climate Study Group. Influence of personal characteristics, job-related factor and psychosocial factors on the sick building syndrome. *Scand. J. Work Environ. Health* **15,** 286–295.

85. Ashford, N. A. and Miller, C. S. (1992) *Chemical Exposures. Low Levels and High Stakes.* Van Nostrand Reinhold, New York.

86. Gilbert, A. N., Sabini, J., and Knasko, S. C. (1997) Sex differences in task performance associated with attention to ambient odor. *Arch. Environ. Health* **52,** 195–199.

87. Roht, L. H., Vernon, S. W., Weir, F. W., Pier, S. M., Sullivan, P., and Reed, L. J. (1985) Community exposure to hazardous waste disposal sites: assessing reporting bias. *Am. J. Epidemiol.* **122,** 418–433.

88. Ooi, P. L. and Goh, K. T. (1997) Sick building syndrome: an emerging stress-related disorder? *Intl. J. Epidemiol.* **26,** 1243–1249.

89. Benignus, V. A. (1993) Importance of experimenter-blind procedure in neurotoxicology. *Neurotoxicol. and Teratol.* **15,** 45–49.

90. Carroll, K. M., Rounsaville, B. J., and Nich, C. (1994) Blind man's bluff: effectiveness and significance of psychotherapy and pharmacotherapy blinding procedures in a clinical trial. *J. Consult. Clin. Psychol.* **62,** 276–280.

91. Margraf, J., Ehlers, A., Roth, W. T., Clark, D. B., Sheikh, J., Agras, W. S., and Taylor, C. B. (1991) How "blind" are double-blind studies? *J. Consult. Clin. Psychol.* **46,** 184–187.

92. Beatty, W. W. (1972) How blind is blind? A simple procedure for estimating observer naivete. *Psychol. Bull.* **78,** 70–71.

93. Ney, P. G., Collins, C., and Spensor, C. (1986) Double blind: double talk or are there ways to do better research. *Med. Hypothesis* **21,** 199–126.

94. Oxtoby, A., Jones, A., and Robinson, M. (1989) Is your "double-blind" design truly double-blind? *Br. J. Psychiatry* **155,** 700–701.

Index

DATE DUE

DEMCO INC 38-2971